Case Studies in Critical Care Medicine

Second Edition

Roy D. Cane, M.B.B.Ch., F.F.A.(S.A.)

Professor of Clinical Anesthesia
Northwestern University Medical School
Chicago, Illinois

Barry A. Shapiro, M.D.

Professor of Clinical Anesthesia
Northwestern University Medical School
Chicago, Illinois

Richard Davison, M.D.

Associate Professor of Medicine
Northwestern University Medical School
Chicago, Illinois

YEAR BOOK MEDICAL PUBLISHERS, INC.
CHICAGO • LONDON • BOCA RATON • LITTLETON, MASS.

1 2 3 4 5 6 7 8 9 0 Y R 94 93 92 91 90

Library of Congress Cataloging-in-Publication Data

Case studies in critical care medicine / [edited by] Roy D. Cane,
  Barry A. Shapiro, Richard Davison. — 2nd ed.
     p. cm.
   Includes bibliographical references.
   ISBN 0-8151-1424-9
   1. Critical care medicine—Case studies. I. Cane, Roy D.
  II. Shapiro, Barry A., 1937- . III. Davidson, Richard, 1937- .
   [DNLM: 1. Critical Care. WX 218 C337]
  RC86.8.C43 1990   90-12096
  616'.028—dc20   CIP
  DNLM/DLC
  for Library of Congress

Sponsoring Editor: Bethany L. Caldwell
Assistant Director, Manuscript Services: Frances Perveiler
Production Project Coordinator: Yvette L. Sellers/Karen Halm
Proofroom Supervisor: Barbara M. Kelly

In Memory of Joyce Ann Cane
1940–1989

CONTRIBUTORS

James F. Bresnahan, S.J., J.D., LL.M., Ph.D.
Lecturer in Medicine
Northwestern University Medical School
Chicago, Illinois

Roy D. Cane, M.B.B.Ch., F.F.A.(S.A.)
Professor of Clinical Anesthesia
Northwestern University Medical School
Chicago, Illinois

Christina Chomka, M.D.
Assistant Professor of Clinical Anesthesia
Northwestern University Medical School
Chicago, Illinois

Richard Davison, M.D.
Associate Professor of Medicine
Northwestern University Medical School
Chicago, Illinois

Benjamin Esparaz, M.D.
Fellow in Hematology/Oncology
Northwestern University Medical School
Chicago, Illinois

Daniel Fintel, M.D.
Assistant Professor of Medicine
Northwestern University Medical School
Chicago, Illinois

Jeffrey I. Frank, M.D.
Chief Resident in Neurology
Northwestern University Medical School
Chicago, Illinois

Anthony Giambardino, M.D.
Fellow in Anesthesia
Northwestern University Medical School
Chicago, Illinois

Jeffrey Glassroth, M.D.
Professor of Medicine
Northwestern University Medical School
Chicago, Illinois

David Green, M.D.
Professor of Medicine
Northwestern University Medical School
Chicago, Illinois

Scott L. Heller, M.D.
Assistant Professor of Clinical Neurology
Northwestern University Medical School
Chicago, Illinois

Kerry Kaplan, M.D.
Attending Cardiologist
Mease Hospital
Safety Harbors, Florida

Frank A. Krumlovsky, M.D.
Associate Professor of Medicine
Northwestern University Medical School
Chicago, Illinois

Paul S. Mesnick, M.D.
Assistant Professor of Clinical Anesthesia
Northwestern University Medical School
Chicago, Illinois

Nancy A. Nora, M.D.
Fellow in Nephrology-Hypertension
Northwestern University Medical School
Chicago, Illinois

William T. Peruzzi, M.D.
Associate in Clinical Anesthesia
Northwestern University Medical School
Chicago, Illinois

John P. Phair, M.D.
Professor of Medicine
Northwestern University Medical
  School
Chicago, Illinois

Barry A. Shapiro, M.D.
Professor of Clinical Anesthesia
Northwestern University Medical
  School
Chicago, Illinois

**Donald M. Sinclair, M.B.B.Ch.,
F.F.A.(S.A.)**
Associate Professor of Clinical
  Anesthesia
Northwestern University Medical
  School
Chicago, Illinois

Tod B. Sloan, M.D., Ph.D.
Associate Professor of Anesthesia and
  Neurosurgery
University of Texas Health Sciences
  Center
San Antonio, Texas

M. Christine Stock, M.D.
Assistant Professor of Anesthesiology
  and Internal Medicine
Emory University Medical School
Atlanta, Georgia

Mark Stolar, M.D.
Assistant Professor of Clinical Medicine
Northwestern University Medical
  School
Chicago, Illinois

Arvydas Vanagunas, M.D.
Assistant Professor of Clinical Medicine
Northwestern University Medical
  School
Chicago, Illinois

Richard M. Vazquez, M.D.
Assistant Professor of Surgery
Northwestern University Medical
  School
Chicago, Illinois

Jeffrey Vender, M.D.
Associate Professor of Clinical
  Anesthesia
Northwestern University Medical
  School
Chicago, Illinois

PREFACE

Critically ill patients differ from other patients, not because of specific pathologies or therapies, but because of their unstable clinical condition which mandates the frequent reevaluation of the patient's physiologic homeostasis and adjustment of therapy. Critical care practitioners are continually required to integrate a plethora of physiologic data and make frequent therapeutic decisions. In our opinion, conventional texts do not readily convey to the reader this process of decision analysis. The case study format of this book represents an attempt to reflect the process of decision making and hopefully better instruct the reader in the application of this process in the management of critically ill patients.

We have chosen topics that describe the major problems encountered in adult intensive care units. Case histories were selected to present a mix of surgical and medical patients though obviously the principles of therapy and monitoring apply equally well to all critically ill patients. This text makes no pretense of addressing the entire body of knowledge of critical care medicine. Rather, we have focused on clinically relevant material and its application in decision analysis and management of critically ill patients.

In this second edition the range of topics has been expanded to cover those subjects in which newer technology has added new dimensions to the care of critically ill patients (clinical blood gas monitoring, alternate forms of mechanical ventilatory support). New chapters on pain control and symptom management, non-traumatic coma, acute endocrine emergencies, and ethical aspects of critical care medicine have been added. The discussion of neurosurgical problems, myocardial ischemic conditions, and coagulopathies in the critically ill patient have been expanded.

With these additions, the topics cover problems that occur with frequency in critically ill patients and in which there is, in most instances, a reasonable body of clinically relevant information.

The earlier chapters deal with therapeutic modalities that have an application to various pathologies and with simpler clinical problems involving single organ systems. The later chapters are devoted to more complex specific therapies and the clinical problem of multi-organ system disease.

Pediatric critical care has been excluded due to limitations of space and the existence of other pediatric case study texts. We chose not to address multiple trauma or burns as specific subjects because outside of the elements of cardiopulmonary support and fluid therapy, the management of these patients is a surgical, not critical care problem. These elements of therapy and support have been discussed in this text, although not necessarily in the context of patients with traumatic disease.

We wish to thank the contributing authors for their chapters. Thanks are due to our colleagues, in particular Drs. Edward Brunner, Roy Patterson, Jeff Glassroth, Chris Chomka, Bill Peruzzi, and Dan Fintel for their unfailing support of our endeavours. We thank Kelly Quinn, Xenia Ruiz, and Joan Woods for secretarial assistance in the preparation of the manuscript.

Roy D. Cane, M.B., B.CH.(RAND), F.F.A.(S.A.)
Barry A. Shapiro, M.D.
Richard Davison, M.D.

CONTENTS

1 / Clinical Blood Gas Monitoring

CHRISTINA CHOMKA, M.D.

The practice of critical care medicine is rapidly changing as new technology and more elaborate monitors are introduced into the marketplace. The usefulness of any patient monitor depends on its ability to provide accurate values and rapidly respond to changes, allowing for early detection of fluctuations from baseline. The dangers of hypoxemia, hypercarbia, and hyperoxia are well recognized in the intensive care setting, as can be attested to by the frequency of arterial blood gas sampling. Although long recognized as the "gold standard" of assessment of oxygen and carbon dioxide tensions, the test provides for only intermittent determinations, frequently missing transient but potentially harmful fluctuations.

In recent years much emphasis has been placed on the use of continuous, non-invasive monitoring.[1] Pulse oximeters, transcutaneous oxygen and carbon dioxide electrodes, and end-tidal CO_2 monitors have been marketed as being essential for assessing the adequacy of oxygenation or ventilation. In order to properly interpret the values generated by these monitors, one must be familiar with their mode of action, values that are actually being measured, and limitations of the system.[2]

Our ultimate goal is to maintain cellular viability by ensuring adequate oxygen delivery as well as carbon dioxide elimination. Because oxygen delivery is equal to oxygen content $[(Hb \times O_2 \text{ sat} \times 1.34) + (0.003 \times Pao_2)]$ times the cardiac output, it is apparent that multiple factors can be responsible for cellular hypoxia. Individual monitors can inform us of some aspect of this equation. By integrating the results of multiple monitors, one can potentially have an on-line, real-time assessment of the adequacy of oxygen delivery.

PULSE OXIMETRY

Pulse oximeters are presently used widely to monitor arterial oxygen saturation. Of all of the monitors currently available to monitor oxygenation, the pulse oximeter is probably the easiest to use; because it is factory precalibrated and noninvasive, it can be put into use instantly without the need for warm-up time.[3] Oximetry relies upon absorption or reflectance spectroscopy and incorporates the principles of the Beer-Lambert law for determination of oxyhemoglobin saturation because the absorption spectra of oxygenated and reduced hemoglobin are different.[4]

1

Developed in the 1940s by Millikan, the initial oximeter required exsanguination of the site to be monitored in order to establish a baseline and subsequent heating of the site to arterialize the blood.[5] Hemoglobin saturation was measured by trans-illuminating a capillary bed with two wavelengths. A photodetector measured the transmitted light. The saturation of the arterial blood was related to the difference between the absorbent signal of the arterialized sample and the baseline. Because of technical difficulties in their usage, the initial oximeters had limited clinical applications.[6, 7]

In the 1970s Nakajima and colleagues made a discovery that transformed the oximeter into a clinically useful tool.[8] They recognized that the pulsatile absorbancies of the red and infrared light transmitted correlated with hemoglobin saturation, with red light being more absorbed at 660 nm by reduced hemoglobin and infrared light being more absorbed by oxygenated hemoglobin at 990 nm. By positioning any vascular bed between a two-wavelength light source and detector, hemoglobin saturations can be measured. The baseline is determined by absorption due to non-pulsatile arterial blood, venous and capillary blood, and tissue. Arterial absorption is a calculation of the ratio of the pulse-added absorption to the baseline absorbancies at the two wavelengths.[9]

With only two wavelengths being measured, the pulse oximeter is only able to distinguish two hemoglobin moieties within the blood—oxyhemoglobin and reduced hemoglobin. If other hemoglobins are present within the blood (i.e., methemoglobin, carboxyhemoglobin), they will be incorporated into the oxyhemoglobin and reduced hemoglobin measurement, thereby generating erroneous saturations.[10, 11] In fact, any substance within the blood that absorbs light at the red and infrared wavelengths of the pulse oximeter may cause measurement error. Dyes such as methylene blue, indigo carmine, and indocyanine green can all cause transient reductions in oxygen saturation.[12, 13] Pulse oximeter saturation can also be affected by room light interference.[14, 15] Although measures have been taken to correct for this interference by rapid averaging and subtraction of the ambient light signal, unrecognized errors can occur. The easiest remedy of this situation would be an opaque protective covering of the sensor site. Additional problems can be caused by motion artifact or weak signals caused by thready pulses.[16] To more accurately interpret the values, a pulse waveform or signal strength indicator should be incorporated into the monitors so that erroneous readings can be ignored.

The use of oximetry probes is not entirely without risk, although they are significantly safer than transcutaneous or intra-arterial probes. Skin damage, with the extreme situation being necrosis of the digit to which the probe had been applied, has been reported in situations of prolonged use with poor peripheral circulation secondary to low-flow states or the use of vasoconstricting drugs.[17]

Currently available pulse oximeters have a reported accuracy of $\pm 2\%$ in the 70% to 100% saturation range and $\pm 3\%$ down to the 60% saturation range, assuming minimal concentrations of dyshemoglobin species.[18-20] Below this range saturations correlate poorly with those obtained with in vitro co-oximeter measurements, significantly overestimating the actual oxygen saturation. Studies have revealed superior accuracy of the ear oximeter to that of the finger oximeter, which in part may be related to differences in transit time.

The greatest advantages of pulse oximetry are its ease of application and ability to provide continuous saturation readings. Because significant reductions in arterial saturation may occur before cyanosis becomes clinically apparent, the pulse oximeter can act as an early-warning monitor of potentially life-threatening desaturation. The primary limitations of this monitoring device, aside from the technical aspects, relate to the fact that oxygen saturation, and not oxygen tension or oxygen delivery, is measured. In view of the sigmoidal shape of the oxyhemoglobin dissociation curve, major changes in oxygen tension may occur (especially in a patient receiving supplemental oxygen) with minimal fluctuation of the oxygen saturation. In addition, one cannot equate an acceptable saturation with adequate perfusion because the device will function as long as a pulse is present. A signal strength indicator or pulse waveform may help qualitate peripheral perfusion. Vascular pulsations that are markedly reduced or absent will incapacitate the monitor. Pulse oximetry can be applied to the ear, digits, bridge of the nose, nasal septum, or temple over the temporal artery.

TRANSCUTANEOUS MONITORS

Transcutaneous gas exchange has been recognized for more than 100 years, since the initial work of von Gerlach in measuring oxygen and carbon dioxide exchange between the skin and air.[21] Numerous obstacles had to be overcome such as compensating for the oxygen consumption of the skin, variations in gas exchange across the epidermis, and regulating oxygen delivery to the skin before transcutaneous measurements of oxygen tension could be relied upon to reflect arterial oxygen tension. Even with all of the refinements, multiple factors can adversely affect cutaneous blood flow and result in erroneous tension readings. It is the recognition of the factors that affect transcutaneous readings that makes this a clinically useful tool. Unlike oximeters that monitor hemoglobin saturation, transcutaneous monitors measure actual gas tensions. A falling $Ptco_2$ at high oxygen tensions may be indicative of undesirable changes long before arterial hemoglobin saturation actually changes.

Clark's discovery of the polarographic oxygen electrode in 1956 along with the introduction of the Severinghaus carbon dioxide electrode in 1958 provided the technologic basis for continuous transcutaneous measurement of oxygen and carbon dioxide that diffuse to the skin surface from the dermal capillary bed beneath. Currently utilized transcutaneous electrodes are essentially miniaturized versions of both the Clark and Severinghaus electrodes.[22] After electrode calibration and special site preparation allowing for airtight electrode positioning, diffusion of gases to the surface of the skin is produced through local hyperemia secondary to heating of the electrode site to 43 to 45°C. Cutaneous blood flow is temperature dependent, with the greatest increases in flow occurring at skin temperatures between 35 and 45°C and maximal dilatation occurring around 45°C. Above this temperature complications to the skin are significant without further increases in blood flow.[23] In addition, the stratum corneum, which provides the mechanical strength of the epidermis, liquefies at temperatures >41°C, and this increases the diffusion of gases between 100 and 1,000 times through this barrier.[24]

Fortunately, the initial clinical application of the transcutaneous oxygen electrode was in the neonatal population, in which, after heating of the skin to 44°C, close correlation was observed between transcutaneous and arterial oxygen tensions. It is only in the neonatal population that arterial blood actually comes in contact with the epidermis; in adults, perpendicular capillary loops approach the epidermis, and oxygen delivery occurs by diffusion. Subsequent studies in hemodynamically unstable neonates revealed that $Ptco_2$ significantly underestimated Pao_2.[25] Application to the adult population proved less rewarding. In hemodynamically stable adult patients, $Ptco_2$, although trending Pao_2, was only 80% of the actual value.[26] Under conditions of hemodynamic stability, rapid alterations in arterial Po_2 will be qualitatively tracked by $Ptco_2$; however, a 95% response time ranging from 8 to 90 seconds has been reported, depending on the magnitude of the change.[27] Because the electrodes measure oxygen that diffuses through the skin, skin tissue rather than arterial oxygen tension is measured. Factors influencing the oxygen delivery to the skin, such as cardiac output and regional perfusion, will be reflected in the transcutaneous measurement as well as the Pao_2. Human and animal studies confirm this fact inasmuch as it has been documented repeatedly that $Ptco_2$ tracks Pao_2 during hypoxemia and cardiac output during shock.[28, 29]

This improved understanding of the physiology of transcutaneous monitoring has prompted an increased use in adults. A monitor that at one time was considered useless in situations of altered perfusion is now being applied more frequently to critically ill patients, specifically those at risk for cardiopulmonary compromise, or to regional alterations in perfusion (e.g., skin flaps, extremities distal to balloon pump insertion).[30, 31]

Initial work performed by Tremper and Shoemaker in 1980 in critically ill patients found that $Ptco_2$ followed Pao_2 until the cardiac index (CI) fell below 2 L/min/m², at which point the $Ptco_2$ values became flow dependent.[32] He subsequently defined a transcutaneous index $(Ptco_2/Pao_2)$ to assess the degree of peripheral perfusion deficit. Patients with a CI > 2.2 L/min/m² had a transcutaneous index of 0.79 ± 0.12; as the CI fell to 2.0 L/min/m², the index decreased to 0.49; and at a CI of 1.0 L/min/m² the transcutaneous index was 0.12.[32] It was apparent that as the CI fell to shock levels, the $Ptco_2$ values correlated with the CI.

The transcutaneous CO_2 electrode was also used initially as a neonatal monitor. Although transcutaneous electrodes respond to $Paco_2$ changes when heated to a lower temperature than required for $Ptco_2$ monitoring, analysis at 44°C allows for a faster response time, with 95% response occurring at 3.5 minutes.[33] Heating of the skin by the sensor increases the Pco_2 at the skin surface by approximately 23 ± 11 mm Hg, but despite this difference in absolute value, the $Ptcco_2$ trends the $Paco_2$ accurately.[34] Because the $Ptcco_2$ averages 140% to 160% of the $Paco_2$, many manufacturers have programmed correction factors into the $Ptcco_2$ monitors, thereby producing transcutaneous CO_2 values comparable to arterial CO_2 values. As with $Ptco_2$ values, $Ptcco_2$ becomes flow dependent and does not trend $Paco_2$ at a CI below 1.5 L/min/m².

Transcutaneous CO_2 electrodes are effective monitors of the adequacy of ventilation, without needing to have the patient intubated as with capnography. Rapid titration of ventilator changes can also be performed. More recent applications include continuous, noninvasive monitoring of fetal acid-base status during labor and delivery with electrode placement on the fetal scalp.

Combined electrodes measuring both $Ptco_2$ and $Ptcco_2$ are currently available. Sensor sites should be changed every 4 hours to minimize the risk of first-degree skin burns. Whereas $Ptcco_2$ electrode calibration should be carried out every 4 hours, $Ptco_2$ electrode calibration is required only every 24 hours; however, a drift check should be performed every 4 hours.

END-TIDAL CO$_2$

Capnography, the measurement of carbon dioxide in the respiratory gases, currently can be measured either by infrared absorption or mass spectrometry. The infrared analyzer passes a beam with a wavelength of 4.3 μm through a sample of gas, and the transmitted light intensity is compared with that of a reference beam. Carbon dioxide's maximal absorption for infrared light occurs around 4.3 μm; thus, to measure the carbon dioxide concentration accurately, the infrared beam must be filtered carefully to avoid measurement of other gases (i.e., N_2O) with absorption peaks close to that of carbon dioxide.[35]

Most infrared analyzers are sidestream analyzers aspirating small amounts of gas from the breathing circuit close to the patient and passing the gas through small-bore tubing to a remote analyzer. The sampling rate is usually 150 cc/min with an average delay of approximately 100 ms. This sampling method adds little weight or dead space to the breathing circuit, but care must be taken to prevent clogging of the sampling tubing with secretions or condensation.

Gas analysis can also occur within the breathing circuit itself by using a mainstream analyzer, which places a detector adjacent to the endotracheal tube and allows for very rapid CO_2 determinations (averaging 10 ms). Although rarely affected by secretions because of the large internal diameter used to minimize airway resistance, the analyzer is bulky and heated to prevent condensation; thus endotracheal tube displacement and patient burns can occur if the system is not well supported.[36]

An alternate means of CO_2 analysis is through mass spectrometry. The gas sample is aspirated into a high-vacuum chamber in which an electron beam ionizes and fragments its components. These are then accelerated through an electric field into a strong magnetic field that deflects the ionic fragments into an arch, the diameter of which is dependent on the charge-to-mass ratio of the fragments. Detector plates are positioned according to the deflection arches of the substances to be measured. As fragments hit the detector, an electric current is generated from which the concentration of the gas to be measured can be calculated. Not only CO_2 but multiple gas components as well can be simultaneously analyzed.[37]

Mass spectrometers tend to be large and expensive; thus they are frequently used to monitor more than one patient, thereby allowing for only intermittent monitoring. Because they are sidestream analyzers, they are subject to the same line blockage problems associated with the sidestream infrared capnometers.[38] The exhaled CO_2 waveform in a healthy individual is nearly a square wave and can be divided into three phases: phase 1, exhaled gas from anatomic dead space; phase 2, exhaled gas

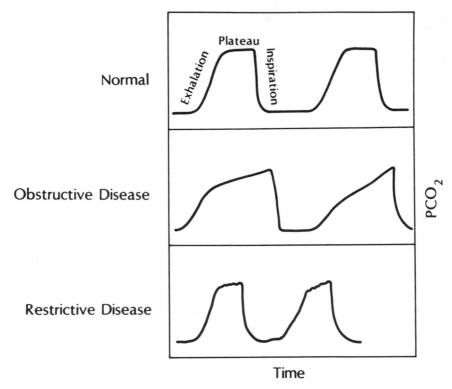

Normal

Obstructive Disease

Restrictive Disease

PCO_2

Exhalation

Plateau

Inspiration

Time

FIG 1–1.

The normal capnograph pattern shows a sharply rising exhalation slope with a clearly iden-
tifiable plateau. Inspiration is seen as an abrupt decrease in CO_2 to baseline. Obstructive
disease generally produces a prolonged exhalation slope with a difficult-to-identify plateau.
Restrictive disease generally provides a "choppy" plateau. (From Shapiro BA, Harrison RA,
Cane RD, et al: *Clinical Application of Blood Gases*, ed 4. Chicago, Year Book Medical
Publishers, Inc, 1989. Used by permission.)

composed of progressively more alveolar gas; and phase 3 (the alveolar plateau),
exhaled gas from alveoli, both perfused and nonperfused.

The end-tidal CO_2 concentration is defined as the maximal concentration of exhaled CO_2 and is usually 1 to 2 mm Hg less than the arterial CO_2 tension because
it reflects the CO_2 concentrations of both perfused and nonperfused (dead space)
alveoli. Abnormalities in ventilation, circulation, and metabolism can be reflected
in the capnogram that is generated.[39, 40] It is therefore important that in addition to
a numerical display of the end-tidal CO_2 concentration a waveform be displayed to
facilitate diagnosis.

Figure 1–1 displays a normal capnogram and those associated with obstructive
and restrictive lung disease. Note the gradual rise of the alveolar plateau that is
produced by increased alveolar dead-space ventilation from chronic obstructive pulmonary disease (COPD) in the obstructive disease example.

Figure 1–2 shows the effect of a fall in cardiac output on the capnogram. Figure 1–3 shows a capnogram displaying cardiogenic oscillations on the tracing.[41]

Capnography provides a continuous, noninvasive means of monitoring CO_2 in intubated patients. Clinical judgment is required to ascertain whether reductions in end-tidal CO_2 are a result of excessive CO_2 elimination or increased dead-space ventilation. Capnography can also be used during cardiopulmonary resuscitation to assess the adequacy of perfusion.[42] Reductions in PETCO$_2$ during cardiopulmonary resuscitation (CPR) are associated with comparable reductions in cardiac output, whereas increases in PETCO$_2$ during successful resuscitation are associated with cor-

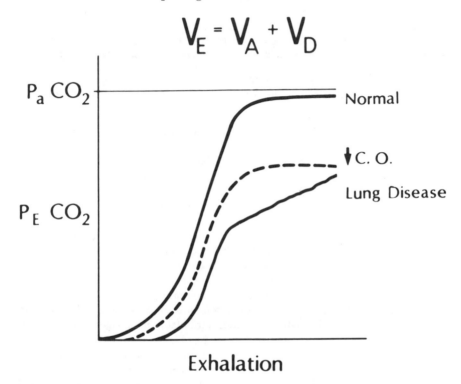

FIG 1–2.
Total ventilation (VE) is composed of both alveolar ventilation (VA) and dead-space ventilation (VD). Paco$_2$ is considered the best reflection of alveolar ventilation. The end-tidal Pco$_2$ (PETCO$_2$) is the expired Pco$_2$ (PECO$_2$) at the end of the plateau. An increased VD will be manifested as an increased P(a-ET)co$_2$ gradient. The two most common causes of increased dead-space ventilation are decreased cardiac output and lung disease. A decreased pulmonary perfusion will result in more alveoli having a lower Pco$_2$; the net result is a decreased expired Pco$_2$ but no change in the lung-emptying pattern. This is depicted as the *dashed curve* with a shape similar to the normal. Lung disease will involve changing lung-emptying patterns and thus a change in the curve. (From Shapiro BA, Harrison RA, Cane RD, et al: *Clinical Application of Blood Gases,* ed 4. Chicago, Year Book Medical Publishers, Inc, 1989. Used by permission.)

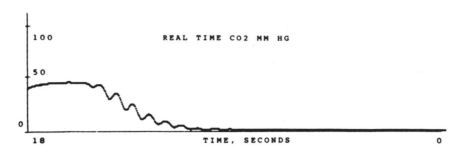

FIG 1-3.
Capnogram with pronounced cardiogenic oscillations. (From Gravenstein JS, Paulus DA, Hayes TJ: *Capnography in Clinical Practice.* Boston, Butterworths, 1989. Used by permission.)

responding increases in cardiac output. The efficacy of chest compressions as well as the adequacy of the restored circulation can be assessed by tracking $PETCO_2$.[43-45]

PULMONARY ARTERY OXIMETRY

Mixed venous oxygen content ($C\bar{v}O_2$) is a global measure of the adequacy of oxygen supply to oxygen demand. If oxygen delivery is decreased in the face of constant oxygen consumption, the $C\bar{v}O_2$ will be lowered as a result of increased oxygen extraction from the arterial blood. If oxygen consumption increases without a commensurate increase in oxygen delivery, the $C\bar{v}O_2$ will also be decreased.[46]

Previous work has documented the correlation of $C\bar{v}O_2$ to cardiac output in the perioperative as well as the acute myocardial infarction period.[47, 48] It was not until 1981, however, that a noncumbersome, reliable system was developed for intrapulmonary monitoring that utilized a pulmonary artery catheter and fiber-optic technology developed earlier for umbilical artery monitoring.

By using a selected three-wavelength system instead of a system with two wavelengths, there was less fluctuation in values attributable to changes in hematocrit, pH, blood flow, and temperature.[49]

The oximetric catheter employs reflectance spectrophotometry, with the light transmitted to the blood via a fiber-optic monofilament and reflected back in a separate fiber-optic monofilament to the photodetector. The percent saturation of oxyhemoglobin is calculated by microprocessor technology. In vitro calibration of the catheter is required before insertion, and in vivo calibration can be performed if blood is withdrawn from the pulmonary artery and measured in a co-oximeter as the control. The system appears stable, with a drift of less than 1% per 24 hours; therefore, once-a-day calibration appears adequate.

In healthy individuals breathing room air, the mixed venous oxygen saturation ($S\bar{v}O_2$) ranges between 68% and 77%. At lower oxygen tensions a near-linear relationship exists between saturation and tension.

Reductions in $S\bar{v}O_2$ can result from decreased arterial saturation, increased oxygen consumption, decreased cardiac output, or decreases in hemoglobin. Although $S\bar{v}O_2$

is not a specific monitor for cardiac output, assuming normal arterial oxygenation and hemoglobin concentration, a fall in $S\bar{v}O_2$ indicates that cardiac output is inadequate for the body's needs. Cardiopulmonary instability has rarely been associated with an $S\bar{v}O_2$ greater than 60%, whereas saturations <40% are frequently associated with hypotension, vasoconstriction, dysrhythmias, and cardiac arrest.[50, 51]

Monitoring $S\bar{v}O_2$ provides little useful information with regard to the adequacy of cardiac output in clinical situations when either anatomic (arteriovenous [AV] fistula) or physiologic shunting exists. In disease states such as hepatitis, sepsis, pancreatitis, or certain drug intoxicated states, $S\bar{v}O_2$ values may be elevated despite clinical evidence of ongoing anaerobic metabolism.

The major question that persists is whether continuous monitoring of $S\bar{v}O_2$ is cost effective in reducing the number of arterial and mixed venous blood gases in addition to decreasing the incidence of potentially adverse hemodynamic effects, length of intensive care unit (ICU) stay or mortality.[52–55] Although $S\bar{v}O_2$ may indicate a failure of the oxygen transport system, it will not determine the source of imbalance between oxygen delivery and consumption, nor will it detect regional perfusion abnormalities. With changes in $S\bar{v}O_2$ further testing is frequently required before the appropriate intervention can be performed.[56]

CASE STUDY

A 70-year-old woman came to the emergency room complaining of a 3-day history of progressive shortness of breath, shaking, chills, and malaise. She was a 60-pack-a-year smoker. Her COPD symptoms had gradually increased, necessitating the addition of steroids to her regimen of aminophylline, aerosolized albuterol, and atropine. Her past medical history was also significant for a myocardial infarction 3 years previously, after which the patient was symptom free with isosorbide dinitrate (Isordil) and diltiazem treatment. She denied any other problems.

Physical examination revealed a tachypneic woman who had an increased anteroposterior (AP) chest diameter, breathed at a rate of 32 breaths per minute, and used her accessory ventilatory muscles. She was unable to complete a sentence without pausing to catch her breath. Pulmonary auscultation was remarkable for shallow ventilatory efforts with diffuse expiratory wheezing and bronchial breath sounds at both bases. Both bases were also dull to percussion. Her blood pressure was 145/85 mm Hg, the heart rate was 125/min, and heart tones were distant, but no S_3 was appreciated.

An arterial blood gas measurement obtained before initiation of oxygen therapy revealed a pH of 7.46, PcO_2 of 38 mm Hg, and PaO_2 of 54 mm Hg. Her complete blood cell count (CBC) was remarkable for a white cell count of 18,000/mm³ with 22% band neutrophils. Chest x-ray examination showed bibasilar patchy infiltrates.

An FIO_2 of 0.4 was initiated via a high-humidity face mask, and the patient was transferred to the ICU for close observation for impending ventilatory failure and aggressive bronchial hygiene therapy. An antibiotic regimen consisting of erythromycin and ceftazidime was started pending results of a sputum Gram stain, culture, and determination of sensitivities. A finger pulse oximeter registered a saturation of 91% during transport to the ICU.

A transcutaneous electrode was also placed in the ICU to monitor the patient's ventilation. Initial readings revealed a $PtcO_2$ of 42 mm Hg and a $PtcO_2$ of 58 mm Hg.

During the first bronchial hygiene treatment, which consisted of aerosolized albuterol and atropine followed by ultrasonic nebulization and chest physical therapy, the patient became disoriented. The $PtcO_2$ fell to 44 mm Hg and the $PtcCO_2$ rose to 56 mm Hg. An arterial blood gas measurement was obtained to confirm the transcutaneous values, which revealed a pH of 7.32, a $PaCO_2$ of 62 mm Hg, and a PaO_2 of 52 mm Hg. At this point it was elected to intubate and ventilate the patient.

A blind nasal intubation was performed successfully after cocainization of the nares, and the patient was placed on full ventilatory support at a rate of 8 breaths per minute and a tidal volume of 1 L. Initially, $PETCO_2$ monitoring revealed a capnogram consistent with COPD; in the next hour the $PETCO_2$ fell from 56 to 37 mm Hg. This was associated with a reduction in $PtcO_2$ to 34 mm Hg despite a pulse oximeter saturation reading of 94%. An arterial blood gas measurement obtained on an FIO_2 of 0.5 revealed a pH of 7.34, a $PacO_2$ of 46 mm Hg, and a PaO_2 of 48 mm Hg.

Discussion

The correlation of transcutaneous and end-tidal CO_2 monitors to arterial blood gas tensions is dependent on an adequate cardiac output to maintain good peripheral perfusion and minimize dead-space ventilation. In this instance, the disparity progressed while the patient was being mechanically ventilated. It is not unusual to see hypotension develop after initiation of positive-pressure ventilation in patients who are marginally hydrated. Positive-pressure ventilation increases the intrathoracic pressure, thereby impairing venous return to the heart. In addition, by taking over the patient's work of breathing, circulating catecholamines may be significantly reduced, thereby leading to a further reduction in cardiac output.

The calculated transcutaneous index in this patient was 0.53, which corresponds to a CI in the range of 2 $L/min/m^2$ (moderate shock).

CASE STUDY CONTINUED

The patient was hydrated, receiving 1.5 L of normal saline over the next hour, with a gradual increase in both $PETCO_2$ and $PtcO_2$ values. An arterial blood gas measurement obtained after volume infusion revealed a pH of 7.38, a $PacO_2$ of 42 mm Hg, and a PaO_2 of 72 mm Hg, with corresponding $PtcO_2$ and $PETCO_2$ values of 54 and 38 mm Hg, respectively. Two days after admission sputum cultures grew *Legionella,* and ceftazidime therapy was discontinued.

The patient's condition deteriorated on the fourth day of therapy, with temperatures to 39°C, a decrease in blood pressure to 70/40 mm Hg, and oliguria. The transcutaneous index and $P(a-ET)CO_2$ were 0.72 and 3 mm Hg, respectively. An oximetric pulmonary artery catheter was inserted to optimize fluid therapy and assess cardiac function. Initial mixed venous saturations were 77%, with a CI of 3.0 $L/min/m^2$ and a calculated systemic vascular resistance of 800 dynes. Blood pressure was restored to 110/80 mm Hg after infusion of 3 L of normal saline.

Discussion

The placement of a pulmonary artery catheter helped to confirm the diagnosis of early septic shock and allowed for rapid restoration of blood pressure without necessitating initiation of inotropic therapy. Unfortunately, in the face of sepsis, the mixed venous saturations may not correlate with fluctuations in cardiac output because of local AV shunting or abnormalities in cellular oxygen uptake.

CASE STUDY CONTINUED

Results of blood cultures revealed *Staphylococcus epidermidis* sensitive to oxacillin in the blood. The patient was appropriately treated and improved clinically in the next 3 days. The pneumonia also appeared to be resolving both radiologically and clinically, with the patient requiring only an FiO_2 of 0.35 to maintain $Ptco_2$ in the 60 mm Hg range.

On the sixth hospital day the patient tolerated a reduction in ventilatory support to a rate of two breaths per minute; however, the $PETCO_2$ rose to 50 mm Hg when the patient fell asleep. Arterial blood gas analysis revealed a pH of 7.36, a Pco_2 of 54 mm Hg, and a po_2 of 68 mm Hg. Electrolytes were checked, and K^+ was found to be reduced to 2.9 mEq/L. With K^+ supplementation the patient's acid-base status was corrected. The patient tolerated withdrawal of ventilatory support and was extubated on the eighth hospital day.

Discussion

Our goal thus far has been to attempt to correlate the accuracy of applied monitors to that of the "gold standard," arterial blood gas values. Patient factors such as cardiac output, regional perfusion abnormalities, alterations in hemoglobin (both type and amount), as well as technical problems may lead to errors in extrapolating to arterial tensions. The ideal monitor would be minimally invasive and provide continuous, real-time values of intravascular gas tensions.

CONTINUOUS BLOOD GAS MONITORING

Numerous intravascular oxygen electrodes have been developed, but most have been unsatisfactory for routine clinical use because of their size, response, or instability. Miniaturized Clark electrodes or isolated platinum electrodes have been correlating well with arterial oxygen tensions; however, technical problems such as clot formation, sensor drift, temperature alterations, and the need for in vitro and in vivo calibration have prompted a search for more dependable monitors.[57-59]

The recent application of optical fluorescence to intravascular monitoring may solve many of the problems associated with the larger polarographic devices.[60] An optode using photoluminescence quenching to measure Po_2 continuously both in animals and anesthetized patients has correlated well with conventional Pao_2 measurement. Intra-arterial fiber-optic sensors inserted into 22-gauge needles have also correlated well with reference electrodes under varying pH ranges. A blood gas monitoring system based on optical fluorescence is currently being used to simultaneously monitor pH, Pco_2, and Po_2 in the extracorporeal cardiopulmonary bypass circuit.

Similar technology is being miniaturized to an intra-arterial system continuously measuring pH, pco_2, and po_2. A three-fiber optode with dyes encapsulated at the tip can be inserted into a 20-gauge catheter without compromising blood pressure monitoring or blood withdrawal. A distally placed thermocouple gives a reading of the temperature at the probe tip, and this allows for correction of solubilities and fluorescent intensities to the appropriate temperature and subsequent calculation of blood gas values at 37°C. Linear regression analysis of data generated both in animals and humans reveals excellent correlation between directly measured intra-arterial values and conventional arterial blood gas analysis.[61] Although still only an investigational tool, the applications of this technology are limitless, assuming it will be available at a reasonable cost.

ACID-BASE IMBALANCE

Continuous intravascular pH monitoring combined with $Paco_2$ assessment will allow for rapid diagnosis and treatment of acute acid-base imbalance. Acid-base balance is a function of respiratory and metabolic components. By knowing the pH and Pco_2 one can easily calculate the metabolic component because for every 10 mm Hg increase in Pco_2 above baseline, the pH decreases by 0.05 units and for every 10 mm Hg decrease in pco_2 the pH increases by 0.1 units. The difference between the arterial pH and the predicted pH represents a deviation from normal buffer base status, in other words, a metabolic derangement. A metabolic pH change of 0.15 reflects a 10 mEq/L change from normal buffer status.

Knowledge of the acid-base status is particularly important in critically ill patients in whom significant deviations from baseline may be associated with cellular enzyme system dysfunction, myocardial and nervous system electrophysiologic abnormalities, electrolyte imbalances, and decreased responsiveness to exogenous catecholamines.

Metabolic acidosis results from a reduction of blood base, accumulation of nonvolatile blood acid, or a combination of the two. It is usually associated with compensatory alveolar hyperventilation unless the pulmonary system is unable to respond to the demand. Frequent etiologies of metabolic acidosis include excessive lactate generation, ketoacidosis, renal failure, or drug ingestion (salicylates, methanol, or ethylene glycol).

Metabolic alkalosis occurs frequently in critically ill patients. Although not as life-threatening as acidosis, if left uncorrected it can be associated with significant electrolyte abnormalities. Hypokalemia frequently contributes to the alkalemia and may result in muscular weakness as well as cardiac dysrhythmias. Alveolar hypoventilation does not usually occur as a compensatory mechanism in the alert individual; however, it may occur in the severely debilitated, comatose, or semicomatose patient.[62] Other causes of metabolic alkalosis include nasogastric suction or vomiting, steroid administration, or excessive bicarbonate administration.

FUTURE APPLICATIONS

Continuous blood gas monitoring used in conjunction with noninvasive monitors potentially can provide us with cardiopulmonary data previously available only after insertion of a pulmonary artery catheter.

Assessment of the arterial–end-tidal carbon dioxide [$P(a\text{-}ET)co_2$] gradient can inform us of changes in physiologic dead-space ventilation. The primary factors responsible for altering this gradient are changes in cardiac output or pulmonary pathology. Pulmonary pathology usually affects lung emptying, thereby altering the configuration of the capnogram. If the $P(a\text{-}ET)co_2$ gradient increases without a change in the configuration of the capnogram, one can assume that the change is the result of a reduction in the cardiac output. By continuously monitoring the gradient one can potentially titrate fluids or pharmacologic support in response to alterations in cardiac output.

The arterial-transcutaneous oxygen gradient can similarly be continually monitored as a reflection of cardiac output. Skin perfusion is cardiac output dependent. As discussed previously, Tremper has defined a transcutaneous oxygen index to assess the degree of peripheral perfusion deficit. A low transcutaneous oxygen index has been associated with hypovolemia in acutely traumatized patients despite the presence of a normal blood pressure.

The use of dual oximetry (arterial and pulmonary artery) allows for continuous calculation of the oxygen extraction index $(O_2EI = Sao_2 - S\bar{v}o_2/Sao_2)$.[63] This index appears to correlate better with total body oxygen utilization than pulmonary artery oximetry alone does.

The ventilation-perfusion index

$$VQI = 100 \times \frac{1.32 \times Hb \times (1 - Sao_2) + 0.0031 \times Pao_2}{1.32 \times Hb \times (1 - S\bar{v}o_2) + 0.0031 \times Pao_2}$$

also calculated from dual co-oximetry measurements, appears qualitatively to reflect intrapulmonary shunting under all circumstances and quantitatively reflects the shunt when Pao_2 values are less than 100 mm Hg.[64]

Proper application of the currently available or soon-to-be-released technology in the critical care setting will allow us to monitor our patients continuously and intervene with appropriate therapy before the manifestation of hemodynamic or respiratory instability. Simultaneous continuous monitoring of arterial blood gases, transcutaneous oxygen tension, and $Petco_2$ will provide the critical care physician with a moment-to-moment reflection of alterations in cardiac output, peripheral perfusion, and gas exchange. Early recognition of changes allowing for rapid intervention and titration of therapy to desired end points will most certainly prove beneficial to the critically ill patient.

REFERENCES

1. Eichorn JH, Cooper JB, Cullen DJ, et al: Standards for patient monitoring during anesthesia at Harvard Medical School. *JAMA* 1986; 256:1017–1020.
2. Block FE: Do we monitor enough? We don't monitor enough. *J Clin Monit* 1986; 2:267–269.
3. Yelderman M, New W: Evaluation of pulse oximetry. *Anesthesiology* 1983; 59:349–352.
4. Taylor MB, Whitwam JG: The current status of pulse oximetry. *Anaesthesia* 1986; 41:943–949.
5. Millikan GA: The oximeter, an instrument for measuring continuously the oxygen saturation of arterial blood in man. *Rev Sci Instr* 1942; 13:434.
6. Millikan GA: Continuous measurement of blood oxygen, in Glasser O (ed): *Medical Physics*, vol 1. Chicago, Year Book Medical Publishers, Inc, 1944.
7. Wood EH, Sutterer WF, Cronin L: Oximetry, in Glasser O (ed): *Medical Physics*, vol 3. Chicago, Year Book Medical Publishers, Inc, 1960.
8. Nakajima S, Hirai Y, Takase H, et al: Performances of new pulse wave earpiece oximeter. *Respir Circ* 1975; 23:41–45.
9. Severinghaus JW, Astrup PB: History of blood gas analysis. IV: Oximetry. *J Clin Monit* 1986; 2:270.
10. Barker SJ, Tremper KK, Hufstadler S, et al: The effects of carbon monoxide inhalation on noninvasive oxygen monitoring. *Anesth Analg* 1986; 65(suppl):12.

11. Pologe JA, Raley DM: Effects of fetal hemoglobin on pulse oximetry. *J Perinatol* 1987; 7:324–326.
12. Scheller MS, Unger RJ, Kelner MJ: Effects of intravenously administered dyes on pulse oximetry readings. *Anesthesiology* 1986; 65:550–552.
13. Sidi A, Rush WR, Paulus DA, et al: Effect of fluorescein, indocyanine green, and methylene blue on the measurement of oxygen saturation by pulse oximetry (abstract). *Anesthesiology* 1986; 65:132.
14. Eisele JH, Downs D: Ambient light affects pulse oximeters. *Anesthesiology* 1987; 67:864–865.
15. Siegel MN, Gravenstein N: Preventing ambient light from affecting pulse oximetry. *Anesthesiology* 1987; 67:280.
16. Lawson D, Norley I, Korbon G, et al: Blood flow limits and pulse oximeter signal detection. *Anesthesiology* 1987; 67:599–603.
17. Berge KH, Lanier WL, Scanlon PD: Ischemic digital skin necrosis: A complication of the reusable Nelcor pulse oximeter probe (letter). *Anesth Analg* 1988; 67:712–713.
18. *Nellcor N100 Technical Manual*. Hayward, Calif, Nellcor Corp, 1983.
19. *Ohmeda Biox 3740 Pulse Oximeter Operating Manual*. Louisville, Colo, BOC Health Care, 1988.
20. Cecil WT, Thorpe KJ, Fibuch EE, et al: A clinical evaluation of the accuracy of the Nellcor N100 and the Ohmeda 3700 pulse oximeters. *J Clin Monit* 1988; 4:31–36.
21. Lubbers D: History of transcutaneous P_{O_2} measurement. *Crit Care Med* 1981; 9:693.
22. Lubbers D: Theory and development of transcutaneous oxygen pressure measurement. *Int Anesthesiol Clin* 1987; 25:3.
23. Hertzmann AB: Vasomotor regulation of the skin. *Physiol Rev* 1959; 39:280–306.
24. Tremper KK, Waxman KS: Transcutaneous monitoring of respiratory gases, in Nochomovitz ML, Cherniack NS (eds): *Noninvasive Respiratory Monitoring*. New York, Churchill Livingstone, Inc, 1986, pp 1–28.
25. Peabody JL, Willis MM, Gregory GA, et al: Clinical limitations and advantages of transcutaneous oxygen electrodes. *Acta Anaesthesiol Scand* 1978; 68:76–82.
26. Gothgen I, Jacobsen E: Transcutaneous oxygen tension measurement I. Age variation and reproducibility. *Acta Anaesthesiol Scand Suppl* 1978; 67:66–70.
27. Abu-Osba Y, Thach B, Brouillette R: Evaluation of response time of a transcutaneous oxygen tension electrode. *Pediatr Res* 1981; 15:143–146.
28. Tremper KK, Waxman K, Shoemaker WC: Effects of hypoxia and shock on transcutaneous P_{O_2} values in dogs. *Crit Care Med* 1979; 7:526–531.
29. Rowe MI, Weinberg G: Transcutaneous oxygen monitoring in shock and resuscitation. *J Pediatr Surg* 1979; 14:773–778.
30. Tremper KK, Shoemaker WC: Continuous CPR monitoring with transcutaneous oxygen and carbon dioxide sensors. *Crit Care Med* 1981; 9:417–418.
31. Achanes BM, Black KS, Lilke DK: Transcutaneous P_{O_2} in flaps: A new method of survival prediction. *Plast Reconstr Surg* 1980; 65:738.
32. Tremper KK, Shoemaker WC: Transcutaneous oxygen monitoring of critically ill adults, with and without low flow shock. *Crit Care Med* 1981; 9:706–709.
33. Tremper KK, Menteles RA, Shoemaker WC: Effects of hypercarbia and shock on transcutaneous carbon dioxide at different electrode temperatures. *Crit Care Med* 1980; 8:608.
34. Tremper KK, Shoemaker WC, Shippy CR, et al: Transcutaneous P_{CO_2} monitoring on adult patients in the ICU and operating room. *Crit Care Med* 1981; 9:752.
35. Ammann EB, Galvin RD: Problems associated with the determination of carbon dioxide by infrared absorption. *J Appl Physiol* 1968; 25:333–335.
36. Gravenstein JS, Paulus DA, Hayes TJ: *Capnography in Clinical Practice*. Boston, Butterworths, 1989.
37. Hill NC: *Introduction to Mass Spectrometry*. London, Heyden, 1966.
38. Gravenstein JS, Gravenstein N, et al: Pitfalls with mass spectrometry in clinical anesthesia. *Int J Comput Monit* 1984; 1:27–34.
39. Hoffbrand BI: The expiratory capnogram: A measure of ventilation inequalities. *Thorax* 1966; 21:518.
40. Hatle L, Rokseth R: The arterial to end-expiratory carbon dioxide tension gradient in acute pulmonary embolism and other cardiopulmonary diseases. *Chest* 1974; 66:352.
41. Arieli R: Cardiogenic oscillations in expired gas: Origin and mechanism. *Respir Physiol* 1983; 52:191–204.
42. Weil MH, Bisera J, Trevino R, et al: Cardiac output and end-tidal carbon dioxide. *Crit Care Med* 1985; 13:907–909.
43. Trevino R, Bisera J, Weil MH, et al: End-tidal CO_2 as a guide to successful cardiopulmonary resuscitation: A preliminary report. *Crit Care Med* 1985; 13:910–911.
44. Garnett AR, Ornato JP, Gonzalez E, et al: End-tidal carbon dioxide monitoring during cardiopulmonary resuscitation. *JAMA* 1987; 257:512–515.

45. Lepilin MG, Vasilyev A, Bildinov O, et al: End-tidal carbon dioxide as a noninvasive monitor of circulatory status during cardiopulmonary resuscitation: A preliminary clinical study. *Crit Care Med* 1987; 15:958–959.
46. Schweiss J: Mixed venous hemoglobin saturation: Theory and application. *Int Anesthesiol Clin* 1987; 25:3.
47. Muir AL, Kirby BJ, King AJ, et al: Mixed venous oxygen saturation in relation to cardiac output in myocardial infarction. *Br Med J* 1970; 4:276–278.
48. Parr G, Blackstone E, Kirklin J: Cardiac performance and mortality early after intracardiac surgery in infants and children. *Circulation* 1975; 51:867.
49. Divertie MB, McMichan JC: Continuous monitoring of mixed venous oxygen saturation. *Chest* 1984; 85:423–428.
50. Krauss XH, Verdouw PD, Hugenholtz PG, et al: On-line monitoring of mixed venous oxygen saturation after cardiothoracic surgery. *Thorax* 1975; 30:636.
51. Martin WE, Cheung PW, Johnson CC, et al: Continuous monitoring of mixed venous oxygen saturation in man. *Anesth Analg* 1973; 52:784–793.
52. Schmidt CR, Frank LP, Forsythe SB, et al: Continuous SvO₂ measurement and oxygen transport patterns in cardiac surgery patients. *Crit Care Med* 1984; 12:523–527.
53. Boutros AR, Lee C: Value of continuous monitoring of mixed venous blood oxygen saturation in the management of critically ill patients. *Crit Care Med* 1986; 14:132–134.
54. Orlando R: Continuous mixed venous oximetry in critically ill surgical patients. *Arch Surg* 1986; 121:470–471.
55. Norfleet E, Watson C: Continuous mixed venous oxygen saturation measurement: A significant advance in hemodynamic monitoring? *J Clin Monit* 1985; 1:245–258.
56. Jastremski MS, Chelluri L, Beney KM, et al: Analysis of the effects of continuous on-line monitoring of mixed venous oxygen saturation on patient outcome and cost-effectiveness. *Crit Care Med* 1989; 17:148–153.
57. Katayama M, Murray GC, Uchida T, et al: Intra-arterial continuous PO₂ monitoring by an ultra-fine microelectrode. *Crit Care Med* 1987; 15:357.
58. Bratanow N, Polk K, Bland R, et al: Continuous polarographic monitoring of intra-arterial oxygen in the perioperative period. *Crit Care Med* 1985; 13:859–860.
59. Green GE, Hassell KT, Mahutte CK: Comparison of arterial blood gas with continuous intra-arterial and transcutaneous PO₂ sensors in adult critically ill patients. *Crit Care Med* 1987; 15:491–494.
60. Gehrich JL, Lubbers DW, Opitz N, et al: Optical fluorescence and its application to an intravascular blood gas monitoring system. *IEEE Trans Biomed Eng* 1986; 33:117–132.
61. Shapiro BA, Cane RD, Chomka CM, et al: Preliminary evaluation of an intra-arterial blood gas system in dogs and humans. *Crit Care Med* 1989; 17:455–460.
62. Jarboe TM, et al: Ventilatory failure due to metabolic alkalosis. *Chest* 1972; 61:615.
63. Rasanen J, et al: Oxygen tensions and oxyhemoglobin saturations in the assessment of pulmonary gas exchange. *Crit Care Med* 1987; 15:1058.
64. Bandala LC, Cane RD, Shapiro BA: Validation of VQI in critically ill patients. *Crit Care Med* 1989; 17(suppl):21.

2/Monitoring Cardiovascular Dynamics

BARRY A. SHAPIRO, M.D.

The maintenance of internal respiration (oxygen and carbon dioxide exchange between blood and tissue) depends upon adequate blood flow through systemic capillaries, or perfusion. Despite impressive technical advances in cardiovascular monitoring, the clinical assessment of acceptable tissue perfusion still depends on subjective criteria such as the level of consciousness and sensorium, appreciation of the amplitude of a palpated peripheral pulse, the status of capillary filling, the status of skin temperature and color, and serial monitoring of urine output.

Tissue perfusion requires adequate circulation that is dependent upon generation of adequate ventricular pressure, which in turn is dependent upon appropriate venous conductance. Although reasonably reliable quantification of cardiac output is clinically available, we often rely upon pressure measurements to guide therapy. Vascular resistance and ventricular pressure generation are important factors to be considered in maintaining adequate flow and minimal myocardial work. Bedside assessment of cardiovascular function depends upon the thorough understanding of physiologic factors affecting flow. This is best approached by a functional analysis of factors affecting blood volume, vascular space, and myocardial function.

DISTRIBUTION OF TOTAL BODY WATER

Total body water is generally expressed as a percentage of body weight. Several studies have shown that approximately 70% of lean body mass consists of water.[1] Fat tissue has a much lower water content per gram than other tissue, resulting in a lower than predicted total body water content in people with excessive fat tissue.[2] Representative mean values of total body water are 60% for lean men and 50% for lean women.[3]

As illustrated in Figure 2–1, total body water expressed in liters constitutes approximately 60% of the total body weight in kilograms. In the adult the intracellular fluid compartment constitutes approximately 40% of the ideal body weight, whereas the extracellular fluid compartment accounts for 20%. The extracellular fluid is distributed between the intravascular space (plasma volume) and the interstitial fluid space. The balance between intravascular and interstitial volume is determined largely by the presence of albumin and globulins, which exert a colloid osmotic pressure

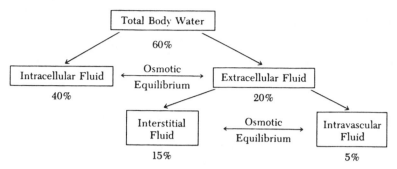

FIG 2–1.
Body fluid compartments with water percentages expressed as a percentage of ideal body weight.

(oncotic pressure). Approximately 5% of the ideal body weight is due to intravascular water, excluding the red blood cell mass, and 15% is due to interstitial fluid. An example of the distribution of fluid volumes within the various compartments is given in Table 2–1.

Primary Blood Volume Deficiency

Inadequate blood volume frequently results from acute blood loss. An acute blood loss of up to 10% (the amount of blood given by a blood donor) can readily be tolerated by most patients without adverse cardiovascular effects. Blood loss between 10% and 20% is usually not associated with significant signs of cardiovascular distress when the patient is supine. However, orthostatic changes, physical exertion, or the administration of vasodilating drugs often cause tachycardia and hypotension. An acute blood loss between 20% and 40% is usually associated with signs of cardio-vascular distress including hypotension, tachycardia, marginal peripheral circulation, and inadequate tissue perfusion.[4] Once acute blood loss exceeds 40%, inadequate

TABLE 2–1.

Representative Fluid Volumes

Measured Parameters	Male Abs Value (% Body Weight)	Female Abs Value (% Body Weight)
Weight (kg)	80	55
Total body water (L)	48.0 (60)	2.75 (50)
Intracellular fluid (L)	32.0 (40)	18.7 (34)
Extracellular fluid (L)	16.0 (20)	8.8 (16)
Interstitial (L)	12.0 (15)	6.3 (11.5)
Intravascular (blood volume, mL)	6,000 (7.5)	3,575 (6.5)
Plasma volume (mL)	4,000 (5.0)	2,475 (4.5)
RBC mass volume (mL)	2,000 (2.5)	1,100 (2.0)

tissue perfusion is likely to persist despite appropriate volume replacement ("irreversible shock").

Other common causes of primarily decreased intravascular volume are dehydration and extravascular third-space sequestration. Endothelial cell dysfunction may lead to increased permeability and loss of protein from the intravascular compartment. The consequent inability to maintain adequate oncotic pressure gradients results in a primary decrease in blood volume.

Secondary Blood Volume Deficiency

Inadequate perfusion is often related to an absolute increase in the intravascular space. This phenomenon is frequently referred to as a secondary or *relative hypovolemia*.

The major arteries contain 5% to 10% of the blood volume. Arterioles are responsible for regional adjustments in the distribution of perfusion because of their ability to significantly vary resistance. The microcirculatory bed (capillaries) contains 25% to 30% of the blood volume. The distribution to individual capillary beds is greatly determined by the precapillary and postcapillary sphincters, which are subject to changes in smooth muscle tone secondary to the autonomic nervous system, endogenous circulatory hormones, and tissue metabolites.[5]

VENOUS CAPACITANCE

Approximately two thirds of the total blood volume normally resides in the venous system. The high "capacitance" of these vessels refers to their ability to significantly alter their blood volume with minimal pressure changes by autonomic nervous system—mediated changes in smooth muscle tone.

A decrease in venous tone leads to a significant increase in the vascular space. If this occurs in conjunction with a "normal blood volume," a state of *relative hypovolemia* exists. This is frequently observed in patients with sepsis, acute spinal cord injury, and regional anesthetic blockade. Relative hypovolemia may also exist in patients who are aggressively treated with vasodilator drugs. The recognition of the relationship between vascular volume and vascular space is of vital importance.

VASCULAR VOLUME/VASCULAR SPACE RELATIONSHIP

Blood flow from the peripheral veins to the atrium is dependent upon a pressure gradient primarily developed by the contraction of venous smooth muscle (venous tone). Whenever the venous system contains a blood volume within its range of storage capacity, a state of *relative normovolemia* exists; when the blood volume exceeds storage capacity, a *relative hypervolemia* exists; when the blood volume is below its range of storage capacity, a *relative hypovolemia* exists.

Figure 2–2 illustrates the relationship between changes in atrial pressure and flow as venous blood volume changes. Any time the blood volume in the venous system is below its maximum capacitance or above its minimum capacitance, reasonable blood volume changes are well tolerated. Volume additions made when maximum capacitance is exceeded result in large pressure changes with very little increase in venous return. Volume removal when minimum capacitance exists results in a marked decrease in venous return.

Venous return can be improved by at least two mechanisms: (1) increased driving pressure accomplished by an increase in venous tone while the volume remains unchanged and (2) improved venous conductance associated with a reduction in venous tone after the addition of volume. The first mechanism is the most common initial response of the critically ill patient in an attempt to improve or maintain venous return; the second mechanism is the therapeutic approach most often used by the clinician in attempting to improve venous return.

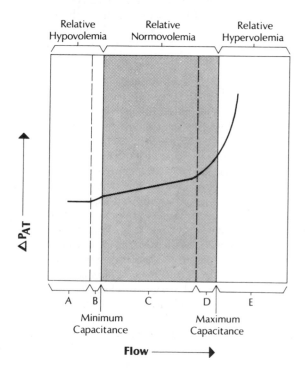

FIG 2–2.
Model depicting the theoretic relationship between venous flow and the change in atrial pressure resulting from a specific fluid load (ΔPAT). Changes in ΔPAT are routinely measured by a CVP catheter for the right atrium and PAOP for the left atrium. (From Shapiro BA, Harrison RA, Trout CA: *Clinical Applications of Respiratory Care,* ed 2. Chicago, Year Book Medical Publishers, Inc, 1979. Used by permission.)

MYOCARDIAL FUNCTION

Heart Rate

Tachycardia (>100/min) is most frequently associated with sympathetic stimulation. In the critically ill patient, insults such as hypoxemia, acidemia, hypercarbia, hyperthermia, and acute decreases in blood volume are common causes of tachycardia. Atropine-like and β-adrenergic drugs can produce pronounced tachycardia. In the elderly or critically ill patient with preexisting heart disease, an increase in heart rate to >140/min often limits ventricular filling time to the extent that cardiac output declines. Increased heart rate is associated with increases in myocardial oxygen consumption.

Bradycardia (<50/min) usually decreases cardiac output because further increases in stroke volume (SV) are limited. Myocardial hypoxia is a potentially lethal cause of bradycardia. Common causes of bradycardia in the critically ill patient are conductance disturbances, hypothermia, β-blockers, calcium channel blockers, and anticholinesterase agents.

Contractility

Contractility can be defined as the shortening capacity and force-generating potential of the myocardial muscle fibers making up the ventricular wall. Contractility remains an extremely difficult entity to evaluate quantitatively.[6] Diminished contractility (negative inotropism) is associated with hypoxia, acidosis, hypercarbia, poor myocardial perfusion, β-blocking agents, calcium channel blockers, and some anesthetic agents. Improved contractility (positive inotropism) is clinically correlated with enhanced states of tissue oxygenation, the acid-base environment, and improved myocardial perfusion. Drugs such as the β-adrenergic catecholamines, digitalis, and calcium chloride are associated with an increase in contractility. Increased myocardial contractility is always associated with increased myocardial oxygen demands.

The majority of experimental work quantitating myocardial contractility are in vitro studies relating contractility to the velocity of muscle shortening (dl/dt), rate of pressure development (dP/dt), and maximum velocity of muscle shortening (V_{max}).[7] A decreased ejection fraction (SV: end-diastolic volume) has been correlated with a decrease in contractility.[8] Gated cardiac blood pool studies, although very dependent on afterload and somewhat dependent on preload, provide a dependable bedside assessment of overall ventricular function.[9]

Preload

Preload is defined as the loading force or the end-diastolic volume distending the relaxed ventricular wall. Assuming constant myocardial compliance, as end-diastolic volume is increased, end-diastolic pressure must increase. Figure 2–3 clearly demonstrates that as the end-diastolic pressure (preload) is increased, SV is correspondingly increased until a point is reached where further increases in preload result in

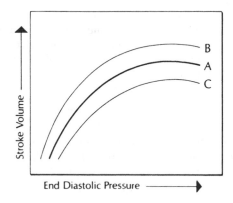

FIG 2–3.
Frank-Starling relationship where end-diastolic pressure is directly proportional to end-diastolic volume. *Curve A* represents normal contractility; *curve B,* increased contractility; and *curve C,* decreased contractility. (From Shapiro BA, Harrison RA, Trout CA: *Clinical Application of Respiratory Care,* ed 2. Chicago, Year Book Medical Publishers, Inc, 1979. Used by permission.)

a decrease in SV. There are an infinite number of pressure-volume curves, each one related to a different state of myocardial contractility.[10]

Afterload

Afterload can be defined as the force or tension developed in the ventricular wall to overcome impedance to flow in the ventricular outflow tract. Factors causing impedance include valvular/vascular wall distensibility, major artery wall compliance, and arteriolar resistance.

Acute afterload increases are associated with increased myocardial oxygen consumption. The most common cause of an acute afterload increase is increased vascular resistance. Two common factors are valvular disease and increased blood viscosity.[11]

BEDSIDE ASSESSMENT OF CARDIOVASCULAR FUNCTION

Tissue perfusion depends upon adequate circulation, which is dependent upon adequate ventricular contractility, preload, and afterload. Proper utilization of arterial, central venous pressure (CVP), and balloon-tipped pulmonary artery (PA) catheters allows the preload and afterload function of both ventricles to be monitored.

Contractility Assessment

The history and physical examination will usually determine the patient with a high probability of primary myocardial dysfunction—myocardial ischemia, ventricular failure, and valvular disease. Negative inotropic factors such as acidemia, alkalemia, hypercarbia, hypoxemia, and sepsis must be evaluated. Once primary and obvious secondary factors leading to negative inotropism have been reasonably ruled out, further evaluation of the circulation and myocardial function depend upon appropriate assessment and support of venous return.

Afterload Assessment

Under most circumstances an arterial catheter properly placed in a brachial or radial artery will measure pressures that are quantitatively close to the aortic root pressure. PA catheters provide access for measurement of PA pressures and hence right ventricular afterload.

Preload Assessment

The clinical assessment of venous return cannot be ascertained from a single pressure reading obtained from a CVP or PA catheter. Since neither the state of venous tone nor the degree of peripheral-to-CVP gradient can be measured, the only alternative approach is to make serial measurements of pressure after manipulation of the volume status. This concept is embodied in the *fluid challenge principle*.

A fluid challenge consists of the administration of a finite volume over a short interval followed by correlation of serial pressure changes in either CVP or pulmonary artery occluded pressure (PAOP) readings with clinical and physiologic assessment of changes in the systemic circulation and tissue perfusion status. The following guidelines are a useful systematic approach for the application of the fluid challenge principle.

Step 1.   Obtain general clinical, hemodynamic, and laboratory baseline values, especially PAOP or CVP measurement.

Step 2.   Give from 50 to 200 mL of appropriate volume (crystalloid, colloid, or blood) within 10 minutes. The amount and type of volume are dependent upon the appraisal of the patient's clinical status.

Step 3.   Observe for improvement in blood pressure (BP), pulse, and peripheral tissue perfusion. Examination of the chest for evidence of pulmonary edema is essential.

Step 4.   Evaluate the change in PAOP or CVP measurement and continue as outlined under conditions listed in Table 2–2.

TABLE 2–2.

Guidelines for Volume Administration When Using a Fluid Challenge Principle

Conditions	ΔPAOP	ΔCVP
Add additional volume	≤3 mm Hg	≤2 cm H_2O
Do not add additional volume	≥7 mm Hg	≥5 cm H_2O
Wait 10 min, add smaller volume, and repeat evaluation	Between 3 and 7 mm Hg	Between 2 and 5 cm H_2O

Once the assessment of vascular volume to vascular space is completed, then the assessment of primary myocardial function is more meaningful. If necessary, more direct pharmacologic support of the myocardium can be instituted.

Cardiac Output Measurement

In the late 19th century, Adolph Fick described a procedure whereby the concentration of a dissolved substance in the blood (in the initial description the substance was oxygen) could be used as an indicator for determining the amount of blood flow.[12] This concept has subsequently become known as the Fick principle and, with oxygen as the dissolved substance, is described by the Fick equation. This approach has remained the standard against which newer techniques are compared. The capability of directly measuring circulation (cardiac output) has provided the clinician with an important direct link to the assessment of cardiovascular function.

Thermal Dilution Technique

This is accomplished by using a PA flotation catheter with an injection port approximately 30 cm from the distal end and a thermister located at the distal end. The thermister, a device capable of sensing changes in temperature, is normally in one of the branches of the PA. The proximal port normally resides within the right atrium and is used for injection of an iced solution of which the temperature is known. Recently use of room-temperature injectate has become more popular.

The "cold injected" can be measured by knowing the volume of injectate, the specific heat of the solution, and the temperature difference between the solution and the patient's blood. The thermister measures the changes in blood temperature from the baseline value as the cold solution ejected by the right ventricle passes the catheter tip. Therefore, because the amount of "cold injected" and the time duration and magnitude of temperature changes have all been measured, the cardiac output can be calculated.[13]

Two distinct advantages of thermodilution are the availability of repeated measurements without the need for repeated blood sampling and less artifact due to the phenomenon of recirculation because of the close proximity of the sampling site to the injection site. Some of the disadvantages in the technique are related to potential incomplete mixing of the cold solution in the right ventricle; variations in the rate of injection; inaccurate sampling by the thermister in the catheter tip because of malposition; and varying losses of the "injected cold" into adjacent cardiac, vascular, and pulmonary tissues.

Derived Indices of Cardiovascular Hemodynamics

Additional information relating to cardiovascular function can be obtained by combining two or more of the measured parameters, thus deriving a new index of function.[14] Often the combination of several independent physiologic measurements will provide insight into specific aspects of myocardial function or cardiovascular relationships that are not as readily apparent by looking at a series of isolated measurements.

Cardiac Index

The cardiac index (CI) is a calculation used to relate cardiac output to body size.

$$CI = \frac{\text{cardiac output (L/min)}}{\text{body surface area (m}^2)}$$

The normal range for CI is 2.7 to 4.3 $L/m^2/min$ with a mean of 3.5 $L/m^2/min$.

Stroke Volume, Stroke Work, and Stroke Work Index

Stroke volume.—The SV is calculated by dividing the measured cardiac output by the heart rate.

Stroke work.—Estimation of myocardial work is important since increases are associated with increased myocardial oxygen demands.[15] Even under resting conditions myocardial oxygen extraction is very large; therefore, significant increases in myocardial work present the possibility of myocardial ischemia unless myocardial blood flow can be augmented. The myocardial work per contraction can be estimated by multiplying the SV by the pressure during systole minus the left ventricular end-diastolic pressure. In practice, stroke work (SW) is obtained by multiplying mean arterial pressure (MAP) minus PAOP by SV.

$$SW = (MAP - PAOP)\,(SV)$$

Stroke work index.—The stroke work index (SWI) is obtained by dividing SW by the body surface area (BSA).

$$SWI = \frac{SW}{BSA}$$

Rate-Pressure Product

The term *rate-pressure product* (RPP) represents a simplified approach extrapolated from the experimentally determined tension index relating ventricular wall tension and systolic intervals to myocardial oxygen consumption. In brief, it uses the well-established relationship that increased heart rate and increased systolic pressure (increased afterload) cause increases in myocardial oxygen consumption. The only advantage to this index is that it does not require sophisticated monitoring equipment.

$$RPP = (\text{heart rate})\,(\text{systolic BP})$$

Values >12,000 are interpreted as indicative of significantly increased myocardial work and increased myocardial oxygen demands.

Systemic and Pulmonary Vascular Resistance

The resistance to flow in arteries can be expressed in the following manner:

$$\text{Resistance} = \frac{\text{arterial pressure} - \text{atrial pressure}}{\text{cardiac output}}$$

Because the two ventricular pumps exist in a series arrangement with two markedly different pressures but the same average flow (cardiac output), the resistances of the two vascular beds are normally quite different.

Resistance calculations require deriving the driving pressure (pressure drop) across the circuit. For systemic vascular resistance (SVR) this is equal to the aortic root pressure (MAP) minus the right atrial pressure (CVP); for pulmonary vascular resistance (PVR) this is equal to the pulmonary artery root pressure (mean PA pressure) minus the left atrial pressure (PAOP). The units of vascular resistance are expressed in dynes sec/cm^{-5}. In clinical practice, pressure is measured in mm Hg and cardiac output in liters per minute. By using these values and taking into account the various conversion factors, the proper units can be arrived at by introducing the number 80 into the basic equation.

$$\text{SVR} = \frac{\text{MAP (mm Hg)} - \text{CVP (mm Hg)}}{\text{cardiac output (L/min)}} \times 80$$

$$\text{PVR} = \frac{\text{PA (mm Hg)} - \text{PAOP (mm Hg)}}{\text{cardiac output (L/min)}} \times 80$$

Representative mean values and the normal range of values are given in Table 2–3.

TABLE 2–3.

Normal Values for Systemic Vascular Resistance (SVR) and Pulmonary Vascular Resistance (PVR)

	Mean (Dynes Sec/Cm^{-5})	Range (Dynes Sec/Cm^{-5})
SVR	1,200	1,000–1,600
PVR	60	50–160

Tissue Perfusion

Recently developed transcutaneous oxygen tension monitors can provide information regarding skin blood flow. A transcutaneous Po_2 index has been evaluated and found to correlate with cardiac output (see Chapter 1).

CASE STUDY

A 27-year-old male passenger pulled from the right front seat of a high-speed, head-on collision arrived in the emergency room via paramedic vehicle. He had been found conscious with his seat belt fastened. An 18-gauge intravenous (IV) line was secured in the right forearm with normal saline running at a rapid rate. An oxygen mask was in place, and the man was speaking incoherently. His skin was clammy and sweaty but not mottled. The hands and feet were cold to the touch.

His BP was 90/? mm Hg; pulse rate, 130/min and regular; and respiratory rate (RR), 35/min. The patient was moving all four extremities and his head without difficulty. No apparent head, neck, or chest trauma was observed. Lung sounds were equal bilaterally and shallow, and no flailing or paradoxical movements were noted. Auscultation of the heart revealed normal S_1 and S_2; no S_3, S_4, or murmurs were noted. The abdomen was tense and tender and no bowel sounds were heard.

Peritoneal lavage documented the presence of intra-abdominal bleeding. Blood specimens for type and crossmatch, complete blood cell count (CBC), and SMA-6 were obtained. A CVP catheter was positioned via the right subclavian route, and then a third IV line (14-gauge) was placed in the left antecubital fossa. A urinary catheter was inserted and 800 mL of blood-tinged urine evacuated. A radial arterial puncture was accomplished and a specimen for blood gas analysis obtained.

Over the next 10 minutes the systolic BP dropped to 60 mm Hg palpable, and the CVP dropped from 5 to 1 cm H_2O. The patient became unresponsive with irregular respirations. The trachea was orally intubated with a 9 mm endotracheal tube and positive-pressure ventilation (PPV) commenced via a self-inflating hand ventilator with a reservoir hose and >15-L/min oxygen flow. The BP was now 40 mm Hg palpable, and the electrocardiographic (ECG) monitor showed a sinus tachycardia.

Discussion

It must be assumed that the inadequate perfusion status is due to a primary blood volume deficiency, i.e., intra-abdominal bleeding. Volume resuscitation is essential. The importance of having inserted the two additional IVs prior to vascular collapse is obvious. There is no indication for vasopressors at this time.

It should be noted that the perfusion status significantly deteriorated when PPV was instituted. This is undoubtedly secondary to decreased venous return and is another reason for rapid volume replacement.

All three IVs should be used to reestablish an adequate blood volume. Of course, blood should be administered as soon as it is available. In the interim, combinations of colloid and crystalloid solutions are appropriate, depending upon availability.

CASE STUDY CONTINUED

Normal saline was administered through the CVP and 18-gauge line while a hetastarch solution was administered through the 14-gauge line. Fifteen minutes later after 2.5 L of saline and 1.5 L of colloid had been administered, the patient's BP was 90/40 mm Hg; pulse rate, 125/min (sinus tachycardia); RR, 10/min by hand ventilator (tidal volumes [V_T], approximately 1.2 L, and FIO_2, 0.6 to 0.7); CVP, 5 cm H_2O; and urine output, 8 cc in the past 10 minutes. His extremities were still cold, with thready peripheral pulses. The abdomen was very tense. The patient began to move his extremities violently and tried to extubate himself. Three people were required to keep him still.

Discussion

Following successful resuscitation of acute hypovolemic shock, the patient often becomes uncooperative and confused due to reestablished cerebral perfusion. This raises the circulating catecholamine level, which increases venous tone, vascular resistance, and myocardial contractility. This sympathetic response is contributing to the maintenance of perfusion and BP. Any sedation would be expected to diminish the level of sympathetic tone and therefore increase the vascular space, thereby creating a relative hypovolemia.

Sedation is essential to allow stabilization and transport to the operating room. Several assumptions are reasonable: (1) this patient's myocardium is strong; (2) tamponade within the abdomen has probably occurred, and further hemorrhage will be slight until the abdomen is surgically opened; and (3) further volume administration to compensate for venodilation is not a problem.

Tranquilizing agents such as the benzodiazepines have unreliable relationships between dose and central nervous system (CNS) and respiratory depression. Furthermore, these drugs are not reversible and have unpredictable cardiovascular side effects. By contrast, morphine sulfate has a well documented and consistent relationship between dose and CNS and respiratory depression, has no direct myocardial depressant properties, is known to be a venodilator, and is completely reversible. These pharmacologic factors make morphine the drug of choice in this circumstance.

CASE STUDY CONTINUED

Morphine sulfate was administered in IV aliquots of 2 mg to a total of 12 mg in 10 minutes. IV fluid was administered to maintain a CVP >5 cm H_2O and a BP >80 systolic. A total of 1.5 L of normal saline was administered in 10 minutes during morphinization. The patient was quiet and unconscious if not stimulated. Ventilation was easily controllable, and the vital signs were now a BP of 85/50 mm Hg, a pulse rate of 122/min (sinus tachycardia), an RR of 10/min (FIO_2 approximately 0.7), a CVP of 6 cm H_2O, and a urine output of 6 cc in 10 minutes. The extremities were still cold. Arterial blood gas analysis revealed a pH of 7.32, a PCO_2 of 45 mm Hg, and a PO_2 of 277 mm Hg.

Blood was now available, and 2 units were started through blood warmers. In the next 20 minutes, 4 units of whole blood and 1 L of crystalloid were administered, which resulted in a BP of 110/60 mm Hg, a pulse rate of 105/min (sinus tachycardia), an RR of 10/min, a CVP of 12 cm H_2O, and a urine output of 30 cc in 20 minutes. The extremities were warmer with good pulses. The abdomen was still very tense. The patient was transported to the operating room for a laparotomy.

Approximately 3 L of blood was suctioned from the abdomen. A liver laceration was oversewn and a lacerated spleen removed. No other abnormalities were found in the abdomen.

Upon arrival in the surgical intensive care unit following surgery the patient had received the following IV fluids:

Blood, whole	2,000 mL (4 units)
Blood, packed cells	2,500 mL (10 units)
Hetastarch	3,000 mL
Crystalloid, saline	5,500 mL
Crystalloid, 0.2% saline	1,500 mL
Total	14.5 L

Fluid losses for the same time period were:

Estimated blood loss	5,000 mL
Urine output	1,700 mL
Total	6.7 L

The BP was 125/70 mm Hg (arterial line); pulse rate, 100/min (no dysrhythmia); and RR, 10/min on the mechanical ventilator (VT, 1,200 mL; FIO_2, 0.35; positive end-expiratory pressure [PEEP], 5 cm H_2O) with no spontaneous ventilatory efforts. A narcotic anesthetic had been used, and a nondepolarizing muscle relaxant had not been reversed. The patient's temperature was 36°C, CVP was 9 cm H_2O, the extremities were warm and dry, the hemoglobin content was 11 gm/dL, pH was 7.41, PCO_2 was 36 mm Hg, and PO_2 was 77 mm Hg.

Over the next 5 hours the patient spontaneously underwent diuresis, breathed spontaneously, and maintained acceptable perfusion and gas exchange. He was removed from ventilatory support and extubated 12 hours postoperatively. The subclavian catheter was removed 36 hours postoperatively.

On the third postoperative day, there were no bowel sounds heard, and he became hypotensive and exhibited tachycardia. Assessment of intake and output revealed a reasonable balance; however, his weight was 2 kg less than his presumed weight prior to the accident. He required 3 L of saline to maintain adequate BP throughout the day, and his urine output remained >50 mL/hour. Electrolyte concentrations were within normal limits; however, total serum protein levels were decreased. An abdominal x-ray film revealed a dilated fluid-filled small bowel without air-fluid levels.

Because the CVP catheter had been removed, it was elected to place a pulmonary artery catheter for further fluid and cardiovascular management. His BP was 110/80 mm Hg; MAP, 90 mm Hg; pulse, 120/min and regular; RR, 22/minute and regular; core temperature, 37.2°C; right atrial pressure, 4 mm Hg; right ventricular pressure, 18/0 mm Hg; PA pressure, 16/9 mm Hg; PAOP, 7 mm Hg; CI, 2.2 L/min; cardiac output, 4.6 L/min; and SVR, 1,520 dynes sec/cm^{-5}.

Discussion

Third-space fluid in the small bowel is the most likely explanation for the hypotension, i.e., a relative hypovolemia (normal or contracted vascular space with diminished vascular volume). Although total body water may be normal at this juncture, much of it is sequestered in the small bowel, thus creating an extracellular (and intracellular) fluid deficit.

The key concept to supportive therapy is to administer adequate fluid to sustain perfusion (ensure adequate preload) while ensuring adequate myocardial contractility. Once the small bowel fluid begins to mobilize, adequate diuresis must be ensured to prevent relative hypervolemia.

PA hemodynamic monitoring is essential if the myocardial status is doubtful or sepsis is suspected. Because neither is true in this case, CVP monitoring would be acceptable. However, because a new central access was necessary, the placement of a PA catheter is acceptable and justifiable.

The inadequate cardiac output is most likely due to an inadequate preload. The increased SVR and tachycardia reflect increased sympathetic tone. Appropriate fluid loading should increase venous conductance and improve cardiac output.

At least 50% of the administered solution should be colloid because the bowel preferentially sequesters protein.

CASE STUDY CONTINUED

Two hundred milliliters of hetastarch solution was administered over a period of 3 minutes without change in vital signs or PAOP. This was repeated twice without measurable changes in hemodynamics. After a total of 800-mL fluid challenge, the heart rate decreased to 105/min, and the cardiac output increased to 5.8 L/min. No change in MAP or PAOP was noted, and SVR was reduced to 1,120 dynes sec/cm^{-5}.

Another 200 mL of colloid was administered and rapidly resulted in a heart rate of 95/min, the PAOP increasing to 11 mm Hg and the cardiac output to 7.2 L/min (CI, 3.5 L/min). The mean arterial pressure was 95 mm Hg with an SVR of 1,100 dynes sec/cm^{-5}. Further fluid administration was titrated to maintain the PAOP at approximately 11 mm Hg.

A positive balance of 6 L over the next 48 hours ensued while perfusion and hemodynamics were maintained. Thereafter, the patient began to undergo diuresis (urine output, >200 mL/hr), and IV fluids were decreased to a minimum. Eleven-liters negative balance ensued over a period of 72 hours with excellent perfusion and maintained hemodynamics. The patient made an uneventful recovery.

REFERENCES

1. Widdowson E, McCance RA, Spray CLM: The chemical composition of the human body. *Clin Sci* 1951; 10:113–125.
2. Keys A, Brazek J: Body fat in adult man. *Physiol Rev* 1953; 33:245–325.
3. Schloerb PR, Friis-Hanson BJ, Edelman IS, et al: The measurement of total body water in the human subject by deuterium oxide dilution with considerations of dynamics on deuterium distribution. *J Clin Invest* 1950; 29:1296–1310.
4. Walcott WW: Blood volume in experimental hemorrhagic shock. *Am J Physiol* 1945; 143:247–261.
5. Fulton GP, Lutz BR, Callahan AB: Innervation as a factor in control of microcirculation. *Physiol Rev* 1960; 40(suppl 4):57.
6. Weissler A, Harris WS, Schoenfeld CD: Bedside techniques for the evaluation of ventricular function in man. *Am J Cardiol* 1969; 23:577–583.
7. Ross J Jr, Covell JC, Sonnenblick EH, et al: Contractile state of the heart characterized by force-velocity relations in variably afterloaded and isovolemic beats. *Circ Res* 1966; 18:149–163.
8. Dodge HT, Baxley WA: Left ventricular volume and mass and their significance in heart disease. *Am J Cardiol* 1969; 23:528–537.
9. Schelbert HR, Verba JW, Johnson AD, et al: Nontraumatic determination of left ventricular ejection fraction by radionuclide angiocardiography. *Circulation* 1975; 51:902–909.
10. Sarnoff SJ: Symposium on regulation of performance of heart; myocardial contractility as described by ventricular function curves; observations on Starling's law of heart. *Physiol Rev* 1955; 35:107–122.
11. Haynes RH, Burton AC: Role of the non-Newtonian behavior of blood in hemodynamics. *Am J Physiol* 1959; 197:943–950.
12. Fick A: Uber die messung des blutquantuns in dem herzventribeln. *Sitzungsb du physmed Ges zu Wurzburg* 1870; 16.
13. Weisel RD, Berger RL, Hechtman HB: Measurement of cardiac output by thermodilution. *N Engl J Med* 1975; 292:682–684.
14. Sonnenblick EH, Strobeck JE: Current concepts in cardiology: Derived indexes of ventricular and myocardial function. *N Engl J Med* 1977; 296:978–982.
15. Sonnenblick EH, Shelton CL; Myocardial energetics: Basic principles and clinical implications. *N Engl J Med* 1971; 285:668–675.

3/Detrimental Work of Breathing

ROY D. CANE, M.B.B.CH.

The ventilatory pump creates transpulmonary pressure gradients by cyclic muscle contractions that require energy expenditure (i.e., work). This work of breathing (WOB) not only provides for alveolar ventilation, it also promotes an efficient pulmonary gas distribution in relation to pulmonary perfusion and maintains cardiac function by augmenting venous return to the right atrium. Thus WOB can be considered beneficial to the maintenance of cardiopulmonary homeostasis. Increased WOB, provided it is accomplished within the limits of cardiopulmonary reserves, will also have a beneficial effect on cardiopulmonary homeostasis. However, if the increased WOB places demands on the cardiopulmonary system that exceed functional reserves, the result is often a deterioration in cardiopulmonary homeostasis. Such levels of WOB can be considered detrimental.

Extreme degrees of detrimental WOB are recognized clinically as acute respiratory distress (i.e., tachypnea, tachycardia, dyspnea, hypertension, intercostal retraction, the use of accessory muscles of ventilation, diaphoresis, and mental status changes). The patient is often described as appearing "fatigued" or "tired out." Lesser degrees of detrimental WOB undoubtedly exist but are difficult to recognize clinically or to quantitate.

Because support of cardiopulmonary homeostasis is a basic tenet of critical care medicine, the concept of detrimental WOB is key to the appropriate management of disorders of ventilation, oxygenation, and perfusion. This chapter considers those factors relevant to the clinical manifestation of detrimental WOB and delineates a clinical approach to management.

DETERMINANTS OF MUSCULAR WORK FOR THE VENTILATORY MUSCLES

Mechanical work is accomplished when a force applied to an object results in movement of the object. The amount of work is reflected by the product of the force applied and the distance moved.

$$\text{Work} = \text{force} \times \text{distance}$$

For spontaneous ventilation the mean pressure generated by the ventilatory muscles represents the force, and the tidal volume (V_T) represents the distance:

$$Work = P \times V_T$$

The ventilatory muscle work load is primarily dependent on the required minute volume, the airway resistance, and the pulmonary compliance. Interaction of these factors determines the pattern of breathing and ventilatory muscle efficiency.

Minute Volume

The relationship of minute volume to WOB is shown in Figure 3–1,A. Under normal physiologic conditions ventilatory muscle oxygen consumption (Vo_2vent) accounts for approximately 5% of the total oxygen consumption (Vo_2tot).[1, 2] As minute volume increases, Vo_2vent increases at a faster rate than Vo_2tot does, i.e., the ventilatory muscle efficiency is less at higher minute volumes, and the ratio of Vo_2vent/Vo_2tot increases.[3–5] The dashed curve in Figure 3–1 shows this relationship for patients with cardiopulmonary disease.[4, 6] This exponential increase in Vo_2vent/Vo_2tot in patients with cardiopulmonary disease[7, 8] probably results in increasing diversion of the oxygen supply to the ventilatory muscles at the expense of other tissues, a situation clearly detrimental to the maintenance of tissue oxygenation.

The minute volume required to maintain eucapnia is determined by carbon dioxide production (Vco_2) and dead-space ventilation. Approximately one third of inspired gas does not participate normally in gas exchange with pulmonary blood because it lies within conducting airways (anatomic dead space) or ventilates nonperfused or underperfused alveoli (alveolar dead space). Lung and cardiac disease can increase dead-space ventilation. The greater the dead-space ventilation, the greater will be the required minute volume to maintain eucapnia for any given Vco_2.

Vco_2 is proportional to the metabolic rate. Any factors that increase the metabolic rate will increase Vco_2 and hence the required minute volume. Examples of clinical circumstances commonly encountered in critically ill patients that will increase the metabolic rate include fever, sepsis, acute metabolic responses to physiologic stress, hyperalimentation, etc.

There are three principal causes of increases in minute volume over and above that required to maintain eucapnia:

1. Arterial hypoxemia
2. Arterial acidemia
3. Central nervous system (CNS) disorders

Arterial Hypoxemia

Acute reduction in the arterial Po_2 below a threshold stimulates the peripheral chemoreceptors of the carotid and aortic bodies. This in turn stimulates the activity of the respiratory center, which results in an increased rate and depth of breathing and hence increased minute volume. Reductions in arterial oxygen content secondary

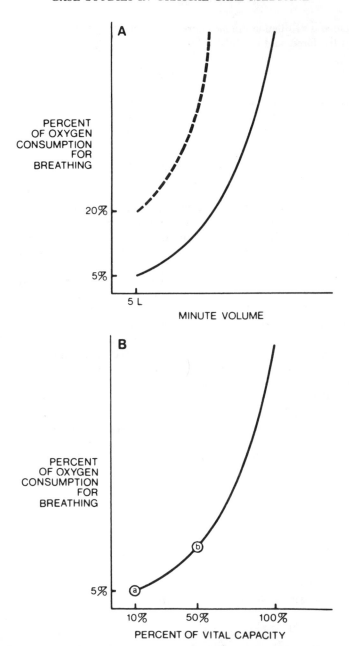

FIG 3–1.
A, WOB in relation to minute volume of ventilation. The *dashed line* represents a patient with cardiopulmonary disease. **B,** WOB in relation to VT expressed as a percentage of vital capacity (VC): a = a VT of 500 mL with a VC of 5 L; b = a VT of 500 mL with a VC of 1 L. (From Shapiro BA, Harrison RA, Cane RD, et al: *Clinical Application of Blood Gases,* ed 4. Chicago, Year Book Medical Publishers, Inc, 1989. Used by permission.)

to anemia or the presence of abnormal forms of hemoglobin will also stimulate the carotid bodies, although to a lesser extent than hypoxemia. It is important to remember that patients with significant hypoxemia invariably have cardiopulmonary disease, which in itself results in increased WOB prior to that induced by the hypoxemia. This combination of factors that increases WOB puts these patients at greater risk of developing detrimental WOB.

Arterial Acidemia

Low arterial pH stimulates the ventilatory drive via chemoreceptors of the carotid and aortic bodies with a resultant increase in minute volume. In circumstances where the acidemia is secondary to hypoxemia and/or inadequate tissue perfusion, the patient usually has underlying cardiopulmonary disease, which in itself contributes to an increased WOB. The combination of cardiopulmonary disease and arterial acidemia has a large impact on WOB.

Noncardiopulmonary causes of arterial acidemia (e.g., diabetes mellitus or renal disease) may or may not be related to cardiopulmonary disease and therefore will not necessarily be associated with preexisting increased WOB; hence, these patients are less likely to have difficulties handling the required WOB.

Central Nervous System Disorders

There are many circumstances, ranging from psychological factors such as anxiety to serious intracranial pathology (e.g., infections, trauma, cerebrovascular accidents, and tumors), in which CNS stimulation results in hyperventilation. CNS dysfunction secondary to hepatic or renal disease, so-called metabolic encephalopathy, is commonly associated with hyperventilation.

Hyperventilation induced by the CNS does not appear to be commonly associated with detrimental WOB per se unless the patient has preexisting cardiopulmonary disease that has resulted in acute increases in WOB or chronic impairment of ventilatory reserve.

Airway Resistance

Gas flow in the airways is a result of the transairway pressure gradient between the mouth and alveoli that is generated by the ventilatory pump. Resistance to this flow equals the pressure gradient divided by the flow.

$$R = \frac{P}{F}$$

The relationship between flow and pressure is further affected by the nature of the flow, which can be laminar or turbulent. Under circumstances of laminar flow the flow rate for any given constant pressure gradient is mainly determined by the fourth power of the radius of the tube as defined by the law of Poiseuille.[9] Small reductions in airway diameter can produce significant increases in airway resistance.

With turbulent flow the density of the gas becomes an important determinant of resistance. If all other factors are equal, resistance will be higher with turbulent flow than with laminar flow. In the tracheobronchial tree laminar and turbulent flow usually coexist. Resistance to gas flow in the airway is therefore a function of the inspiratory flow rate, airway diameter, and density of the inspired gas.

The pressure gradient and hence the work generated by the ventilatory pump has to be sufficient to overcome the resistance to gas flow through the airway. Given that resistance is a flow-dependent phenomenon, any factors (e.g., rapid patterns of breathing) that result in increased gas flow rates increase airway resistance and WOB. Decreases in airway diameter (e.g., bronchoconstriction; bronchial mucosal edema; presence of secretions, foreign bodies, or tumors in the airway) increase WOB. Gas density, although usually constant, can be increased by the aerosolization of water or saline into the inspiratory gas for bronchial hygiene treatments or as a vehicle for the pulmonary administration of medications.

Compliance

A force greater than the balance of elastic forces of the lung and chest wall must be generated to achieve airflow into the lungs. The greater the elastic forces of the lung (lower compliance), the greater the force required to achieve ventilation, and the greater will be the WOB. Most acute pathology of the lung parenchyma results in a decline in lung compliance and increased WOB. Any factors that restrict chest wall and diaphragmatic movement have a similar effect.

Some of the energy expended for inspiration is "stored" in the elastic tissues of the lung and chest wall as elastic recoil energy, and this provides most of the required energy for expiration. When expiration is passive, WOB is almost entirely related to inspiration. However, when the expiratory muscles actively contract (e.g., minute volumes >20 L/min with normal lungs or lower minute volumes in diseased lungs with significantly increased airway resistance), the WOB will be determined by both inspiration and expiration.

Pattern of Breathing

If a constant minute volume is maintained, the work required to overcome elastic forces varies directly with V_T and is greater with deep, slow breathing patterns. The work required to overcome airway resistance varies directly with the inspiratory flow rate and is increased with rapid, shallow breathing patterns. Figure 3–2 shows a theoretical plot of total WOB vs. differing breathing patterns associated with a constant minute volume. For any given combination of airway resistance and lung/chest wall compliance there is an optimal pattern of breathing that is associated with the lowest possible WOB. It has been demonstrated that human subjects and animals tend to select breathing frequencies that are close to theoretically ideal patterns requiring the least possible WOB.[10] A similar response is commonly seen in patients with pulmonary disease. When compliance decreases, the respiratory rate increases, and V_T decreases; when airway resistance increases, the respiratory rate decreases,

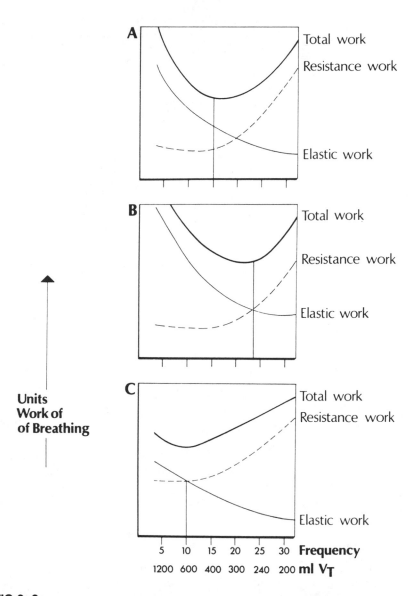

**Units
Work of
of Breathing**

FIG 3–2.
Graphic representation of the relationship between total WOB and different patterns of breathing associated with the same minute ventilation. Total work is the sum of resistance and elastic work. Note that there is a ventilatory pattern that requires the least work. **A,** normal compliance and airway resistance; **B,** decreased compliance and normal airway resistance; **C,** increased airway resistance and normal compliance. (From Shapiro BA, Harrison RA, Kacmarek RM, et al: *Clinical Application of Respiratory Care,* ed 3. Chicago, Year Book Medical Publishers, Inc, 1985. Used by permission.)

and VT increases. Therefore, provided CNS factors such as anxiety do not override these mechanisms, the clinician can assume that a ventilatory pattern in any patient with lung disease is determined by a need for minimal energy expenditure rather than efficient physiologic ventilation.

Muscle Efficiency

The biochemical events that occur in a contracting ventilatory muscle are of little practical significance to clinicians. Of importance to clinicians are those factors that affect ventilatory muscle efficiency and WOB and are amenable to therapeutic manipulation. In this context ventilatory muscle efficiency can be considered in terms of the muscle fiber length at the initiation of a contraction, energy supply to the muscle from intrinsic energy stores and blood flow, and the mechanical circumstances in which the muscle activity occurs. For this discussion, ventilatory muscle efficiency will be considered in terms of the relationship between the amount of work performed and the energy cost of that work. Thus, efficient ventilatory muscle function generates a required minute volume for the lowest possible energy cost. Impairment of ventilatory muscle efficiency results in a higher energy cost for the maintenance of a required minute volume.

Ventilatory Muscle Fiber Length

The force generated by a skeletal muscle during contraction is partially dependent on the muscle fiber length at the initiation of a contraction. All skeletal muscles have an optimal position on their force-length curve for energy-efficient contractions. For the ventilatory muscles lung volume is the primary determinant of muscle fiber length and hence is an important factor in force-length relationships.

The force generated by the diaphragm can be assessed by measurement of the transdiaphragmatic pressure during a diaphragmatic contraction induced by phrenic nerve stimulation. It has been shown that the transdiaphragmatic pressure generated for a given phrenic nerve stimulation decreases linearly as lung volume increases from functional residual capacity.[11] This is believed to result from shorter diaphragm muscle fibers secondary to the increase in lung volume, which places the fibers in a disadvantageous circumstance with respect to their force-length relationships.

Energy Supply

The contracting muscle consumes oxygen and energy in the form of adenosine triphosphate (ATP). Generation of ATP by a muscle occurs by several processes including phosphorylation of adenosine diphosphate (ADP), oxidative phosphorylation of fatty acids, and anaerobic glycolysis. To maintain these processes the muscle must have a supply of phosphate, fatty acids, and glucose. Skeletal muscles contain creatine phosphate, fat, and glycogen stores, which provide the substrate for these biochemical reactions. Starvation and/or catabolic states are associated with depletion of these intramuscular stores and can have a negative impact on the ability of the muscle to generate a constant supply of ATP.[12] Intramuscular concentrations of ATP have been shown to be low in patients with chronic obstructive pulmonary disease (COPD) and marginal nutrition, a possible factor in the increased susceptibility of these patients to experience ventilatory failure when stressed.[13] Serum concentrations of phosphate <1.5 mg/dL are associated with ventilatory failure.[14] The clinical observation that some patients, committed to mechanical ventilatory support during an acute catabolic illness, are unable to be weaned from ventilatory support until their nutritional status has been restored to premorbid levels stresses the importance of muscle energy storage on maintenance of muscle efficiency.

Muscle blood flow, responsible for the delivery of oxygen and energy substrates to the ventilatory muscles, is essential for maintenance of ventilatory muscle function.[15] Therefore, an adequate arterial oxygen content and cardiac output are essential to the maintenance of ventilatory muscle function. Because muscle perfusion occurs primarily during muscle diastole, the breathing pattern of a patient may have an impact on oxygen delivery. The higher the respiratory rate, the lesser the available time for muscle perfusion and oxygen and energy substrate delivery.

Ventilatory Muscle Mechanics

Diaphragm.—The diaphragm consists of a central tendon connecting two muscular hemidiaphragms whose fibers arise from the first three lumbar vertebral bodies and the inner surfaces and upper margins of the lower six ribs. The fibers of the costal part of the diaphragm are directed upward, parallel to the long axis of the thorax, and are apposed directly to the inner surface of the lower part of the thoracic cage. The central zone of each hemidiaphragm is domed upward. During diaphragmatic contraction the costal fibers shorten and displace the dome axially downward, which results in (1) a decrease in intrathoracic pressure, which in turn will increase lung volume if the airway is open, (2) an increase in abdominal pressure, and (3) displacement of the lower rib cage. If the descent of the dome of the diaphragm is opposed by increasing abdominal pressure, the shortening of the costal fibers results in an upward and outward movement of the lower rib cage. Thus it is clear that the area of apposition between the diaphragm and chest wall is crucial to diaphragmatic action. Decreasing lung volume below functional residual capacity (FRC) increases the area of apposition and increases displacement of the rib cage by diaphragmatic contraction. Conversely, increasing the lung volume decreases the area of apposition and reduces the action of the diaphragm on the rib cage.[16] A reduction in rib cage displacement results in a smaller change in lung volume and less ventilation. To maintain ventilation as the zone of apposition decreases, greater force has to be generated by the diaphragm, hence WOB is increased. Extreme flattening of the diaphragm, as is seen in severe hyperinflation, may abolish the area of diaphragm and chest wall apposition and result in an inward displacement of the rib cage with diaphragmatic contraction.

The mechanical advantage of a rising intra-abdominal pressure on diaphragmatic contraction is also important. Loss of intra-abdominal pressure secondary to paralysis of abdominal wall musculature results in greater downward displacement of the dome of the diaphragm and less effective elevation of the lower portion of the rib cage.

Expansion of the lower part of the rib cage is less in the supine than in the upright position.[16] Although the exact mechanism for this difference is unclear, it probably explains the clinical observation that patients breathe more comfortably in an upright or semi-upright position.

Chest wall.—The chest wall is a syncytium composed of ribs, sternum, intercostal muscles, and fibrous membranes and is attached posteriorly to the vertebral column. The actions of inspiratory muscles on the chest wall depend on the movement of the ribs around the axes of their articulation with the vertebral bodies. Any muscle contraction that elevates the ribs results in an increase in the anteroposterior and transverse diameters of the rib cage. The upper ribs have shorter cartilaginous attachments and articulations with the sternum than do the lower ribs and hence tend to move to a lesser degree. The change in pleural pressure secondary to rib displacement is therefore usually greater with movement of the lower ribs than with the upper ribs. Factors that interfere with rib movement (e.g., external compression, abnormal rib anatomy, extreme hyperinflation of the chest) require greater force to be generated by the ventilatory muscles to achieve a given transpulmonary pressure and therefore result in increased WOB.

The external intercostal muscle fibers run obliquely downward and forward, with the lower rib insertion further from the axis of rotation than the upper rib insertion, which on contraction results in a greater torque on the lower than the upper rib, thus in a net upward movement of the rib. Hence they act as inspiratory muscles. Conversely, the internal intercostal muscle fibers run obliquely downward and backward, with the upper rib insertion further from the point of rotation than the lower rib insertion. Contraction produces a greater force on the upper rib, and this results in a net downward movement of the rib. Hence they act as expiratory muscles.

Accessory muscles.—The major accessory muscles are the scalene, sternomastoid, trapezius, and pectoralis muscles. Although they are not normally active during resting ventilation, they are capable of elevating the rib cage and can provide a degree of inspiratory action.

MEASUREMENT OF THE WORK OF BREATHING

Measurement of aspects of ventilatory muscle metabolism (oxygen consumption, electromyography) or of the pressures and flows generated by the ventilatory muscles provide means for quantifying WOB.

Oxygen Consumption (V_{O_2})

Measurement of the change in V_{O_2} after an induced change in ventilatory demand quantitates the oxygen cost of breathing and provides a reflection of WOB. For example, the change in measured V_{O_2} of a patient initially assessed on full ventilatory support and then when ventilating spontaneously would be caused by WOB, provided no change in metabolic rate due to nonventilatory work had occurred between the two measurement points. In the critical care area this approach has not proved to be useful for several reasons. First, stability of the metabolic rate is unusual in critically ill patients. Second, the measurement technique has to be extremely sensitive and accurate because the Vo_2 of WOB is a small part of the total Vo_2 and, furthermore, high FIo_2s, commonly used in the management of critically ill patients, result in very small differences in inspiratory and expiratory O_2 concentrations. The available equipment lacks this high degree of accuracy and sensitivity.[17] Third, interfacing the patient and monitor to ensure reliable sampling of true mixed expired gas is technically difficult in the clinical setting.

The Vo_2 can be calculated from the product of cardiac output and the arteriovenous oxygen content difference. However, this approach is subject to considerable error because measurement of cardiac output is imprecise and derivation of blood oxygen content is susceptible to multiplicative arithmetic errors. It also requires a mixed venous blood sample, which is not readily available in all patients.

Electromyography of Ventilatory Muscles

The integrated electromyogram of the ventilatory muscles provides an indirect measure of the intramuscular tension and metabolic activity and correlates with Vo_2 of the muscle.[18] Although this is a useful research tool, its application to critically ill patients is limited for technical reasons. Furthermore, the magnitude of the integrated electromyogram varies widely from patient to patient.

Pressure and Flow Measurements

The work of breathing can be determined from the relationship between the volume change induced in the lung by a pressure gradient (ΔP). This approach is easily applied to measure the mechanical work applied across the thorax ($\Delta P = P_{airway} - P_{atmospheric}$) or lung ($\Delta P = P_{airway} - P_{intrapleural}$) when a patient's lung is passively inflated with a known volume of gas. Unfortunately, this approach cannot be applied if the patient is actively breathing because the pressure of interest is that generated in the muscle, which is not amenable to easy measurement. Various mathematical approaches based on pressure and flow measurements have been used to evaluate spontaneous WOB through mechanical ventilator circuits.[18] Unfortunately, these are not readily applied to the spontaneously ventilating critically ill patient.

DETRIMENTAL WORK OF BREATHING
Diagnosis of Detrimental Work of Breathing

From the above discussion it is apparent that the bedside measurement of WOB in the spontaneously ventilating critically ill patient is not a clinical reality at this time. The clinician has to rely on clinical judgments of WOB and its impact on cardiopulmonary function. The concept of detrimental WOB describes a clinical picture of progressively increasing WOB manifested by progressive increases in the respiratory rate, heart rate, and systolic blood pressure; onset of diaphoresis; and mental confusion, delirium, or even obtundation. Patients able to communicate invariably complain of dyspnea. The progression of clinical signs is an important element in the diagnosis of detrimental WOB. An isolated observation of tachypnea or tachycardia, although possibly related to detrimental WOB, cannot be used to make the diagnosis. Any patient with pathology that results in an increase in WOB is susceptible to the development of detrimental WOB.

Clinical Conditions Associated With Increased Work of Breathing

Ventilatory Reserve

The mechanical efficiency of the ventilatory pump is poor. In the resting state about 10% of the energy consumed is used to achieve gas exchange, the other 90% being lost as heat.[19] Pulmonary disease further reduces this mechanical efficiency. However, despite this, most individuals have some reserve of ventilatory power.

Figure 3–1,A shows the relationship between WOB and minute ventilation. As discussed above, increases in minute ventilation cause an exponential increase in WOB. Assuming a relatively constant respiratory rate, increases in minute volume are caused by increases in VT. Graphic representation of WOB vs. VT expressed as a percentage of VC produces a curve similar to the relationship of WOB and minute volume (Fig 3–1,B). Thus it is obvious that the greater the portion of the vital capacity used for each VT, the greater is the WOB, and the lesser is the patient's ability to increase VT to meet any increase in ventilatory demand secondary to acute illness and physiologic stress. Hence VC may be used as an expression of the ventilatory reserve. Although this is a greatly oversimplified view of ventilatory reserve, it has the merit of being qualitatively reliable and readily applicable to the clinical care of patients.

Reduction of ventilatory reserve secondary to chronic cardiopulmonary disease predisposes to development of detrimental WOB. Clinically, patients required to generate VT of >40% to 50% of their VC commonly manifest detrimental WOB.

Development of detrimental WOB should be anticipated in any clinical circumstance where ventilatory demand is increased concomitantly with a reduction in ventilatory reserve. Ventilatory demand is directly increased by hypoxemia and metabolic acidemia. Common conditions associated with increased ventilatory demand secondary to increased metabolic demand include sepsis, acute physiologic stress, and provision of hyperalimentation. Ventilatory reserve is decreased in all forms of chronic lung disease, in most forms of acute cardiopulmonary disease, and following thoracoabdominal surgery.

Impending Ventilatory Failure

The clinical assessment of increased WOB in a patient with compromised ventilatory reserve and worsening acute cardiopulmonary pathology suggests that acute ventilatory failure is probably inevitable. This circumstance, termed impending ventilatory failure, is an example of significantly detrimental WOB. It is not unusual for patients in this situation to maintain acceptable blood gas values by increasing cardiopulmonary work. However, if no therapeutic interventions are made, acute ventilatory failure (rising $PaCO_2$ and falling pHa) will ensue.

Ventilatory Muscle Fatigue

Any skeletal muscle can be overworked to the point that it fails to maintain function. Fatigue may be defined as the inability of the muscle to sustain a required force.[20] Ventilatory muscle fatigue may be defined as the inability of the inspiratory muscles to continue to generate sufficient transpulmonary pressure to maintain adequate alveolar ventilation. Ventilatory muscle fatigue has been the focus of considerable investigation, well summarized by Roussos and Macklem.[20] The causes and sites of failure of the ventilatory pump and the metabolic changes in the ventilatory muscles under conditions of fatigue are of little practical significance to the critical care practitioner. Conceptualizing ventilatory muscle fatigue as a consequence of circumstances where ventilatory muscle energy demands exceed energy supply provides a clinically relevant approach that focuses attention on those factors amenable to therapeutic intervention. Table 3–1 summarizes factors relating to energy supply and demand for the ventilatory muscles.

The diagnosis of ventilatory muscle fatigue is readily made in the research laboratory by various techniques (e.g., measurement of the integrated electromyogram of the inspiratory muscles, measurement of transdiaphragmatic pressures, measurement of mouth pressures under differing conditions of inspiratory work load, etc.); however, these techniques are not readily applied to critically ill patients. Patients

TABLE 3–1.

Factors Related to the Development of Ventilatory Muscle Fatigue

Energy Demand	Energy Supply
Work of breathing	Muscle blood flow
Minute volume	Cardiac output
Compliance	Respiratory pattern
Resistance	Distribution of perfusion
Respiratory pattern	
	Energy substrate supply
Muscle efficiency	Blood glucose
Lung volume	Blood fatty acids
Nutritional state	Serum phosphorus
Fiber length	
Atrophy	Energy stores
Neuromuscular disease	Muscle glycogen
	Muscle ATP
	Muscle creatine phosphate
	Arterial oxygen content
	Hemoglobin concentration
	Oxygen saturation

with ventilatory muscle fatigue show the clinical signs of detrimental WOB. Under conditions of ventilatory muscle fatigue a patient may alternate the inspiratory work between the two principal inspiratory muscles, i.e., the diaphragm and the external intercostal muscles, which results in alternating paradoxical chest and abdominal wall movement. Measurement of airway pressure at the mouth allows for objective measurement of ventilatory muscle power in many critically ill patients. An inspiratory work load that requires the patient to generate a mouth pressure with each breath >40% of the maximal mouth pressure that the patient can generate will invariably be associated with ventilatory muscle fatigue.

Detrimental WOB and Airway Pressure Therapy

The work of breathing has been measured in patients undergoing various modes of mechanical ventilatory support. The assist and intermittent mandatory ventilation (IMV) modes (see Chapter 4) may be associated with significantly increased WOB when compared with control mode.[21-23] With the assist mode of ventilatory support, the required work, which varies with exhaled VT and delivered gas flow rate, persists into the mechanical phase of inspiration and reaches levels sufficient to compromise ventilatory reserve.[22] The IMV mode is associated with a greater energy demand than is the assist mode.[23] These increases in WOB may compromise recovery of ventilatory muscle function in patients with ventilatory muscle fatigue who are managed with the assist or IMV modes of mechanical ventilatory support.[16]

The application of continuous positive airway pressure (CPAP) is also associated with increased WOB.[24] The work of breathing depends on the technique (continuous flow vs. demand flow) and the relationship between the patient's inspiratory flow requirement and the actual delivered flow. If the delivered flow is greater than the patient's flow requirement, and there is no significant time lag in delivery of the flow, the increase in WOB is small.[24] At any given flow rate, continuous flow systems are associated with lesser increases in WOB than are demand flow systems.[25-27]

TREATMENT OF DETRIMENTAL WORK OF BREATHING

Treatment of detrimental WOB may be approached in several ways depending on the underlying cause. In principle, detrimental WOB develops when there is an imbalance between the inspiratory work load and the capacity of the ventilatory pump to handle that work load. Therapy should be directed at reducing the inspiratory work or improving the ventilatory muscle efficiency. Table 3–2 lists the major factors that are amenable to acute therapeutic manipulation. Mechanical ventilatory support allows for total to partial ablation of the inspiratory work load by provision of full or partial ventilatory support (see Chapters 4 and 5). However, mechanical ventilatory support is not without potential complications. Consideration of the factors increasing the ventilatory work load or reducing ventilatory muscle efficiency may enable the clinician to favorably manipulate WOB without committing the patient to mechanical ventilatory support. The following case studies illustrate this approach.

TABLE 3–2.

Factors Related to Detrimental Work of Breathing and Their Therapy

Factor	Therapy
Increased work load	
Hypoxemia	Increase F_{IO_2}/PEEP*
Acidemia	Treat cause, e.g., diabetic acidosis
	Bicarbonate therapy[†]
Fever, sepsis	Cooling, antipyretics
Hyperalimentation	Decrease calorie supply[‡]
	Add lipids to calorie source[‡]
High airway resistance	Treat bronchospasm
	Bronchial hygiene therapy to remove secretions
	Diuresis for bronchial edema associated with CHF*
	Artificial airway for upper airway narrowing
Low lung compliance	Diuresis if hemodynamic pulmonary edema, treat CHF
	PEEP/CPAP* for noncardiogenic pulmonary edema[§]
	PEEP/CPAP for acute restrictive pulmonary pathologies
	Bronchial hygiene therapy for atelectasis, retained secretions
Decreased muscle efficiency	
Muscle fiber length	PEEP/CPAP to increase lung volume
	Bronchodilators, expiratory resistance for hyper-inflation
Restricted chest wall movement	Change body position, remove constricting dressings, etc.
Decreased muscle perfusion	Treat cardiac failure
Decreased O_2 supply	Correct hypoxemia/anemia
Decreased energy supply	Correct hypoglycemia
Decreased energy stores	Correct hypophosphatemia, hyperalimentation[¶]
Muscle weakness	Correct electrolyte problems, muscle training[¶]

*PEEP = positive end-expiratory pressure; CHF = congestive heart failure; CPAP = continuous positive airway pressure.
[†]Because bicarbonate therapy represents a CO_2 load, this approach may not be appropriate if muscle fatigue or impending ventilatory failure is suspected.
[‡]See Chapter 7.
[§]See Chapter 18.
[¶]These therapies do not produce immediate results and usually have to be provided in conjunction with some mechanical ventilatory support.

CASE STUDY 1

A 32-year-old, 65-kg woman with a history of asthma came to the emergency room with complaints of shortness of breath and a "tight" feeling in her chest. She was taking an oral form of theophylline but recently had felt "so well" that she spontaneously omitted several doses. She had recently acquired a cat as a pet. On examination she was noted to be sitting up, leaning forward, and supporting herself on her outstretched arms. She was breathing 16 times per minute with a VT of 425 mL. She was unable to perform a VC maneuver. She was using accessory muscles of ventilation and was actively contracting her abdominal musculature during expiration. Her heart rate was 125/min with sinus rhythm; her blood pressure was 150/85 mm Hg. She had a temperature of 39°C. She denied any preceding fevers, cough, or sputum production. Auscultation of the chest revealed diffuse inspiratory and expiratory wheezing over both lung fields and a markedly prolonged expiratory time. The rest of the physical examination was noncontributory. Arterial blood gas (ABG) analysis on room air revealed a pH of 7.36, a Pco_2 of 48 mm Hg, and a Po_2 of 68 mm Hg. Chest x-ray films showed evidence of hyperinflation with no infiltrates. A complete blood cell count (CBC) with a differential white blood cell (WBC) count was unremarkable except for a mild increase in eosinophils. Serum electrolyte levels were within normal limits. An intravenous (IV) line was established and a theophylline infusion started at a rate of 0.9 mg/kg/hr. She was administered 40% oxygen by face mask and given 0.3 mg of epinephrine subcutaneously. A respiratory therapist was called to administer albuterol, 25 mg, by aerosol. During the course of the physical examination and before administration of albuterol the patient's heart rate increased to 140/min, and she complained of increasing shortness of breath.

Discussion

This patient had an acute exacerbation of asthma. The preliminary clinical assessment was consistent with an elevated WOB that can be considered detrimental because her heart rate and complaints of dyspnea increased during physical examination. The ABG analysis and physical examination were consistent with a diagnosis of impending ventilatory failure (stage III of asthma). The primary factor responsible for the detrimental WOB appears to be worsening of her asthma and an acute increase in airway resistance. Endotracheal intubation is particularly hazardous in patients with reactive airway disease. Every reasonable attempt to break the bronchospasm pharmacologically, thereby avoiding intubation and mechanical ventilation, is justified. The patient had been taking an oral theophylline preparation, thus it is advisable to omit or administer a reduced loading dose before initiation of a continuous IV infusion. The dosage can be adjusted after checking a serum theophylline level.

CASE STUDY 1 CONTINUED

After initiation of oxygen therapy, administration of epinephrine subcutaneously, and delivery of albuterol, her respiratory rate was 14/min; heart rate, 128/min; and blood pressure, 140/80 mm Hg. Repeat ABG analysis or an Fio_2 of 0.4 showed pH 7.37; Pco_2, 46 mm Hg; and Po_2, 165 mm Hg. She reported that her shortness of breath was improved. After administration of 100 mg of hydrocortisone IV and a second aerosol albuterol treatment her heart rate declined to 100/min with a blood pressure of 125/80 mm Hg. She could now sit in a semi-supine position and breathe 14 times per min without the use of accessory muscles. She stated that her breathing was only mildly uncomfortable. Auscultation of the chest at this time revealed diminished yet still diffuse inspiratory and expiratory wheezing. Repeat

ABG analysis with 2 L O_2 by nasal cannula revealed a pH of 7.39, a P_{CO_2} of 41 mm Hg, and a P_{O_2} of 110 mm Hg. She was referred to a pulmonologist for long-term management of her asthma.

Discussion

Combined treatment of epinephrine, albuterol, aminophylline, and hydrocortisone reduced the patient's airway resistance and decreased her WOB. Correction of the mild hypoxemia probably contributed to the reduction in ventilatory work load and thereby further ameliorated her detrimental WOB.

CASE STUDY 2

A 62-year-old, 56-kg man with a long-standing history of COPD with chronic CO_2 retention was admitted with a history of worsening shortness of breath, increased sputum production for the past 3 days, and fevers. On examination he was noted to be cachectic and mildly cyanotic around the lips and fingertips. He had difficulty completing a sentence without pausing to take a breath. He was breathing with the use of accessory muscles at a rate of 19 breaths per minute. His VC was 700 mL, with a V_T of 280 mL. His heart rate was 125/min, with atrial fibrillation. Blood pressure was 130/90 mm Hg, and temperature was 40°C. A spontaneously produced sputum sample was grossly purulent. Examination of the chest revealed a barrel shape, with diminished air entry and expiratory wheezing. Cardiovascular examination was remarkable for tachycardia and an irregular rhythm. There was no evidence of heart failure. Arterial blood gas analysis showed a pH of 7.50, a P_{CO_2} of 49 mm Hg, and a P_{O_2} of 48 mm Hg. The CBC revealed a hemoglobin concentration of 16 g/dL and a WBC count of 16,000/mm³ with a left shift. Other than an elevated bicarbonate concentration and a phosphorus of 1.8 mg/dL his serum electrolytes were within reasonable limits. A chest x-ray film showed hyperinflation, flattening of the hemidiaphragms, and a right lower lobe infiltrate. A regimen of appropriate antibiotics for a community-acquired pneumonia was instituted and oxygen was administered by face mask on an Fi_{O_2} of 0.24. His shortness of breath persisted, and his respiratory rate increased to 22/min. Occasional ventricular ectopic beats were noted on the electrocardiographic (ECG) monitor. His blood pressure was 140/90 mm Hg. Repeat ABG analysis showed a pH of 7.50, a P_{CO_2} of 46 mm Hg, and a P_{O_2} of 52 mm Hg.

Discussion

This patient was hospitalized with factors that lead to increased ventilatory demand, i.e., hypoxemia and fever. His COPD resulted in a chronically increased WOB by several means: flattening of the diaphragm, which decreases its mechanical efficiency; hyperinflation, which adversely affects inspiratory muscle fiber length; and increased airway resistance. The patient's marginal nutritional status, a common finding in patients with COPD, may have caused diminished ventilatory muscle efficiency by a reduction in muscle phosphate and energy substrate storage. In addition to these factors that had chronically reduced his ventilatory reserve, the acute pneumonia further reduced it. This increased ventilatory demand, combined with a reduced ventilatory reserve and ventilatory muscle efficiency, made him particularly susceptible to the development of detrimental WOB.

The initial blood gas analysis revealed acute alveolar hyperventilation superimposed on chronic ventilatory failure and severe hypoxemia. The hypoxemia was the most likely cause of the current alveolar hyperventilation. Given a chronically compromised ventilatory reserve and diminished ventilatory muscle efficiency, the patient's ability to maintain this hyperventilation for a significant length of time was severely limited. Two possible therapeutic approaches are possible: (1) Place the patient on full ventilatory support to completely remove his WOB and treat the pneumonia, or (2) reduce his inspiratory work, thereby ameliorating detrimental WOB, and maintain spontaneous ventilation while treating the pneumonia. Given that a combination of chronic lung disease and impaired nutrition commonly leads to difficulties in weaning from ventilatory support (see Chapter 4), it is reasonable to attempt to manipulate the WOB and avoid mechanical ventilatory support. It is imperative that the patient be very closely monitored for the onset of acute ventilatory failure during these therapeutic maneuvers. His ventilatory demand can be reduced by appropriate oxygen therapy and aggressive treatment of his fever with antipyretics and a cooling blanket. The acute effects of the pneumonia on lung mechanics can be improved by meticulous bronchial hygiene therapy to facilitate removal of secretions. Airway resistance could possibly be reduced by the use of systemic or aerosolized bronchodilators. Improvement of the patient's nutritional status, while clearly desirable, takes time. The mild hypophosphatemia, a possible contributor to ventilatory muscle weakness, can be corrected easily. The use of theophylline in a patient such as this has two aims: (1) bronchodilation, and (2) enhanced contractility of the diaphragm. Theophylline can exert a positive inotropic effect on the diaphragm at serum concentrations within the normal therapeutic range.[28]

CASE STUDY 2 CONTINUED

The FIO_2 was increased to 0.28 and an acetaminophen (Tylenol) suppository administered. The patient was placed under a cooling blanket. A theophylline infusion at 0.5 mg/kg/hr was started. The patient was given albuterol, 25 mg, by aerosol, and chest physical therapy (postural drainage with percussion and vibration of the chest wall over the right lower lung field) was initiated, which resulted in mobilization of large amounts of secretions. Phosphorus, 20 mEq, was added to the IV solution. Repeat assessment of the patient revealed a respiratory rate of 18/min, a blood pressure of 130/85 mm Hg, and a heart rate of 110/min. No further ectopic beats were noted on the ECG monitor. His temperature declined to 39°C, and ABG analysis showed a pH of 7.42, a PCO_2 of 56 mm Hg, and a PO_2 of 62 mm Hg. The patient stated that he felt more comfortable.

Discussion

The overall clinical assessment of the patient after these interventions was encouraging in that he felt more comfortable and his vital signs suggested an improved cardiopulmonary status. However, it is important to continue close monitoring because the rise in $PaCO_2$ may not reflect a return toward baseline but, rather, evolving acute ventilatory failure.

CASE STUDY 2 CONTINUED

Repeat ABG analysis half an hour later revealed a pH of 7.39, a Pco_2 of 60 mm Hg, and a Po_2 of 61 mm Hg. Vital signs were essentially unchanged. The regimen of oxygen therapy, antibiotics, temperature control, and bronchodilator and bronchial hygiene therapy was continued. On the next day the patient was breathing at 16/min with a heart rate of 100/min and a blood pressure of 125/85 mm Hg. He complained of hunger, and a light oral diet was initiated. Oxygen therapy was continued via nasal cannula to enable eating. On 2 L/min of O_2 his pHa was 7.39, his $Paco_2$ was 60 mm Hg, and his Pao_2 was 59 mm Hg. He was afebrile. During the ensuing 3 days his WBC count normalized, he remained afebrile, sputum production diminished, and he was weaned from oxygen with maintenance of appropriate arterial oxygenation.

CASE STUDY 3

A 42-year-old, 74-kg man was admitted to the ICU after laparotomy for vagotomy and pyloroplasty. The patient had a history of pulmonary fibrosis. Preoperative assessment of pulmonary function revealed a pattern of restrictive lung function with VC of 1.6 L. The patient's resting respiratory rate was 18 breaths per minute, and he had a pHa of 7.41, a $Paco_2$ of 40 mm Hg, and a Pao_2 of 75 mm Hg on room air.

On admission to the ICU he had the following vital signs: heart rate of 82/min in sinus rhythm, blood pressure of 115/75 mm Hg, respiratory rate of 17 breaths per minute, and temperature of 38.4°C. He was drowsy and complained of mild discomfort from the surgical incision. He had been left intubated after surgery because it was anticipated that he might require ventilatory assistance in the immediate postoperative period. The ABG analysis on an Fio_2 of 0.4 revealed a pH of 7.36, a Pco_2 of 45 mm Hg, and a Po_2 of 126 mm Hg. His VC was 1.2 L, with a V_T of 350 mL. He was given 2 mg of morphine IV for analgesia.

Discussion

Thoracoabdominal surgery is well known to produce a pattern of restrictive lung function in the immediate 24 to 36 hours postoperatively, with a major reduction in VC and a minor reduction in FRC. Characteristically, the VC will be decreased by approximately 75% for upper abdominal or lateral thoracic surgery and 50% for lower abdominal surgery. This loss of VC is progressive and reaches the nadir 12 to 14 hours post surgery. Because this patient had restricted lung function and a chronically compromised ventilatory reserve preoperatively, with a VC of only 1.6 L, he clearly was at risk for the development of ventilatory difficulties in the postoperative period. The restrictive effects of thoracoabdominal surgery are not fully understood; factors including chest and abdominal wall pain, possible discoordinate diaphragmatic action, and pressure from serous fluid accumulation in the surgical wound are thought to play roles in its genesis. The blood gas picture on admission to the ICU is consistent with a spontaneously breathing patient following general anesthesia.

CASE STUDY 3 CONTINUED

Continuous positive airway pressure (CPAP) of 5 cm H_2O was started via the endotracheal tube. Frequent small doses of morphine were given IV to keep the patient as pain free as possible without significant depression of the central respiratory drive. His VC was monitored two hourly. Four hours after ICU admission he was breathing 22 times per minute with a VT of 300 mL and a VC of 1.0 L. The ABG values at $+5$ cm H_2O of CPAP and an FIO_2 of 0.4 were a pH of 7.40, a PCO_2 of 41 mm Hg, and a PO_2 of 105 mm Hg. Six hours post admission he was breathing at 25 times per minute, his VC was 850 mL, heart rate was 95/min, blood pressure was 125/75 mm Hg, and temperature was 39°C. Blood gas analysis showed a pH of 7.39, a PCO_2 of 42 mm Hg, and a PO_2 of 95 mm Hg (FIO_2 = 0.4). He had received several doses of morphine and reported mild wound discomfort. Increasing CPAP to $+10$ cm H_2O resulted in no change in the patient's pattern of breathing.

Discussion

In intubated patients, particularly those with preexisting restricted lung function, the FRC tends to decrease when the airway is at ambient pressure secondary to a loss of glottic function. Application of $+5$ cm H_2O of CPAP to the airway usually helps to stabilize the FRC. The patient under consideration had signs of increasing loss of VC and declining lung compliance, as evidenced by an evolving pattern of rapid, shallow breathing. Application of CPAP may increase intrathoracic gas volume and thereby improve lung compliance and reduce WOB. A lack of change in this patient's breathing pattern after an increase in CPAP to $+10$ cm H_2O suggested that his fibrotic lungs were not readily expanded by this maneuver. The progressive change in his vital signs was consistent with increasing WOB secondary to loss of ventilatory reserve, which, if not addressed, would in all probability lead to further disruption of his cardiopulmonary homeostasis.

CASE STUDY 3 CONTINUED

Because the patient's VC was anticipated to fall even more in the next 6 to 8 hours, it was decided to provide mechanical ventilatory assistance. Pressure support ventilation (PSV) was started at a level of 5 cm H_2O. This was increased in increments of 5 cm H_2O and titrated against the spontaneous respiratory rate. (See Chapter 5 for a discussion of PSV.) At 20 cm H_2O of PSV and $+5$ cm H_2O of CPAP he was breathing 16 times per minute with a heart rate of 80/min, and blood pressure of 115/75 mm Hg. Blood gas values on an FIO_2 of 0.4 were pH, 7.41; PCO_2, 39 mm Hg; and PO_2, 120 mm Hg. The patient remained stable at this level of partial ventilatory support overnight. The next morning he had a VC of 1.1 L and no complaints of pain. Pressure support ventilation was decreased in increments of 5 cm H_2O without any major changes in his vital signs. At 5 cm H_2O of PSV and 5 cm H_2O of CPAP he had a respiratory rate of 18/min, heart rate of 78/min, and blood pressure of 120/75 mm Hg. His pHa and $PaCO_2$ were essentially unchanged, and his PaO_2 with the same oxygen concentration had increased to 145 mm Hg. Twenty hours postoperatively his VC had increased to 1.3 L. The patient was extubated and made an uneventful recovery.

Discussion

Provision of partial ventilatory support to this patient diminished the WOB and prevented further development of detrimental WOB. Partial ventilatory support can be provided by several ventilatory modes, IMV, synchronized intermittent mandatory ventilation (SIMV), or PSV. The desirability of one mode over another is based largely on physician preference because there are no data comparing the different modes with respect to provision of partial ventilatory support and the associated WOB. Theoretically, PSV may offer advantages over the other two modes in a patient with restricted lung function in that it provides assistance with every breath and the airway pressure will not be significantly higher than the preset PSV level. It is acceptable practice to extubate a patient from 5 cm H_2O of PSV because this level of support probably does no more than ameliorate the increased WOB secondary to the airway resistance of the endotracheal tube.

CASE STUDY 4

A 66-year-old, 65-kg man with a history of coronary artery disease and two previous myocardial infarctions was admitted with substernal chest pain and shortness of breath. He was afebrile and diaphoretic, with a heart rate of 95/min in sinus rhythm, blood pressure of 90/70 mm Hg, respiratory rate of 30 breaths per minute, and a V_T of 320 mL. He used accessory muscles of ventilation. Auscultation of the chest revealed normal heart sounds, diminished air entry at both bases, and rales two thirds of the way up on both lung fields posteriorly. The ECG findings were consistent with myocardial ischemia. A chest x-ray film showed diffuse bilateral hilar infiltrates, prominent vascular markings, and blunting of both costophrenic angles. Blood gas analysis on an F_{IO_2} of 0.4 by face mask revealed a pH of 7.49, a P_{CO_2} of 30 mm Hg, and a P_{O_2} of 62 mm Hg. The F_{IO_2} was increased to 0.6, a nitroglycerin infusion was started, and the patient was given 8 mg of morphine IV in 2-mg increments, with relief of the substernal pain. Repeat ABG analysis showed a pH of 7.41, a P_{CO_2} of 37 mm Hg, and a P_{O_2} of 82 mm Hg. His blood pressure was still 90/75 mm Hg with a heart rate of 92/min. Breathing remained labored at a rate of 28 breaths per minute with a V_T of 260 mL. A Foley catheter was inserted and 10 mg of furosemide given IV. A dopamine infusion at a rate of 2 μg/kg min was started. A pulmonary artery catheter demonstrated a pulmonary artery occluded pressure of 28 mm Hg and a cardiac index of 2.1 L/min/m².

Discussion

This patient with acute myocardial ischemia and left ventricular failure had an initial blood gas picture of alveolar hyperventilation with moderate hypoxemia. Correction of the hypoxemia by increasing the F_{IO_2} resulted in decreased alveolar ventilation secondary to lower V_T, although the patient remained tachypneic. The persistence of tachypnea with a lower V_T probably reflects the low lung compliance secondary to cardiogenic pulmonary edema. Given that an elevated WOB places additional stress on myocardial function, steps to improve lung compliance may be beneficial.

CASE STUDY 4 CONTINUED

The patient was treated by 5 cm H_2O CPAP by face mask with an F_{IO_2} of 0.6 and vigorous diuretic therapy continued. Repeat ABG analysis with the CPAP mask in place showed a pH of 7.41, a P_{CO_2} of 39 mm Hg, and a P_{O_2} of 125 mm Hg. His respiratory rate at this time was 22 breaths per minute with a V_T of 395 mL. Several hours laters, after diuresis of 1,500 mL, the PAOP was 17 mm Hg; cardiac index, 2.9 L/min/m²; blood pressure, 105/80 mm Hg;

and heart rate, 84/min. His respiratory rate was now 14 breaths per minute, and the patient appeared comfortable. Blood gas analysis revealed a pH of 7.43, a P_{CO_2} of 40 mm H g, and a P_{O_2} of 185 mm Hg at $+5$ cm H_2O of CPAP, and an F_{IO_2} of 0.5. The mask CPAP was withdrawn and O_2 therapy continued by nasal cannula at a flow of 3 L/min. After this change in O_2 therapy the patient had a respiratory rate of 16 breaths per minute and unchanged cardiac parameters. Repeat ABG analysis showed a pH of 7.44, a P_{CO_2} of 40 mm Hg, and a P_{O_2} of 86 mm Hg.

Discussion

Application of CPAP to the airway usually results in an increase in intrathoracic gas volume with a consequent improvement in lung compliance. The reduction in respiratory rate and increase in V_T demonstrated by the patient after initiation of CPAP is consistent with improved pulmonary compliance. Mask CPAP is a reasonable temporizing step in this clinical circumstance while diuresis is achieved.

REFERENCES

1. Campbell EJM, Westlake EK, Cherniack RM: The oxygen consumption and efficiency of the respiratory muscles of young male subjects. *Clin Sci* 1959; 18:55–64.
2. Levison H, Cherniack RM: Ventilatory cost of exercise in chronic obstructive pulmonary disease. *J Appl Physiol* 1968; 25:21–27.
3. Bartlett R, et al: The oxygen cost of breathing. *J Appl Physiol* 1958; 12:413.
4. Cherniack RM: The oxygen consumption and efficiency of the respiratory muscles in health and emphysema. *J Clin Invest* 1959; 38:494–499.
5. Robertson CH, Pagel MA, Johnson RI: The distribution of blood flow, oxygen consumption and work output among the respiratory muscles during unobstructed hyperventilation. *J Clin Invest* 1977; 59:43–50.
6. Fritts HW, Filler J, Fishman AP, et al: The efficiency of ventilation during ventilatory hyperpnea: Studies in normal subjects and in dyspneic patients with either chronic pulmonary emphysema or obesity. *J Clin Invest* 1959; 38:1339–1348.
7. Robertson CH, Foster GH, Johnson RL: The relationship of respiratory failure to the oxygen consumption of lactate production by and distribution of blood flow among respiratory muscles during increasing inspiratory resistance. *J Clin Invest* 1977; 59:31–42.
8. Rochester DF, Betini G: Diaphragmatic blood flow and energy expenditure in the dog, effects of inspiratory airway resistance and hypercapnia. *J Clin Invest* 1976; 57:661–672.
9. Briscoe W, et al: Alveolar ventilation at very low tidal volumes. *J Appl Physiol* 1954; 7:27.
10. McCutcheon FH: Atmospheric respiration and complex cycles in mammalian breathing mechanisms. *J Cell Physiol* 1953; 41:291.
11. Danon J, Druz WS, Goldberg NB, et al: Function of the isolated paced diaphragm and the cervical accessory muscles in C_1 quadriplegics. *Am Rev Respir Dis* 1979; 119:909–919.
12. Gertz I, Hedenstierna G, Hellers G, et al: Muscle metabolism in patients with chronic obstructive lung disease and acute respiratory failure. *Clin Sci Mol Med* 1977; 52:395–403.
13. Campbell JA, Hughes RL, Sahgal V, et al: Alterations in intercostal muscle morphology and biochemistry in patients with obstructive lung disease. *Am Rev Respir Dis* 1980; 122:679–686.
14. Newman JH, Neff TA, Ziporin P: Acute respiratory failure associated with hypophosphatemia. *N Engl J Med* 1977; 296:1101.
15. Aubier M, Trippenbach T, Roussos C: Respiratory muscle fatigue during cardiogenic shock. *J Appl Physiol* 1981; 51:499–508.
16. De Troyer A, Loring SH: Action of the respiratory muscles, in Fishman AP, Macklem PT, Mead J (eds): *Handbook of Physiology—The Respiratory System III.* Baltimore, Waverly Press, 1986, pp 443–461.
17. Campbell SM, Kudsk KA: "High tech" metabolic measurements: Useful in daily clinical practice? *JPEN J Parenter Enteral Nutr* 1988; 12:610–612.
18. Marini JJ: Work of breathing, in Kacmarek RM, Stoller JK (eds): *Current Respiratory Care.* Philadelphia, BC Decker, Inc, 1988, pp 188–194.
19. Peters R: The energy cost (work) of breathing. *Ann Thorac Surg* 1969; 7:51.

20. Roussos C, Macklem PT: Inspiratory muscle fatigue, in Fishman AP, Macklem PT, Mead J (eds): *Handbook of Physiology—The Respiratory System III*. Baltimore, Waverly Press, 1986, pp 511–527.

21. Marini JJ, Capps JS, Culver BH: The inspiratory work of breathing during assisted mechanical ventilation. *Chest* 1985; 87:612–618.

22. Marini JJ, Rodriguez RM, Lamb V: The inspiratory workload of patient-initiated mechanical ventilation. *Am Rev Respir Dis* 1986; 134:902–909.

23. Savino JA, Dawson JA, Agarwal N, et al: The metabolic cost of breathing in critical surgical patients. *J Trauma* 1985; 25:1126–1133.

24. Katz JA, Kraemer RW, Gjerde GE: Inspiratory work and airway pressure with continuous positive airway pressure delivery systems. *Chest* 1985; 88:519–526.

25. Gibney RTN, Wilson RS, Pontoppidan H: Comparison of work of breathing on high gas flow and demand valve continuous positive airway pressure systems. *Chest* 1982; 82:692–695.

26. Op't Holt TB, Hall MW, Bass JB, et al: Comparison of changes in airway pressure during continuous positive airway pressure (CPAP) between demand valve and continuous flow devices. *Respir Care* 1982; 27:1200–1209.

27. Henry WC, West GA, Wilson RS: A comparison of the oxygen cost of breathing between a continuous flow CPAP system and a demand flow CPAP system. *Respir Care* 1983; 28:1273–1281.

28. Murciano D, Auclair M-H, Pariente R, et al: A randomized, controlled trial of theophylline in patients with severe chronic obstructive pulmonary disease. *N Engl J Med* 1989; 320:1521–1525.

4/ Conventional Mechanical Ventilation

BARRY A. SHAPIRO, M.D.
ROY D. CANE, M.B.B.CH.

Consistently successful techniques for positive-pressure ventilation (PPV) were developed in the 1920s in conjunction with general anesthesia and endotracheal intubation. Negative-pressure methods of providing ventilatory support developed outside the operating room primarily because of the unavailability of endotracheal intubation and the desire to avoid tracheostomy.[1] Because access to the patient's body was less important on the wards than in the operating room, the negative-pressure ventilator (iron lung) gained enormous popularity for supporting polio victims.[2]

The disadvantages of inaccessibility of patients ventilated with an iron lung became apparent during World War II. This in conjunction with improved survival of polio patients in the 1950s who were managed with PPV firmly established the superiority of positive-pressure techniques and ushered in the age of modern mechanical ventilatory support. More than 35 years of experience have shown that positive-pressure ventilators are more powerful and flexible, and more universally applicable, than are negative-pressure ventilators.

INDICATIONS FOR POSITIVE-PRESSURE VENTILATION

The primary purpose of mechanical ventilation is support of cardiopulmonary homeostasis. Innumerable specific diseases impact on cardiopulmonary homeostasis and reserves. Consideration of indications for mechanical ventilatory support by pathology would result in lengthy useless lists. Classification of indications for PPV is best stated in terms of cardiopulmonary pathophysiology. There are three major categories of disturbed cardiopulmonary homeostasis amenable to mechanical ventilatory support.

1. Apnea
2. Acute ventilatory failure
3. Impending acute ventilatory failure

Apnea

An absence of spontaneous ventilation (apnea) necessitates mechanial support of ventilation.

Acute Ventilatory Failure

Acute ventilatory failure describes a situation in which the pulmonary system fails to meet the patient's CO_2 excretion demands. Alveolar ventilation represents that portion of the gas moving in and out of the pulmonary system that undergoes molecular gas exchange (respiration) with pulmonary blood; dead-space ventilation represents the ventilated gas that does not respire. Because inadequate alveolar ventilation may be attributable to an increased physiologic dead space, simple clinical observation or measurement of minute ventilation does not necessarily reflect the adequacy of CO_2 excretion. Assessment of the adequacy of alveolar ventilation can be best accomplished by a measurement of CO_2 in the arterial blood.[3] Inadequate alveolar ventilation (arterial carbon dioxide above an acceptable limit) reflects a failure to remove carbon dioxide adequately by means of the lungs. When such a "ventilatory failure" is accompanied by acidemia (arterial pH below an acceptable limit), the failure must be of recent origin (acute) and, therefore, a direct threat to cardiopulmonary homeostasis. Ventilatory failure is traditionally termed "respiratory acidosis."

Acute ventilatory failure may be defined arbitrarily as an arterial P_{CO_2} above 50 mm Hg coincidental with an arterial pH below 7.30.

Impending Acute Ventilatory Failure

In the absence of acute ventilatory failure, clinical assessment of (1) the work of breathing, (2) the pathogenesis of the disease process, or (3) the patient's cardiopulmonary reserves can result in the clinical judgment that acute ventilatory failure is inevitable or highly probable. This is often encountered when the work of breathing becomes detrimental to the maintenance of cardiopulmonary homeostasis (see Chapter 3). At times this clinical impression of the patient appearing to be "tiring" or "fatiguing" may be documented by sequential blood gas measurements revealing increasing P_{CO_2} values and decreasing pH values. It is not unusual, however, for patients to manifest increasing cardiopulmonary work (increasing respiratory rate, heart rate, and systolic blood pressure (BP); onset of diaphoresis, dyspnea, and confusion) while maintaining acceptable blood gas measurements. Such circumstances may be considered impending ventilatory failure.

PATHOGENESIS OF ACUTE VENTILATORY FAILURE

Respiration is the exchange of gas molecules (O_2 and CO_2) across permeable membranes. Respiratory failure traditionally refers to inadequate molecular gas exchange at the pulmonary level. Because pulmonary gas exchange involves both bulk

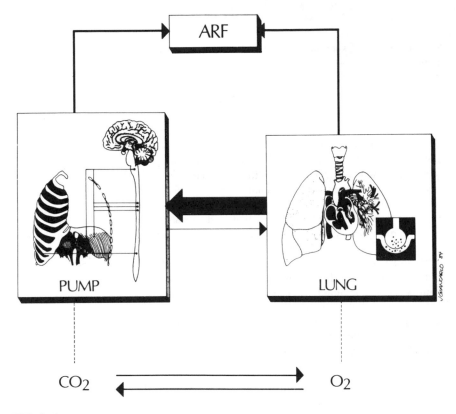

FIG 4–1.
A schematic representation of the pathogenesis of acute respiratory failure *(ARF)*. The ventilatory pump is composed of the chest cage, the ventilatory muscles, and the nervous system elements involved in respiration. The pump primarily effects carbon dioxide excretion *(CO₂)*. The lung involves the elements that allow inspired gas to exchange with pulmonary blood flow and primarily effect blood oxygenation *(O₂)*. The *large arrow* from the lung to the pump represents the fact that lung disease often increases the work of the pump. (From Shapiro BA, Harrison RA, Kacmarek RM, et al: *Clinical Application of Respiratory Care,* ed 3. Chicago, Year Book Medical Publishers, Inc, 1985. Used by permission.)

flow of gas in and out of the lungs (ventilation) and molecular gas exchange across the alveolar-capillary membrane (external respiration), ventilatory failure is a *component* of respiratory failure.

Acute respiratory failure (ARF) can be conceptualized as resulting from one of two primary mechanisms (Fig 4–1): lung failure or pump failure.

Lung Failure

Lung failure is the result of lung pathology that results in either inadequate alveolar gas exchange or inadequate exchange between alveolar gas and pulmonary blood. Such pathology usually manifests itself primarily as an arterial oxygenation deficit because adequate CO_2 excretion may be accomplished by increased work of the ventilatory pump.

An increased work of breathing invariably results from lung failure secondary to one or a combination of (1) hypoxemia resulting in increased ventilatory drive, (2) increased airway resistance, (3) decreased lung compliance, or (4) increased physiologic dead space. If the increased work of breathing is excessive, it may lead to pump failure secondary to ventilatory muscle fatigue.

Pump Failure

The pulmonary system is a to-and-fro valveless pump, alterations in the pulmonary mechanics of which have significant impact on the ability to maintain adequate ventilation. Therefore, an appreciation of normal pulmonary mechanics is essential to the comprehension of the pathogenesis of ARF.

The *transairway pressure gradient* is defined as the difference between the tracheal and alveolar pressure (Fig 4–2). Gas flow into and out of the lungs normally occurs only in response to transairway pressure gradients. Alterations in distribution of inspired gas are primarily the result of changes in airway resistance. The *transpulmonary pressure gradient* (Fig 4–2) is the pressure difference between the tracheal and pleural pressures. Ventilatory muscle contraction alters intrapleural pressure and thereby affects alveolar pressures. The relationships of transairway and transpulmonary pressure gradients to lung volume and pleural pressures are illustrated in Figure 4–3.

OXYGENATION AND POSITIVE-PRESSURE VENTILATION

Hypoventilation creates arterial hypoxemia while breathing room air. Restoration of adequate physiologic ventilation reverses the arterial oxygenation deficit. Hypoxemia coincident with adequate alveolar ventilation (hypoxemic respiratory failure) is seldom improved by the institution of PPV except when decreasing the oxygen cost of breathing will significantly diminish total oxygen consumption.

Most primary arterial oxygenation deficits are best supported by means of oxygen therapy, cardiovascular therapy, bronchial hygiene therapy, positive end-expiratory pressure (PEEP) therapy, or combinations of these techniques. Although any or all of these therapies may be administered in conjunction with the ventilator, none of them *require* the use of a ventilator. Positive-pressure ventilation must be considered a tool for directly relieving or diminishing the work of breathing while only indirectly improving oxygenation.

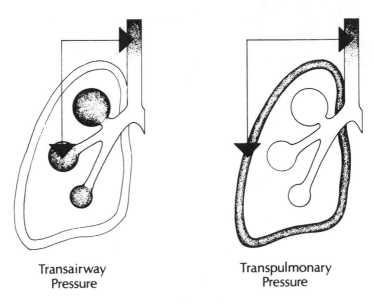

Transairway
Pressure

Transpulmonary
Pressure

FIG 4–2.
Nomenclature of pressure gradients within the pulmonary system. *Left,* pressure gradient of transairway pressure between the airway opening and the alveolus; *right,* pressure gradient of transpulmonary pressure between the airway opening and the pleural space. (From Shapiro BA, Harrison RA, Kacmarek RM, et al: *Clinical Application of Respiratory Care,* ed 3. Chicago, Year Book Medical Publishers, Inc, 1985. Used by permission.)

CAPABILITIES OF POSITIVE-PRESSURE VENTILATION

It cannot be assumed that all patients in ARF or acute respiratory insufficiency will benefit from mechanical support of ventilation. Because the ventilator is a machine that only alters inspiratory airway pressures, a rationale for its application must be based on delineating the conditions in which such airway pressure alteration may be physiologically advantageous.

It may be generalized that a positive-pressure ventilator may beneficially alter physiologic gas exchange by performing three tasks: (1) to provide all or part of the power required for the work of breathing to maintain physiologic ventilation, (2) to manipulate inspiratory airway pressures and flow patterns to improve distribution of ventilation, and (3) to manipulate the ventilatory pattern to improve gas exchange.

Work of Breathing

A ventilator can provide all or part of the energy necessary to move gas into the pulmonary tree. When the patient is unable to provide the energy (or its provision

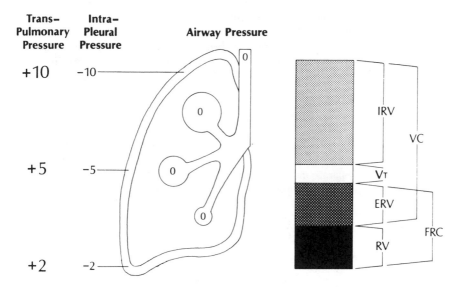

FIG 4–3.
The bar graph depicts normal total lung capacity and normal lung volumes. The lung diagram represents the erect lung and pleural space at functional residual capacity (FRC). Airway pressure and all alveolar pressures are zero (atmospheric). Intrapleural pressures are negative and to a greater degree at the apex than at the base. The numbers are for illustrative purposes and do not necessarily represent actual physiologic measurement. Note that transpulmonary pressure (airway pressure minus intrapleural pressure) is greater at the apex than at the base. This is the primary reason why the alveoli are larger at the apex and smaller at the base of the lung. RV = residual volume; ERV = expiratory reserve volume; V_T = tidal volume; IRV = inspiratory reserve volume; VC = vital capacity. (From Shapiro BA, Harrison RA, Kacmarek RM, et al: Clinical Application of Respiratory Care, ed 3. Chicago, Year Book Medical Publishers, Inc, 1985. Used by permission.)

is detrimental to homeostasis), PPV may maintain or reestablish adequate respiratory gas exchange; however, simply providing PPV does not always improve gas exchange, especially in the presence of relative hypovolemia or left ventricular failure.

Inspiratory Flow Pattern

Inspiratory flow patterns may have a significant effect on the manner in which inspired gases are distributed, especially in the presence of pulmonary disease.[4, 5] Modern ventilators have significant flexibility in altering inspiratory pressures and flow patterns. The most significant of these maneuvers appears to be the end-inspiratory pause (inflation hold).

Ventilatory Pattern

Inspiratory-to-expiratory (I:E) ratios, ventilatory rate, and tidal volume (VT) greatly affect respiration.[6, 7] Ventilators can partially or completely control (or modify) these factors.

VENTILATORY MODES

The term *ventilator mode* usually refers to the capabilities and limitations of the machine and its circuitry. The degree to which a ventilator mode allows patient participation is a separate matter from what the patient may actually be doing.

There are four ventilator modes presently utilized for conventional PPV. Representative airway pressure curves are shown in Figure 4–4.

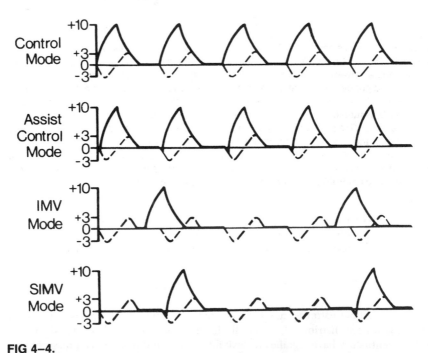

FIG 4–4.
Classic airway pressure curves for various modes of intermittent positive-pressure ventilation superimposed on the normal spontaneous airway pressure curves *(dashed lines). IMV =* intermittent mandatory ventilation; *SIMV =* synchronized IMV. (From Shapiro BA, Harrison RA, Kacmarek RM, et al: *Clinical Applications of Respiratory Care,* ed 3. Chicago, Year Book Medical Publishers, Inc, 1985. Used by permission.)

Control Mode Ventilation

Control mode means that the ventilator and circuitry are totally unresponsive to patient effort or response; the patient is unable to alter or influence any portion of the ventilatory cycle. If inspiratory dynamics are kept constant, the slower the ventilator rate, the lower will be the mean airway pressure.

Assist/Control Mode Ventilation

The ventilator initiates inspiration when the patient creates a sub-baseline pressure in the inspiratory limb of the ventilator circuit. If the patient's ventilatory rate falls below a preset level, the machine will automatically enter the control mode. Because V_T and the flow rate are predetermined, assist/control mode ventilation allows the patient to influence only the ventilator rate.

Intermittent Mandatory Ventilation

Intermittent mandatory ventilation (IMV) consists of a control mode ventilator in conjunction with a circuitry that allows for unhindered, spontaneous ventilation.[8, 9] In other words, the patient spontaneously breathes gas at the same temperature, humidity, and oxygen concentration that the ventilator provides without any increased resistance, while at predetermined intervals a positive-pressure breath is delivered by the ventilator. The positive-pressure breath is completely independent of the patient's spontaneous ventilatory pattern.

To ensure no added impedance to spontaneous ventilation, a circuit should be used that maintains a continuous gas flow past the patient's airway sufficient to meet the patient's peak inspiratory flow requirements (Fig 4–5). Peak inspiratory flow rates can usually be achieved by providing a continuous gas flow equal to at least four times the patient's spontaneous minute volume (MV). A measurable flow exiting the exhalation port of the ventilator circuit during the patient's spontaneous inspiratory efforts usually ensures minimal impedance.

Synchronized Intermittent Mandatory Ventilation

The IMV mode may deliver a mechanical breath upon completion of a spontaneous inspiration. Concern that such "stacking" of breaths could result in greater disruption of cardiopulmonary function led to the development of a technology that would synchronize the positive-pressure breaths with the patients' spontaneous breathing.[10] Subsequent studies demonstrated that "stacking" did not alter intrapleural pressures or disrupt cardiopulmonary function to any significant degree, and therefore, a physiologic advantage to synchronizing the IMV (SIMV) proved to be nonexistent.[11] However, the engineering and manufacturing advantages of such a technology led to its present availability and use.

The SIMV mode is composed of a ventilator in the assist/control mode in con-

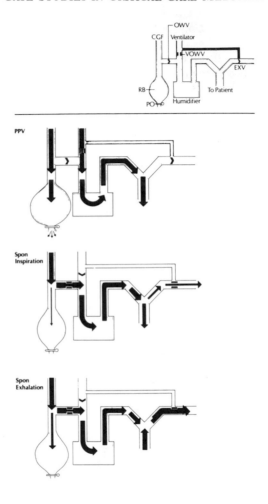

FIG 4–5.

Schematic representation of a continuous-flow IMV system. *CGF* = continuous gas flow source; *RB* = elastic reservoir bag; *PO* = pop-off mechanism, which is an open nipple with an adjustable clamp; *OWV* = one-way valve; *VOWV* = ventilator one-way valve; *EXV* = exhalation valve. The area labeled *PPV* shows gas flow during positive-pressure ventilation. The exhalation valve is closed because the connecting line is pressurized. During this period, all of the continuous gas flow enters the reservoir bag. The area labeled *Spon Inspiration* shows gas flow during active spontaneous inspiration. The majority of the continuous gas flow is to the patient circuit because the pressure in the reservoir bag is maintained slightly above circuit pressure. Gas that does not go to the patient flows through the exhalation valve. The area labeled *Spon Exhalation* shows gas flow during active spontaneous exhalation. Note that more of the continuous gas flow is to the reservoir bag since the patient circuit pressure is above ambient. Reservoir bag pressure should always be maintained slightly above patient circuit pressure. There may be significantly greater flow through the exhalation valve, which may cause an orificial resistor phenomenon and increase the expiratory work of breathing. (From Shapiro BA, Harrison RA, Kacmarek RM, et al: *Clinical Application of Respiratory Care*, ed 3. Chicago, Year Book Medical Publishers, Inc, 1985. Used by permission.)

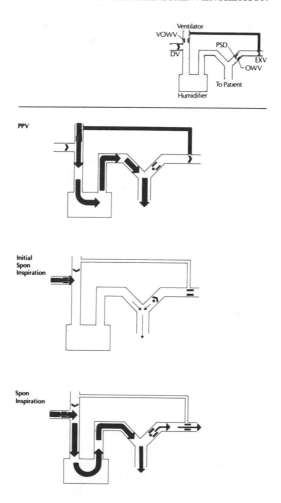

FIG 4–6.

Schematic representation of an SIMV demand flow system. *VOWV* = ventilator one-way valve; *DV* = demand valve device; *PSD* = pressure-sensing device that cycles the ventilator and demand valve mechanism; *OWV* = one-way valve to minimize tubing that must be decompressed to create a sub-baseline pressure; *EXV* = exhalation valve. The area labeled *PPV* shows gas flow during positive-pressure ventilation. The exhalation valve is closed because the connecting line is pressurized. The demand valve mechanism is closed. The area labeled *Initial Spon Inspiration* shows gas flow at the moment the demand valve mechanism opens. Spontaneous inspiratory effort has somewhat decompressed the tubing, and a pressure-sensing device has triggered the demand valve mechanism. The area labeled *Spon Inspiration* shows gas flow after the flow has reached the patient. The demand valve will close at the end of inspiration so that there will not be excessive flow through the exhalation valve during exhalation, as occurs with a continuous flow system. Increased work of breathing with a demand valve system is primarily attributable to inspiratory work generated from opening of the demand valve mechanism to flow reaching the patient. The response time for a demand valve mechanism to open is also a potential problem. (From Shapiro BA, Harrison RA, Kacmarek RM, et al: *Clinical Application of Respiratory Care,* ed 3. Chicago, Year Book Medical Publishers, Inc, 1985. Used by permission.)

junction with a mechanism and circuitry that allows for independent spontaneous ventilation. The patient may spontaneously breathe through the circuitry while at predetermined intervals the next spontaneous breath will by assisted by the machine. Thus, the positive-pressure breath is always in synchrony with the patient's spontaneous ventilatory pattern.

Because a properly functioning continuous flow system does not allow a sub-baseline pressure to be generated in the circuit, demand flow systems were developed for SIMV. When the demand valve is opened, a very high flow of gas enters the system and continues until the valve is closed. Although the first generation of demand valves required the patient to generate significant sub-baseline pressures and were slow to provide adequate inspiratory flow rates, subsequent generations are more sensitive and provide better flow rates.[12]

Figure 4–6 schematically represents an SIMV mode. A pressure-sensing device located near the patient's airway detects the initiation of a spontaneous inspiration and activates either the ventilator or the demand flow device. The major disadvantage of the demand flow system remains the delay in providing adequate gas flow, which results in an increased work of breathing when compared with a continuous gas flow system.[12–14]

PHYSIOLOGIC ALTERATIONS WITH POSITIVE-PRESSURE VENTILATION

The major disadvantages of PPV are related to diminished cardiac output, increased dead-space ventilation and altered diaphragm function.

Diminishment of cardiac output was the first documented disadvantage of PPV.[15, 16] It is well documented that the primary mechanism of this decreased cardiac output is embarrassment to venous return and that appropriate intravenous (IV) fluid administration restores the cardiac output to pre-PPV levels.

Normal V/Q is greatly determined by the fact that gravity favors pulmonary blood flow to the basilar (gravity-dependent) lung and contributes to the existence of a gradation of pleural pressures and alveolar sizes. Spontaneous ventilation favors the distribution of gas to the bases by creating a relatively equal pressure change throughout the pleural space during inspiration. Although the absolute pleural pressures illustrated in Figure 4–3 are exaggerated, the relative differences between apex and base are consistent with normal physiology. This model is useful to illustrate the *relative* changes that occur during spontaneous inspiration. For example, a uniform pleural pressure decrease of 5 units results in an instantaneous transpulmonary pressure gradient change of 10 to 15 at the apex and 2 to 7 at the base. This represents a 33% increase at the apex and a 350% increase at the base, which favors a relatively greater portion of the inspired gas being distributed to the base. During exhalation, the lower compliance of the basilar alveoli results in a relatively greater emptying.

Positive-pressure ventilation increases dead-space ventilation because inspiration occurs without decreases in pleural pressures, thereby losing the relative advantage of the basilar distribution of gas that occurs with spontaneous ventilation. Also, apical lung normally has less airway resistance and higher compliance than basilar lung does, which favors distribution of ventilation to the apical lung in PPV.

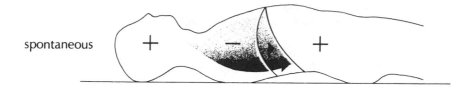

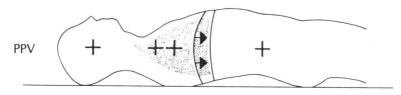

FIG 4–7.

Spontaneous ventilation provides optimal distribution of ventilation in relation to perfusion because of the mechanics of the spontaneously contracting diaphragm. In addition, venous return is optimized because intra-abdominal and intracranial pressures are more positive than intrathoracic pressures are. Positive-pressure ventilation *(PPV)* results in greater air distribution to the non–gravity-dependent portions of lung and potentially hinders venous return because intrathoracic pressure is more positive than intra-abdominal or intracranial pressure is. (From Shapiro BA, Harrison RA, Kacmarek RM, et al: *Clinical Application of Respiratory Care,* ed 3. Chicago, Year Book Medical Publishers, Inc, 1985. Used by permission.)

Altered diaphragm function after abdominal surgery[17, 18] illustrates that proper coordination of muscle fiber contraction is necessary for normal diaphragm function. It has been observed (Fig 4–7) that in a supine position the posterior aspect of the diaphragm normally has a greater excursion than the anterior aspect does during spontaneous ventilation and that this difference is ablated with PPV.[19]

Thus, when PPV replaces spontaneous ventilation, at least two physiologic mechanisms favoring ventilation of the gravity-dependent area of the lung (decreased pleural pressures and diaphragm function) are lost. Further, the increased alveolar pressures of PPV favor pulmonary blood flow to the gravity-dependent portion of the lung even when adequate cardiac output is maintained.[20]

CARDIOVASCULAR STABILIZATION WITH POSITIVE-PRESSURE VENTILATION

Too often, hypotension developing after establishment of an airway and PPV is assumed to be caused by factors such as (1) stress of intubation, (2) delay in accomplishing successful intubation, (3) pharmacologic agents used to facilitate intubation, and (4) inappropriate support of ventilation. Although any of these factors are possible (especially when improperly applied), hypotension often occurs in the absence of these factors and despite the highest degree of skill. Most often, hypotension and dysrhythmia are secondary to either (1) decreased sympathetic tone, (2) decreased venous return, or (3) a combination of these factors.

Autonomic stimulation is common in patients requiring initiation of ventilatory support secondary to hypoxemia, hypercarbia, acidemia, and work of breathing. In conscious patients the physiologic stress is compounded by anxiety and fear. This sympathetic stimulation creates significant degrees of arterial and venous constriction as well as myocardial stimulation. Initiation of PPV usually relieves the work of breathing and significantly reverses hypercarbia, acidemia, and hypoxemia. It is not uncommon for a state of unconsciousness to be induced pharmacologically.

Combinations of loss of consciousness, relief of work of breathing, and improved ventilation and oxygenation often lead to a profound and sudden decrease in sympathetic stimulation. This decrease in sympathetic tone often results in significant arteriolar and venous relaxation. The resultant "relative hypovolemia" may not be compensated immediately because the patient is unable to mobilize extravascular fluid rapidly. In addition, the relative hypovolemia is significant because the intrathoracic positive pressure created by the ventilator accentuates interference with venous return. It is imperative to be aware of the potential for hypotension following the establishment of PPV.

When hypotension is severe, the patient should immediately have both lower extremities elevated 20 to 30 degrees from the horizontal position. The transient increase in "core" blood volume should improve venous return to the heart. Eventual correction of the relative hypovolemia is accomplished by appropriate IV fluid administration. The patient must not be allowed to "fight" the positive pressure and unduly increase intrathoracic pressure.

MAINTENANCE OF POSITIVE-PRESSURE VENTILATION

Patients may be maintained on PPV by one of two major methods: (1) full ventilatory support (FVS) and (2) partial ventilatory support (PVS).[21]

Full Ventilatory Support

When PPV is applied in a manner whereby the ventilator provides all the energy required to maintain effective alveolar ventilation, the patient receives FVS. In other words, FVS is defined as the machine providing enough ventilation so that the patient is not required to expend any energy to maintain ventilatory homeostasis. Full ventilatory support can be provided with any of the four ventilator modes.

Partial Ventilatory Support

Partial ventilatory support (PVS) may be defined as the clinical circumstance in which both the patient and the ventilator contribute physiologically significant roles

toward maintaining ventilatory homeostasis. It allows the patient to breathe spontaneously to whatever extent possible without detriment to homeostasis—the remaining ventilatory requirements are supplied by the ventilator.[22] Partial ventilatory
support can be provided only with the IMV, SIMV ventilator modes, and pressure
support ventilation (see Chapter 5).

A theoretical advantage of PVS centers around the concept that spontaneous
ventilation is a physiologic advantage (improved cardiac output and V/Q) when compared with PPV. If the patient is capable of providing energy for a significant portion
of the required ventilation, it should be advantageous to provide only the remaining
portion by artificial means. Additionally, there is ample evidence to support the
statement that PEEP is best provided in conjunction with as much spontaneous
ventilation as the patient can reasonably provide.[23-25] There is no direct evidence
that spontaneous breathing efforts in conjunction with PPV are detrimental, although
some data suggest this may be so in the severe chronic obstructive pulmonary disease
(COPD) patient.[26] Present data and the preponderant clinical experience support
the thesis that spontaneous ventilation in conjunction with PPV is desirable in most
patients.

Ventilator Rate and Tidal Volume

In adults with normal or acutely diseased lungs, positive-pressure VTs in the range
of 10 to 20 mL/kg delivered within 0.5 to 1.5 seconds demonstrate no significant
differences in mean inspiratory airway pressure.[27, 28]

Thus, positive-pressure ventilators can deliver up to three times a predicted
normal VT without significant increases in the mean inspiratory airway pressure.
More than 30 years of clinical experience has shown that these relatively large VTs
(1) are advantageous in compensating for the increased dead-space ventilation that
accompanies PPV, (2) appear to decrease the incidence of atelectasis when compared
with smaller VTs,[29, 30] and (3) usually are better tolerated by the conscious patient.

It has become standard practice in patients without chronic restrictive pathology
to deliver positive-pressure VTs of 12 to 15 mL/kg. This is almost always in conjunction
with a flow rate that allows the volumes to be delivered in less than 1 second.
Variations from this rule depend upon clinical judgment, physiologic monitoring,
and personal preference.

Ventilator rates of 8/min or greater in conjunction with VTs of 12 to 15 mL/kg
will almost always result in arterial PCO_2s less than 45 mm Hg and should be considered full ventilatory support. Partial ventilatory support is usually present with
ventilator rates of 7/min or less; however, the key factor is that the patient is providing
a physiologically significant degree of spontaneous ventilation.

Recent interest in the work of breathing imposed during PPV has been useful
and enlightening.[31, 32] However, it must be remembered that all work of breathing
is *not* intrinsically bad or undesirable. What we want to avoid is energy expenditure
that detrimentally taxes the cardiopulmonary reserves. This is best noted by clinical
signs of cardiovascular stress (e.g., tachycardia, dysrhythmia, hypertension) and pulmonary stress (e.g., tachypnea, hypopnea, accessory muscle activity, dyspnea, distress). (See Chapter 3 for discussion of detrimental work of breathing.)

Maintenance With Partial Ventilatory Support

In our experience, most patients benefit from FVS for the first several hours while stabilization, diagnostic, and therapeutic procedures are accomplished. Fewer than 20% of our patients require full support for more than the initial 12 hours. Our confidence in the physiologic advantages of PVS is such that we generally seek the lowest ventilator rate the patient will tolerate at the earliest opportunity. This is usually accomplished by decreasing the ventilator rate in increments of 2/min until the patient either shows signs that the work of breathing is stressful (e.g., tachycardia, hypertension, distress, dysrhythmia, hypercarbia, acidemia), or a significant degree of spontaneous ventilation is being accomplished (e.g., a ventilator rate of 4/min). We consider this a reasonable maintenance level until the decision to discontinue ventilatory support is made.

Eucapnic Ventilation

Eucapnic ventilation is the maintenance of an arterial PCO_2 within a "normal" range—defined classically as a PCO_2 between 35 and 45 mm Hg. There are two major considerations mandating eucapnic ventilation: (1) acid-base balance and (2) cerebral blood flow.

Acid-Base Balance

The reasons for maintaining normal ventilation are primarily acid-base and electrolyte considerations. If a person is maintained at an arterial PCO_2 significantly different from his normal range, acute alkalemia or acidemia will result. The kidneys will appropriately respond by holding onto or getting rid of base (HCO_3^-). Normal kidneys will compensate for a ventilatory-induced pH change within 24 to 36 hours. This is most important in patients who chronically retain CO_2 secondary to cardiopulmonary disease. If they are ventilated at a PCO_2 of 40 mm Hg for several days, the kidneys will excrete the "excess" base to correct the sudden "respiratory alkalemia."

When the patient is removed from the ventilator and he assumes his previous baseline arterial PCO_2 of 70 mm Hg, he becomes acidemic secondary to the acute CO_2 rise and the inability of the kidneys to immediately reaccumulate bicarbonate ion. The acute acidemia acts as an additional challenge to his limited cardiopulmonary reserves. Not uncommonly, the patient ends up in severe respiratory and cardiovascular distress because of his inability to maintain ventilation greater than his "normal" baseline state. This generally results in the reinstitution of mechanical ventilation, and the patient is considered a "weaning problem." This "problem" is strictly a result of improper ventilator maintenance.

Cerebral Blood Flow

Acute alveolar hyperventilation results in cerebral vasoconstriction in response to the decreased arterial P_{CO_2}. In most circumstances this leads to a decreased cerebral blood flow. This may be desirable for short periods of time in acute head trauma; however, in the critically ill patient without brain damage this decreased blood flow to the brain is undesirable.

Fighting the Ventilator

The patient's active attempt to restrict inspiration while the ventilator is in the inspiratory cycle results in diminished flow and increased airway pressures. This is referred to as "fighting the ventilator" or being "out of phase." At minimum, this maneuver increases intrathoracic pressure and diminishes effective ventilation. The most common reasons for fighting the ventilator are (1) inadequate ventilation (hypercarbia), (2) acidemia, (3) inadequate oxygenation, (4) central nervous system (CNS) malfunction, and (5) pain or anxiety. Assisting the patient with a hand ventilator or switching to the assist mode for a short time often "settles the patient down." However, these maneuvers should not replace adequate evaluation and treatment of the underlying cause for the patient fighting the ventilator.

Patients often make ventilatory efforts during the expiratory cycle of the ventilator. This phenomenon has little (if any) detrimental effect in most patients. In general, the patient who is "out of phase" during the inspiratory cycle must be manipulated to come into phase; conversely, the patient who is out of phase during the expiratory cycle most often may be left alone if an IMV circuit is provided.

End-Inspiratory Pause (Inflation Hold)

The delivery of volume in early inspiration is a matter that has received a great deal of attention in the past few years.[4, 35, 36] With time-cycled ventilators, it is relatively simple to deliver the inspiratory volume and then hold inspiration (delay expiration) for an additional period. This end-inspiratory pause or inflation hold capability appears to have significant clinical application. In simple terms, the longer the time from gas delivery to end inspiration; (1) the greater the peripheral distribution of gas, and (2) the better the distribution of gas to areas of low V/Q caused by regional airway resistance variance.[4, 37, 38]

"Manual" inflation hold has been used by anesthetists for 50 years to reexpand the retracted lung at the end of chest procedures. This principle was first applied in respiratory care after suctioning procedures to ensure expansion of collapsed lung. Whether the naturally occurring yawn has a similar function is still being debated; however, many investigators believe that the constant-volume hypoventilation of the sleep state leads to miliary atelectasis that is reexpanded upon awakening by the "natural inflation hold"—the yawn.[39]

End-inspiratory pause (inflation hold) is a useful and available airway pressure maneuver to provide the optimal inspiratory alveolar distribution of gas with PPV. With a ventilator rate of 10/min (6-second frequency) and an inspiratory delivery time of 1 second, a 0.5-second inflation hold may be given and still maintain an acceptable I:E ratio. Many clinicians prefer routine use of this airway maneuver.

Inflation hold has its greatest potential clinical application in patients with significant airway resistance,[40] although occasionally it may prove helpful in disease states associated with severely reduced compliance.

Pharmacologic Adjunct With Ventilator Maintenance

Significant sedation of the patient is usually required only to accomplish FVS; however, it is desirable to provide some sedation to most mechanically ventilated patients. The ideal drug to control fighting the ventilator would possess a minimum of eight factors: (1) have a potent central respiratory depressant effect; (2) have minimal cardiovascular side effects; (3) have a potent euphoric effect making consciousness tolerable during the ventilator course; (4) have an analgesic effect because it is not uncommon for these individuals to experience pain; (5) be totally reversible by a pharmacologic agent without dangerous effects of its own; (6) be inexpensive; (7) be clinically familiar to nursing and physician personnel; and (8) have a long, stable shelf life.

Narcotics

Of the drugs available to meet these eight criteria, the narcotics are the closest. We will use morphine sulfate as the best example of a narcotic agent.

It has been well documented that large doses of morphine may be extremely dangerous to the cardiovascular system in the spontaneously breathing patient. However, these adverse effects of cardiac dysrhythmias and hypotension are secondary to ventilatory depression (hypercarbia, hypoxemia, and acidemia). In the well-ventilated, well-oxygenated, acid-base–balanced patient, the only documented cardiovascular effect of large IV doses of morphine is increased venous capacitance.[33, 34] This can be readily compensated by appropriate attention to hemodynamic monitoring and fluid therapy. Morphine sulfate is a good euphoric agent and an excellent analgesic. It is completely reversed by naloxone hydrochloride (Narcan). Morphine sulfate is inexpensive, is familiar in clinical medicine, and has a long shelf life.

Morphine sulfate is an almost-perfect drug for sedating patients requiring ventilatory support. Of course, the patient must have reasonable blood gas values and the airway established before administration of large doses of morphine. In adults, up to 80 mg has been administered IV in the first hour and up to 20 mg each hour for maintenance without untoward effects. If the guidelines are followed, the only problem with the administration of morphine is an increase in the vascular space, which is readily corrected with proper fluid loading. Our usual doses for cardiovascularly stable patients are 10 to 20 mg (0.2 to 0.3 mg/kg) the first hour with 3 to 6 mg (0.05 to 0.1 mg/kg) every hour for maintenance. When providing sedation to patients undergoing PVS, lower doses (1 to 3 mg/hr) are effective. Ideally, the dose should be determined by titration in 1 mg increments to the desired end point.

The decision to sedate a patient to accomplish FVS requires an increased responsibility to evaluate the cardiopulmonary system and tissue oxygenation status. Patients often fight the ventilator because of improper ventilation or CNS hypoxia. Sedation is given only after a careful evaluation of the adequacy of ventilatory and oxygenation support.

Tranquilizers

Diazepam (Valium) has gained great popularity in ventilator care, especially as an adjunct to PVS. It has yet to be documented that Versed (midazolam) has any significant advantages in these patients. The greatest objection to the tranquilizing agents is that they are not predictable central respiratory depressants, not analgesics, and not reversible.

Nondepolarizing Muscle Relaxants

The nondepolarizing muscle relaxants produce motor paralysis by competitive blockage of the neuromuscular junction and are particularly useful in agitated, restless patients when trying to initiate ventilation and gain control without producing significant cardiovascular changes. Humane considerations mandate the use of sedation in conjunction with long-term paralysis by nondepolarizing muscle relaxants.

Pancuronium bromide (Pavulon) is presently the standard nondepolarizing muscle relaxant. Tachycardia has been reported as a common side effect. The usual initial paralyzing dose of pancuronium bromide is 0.1 mg/kg in adults and should be administered by a physician familiar with the drug. Maintenance doses are 1 to 2 mg/hr administered by the intensive care nurse. Reversal should be attempted only by physicians familiar with the process.

CASE STUDY 1

A 47-year-old woman entered the intensive care unit (ICU) after evacuation of a right subdural hematoma sustained in a motor vehicle accident. There were no other apparent injuries. An oral endotracheal tube was in place, and no spontaneous breathing efforts were present.

The patient was placed on volume-cycled PPV with an IMV/SIMV capability. A V_T of 1,000 mL (13 mL/kg) was set to be delivered at a rate of 10/min with an F_{IO_2} of 0.4. The patient had a BP of 140/100 mm Hg and a pulse of 100/min, and electrocardiogram (ECG) showed sinus tachycardia. Arterial blood gas (ABG) analysis revealed a pH of 7.44, a P_{CO_2} of 32 mm Hg, and a P_{O_2} of 110 mm Hg.

The neurosurgeons requested that the P_{CO_2} be maintained at 30 to 34 mm Hg because they were concerned about cerebral edema and wanted to be notified of any change in neurologic status.

Two hours later the patient began to make spontaneous breathing efforts at a rate of 30 to 40/min and to "fight" the positive-pressure breaths. This resulted in a BP of 190/140 mm Hg and a tachycardia to 130/min. Manually assisted ventilation with a self-inflating ventilator and an F_{IO_2} approximately equal to 0.7 did not alter the spontaneous pattern and resulted in a pH of 7.54, a P_{CO_2} of 26 mm Hg, and a P_{O_2} of 340 mm Hg. Spontaneous V_T varied from 100 to 200 mL with poor breath sounds. After 90 seconds of spontaneous breathing, it was clinically obvious that she would not maintain adequate ventilation spontaneously.

Discussion

Central nervous system dysfunction results in a ventilatory pattern that is incompatible with spontaneous ventilation. Hyperventilation with hand assist does not alter the breathing pattern that is typical of "central hyperventilation." It can be anticipated that whether assist/control or IMV modes are used, the patient will fight the positive-pressure breaths because the respiratory center is not responsive to afferent stimuli. Because the spontaneous respiratory efforts are incompatible with adequate maintenance of pulmonary gas exchange, either paralysis or CNS depression is warranted. It is doubtful whether sedatives or narcotics will alter the respiratory pattern short of levels of general anesthesia, a situation that will render neurologic evaluation impossible.

The best solution to this dilemma is to use a nondepolarizing muscle relaxant (e.g., pancuronium [Pavulon]) and temporarily reverse the neuromuscular blockade with edrophonium bromide (Tensilon) when neurologic evaluation is required. Ten to 20 mg. of Tensilon will sufficiently reverse the neuromuscular blockade for 3 to 5 minutes, during which a neurologic examination may be conducted under acceptable, albeit less than ideal conditions. Muscarinic (vagal) stimulation is uncommon with Tensilon but may be blocked with atropine sulfate, which should be readily available.

This is a situation in which full ventilatory support is required, but neither assist/control nor IMV is adequate, i.e., continuous mandatory ventilation (CMV) is required.

CASE STUDY 1 CONTINUED

Five milligrams of Pavulon was administered and within 3 minutes the hemodynamics and ventilatory status had stabilized. The patient was appropriately maintained at a ventilator rate of 8/min. During the next 24 hours the patient required 2 mg of Pavulon on three occasions to maintain CMV.

On two occasions the patient was given 10 mg of Tensilon to allow neurologic assessment by the neurosurgeon. Manually assisted ventilation was administered during these periods, and the patient tolerated the transient reversal of muscular blockade without serious sequelae. At the second examination the neurologic status was markedly improved, and the spontaneous respiratory pattern was noted to be around 20/min. No further Pavulon was administered, and the spontaneous efforts were allowed to return during the next several hours.

Discussion

Discontinuance of Ventilatory Support

Because ventilator therapy is instituted for the purpose of supporting respiratory function while an acute pathophysiologic process is corrected, adequate reversal of that underlying pathology should dictate discontinuance of the therapy. There is no magic way a ventilator can be manipulated to "tease" a patient away from the support before reversal of pathophysiology warrants. Although the dictionary defines the word wean as "to withdraw," the common connotation of the term is "to tease away gradually." This slow, gradual concept is unfortunate when applied to ventilator discontinuance. Therefore, we shall purposely avoid the term "weaning from the ventilator" because the vast majority of patients may be safely removed from the ventilator when the disease process has been adequately reversed. In our experience, more than 80% of patients successfully discontinued from ventilator use do not require a weaning process; rather, they are discontinued from the ventilator within several hours. We prefer to use the term weaning only in reference to those 20% of patients who cannot be discontinued from ventilatory support without gradual maneuvers for more than 12 hours.

Criteria for Discontinuing Positive-Pressure Ventilation

Mechanical support of ventilation must be discontinued at the earliest possible time consistent with patient safety. This should not imply early weaning attempts without rationale as this usually results in unnecessary cardiopulmonary stress without shortening the ventilator course. Everyone is anxious to "get the patient off the ventilator" as soon as possible. What must be realized is that the shortest ventilator course is accomplished by proper maintenance for the necessary period of time.

The procedure of ventilator discontinuance should begin once the following determinations have been appropriately assessed: (1) the underlying indication for ventilatory support is significantly reversed, (2) measurements of the cardiopulmonary reserves are judged adequate for spontaneous ventilation, and (3) general clinical examination and laboratory measurements present no contraindications to maintaining both adequate spontaneous ventilation and cardiopulmonary homeostasis.

Reversal of Indication for Ventilatory Support

The need for ventilatory support is solely a medical judgment. The pathology is often obvious (e.g., pneumonia, heart failure) and readily identifiable; sometimes the working diagnosis is tenuous or unknown. Partial ventilatory support may be helpful in the latter case because the ability to tolerate decreasing ventilator rates assists in evaluation of the overall process.

Assessment of Cardiopulmonary Reserves

Discontinuance of ventilatory support requires the patient to assume the entire work of breathing; however, evaluation of the work of breathing and its impact on cardiopulmonary homeostasis is difficult to assess while the patient is being mechanically ventilated. PVS enables some assessment of the patient's ability to tolerate the work of breathing. The following guidelines have proved to be useful in assessment of cardiopulmonary reserves before discontinuance of PPV: (1) vital capacity (VC) greater than 15 mL/kg is encouraging; however, VC often improves dramatically over several hours of spontaneous breathing. Do not rule out a trial of discontinuance for a VC between 10 and 15 mL/kg. Chronically diseased patients (e.g., chronic obstructive pulmonary disease, quadriplegics) can breathe spontaneously with extremely limited VCs. (2) VTs are often difficult to evaluate before the patient is breathing spontaneously for a period of time. Immediate VTs of greater than 2 mL/kg are encouraging. (3) Spontaneous ventilatory rates of less than 25/min are encouraging; more than this calls for reevaluation. (4) Significant tachycardia on the ventilator is discouraging because the work of breathing places an additional stress on the heart. Again, PVS may prove helpful in these patients. (5) Hypotension on the ventilator is discouraging; hypertension must be evaluated carefully. (6) Cardiac dysrhythmia must be evaluated. (7) The hemoglobin content should be optimized.

Other factors that require consideration because they have potential to increase demand on the ventilatory system include oxygenation status and degree of dead-space ventilation. The following guidelines are suggested: (1) ABG measurements must be acceptable on the ventilator, (2) no evidence of acute increased dead-space ventilation should be present, and (3) the intrapulmonary shunt measurement should be less than 30% and preferably less than 20%.

Discontinuing Positive-Pressure Ventilation

The authors have found the following approach useful in discontinuing ventilatory support.

Some patients manifest obvious indications that there will be no problem discontinuing PPV. In fact, many extubate themselves. Such patients should be removed from the ventilator and extubated shortly thereafter. Most patients do not give this clear-cut picture, and we have found the following method helpful; the factors and techniques are presented as examples and guidelines.

Psychological preparation.—A conscious patient requires careful explanation of the procedure so that the activity willl not be alarming. Patients must understand that initial sensations of dyspnea are expected and not unusual. Forewarning patients of the expected sequence of events results in less apprehension and reassures them that the clinician supervising the program is competent.

The patient must never be "guaranteed" that he will not need further support. It should be explained that this is an "initial" attempt and you must express your confidence in his ability to breathe. Do not express disappointment if he is unsuccessful; simply explain that it was an attempt and there will be others. The patient must not become depressed if the initial attempt fails.

The ventilatory challenge.—An adequate CNS stimulus is essential for maintenance of spontaneous ventilation. This stimulus is provided by the pH of the cerebrospinal fluid (CSF) bathing the floor of the brain's fourth ventricle. Acute changes in blood PCO_2 are reflected immediately in the CSF and therefore affect the pH. Because the CSF does not contain appreciable buffering capabilities, small changes in PCO_2 result in relatively large pH changes.

It can be calculated that a well-oxygenated, 70-kg human at the basal metabolic rate produces enough carbon dioxide in 1 minute to increase the blood PCO_2 by 1 to 2 mm Hg assuming no CO_2 is excreted by the lungs. It may be assumed that the venous, alveolar, and arterial PCO_2 will equilibrate within the first minute of no ventilation and result in a 4- to 6-mm Hg rise in arterial PCO_2. Thus, at basal metabolic rates, 5 minutes without ventilation theoretically would result in no more than a 15-mm Hg rise in arterial PCO_2. This information provides the basis for a safe and predictable approach to ventilator discontinuance—the clinical ventilatory challenge.

The initial step is best accomplished with a manual ventilator delivering 50% to 80% oxygen. This procedure directly and immediately involves you in the process and assures the patient that you can breathe for him at any time if necessary. A positive-pressure breath synchronized with the patient's spontaneous pattern is provided approximately every 30 seconds. If more than one breath every 30 seconds is required or the patient manifests significant detrimental changes in vital signs or clinical appearance, ventilator use should be reinstituted.

After several minutes most patients will not require any positive-pressure breaths. If the patient does well for 5 minutes, he should be attached to an appropriate gas source and observed. Patients with COPD and chronic CO_2 retention may behave as though they require a hypoxic drive to maintain spontaneous ventilation. In such patients, the manual ventilator should be used with an FIO_2 set to give an PaO_2 in the range normally seen in that particular patient.

The patient is allowed to assume his work of breathing while the ECG and BP are closely monitored. Clinical evaluation of the ventilatory pattern, the ventilatory effort, and the cardiovascular system must be continuously accomplished. Any patient stress must evoke immediate and obvious recognition on the physician's part, and that recognition must be obvious to the patient. He must be convinced you are aware and in control! The main criterion and responsibility of the physician during these first attempts at ventilator discontinuance is to decide whether observed distress is physiologic or emotional.

Assessment of vital sign changes.—There are vital sign changes that should be anticipated when a patient assumes spontaneous ventilation: (1) The ventilator has been providing a slower and deeper ventilatory pattern than the patient's natural, spontaneous pattern. When the patient assumes a spontaneous ventilatory pattern with higher respiratory rates (RRs), it should not cause concern so long as the pattern is acceptable and remains consistent with cardiopulmonary homeostasis. (2) The ventilator supports the cardiovascular system significantly, so when the work of breathing is assumed by the patient, it oftens requires some increase in BP and cardiac rate; increases up to 10% of baseline are acceptable. (3) Mild diaphoresis (sweating) is a common feature and should not cause concern unless accompanied by other signs of increased sympathetic discharge or physiologic stress. As long as the vital signs and clinical changes are within acceptable limits, they should not cause concern. Far more important than the immediate vital sign changes is their stability over the next hour or 2.

After 15 to 30 minutes of reasonable clinical stability, vital signs, blood gases, and general clinical status must be reevaluated. It is important to assess what has happened to the VC and the ventilatory pattern over this time.

CASE STUDY 1 CONTINUED

Four hours after the last Pavulon dose, the ventilator rate was decreased to 4/min with an IMV circuit. The patient's spontaneous breathing rate was 20 to 22/min with a V_T of 2 mL/kg. Arterial blood gas values at 30% oxygen were a pH of 7.49, a PCO_2 of 31 mm Hg, and a PO_2 of 120 mm Hg. The ventilator rate was decreased to 2/min, and after 1 hour the patient was placed on a T-piece. Spontaneous ventilation remained adequate. The endotracheal tube remained in place for airway protection and suctioning because the patient was still comatose.

CASE STUDY 2

After a severe myocardial infarction, a previously healthy 53-year-old man was severely hypotensive and required placement of an aortic counterpulsating balloon pump to restore a borderline-acceptable cardiac output (cardiac index [CI] = 2.2 L/min). He complained of dyspnea and was found to have an RR of 35/min and a VT of 400 mL (MV = 14 L). ABG analysis at 0.50 FIO$_2$ showed a pH of 7.32, a PCO$_2$ of 45 mm Hg, and a PO$_2$ of 52 mm Hg.

After explaining the procedure for nasotracheal intubation to the patient and accomplishing adequate topical anesthesia, an 8-mm nasotracheal tube was inserted without incident. Assisted ventilation by a manual self-inflating ventilator (FIO$_2$, approximately 0.70) resulted in abatement of the patient's spontaneous breathing efforts.

Discussion

The significant increase in dead-space ventilation (MV = 14 L with an arterial PCO$_2$ of 45 mm Hg) must be attributed primarily to diminished pulmonary perfusion secondary to the low cardiac output.[3] The increased dead space resulted in an increased ventilatory effort that increased the total oxygen consumption. This increased work of breathing was causing the patient considerable discomfort and anxiety. The decision was made to relieve the work of breathing, thus decreasing oxygen consumption and hopefully improving myocardial function.

The awake nasal intubation allowed airway placement without stress or sedation. If the patient were to become uncooperative during the procedure, small increments of IV morphine or Valium may prove beneficial. However, at the first sign of stress, the nasal intubation should be abandoned and an oral endotracheal tube established following appropriate sedation and paralysis.

The fact that the patient stopped breathing when PPV was initiated is a good indication that the work of breathing was significant. Full ventilatory support can now be administered by either IMV or assist/control techniques. Any decrease in cardiac output may result from decreased venous return and should be treated with an appropriate fluid challenge.

CASE STUDY 2 CONTINUED

The patient was placed on the assist/control mode of ventilation (8/min), a VT of 14 mL/kg, and an FIO$_2$ of 0.40 with resultant arterial blood gas values of pH 7.38, a PCO$_2$ of 39 mm Hg, and a PO$_2$ of 62 mm Hg.

Cardiac output remained unchanged while the ventricular rate significantly decreased. Urine output remained at 45 mL/hr.

Twelve hours later the patient began to make spontaneous breathing efforts at a rate of 12/min. ABG analysis at this point showed a pH of 7.42, a PCO$_2$ of 35 mm Hg, and a PO$_2$ of 63 mm Hg. During the next 6 hours the patient was tapered off the balloon pump with good cardiovascular dynamics and essentially unchanged blood gas values. It was decided to see whether ventilator use could be discontinued.

Discussion

There are at least two reasons why a short transition period of PVS would be more desirable than abrupt discontinuance in this patient: (1) reassumption of the work of breathing may significantly increase myocardial demands, and (2) removal of PPV may result in a significant increase in venous return and precipitate ventricular failure. Although assist/control has adequately provided FVS, the same could have been provided by IMV. The desirability of PVS now requires changing from assist/control to IMV. Although this change is seldom troublesome, it is always time-consuming and requires a period of evaluation once the change is made. This is the main reason why IMV techniques are preferable—not because they are better than assist modes are for full support, but because they can provide both full and partial support.

CASE STUDY 2 CONTINUED

The patient was placed on SIMV at 8/min, and hemodynamic studies, obtained after 30 minutes, revealed a mean arterial pressure (MAP) of 80 mg Hg, a pulse of 95/min, a spontaneous RR of 16/min (V_T, 75 mL), a PPV of 8/min (V_T, 900 mL), a cardiac output of 3.7 L/min (CI, 2.4 L/min), a pH of 7.42, a $Paco_2$ of 37 mm Hg, and a Pao_2 of 64 mm Hg (Fio_2, 0.4).

After explaining the procedure to the patient, the SIMV rate was decreased to 6/min without distress to the patient. Fifteen minutes later the patient had a MAP of 80 mm Hg, a pulse of 95/min, a spontaneous RR of 12/min (V_T, 200 mL), a PPV of 6/min (V_T, 900 mL), a cardiac output of 3.7 L/min (CI, 2.4 L/min), a pulmonary artery occluded pressure (PAOP) of 17 mm Hg, a pH of 7.43, a $Paco_2$ of 36 mm Hg, and a Pao_2 of 61 mm Hg (Fio_2, 0.4).

When the SIMV rate was decreased to 4/min, the patient indicated he was aware of the need to breathe on his own and was reassured. Cardiopulmonary assessment revealed a MAP of 90 mm Hg, a pulse of 102/min, a spontaneous RR of 12/min (V_T, 400 mL), a PPV of 4/min (V_T, 900 mL), a cardiac output of 4.4 L/min (CI, 2.6 L/min), a PAOP of 14 mm Hg, a pH of 7.39, a $Paco_2$ of 39 mm Hg, and a Pao_2 of 56 mm Hg (Fio_2, 0.4).

Discussion

Reassumption of a portion of the work of breathing results in increased myocardial work. The drop in PAOP may be due solely to a diminished mean intrathoracic pressure. However, it is prudent to remain on PVS for a period.

CASE STUDY 2 CONTINUED

The patient continued to improve and 12 hours later was removed from PVS. He was subsequently extubated after remaining in stable condition and breathing spontaneously via the endotracheal tube for another 3 hours.

CASE STUDY 3

A 68-year-old man with a history of pulmonary fibrosis presented to the emergency room with increasing shortness of breath over the preceding 3 days, cough productive of thick yellow sputum, and increasing lethargy.

On examination he was noted to be cachectic (60 kg) and breathing 36 breaths per minute with the use of accessory muscles of ventilation. He was arousable but not oriented to time or place. His BP was 100/60 mm Hg, his pulse rate was 115/min and irregular, and his temperature was 100°F. Ausculation of the chest revealed decreased airway entry in the right base with scattered rhonchi. The liver was slightly enlarged and 2 + pedal edema noted.

Chest x-ray films showed bilateral diffuse interstitial infiltrates with a denser alveolar-type infiltrate in right lower lung field. A small right pleural effusion was seen. The heart appeared enlarged.

Arterial blood gas analysis on supplemental oxygen at 35% revealed a pH of 7.23, a P_{CO_2} of 70 mm Hg, and a P_{O_2} of 53 mm Hg. His hemoglobin content was 11.5 g/dL, and his white blood cell count was 16,000/mm^3 with 10% bands. Blood chemistries showed an elevated bicarbonate and glucose level, electrolytes were within normal limits, the blood urea nitrogen (BUN) concentration was 40 mg/dL, and the creatinine level was 2.2 mg/dL. The ECG showed right ventricular hypertrophy and atrial fibrillation.

A diagnosis of acute and chronic ventilatory failure secondary to pneumonia, cor pulmonale, and dehydration was made. A large-bore IV line was established and rehydration with 5% dextrose in 0.9% saline started. The patient was nasally intubated with a no. 8 endotracheal tube and placed on FVS with a V_T of 700 mL at ten breaths per minute and an F_{IO_2} of 0.5. On initiation of ventilatory support his BP fell to a systolic of 75 mm Hg. Administration of 500 mL of saline and initiation of inotropic support with dopamine at 5 μg/kg/min restored the BP to 100/75 mm Hg. Appropriate antibiotic therapy for a community-acquired pneumonia was commenced. The patient was transferred to the ICU for further management.

Discussion

Initiation of ventilatory support in this patient resulted in a fall in BP. Several mechanisms are probably responsible for this hypotension: (1) absolute hypovolemia secondary to dehydration, (2) arterial vasodilatation secondary to removal of sympathetic stimulation consequent on assuming the work of breathing and correction of hypoxemia and acute acidemia, and (3) reduction in venous return secondary to positive airway pressure. In most patients volume repletion is all that is required to restore BP and tissue perfusion. In this patient it was deemed necessary to initiate inotropic support in addition to volume replacement because of his cor pulmonale and clinical signs of congestive heart failure.

The initial blood gas values clearly indicate that the patient had retained CO_2 secondary to the chronic lung disease. It is essential to titrate the ventilatory support to restore carbon dioxide homeostasis with a pH of 7.40 rather than a "normal" P_{CO_2} of 40 mm Hg.

CASE STUDY 3 CONTINUED

Arterial blood gas analysis 30 minutes after institution of ventilatory support revealed a pH of 7.31, a P_{CO_2} of 67 mm Hg, and a P_{O_2} of 94 mm Hg. The maximum inspiratory pressure was 65 cm H_2O. The ventilatory rate was increased to 14/min, and repeat arterial blood gas analysis showed a pH of 7.39, a P_{CO_2} of 53 mm Hg, and a P_{O_2} of 105 mm Hg. The F_{IO_2} was decreased to 0.4 with a resultant Pa_{O_2} of 75 mm Hg. A nasogastric tube was placed for enteral feedings and appropriate bronchial hygiene therapy started to facilitate removal of secretions. The following day the patient's vital signs were stable, and the dopamine dosage had been reduced to 3 μg/kg/min. Blood urea nitrogen, creatinine, and electrolyte values were within normal limits. The patient remained febrile. The ventilator was set to an IMV mode with a rate of 10/min, and the patient started to spontaneously ventilate at a rate of 14 breaths per minute. This switch to PVS was well tolerated by the patient who exhibited no signs of distress and required very little sedation (1 to 2 mg of morphine sulfate every 2 to 4 hours).

Discussion

In most circumstances increasing alveolar ventilation is best achieved by increases in V_T. However, in this patient with chronic restrictive lung disease delivery of 700 mL V_T was associated with fairly high maximum inspiratory pressure, and hence it was decided to increase the rate rather than V_T to achieve adequate alveolar ventilation. Note that a Pa_{CO_2} of 53 mm Hg is associated with a normal pH and should be considered "eucapnia" for this patient with chronic CO_2 retention. Ventilating this patient to a physiologically normal Pa_{CO_2} would initially result in significant alkalemia, which may have immediate undesirable effects and, if maintained for several days, would result in renal excretion of bicarbonate and a resetting of the patient's acid-base balance around a set point that would require a higher spontaneous MV when ventilatory support is discontinued. Such inappropriate ventilator maintenance in patients with chronic CO_2 retention frequently results in difficulties in discontinuance of ventilatory support.

CASE STUDY 3 CONTINUED

Three days later the patient was afebrile, his white blood cell count had returned to normal, inotrope administration was stopped, and his chest x-ray film showed considerable clearing of the consolidation in the right lower lung field. His oxygenation status had improved with a Pa_{O_2} of 82 mm Hg on 30% oxygen. It was decided to attempt discontinuance of ventilatory support. The patient's VC was 900 mL, and he was breathing between the machine breaths at 14/min with a V_T of 165 mL. In light of his chronic lung disease it was decided to withdraw ventilatory support by decrements in the IMV rate. The IMV rate was decreased to 8/min. The patient's spontaneous rate went up to 20/min, and V_T increased to 185 mL. He remained cardiovascularly stable and was comfortable. ABG analysis revealed a pH of 7.40, a P_{CO_2} of 55 mm Hg, and a P_{O_2} of 78 mm Hg. The IMV rate was further reduced to 6/min. The patient's heart rate increased from 85 to 105/min, systolic BP went up to 135 mm Hg, and the spontaneous ventilatory rate increased to 28/min. The patient indicated that he was aware of his breathing but denied that he was short of breath. Arterial blood gas analysis revealed a pH of 7.38, a P_{CO_2} of 58 mm Hg, and a P_{O_2} of 69 mm Hg. It was decided to leave the ventilator settings at those levels and observe the patient closely for a couple of hours. An hour later the patient's respiratory and heart rate started to increase, his BP fell to a systolic of 90 mm Hg, and he became diaphoretic and complained of dyspnea. Arterial blood gas measurement revealed a pH of 7.34, a P_{CO_2} of 64 mm Hg, and a P_{O_2} of 60 mm Hg. The ventilator rate was increased to 14/min, and the patient's cardiopulmonary function stabilized.

Discussion

When reasonable procedures for discontinuance of ventilatory support are followed and the patient fails to maintain an adequate cardiopulmonary status with spontaneous breathing, complete reevaluation is mandatory. It must be ascertained that narcotics, sedatives, and muscle relaxants have been completely reversed, and the physiologic parameters of cardiopulmonary reserves must be reviewed. If these are in order, the assumption should be made that the patient is either unable to come off the ventilator because the disease is not reversed adequately for the general body reserves or that psychologic dependence exists. In our experience, most weaning problems are caused by either (1) attempts to discontinue ventilation too early in the disease course, (2) improper ventilator maintenance, or (3) preexisting chronic disease or malnutrition that severely limits reserves.

The Difficult-to-Wean Patient

Difficult-to-wean patients are almost always those with chronic cardiopulmonary limitations. For the patient who does not assume ventilator independence readily the techniques of IMV or SIMV are clinically useful. These techniques hold the advantage of allowing the patient to gradually assume more work of breathing. This makes it far more practical (and far less frustrating) to accomplish a weaning process without being limited by the availability of bedside personnel. There still must be appropriate intensive care monitoring, but the process of sequential decreases in the rate of the intermittent ventilation may be beneficial; however, there are no data to support these techniques as being superior to others for accomplishing ventilator discontinuance.[41]

As useful as the IMV and SIMV techniques have proved for the patient truly in need of a weaning process, these techniques are misused for routine ventilator discontinuance. Many physicians "routinely" decrease IMV rates over a period of 24 to 48 hours, a process that unnecessarily prolongs the ventilator course. Because the vast majority of patients do not need a weaning process, they do not need several days of tapering the IMV rate before breathing spontaneously. Both IMV and SIMV are useful weaning techniques for those patients in need of a weaning process; they should not be misused to prolong the time on the ventilator unnecessarily. It is recommended that SIMV not be used at ventilator rates of less than 4/min, as the demand valve may unnecessarily increase the work of breathing.[42]

Improved understanding of ventilatory muscle function has led to development of techniques (isocapnic hyperpnea, inspiratory resistive breathing) specifically designed to increase ventilatory muscle strength and endurance.[43, 44] We have used inspiratory resistive breathing exercises in non-COPD patients with chronically compromised ventilatory reserve whom we have been unable to wean from mechanical ventilatory support. Provided the patient can be stabilized by PVS, it is feasible to introduce an inspiratory resistance into that part of the ventilator circuit through which the patient spontaneously breathes. Providing an appropriate inspiratory workload for 10 to 15 minutes two to three times per day has resulted in improved ventilatory muscle function as manifested by higher VCs and in our opinion facilitated weaning in some of the patients.

Continuous Positive Airway Pressure and Weaning

There are circumstances in which the use of 5 to 10 cm H_2O PEEP aids in the ability to maintain spontaneous ventilation. Theoretical benefits include the maintenance of an improved FRC, improved lung compliance, and a subjective "sensation" of better lung inflation. As a general rule, patients already receiving PEEP therapy should be maintained on 5 to 8 cm H_2O continuous positive airway pressure (CPAP) and extubated from that level.

The possible reasons for failure to discontinue ventilatory support in this patient included chronic cardiopulmonary disease and inadequate nutritional status.

CASE STUDY 3 CONTINUED

Reevaluation of the patient revealed that although he appeared cachetic, his nutritional status was not inadequate. His ventilatory reserve as assessed by measurement of VC appeared adequate (Vc = 15 mL/kg). His acid-base balance, oxygenation status, and airway resistance appeared to be within reasonable limits. His lung compliance was decreased secondary to his pulmonary fibrosis. In light of this it was felt that his myocardial function may have been the limiting factor in assumption of spontaneous breathing. A pulmonary artery catheter was inserted and the following findings noted:

- Right atrial filling pressure—9 mm Hg
- Right ventricular pressure—30/5 mm Hg
- Pulmonary artery pressure—30/18 mm Hg
- PAOP—11 mm Hg
- Thermodilution cardiac output—4.1 L

The ventilator rate was again decreased in increments to 6/min. No significant changes occurred in the pulmonary artery catheter readings until the ventilator rate was decreased below 8/min, at which time the right atrial pressure went up to 18 mm Hg, PAOP increased to 23 mm Hg, and the cardiac ouput fell to 3.4 L/min. Dopamine infusion at a rate of 6 μg/kg/min was started, the right atrial pressure fell to 12 mm Hg, PAOP decreased to 16 mm Hg, and the cardiac output increased to 4.2 L/min. The patient appeared more comfortable and no longer complained of dyspnea. After PEEP of 10 cm H_2O was added to the ventilator settings, the process of discontinuance of ventilatory support continued slowly over the next 12 hours. Cardiac function was continuously monitored and adjusted with fluid therapy and inotropic support. The patient was eventually discontinued from ventilatory support and was stable on CPAP at +10 cm H_2O and inotropes. He was digitalized and then weaned off inotrope usage. The CPAP was decreased to +5 cm H_2O after 12 hours. A day later, the patient was extubated from +5 cm H_2O of CPAP without difficulty.

Discussion

The successful discontinuance of ventilatory support while the patient was receiving inotropic support suggests that cardiac failure secondary to the increased demands on the myocardium from spontaneous breathing was the problem. Dopamine enhances diaphragmatic blood flow and diaphragmatic strength generation in patients with COPD and ARF.[45] Although that may have played a role in this patient, the patient's ventilatory muscle strength, as evidenced by his VC, was adequate, and the clinical signs suggested a primary inability of the heart to assume the work of breathing. Whatever the mechanism, it was clearly advantageous to continue inotropic support during the process of gradual discontinuance of ventilatory support.

REFERENCES

1. Emerson H: Artificial respiration in the treatment of edema of the lungs: A suggestion based on animal experimentation. *Arch Intern Med* 1909; 3:368–371.
2. Drinker P, Shaw LA: An apparatus for the prolonged administration of artificial respiration. I. A design for adults and children. *J Clin Invest* 1929; 7:229–247.
3. Shapiro BA, Harrison RA, Walton JR: *Clinical Application of Blood Gases*, ed. 3. Chicago, Year Book Medical Publishers, Inc., 1982.
4. Dammann JF, McAslan TC: Optimal flow pattern for mechanical ventilation of the lungs. *Crit Care Med* 1977; 5:128.
5. Jansson L, Jonson B: A theoretical study of flow patterns of ventilation. *Scand J Respir Dis* 1972; 53:237.
6. Knelson JH, et al: Effect of respiratory pattern on alveolar gas exchange. *J Appl Physiol* 1970; 29:278.
7. Otis A: The work of breathing. *Physiol Rev* 1954; 34:449.
8. Downs JB, Perkins HM, Modell JH: Intermittent mandatory ventilation: An evaluation. *Arch Surg* 1974; 109:519–523.
9. Downs JG, Klein EF, Desutels D, et al: Intermittent mandatory ventilation: A new approach to weaning patients from mechanical ventilators. *Chest* 1973; 64:331–335.
10. Shapiro BA, Harrison RA, Walton, et al: Intermittent demand ventilation (IDV): A new technique for supporting ventilation in critically ill patients. *Respir Care* 1976; 21:512–525.
11. Hasten RW, Downs JB, Heenan TJ: A comparison of synchronized and non-synchronized intermittent mandatory ventilation. *Respir Care* 1980; 25:554–557.
12. Op't Holt TB, Hall MW, Bass JB, et al: Comparison of changes in airway pressure during continuous positive airway pressure (CPAP) between demand valve and continuous flow devices. *Respir Care* 1982; 27:1200–1209.
13. Gibnew RTN, Wilson RS, Pontoppidan H: Comparison of work of breathing on high gas flow and demand valve continuous positive airway pressure systems. *Chest* 1982; 82:692–695.
14. Henry WC, West GA, Wilson RS: A comparison of the oxygen cost of breathing between a continuous-flow CPAP system and demand flow CPAP system. *Respir Care* 1983; 28:1273–1281.
15. Cournand A, Motley HL, Werko L, et al: Physiologic studies of the effects of intermittent positive pressure breathing on cardiac output in man. *Am J Physiol* 1948; 152:162–174.
16. Werko L: Influence of positive pressure breathing on the circulation in man. *Acta Med Scand* 1947; 193(suppl):1.
17. Ford GT, Whitelaw WA, Rosenal TW, et al: Diaphragm function after upper abdominal surgery in humans. *Am Rev Respir Dis* 1983; 127:431–436.
18. Simonneau G, Vivien A, Sartene R, et al: Diaphragm dysfunction induced by upper abdominal surgery: Role of postoperative pain. *Am Rev Respir Dis* 1983; 128:899–903.
19. Froese AB, Bryan AC: Effects of anesthesia and paralysis on diaphragmatic mechanics in man. *Anesthesiology* 1974; 41:242–255.
20. Watson WE: Observations of physiologic deadspace during intermittent positive pressure respiration. *Br J Anaesth* 1962; 34:502.
21. Shapiro BA, Cane RD: The IMV-AMV controversy: A plea for clarification and redirection. *Crit Care Med* 1984; 12:472–473.
22. Cane RD, Shapiro BA: Mechanical ventilatory support. *JAMA* 1985; 254:87–92.
23. Downs JB, Douglas ME, et al: Ventilatory pattern, intrapleural pressure and cardiac output. *Anesth Analg Curr Res* 1977; 56:88.
24. Shad DM, Newell JAC, Dutton RE, et al: Continuous positive airway pressure versus positive end-expiratory pressure in respiratory distress syndrome. *J Thorac Cardiovasc Surg* 1977; 75:557–562.
25. Venus B, Jacobs HK, Mathru M: Hemodynamic responses to different modes of mechanical ventilation in dogs with normal and acid aspirated lungs. *Crit Care Med* 1980; 8:620.
26. Roussos CH, Fixley M, Gross D, et al: Fatigue of inspiratory muscles and their synergistic behavior. *J Appl Physiol* 1979; 46:897–904.
27. Bergman NA: Effects of varying respiratory waveforms on gas exchange. *Anesthesiology* 1967; 28:390.
28. Maffeo W, Dammann JF: Influence of ventilation parameters on mechanical ventilation of the lungs, in Vogt WG, Mickel MM (eds): Proceedings of the 9th Annual Model and Simulation Conference, Pittsburgh, 1978.
29. Bendixen HH, Bullwinkel B, Hedley-Whyte J, et al: Atelectasis and shunting during spontaneous ventilation in anesthetized patients. *Anesthesiology* 1964; 25:297–301.
30. Massaro GD, Massaro D: Morphologic evidence that large inflations of lung stimulate secretions of surfactant. *Am Rev Respir Dis* 1983; 127:235–236.

31. Marini JJ, Capps JS, Culver BH: The inspiratory work of breathing during assisted mechanical ventilation. *Chest* 1985; 87:612–618.
32. Marini JJ, Rodriguez RM, Lamb V: Bedside estimation of the inspiratory work of breathing during mechanical ventilation. *Chest* 1986; 89:56–63.
33. Lappas D, et al: Filling pressures of the heart and pulmonary circulation of the patient with coronary-artery disease after large intravenous doses of morphine. *Anesthesiology* 1975; 42:153.
34. Lowenstein E: Morphine "anesthesia"—A perspective. *Anesthesiology* 1971; 35:563.
35. Dammann JF, et al: Optimal flow pattern for mechanical ventilation of the lungs. The effect of a sine versus square flow pattern with and without an end-expiratory pause on patients. *Crit Care Med* 1978; 6:293.
36. Fulheihan SF, et al: Effect of mechanical ventilation with end-inspiratory pause on blood gas exchange. *Anaesth Analg* 1976; 55:122.
37. Dolfuss R, et al: Regional ventilation of the lung studied with boluses of xenon. *Respir Physiol* 1967; 2:234.
38. Klocke RA, Farhi EL: Simple method for determination of perfusion ventilation ratio of the underventilated element (the slow compartment) of the lung. *J Clin Invest* 1964; 43:2227.
39. Bartlett RH, Hanson EL, Moore RD: Physiology of yawning and its application to postoperative care. *Surg Forum* 1970; 22:222.
40. Henning RJ, et al: The measurement of the work of breathing for the clinical assessment of ventilator dependence. *Crit Care Med* 1977; 5:264.
41. Schacter EN, Tucker D, Beck GJ: Does intermittent mandatory ventilation accelerate weaning? *JAMA* 1981; 246:1210–1214.
42. Henry WC, West GA, Wilson RS: A comparison of the oxygen cost of breathing between a continuous-flow CPAP system and demand-flow CPAP system. *Respir Care* 1983; 28:1273.
43. Pardy RL, Leigh DE: Ventilatory muscle training. *Respir Care* 1984; 29:278–284.
44. Leigh DE, Bradley M: Ventilatory muscle strength and endurance training. *J Appl Physiol* 1976; 41:508–516.
45. Aubier M, Murciano D, Meau Y, et al: Dopamine effects on diaphragmatic strength during acute respiratory failure in chronic obstructive pulmonary disease. *Ann Intern Med* 1989; 110:17–23.

5/Alternate Forms of Mechanical Ventilation

M. CHRISTINE STOCK, M.D.
ROY D. CANE, M.B.B.CH.

The recent technology explosion prompted a proliferation of mechanical ventilatory modes for adults, children, and neonates. Unfortunately, our ability to develop new and different machines and monitoring systems has exceeded our ability to test these devices scientifically before public marketing. This phenomenon created misunderstanding of the function and purpose of some newer mechanical ventilatory modes. The alternate forms of mechanical ventilation discussed in this chapter have undergone or are undergoing scientific scrutiny.

In this chapter three newer techniques for adult mechanical ventilatory support—high-frequency ventilation (HFV), pressure support ventilation (PSV), and airway pressure release ventilation (APRV)—will be evaluated.

HIGH-FREQUENCY VENTILATION

Historical Perspective

In 1915 Henderson and coworkers[1] demonstrated that tidal volumes (VTs) that were smaller than anatomic dead space promoted gas exchange. Years later Briscoe and colleagues[2] again showed that VTs as low as 60 mL would cause gas exchange if the ventilatory frequency was high. In searching for a research tool that would support ventilation without affecting hemodynamic function, Sjostrand developed high-frequency positive-pressure ventilation (HFPPV).[3] He was the first "modern" physiologist to recognize that the observations of his predecessors could be applied practically.

A useful HFV classification is based on equipment needs and delivery mode (Table 5–1). The generic "HFV" term applies to assisted ventilation delivered at rates four times the normal respiratory rate of the patient.[4] The four major types of HFV are HFPPV, high-frequency oscillatory ventilation (HFOV), high-frequency jet ventilation (HFJV), and high-frequency chest wall oscillation (HFCWO). The first three of these are used clinically to achieve alveolar ventilation. The fourth, HFCWO, is still experimental and probably does not eliminate CO_2 well. However, HFCWO may enhance mucociliary transport and secretion clearance.[5] The following discussion will focus on HFJV exclusively because it is more widely available and successful than are the other forms of HFV.

TABLE 5–1.

Classification of High-Frequency Ventilation

HFV Type*	V_T* (mL/kg)	f* (breaths/min)	Bulk Gas Flow	Mode of Delivery
HFPPV	3–4	60–100	Yes	Tracheal tube
HFOV	1–3	900–3,600	No	Tracheal tube
HFJV	2–4	80–300 (rarely >150)	Yes, plus entrainment	Jet injector
HFCWO	Unknown	180–600	No	Rigid harness

*HFPPV = high-frequency positive-pressure ventilation; HFOV = high-frequency oscillatory ventilation; HFJV = high-frequency jet ventilation; HFCWO = high-frequency chest wall oscillation; V_T = tidal volume; f = ventilatory frequency.

A detailed discussion of the diffusive and convective properties that allow CO_2 elimination and oxygenation during HFV are beyond the scope of this chapter. However, different mechanisms probably operate at frequencies in excess of 600 breaths per minute (bpm) as opposed to those between 60 and 300 bpm.

Gas Exchange

Because the vast majority of clinicians understand mechanical ventilation through the use of conventional ventilation, analogies of HFJV to conventional ventilation can be helpful. These analogies are not mechanistically related, perhaps with the exception of mean airway pressure during HFJV and continuous positive airway pressure (CPAP) during conventional ventilation (Table 5–2). During conventional ventilation, the clinician must choose four basic functions: V_T, ventilatory frequency (f), fraction of inspired oxygen (FIO_2), and CPAP/positive end-expiratory pressure (PEEP) level.

TABLE 5–2.

Analogy of Conventional Ventilation to High-Frequency Jet Ventilation

Determinants	Conventional Ventilation	HFJV
Oxygenation		
Alveolar pO_2	FIO_2	FIO_2
Resting lung volume	CPAP/PEEP	Mean Paw*
Alveolar ventilation (CO_2 elimination)		
Minute ventilation	f*	Jet driving pressure
	V_T*	T_{insp}*
		Entrainment rate

*Mean Paw = mean airway pressure; f = ventilatory frequency; V_T = tidal volume; T_{insp} = percentage of mechanical ventilatory cycle devoted to inspiration.

During conventional ventilation, the primary determinants of arterial oxygenation are FIO_2 and CPAP/PEEP (or possibly, the mean airway pressure). During HFJV, FIO_2 helps to determine arterial oxygenation just as it does during conventional ventilation. The use of CPAP/PEEP to enhance arterial oxygenation during conventional ventilation is analogous to increasing mean airway pressure during HFJV. Mean airway pressure determines the resting lung volume, or functional residual capacity (FRC), during HFJV as PEEP does during conventional ventilation.[6, 7]

Mean airway pressure values obtained during HFJV depend on where pressure is measured in the airway. During HFJV, mean alveolar pressure usually exceeds mean upper airway pressure.[8, 9] Ideally, changes in mean alveolar pressure would reflect the ventilator's influence on resting lung volume. Unfortunately, mean alveolar pressure measurement is technically difficult. Airway pressure in the distal endotracheal tube better approximates alveolar pressure than does the airway pressure measured at the proximal end of the endotracheal tube. A comparison of resting lung volume must be performed by using airway pressures measured in or beyond the distal portion of the endotracheal tube. By using this technique, similar mean airway pressures during conventional and HFJ ventilation result in indistinguishable arterial oxygenation. Thus, arterial oxygenation during either conventional or HFJV appears to be equivalent at a given resting lung volume provided that the lung volume prevents end-expiratory collapse of "most" of the alveoli.[6]

Carbon dioxide elimination during both HFJV and conventional mechanical ventilation is determined primarily by the total gas flow into the lungs, or minute ventilation. Determinants of alveolar ventilation during the two ventilatory methods do not parallel each other as closely as do determinants of arterial oxygenation. During conventional ventilation, ventilatory frequency is one of the primary determinants of CO_2 elimination. This is not usually true during HFJV, in which an increase in ventilatory frequency does not imply an increase in minute ventilation; the opposite may occur.[10] The percentage of time devoted to inspiration with each mechanical breath (T_{insp}), the jet driving pressure, and gas entrainment determine minute ventilation. The HFJV VT depends on ventilatory cycle length (or frequency,) T_{insp}, jet driving pressure, and the rate of entrainment. Because VT varies with the mechanical ventilatory rate and minute ventilation does not, it is more useful to consider CO_2 elimination in terms of minute ventilation rather than VT.

The use of gas entrainment further distinguishes HFJV from conventional techniques. Because CO_2 excretion is determined primarily by total gas flow into the lungs, impeding entrainment usually decreases CO_2 elimination. The volume of gas entrained depends on the jet gas velocity and pressure at the jet nozzle.[11] A greater jet driving pressure increases both gas flow through the jet cannula and gas entrainment. Because entrainment is so essential to HFJV, an oxygen-enriched, blended gas source must be available at the proximal end of the endotracheal tube where the tip of the injector cannula resides. When gas entrainment is small, VT and minute ventilation vary linearly with T_{insp}.[12] As gas entrainment increases, the relationship between T_{insp} (inspiratory-expiratory time ratio) and VT loses linearity.[11, 12] T_{insp} that exceeds 40% to 50% of the total ventilatory cycle time causes gas trapping, which may limit entrainment and thereby decrease CO_2 elimination. The insignificance of ventilatory frequency is illustrated best by example. At 60 bpm, with 25% of every breath spent during inspiration, the total inspiratory time during each minute would be calculated as follows:

$$(\text{Vent cycle length}) \ (f) \ (T_{insp})$$
$$= 1 \text{ second per breath} \times 60 \text{ bpm} \times 0.25$$
$$= 15 \text{ seconds of inspiratory time per minute}$$

If the ventilatory frequency is doubled to 120 bpm and the driving pressure and T_{insp} remain constant, each breath requires 0.5 seconds. If 25% of every breath is inspiratory time, the total amount of inspiratory time is 0.5 seconds per breath × 120 bpm × 0.25, or 15 seconds of inspiratory time per minute. Driving pressure determines the gas flow generated by the ventilator, and T_{insp} determines how long the lungs are exposed to that flow during each minute; therefore, jet driving pressure and T_{insp} are important determinants of minute ventilation and CO_2 elimination.

Equipment

A brief discussion of the HFJV components will aid the understanding of clinical applicability. Starting at the high-pressure gas source, each of the major components of the HFJ ventilator will be discussed.

Currently marketed HFJV devices function at jet driving pressures less than 50 psi.[11, 13] The most useful range of driving pressures is 20 to 35 psi. Once the gas enters the ventilator, it undergoes near-instantaneous gating to provide a nearly perfect square-wave inspiratory waveform.[12, 13] Gating the jet gas stream determines ventilatory frequency and T_{insp}. After gating, the high-pressure gas travels through the inspiratory line, which must be noncompliant (0.005 mL/cm H_2O) and have a small compressible volume.[13] These characteristics will ensure that rapid pressure changes will not cause volume loss in the inspiratory line. Once the gas passes through the inspiratory line, the square wave degrades to a sinusoidal waveform.[12, 14] To minimize this degradation, the shortest practical tubing should be used for the inspiratory line. Further, the inspiratory line's internal diameter should not exceed three to four times the diameter of the injector cannula.

After the gas traverses the inspiratory line, it enters the injector cannula, from which it is delivered to the patient. Investigation of the different characteristics of the injector cannula have revealed that the internal diameter should be 1.5 to 2 mm for the adult. Internal diameters less than 1.5 mm deliver insufficient gas volume to patients with severe respiratory failure and become easily occluded.[11, 14, 15] The length of the injector cannula is relatively insignificant, except when it influences the distance from the injector cannula tip to the entrainment source.[16] The injector cannula usually resides within an endotracheal tube. The ratio of the cross-sectional area of the injector cannula to that of the endotracheal tube should be greater than 1:6. If this ratio falls below 1:6, entrainment is decreased significantly, thus impairing CO_2 elimination.[11, 17] However, very large injector cannulas or very small tracheal tubes may create turbulence, which impairs gas flow to the alevoli. The best position for the injector cannula within the tracheal tube is in the central axis of the tracheal tube lumen. The tip of the injector cannula should reside at the proximal end of the tracheal tube, with the tip near the entrainment source.

In summary, the most common applications of HFV are with a jet device. The Federal Drug Administration guidelines are based on the literature discussed above and include the following:

1. *Ventilatory frequency:* usually >60, always <150 bpm
2. *VT:* not directly determined
3. *Driving pressure:* usually need >12 psi to achieve ventilation, should not require >35 psi; machines will not drive more than approximately 45 psi
4. *Inspiratory time:* inspiratory-to-expiratory (I:E) ratio always ≤1:1 (T_{insp} ≤ 50%), usually <2:3 (T_{insp} < 40%)
5. *Injector cannula:* diameter 1.5 to 2.0 mm, ratio of internal cross-sectional area of injector cannula to tracheal tube always >1:6; central coaxial position in proximal tracheal tube preferable

Special Precautions

High-frequency ventilation poses several special problems that require increased vigilance. These problems are primarily mechanical: occluded exhalation limb, inadequate expiratory time, tracheal injury, and mucus plugging.

Because a relatively high gas flow enters the trachea, occlusion of the exhalation limb can rapidly result in serious barotrauma. The pathway for expired gas includes the tracheal tube. Thus, mucus plugging of the tracheal tube can result in rapid increases in intrathoracic pressure that cause alveolar overdistension, barotrauma, and cardiac output depression.[14, 18] To prevent severe injury, an airway pressure sensor can be connected to a servocontrolled relief valve that opens the patient's circuit to ambient (or to a lower) pressure when circuit pressure exceeds a predetermined level, e.g., 40 cm H_2O. Because mean airway pressure that is measured at the proximal end of the tracheal tube does not reflect mean alveolar pressure or lung volume accurately, airway pressure should be measured at or, preferably, beyond the tip of the tracheal tube. This is especially important in infants and patients with increased lung compliance.

Mucus plugging is a common and insidious problem during HFV. Although HFV may increase mobilization of pulmonary secretions to the more central airways,[19] inadequate humidification will dry secretions and promote mucus plugs. In this and other circumstances, pulmonary secretions are cleared poorly during HFV.[20, 21] Since occlusion of the endotracheal tube with pulmonary secretions is a relatively common and potentially dangerous complication with HFJV, monitoring of the distal airway pressure is important in that it may provide an early warning of this event. Distal mucus plugging can be prevented only by adequate humidification of the inspired gas, adequate systemic hydration of the patient, and suctioning and postural drainage. Cascade or passover humidification is not adequate. If approximately 44 mg H_2O/L jet flow is infused into the jet stream, relative humidity at 37°C will approach 100% if the gas is initially dry.

High-frequency jet ventilation potentially can cause tracheal mucosal damage because of the large volume of gas that is injected into the trachea under high pressure.[22, 23] Especially in the newborn, this type of injury is related to inadequate humidification of the gas jet rather than being a result of the gas jet striking the tracheal mucosa.[24] If jet gas humidification is adequate, tracheal damage should not occur.[25]

An appropriately short T_{insp} is also essential. If the expiratory time is inadequate, gas trapping occurs, and resting lung volume increases. Gas trapping increases intrathoracic pressure, which may cause barotrauma, decrease CO_2 elimination, and depress cardiac output.[26, 27] Gas trapping is more likely when VTs are larger. Therefore, the use of higher jet driving pressures requires shorter T_{insp}.

High-frequency ventilation development was based on intellectual interest stemming from observation of animal physiology. Although this method of ventilation clearly works, after two decades the application of this more complicated form of ventilatory support remains controversial.

PRESSURE SUPPORT VENTILATION (PSV)

Since the advent of microprocessor-controlled mechanical ventilators, many new "modes" of mechanical ventilation have become available. Even though these have been marketed widely, little investigation has been done to determine the efficacy, attributes, complications, or usefulness of these modes. One such mode, PSV, may offer unique advantages over conventional mechanical ventilation and may provide a mechanism that overcomes the increased work of spontaneous breathing.

Pressure support ventilation is a flow-cycled, pressure-limited, positive-pressure ventilatory mode in which each spontaneous inspiratory effort is assisted by mechanically maintaining a predetermined inspiratory pressure plateau throughout inspiration. As a patient begins to inspire, the ventilator delivers a gas flow sufficient to maintain a predetermined supra-ambient inspiratory airway pressure. Gas is delivered at this pressure until the patient's inspiratory flow falls below a predetermined level. Thus, a PSV machine includes a demand valve capable of delivering a high flow of gas during inspiration and a mechanism to detect the patient's inspiratory effort. A feedback loop ensures a constant inspiratory plateau pressure. The ventilator continually monitors the airway pressure and adjusts flow to maintain the same pressure throughout the "plateau phase." Thus, PSV provides an adjustable level of inspiratory pressure assist with every spontaneous inspiratory effort.

This "mode" was designed initially to overcome demand valve inertia. Later, observers noted that with higher levels of pressure support, mechanical ventilation could be achieved by augmenting each VT. Depending on the level of inspiratory pressure assist, ventilatory muscle effort with each breath is reduced partially.[28] Although application of ventilatory support by PSV mode is relatively new, the old Puritan-Bennett PR-2 machine operated under the same principles, although it was not microprocessor controlled.

MacIntyre studied ventilatory muscle work requirements during unassisted and pressure-assisted breaths with PSV.[28] He used a two-compartment mechanical lung simulator so that the ventilatory muscle and lung compartments were linked in series. The muscle compartment was "driven" by a pressure-limited, time-cycled ventilator that supplied an adjustable inspiratory time, expiratory time, and accelerating pressure waveform. While the muscle compartment drove the lung compartment of the model, the lung compartment received PSV from a second mechanical ventilator. Then, the degree of work performed by the muscle compartment was determined at various "spontaneous respiratory rates" and different PSV levels. As the PSV inspiratory plateau pressure level was increased, the "spontaneous" ventilatory rate was decreased so that an alveolar ventilation of 5.5 L/min was achieved at each combination of VT, respiratory rate, and PSV. As the PSV plateau pressure level was increased, PSV augmented alveolar ventilation. A slower "spontaneous" respiratory rate achieved the same alveolar ventilation, and the work of the muscle compartment decreased significantly.

In the same report, MacIntyre studied 15 stable patients who required mechancial ventilatory support in a medical intensive care unit (ICU). He compared synchronized intermittent mandatory ventilation (SIMV) with PSV. During SIMV, patients received VTs of 10 to 15 mL/kg at rates sufficient to maintain $PaCO_2$ under 50 mm Hg. The SIMV mechanical rates are not given, but the author states "most [patients] relied on mechanical ventilation for a majority of their ventilatory requirement." During PSV, the negative inspiratory pressure required to trigger inspiratory flow was -0.5 to -1 cm H_2O. The inspiratory plateau pressure was maintained by the ventilator's servocontrol loop and continuously adjusted inspiratory flow; inspiration ceased when the inspiratory flow fell below 25% of the peak flow. Expiratory airway pressure was the same for both SIMV and PSV.

The initial pressure support level was chosen so that the VT during PSV approximated the mandatory mechanical breath during SIMV. When this was achieved, all mandatory SIMV breaths were stopped, and measurements were repeated. Then measurements were made as the PSV plateau airway pressure was decreased in increments of 5 cm H_2O. The maximum PSV plateau pressure (PSV_{max}) for each patient was defined either as the PSV plateau pressure that resulted in the slowest, regular respiratory rate or as the PSV level that results in a VT volume of 10 to 12 mL/kg body weight.[29] The PSV_{max} ranged from 13 to 41 cm H_2O and resulted in VTs that were similar to SIMV mechanical VTs. Also, PSV_{max} accomplished a lower spontaneous ventilatory rate and lower peak and mean airway pressures when compared with SIMV. There were no differences in hemodynamic variables between the two ventilatory modes. Eight of the nine patients who were fit to respond to questions communicated that PSV_{max} was "clearly more comfortable" than the level of SIMV that provided 87% of their total ventilation. This study compared PSV with SIMV, a technique that uses a demand valve known to increase the work of spontaneous breathing to a greater extent than do other techniques that use a high continuous gas flow.[30] Therefore, it is not surprising that the work of breathing in both the model and the patients was less with PSV, which decreased the work from the demand valve, as compared with SIMV, where the patient must assume all of the work induced by the demand valve. Further study is required to determine the work characteristics of PSV as compared with continuous-flow systems. However, this investigation does demonstrate that increased work caused by the demand valve can

TABLE 5–3.

Pressure Support Ventilation Protocol*

Patient selection†:   Reliable and appropriate respiratory drive
Initial settings‡:
Start with PSV_{max} (minimal ventilatory work)
Reduce PSV as tolerated (respiratory rate reflects tolerance)
Extubate at 5 cm H_2O PSV

*Modified from MacIntyre NR: Respir Care 1988; 33:121–125.
†PSV_{max} > 50 cm H_2O suggests an unstable patient not suitable for the
PSV technique.
‡Back-up controlled ventilation can be set as a safety precaution.

be eliminated by using PSV. Furthermore, it revealed the flow, pressure, and volume characteristics of the PSV mechanical breath.

Patients who receive ventilatory support with PSV can be weaned by decreasing the inspiratory pressure assist from high levels of support to progressively lower levels as the etiology of ventilatory failure resolves.[29] Table 5–3 gives a protocol for ventilatory support and eventual weaning using PSV.[29] Initially, full ventilatory support should unload the ventilatory muscles almost totally: PSV_{max}. Weaning is accomplished by gradually reducing the inspiratory pressure level. A gradual decrease in inspiratory pressure level allows the patient to assume an increasingly greater proportion of the ventilatory work. The rate of weaning is determined from conventional parameters, especially the respiratory rate. Weaning is complete when the level of inspiratory pressure support is that required to overcome the resistance imposed by the tracheal tube. Pressure support can be used with CPAP to overcome tracheal tube resistance and demand valve inertia.

Pressure support ventilation differs from conventional ventilation in several important aspects. First, the work of breathing is assisted with every breath, in contradistinction to conventional ventilation, which alleviates all work of breathing (full ventilatory support) or intermittently requires the patient to perform unassisted spontaneous breaths (partial ventilatory support with intermittent mandatory ventilation [IMV] or SIMV). Thus, during weaning with PSV, work is returned to the patient gradually with every breath as opposed to the intermittent full return of work/breath that occurs when conventional ventilatory support and spontaneous ventilation are intermingled. This more regular support of work load may contribute to the improved comfort reported by patients receiving PSV.[28] Second, because the pressure-volume relationship during PSV is similar to normal spontaneous ventilation, increased muscle efficiency and endurance conditioning may result.[28] PSV has not been compared with conventional ventilation or weaning in any systematic study.

It is tempting to confuse PSV with intermittent positive-pressure breathing (IPPB) or CPAP. Pressure support ventilation is conceptually very similar to IPPB. Most modern ventilators capable of delivering PSV usually offer larger inspiratory flow, more rigorous controls of the plateau airway pressure, and much more extensive ventilatory alarm systems than did the devices originally marketed for delivering IPPB.

The primary therapeutic goal of CPAP administration is the maintenance of expiratory airway pressure above the ambient pressure. To prevent the work of breathing from increasing, airway pressure is maintained as constant as possible during the entire ventilatory cycle. During CPAP, the supra-ambient expiratory airway pressure increases FRC, and the near-constant airway pressure allows the elastic work of breathing to decrease. However, CPAP does not augment alveolar ventilation. In contrast, PSV is a form of pressure-limited ventilation that augments minute and alveolar ventilation but probably does not increase FRC because it does not raise expiratory pressure.[29, 31]

AIRWAY PRESSURE RELEASE VENTILATION

Basis for Development

In contradistinction to HFV and PSV, for which applications were sought after development, APRV was developed with a specific physiologic problem in mind.[32] Patients with decreased lung compliance usually benefit from the application of CPAP. Despite the appropriate use of CPAP to enhance arterial oxygenation and decrease the elastic work of breathing, patients with acute lung injury and decreased lung compliance occasionally manifest ventilatory failure and require augmented alveolar ventilation. Unfortunately, applying conventional ventilation to these patients' stiff lungs results in high peak airway pressures that may impede cardiac output and probably increases the risk of barotrauma.

Ideally, the patient with acute lung injury and ventilatory failure should receive CPAP and mechanical ventilation without creating high peak airway pressures and without impeding cardiac output. HFJV may approach these goals, but Brichant and coworkers[33] and Schuster et al.[34] observed no differences in gas exchange, cardiac function, or outcome of patients with acute lung injury when they were ventilated with HFJV, conventional ventilation, or a combination of these. Peak airway pressures were lower during HFJV than during conventional ventilation. Carlon and coworkers[35] made similar observations; however, the peak airway pressures that they observed during HFJV still exceeded the level of CPAP that was required to maintain oxygenation.

Because a severe decrease in FRC is the underlying physiologic problem during acute lung injury, the first objective of APRV is to apply supportive CPAP and then to augment alveolar ventilation without impeding cardiac function or creating high peak airway pressure. Further, APRV allows unrestricted spontaneous breathing so that ventilation can be supported at the minimally required level.

Equipment

The APRV circuit is a high-flow CPAP system with a release valve in the expiratory limb (Fig 5–1).[36] Opening this release valve for 1.5 to 2 seconds allows circuit and airway pressures to drop from the CPAP level used for support of oxygenation to near-ambient pressure or a lower CPAP level. This brief interruption of CPAP causes

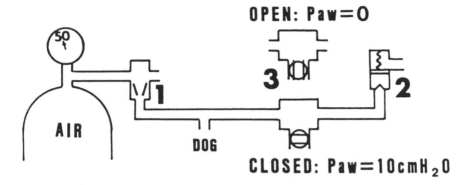

FIG 5–1.
APRV schematically depicted. Air delivered at 50 psi from an H-cylinder passes through a Venturi device *(1)* capable of entraining enough room air to deliver 90 to 100 L/min. This high gas flow proceeds through the inspiratory limb of the circuit to the subject. When the switch in the expiratory limb *(3)* is closed, airway pressure *(Paw)* is equal to the pressure generated by the threshold resistor expiratory valve *(2)*. When the switch is open, gas escapes to the atmosphere at near-ambient pressure or to a predetermined, lower CPAP level. (From Stock MC, Downs JB, Frolicher DA: Airway pressure release ventilation. *Crit Care Med* 1987; 15:462–466. Used by permission.)

airway pressure to fall and thereby allows lung volume to decrease. When the release valve closes, airway pressure increases to the higher CPAP, and lung volume is restored to FRC. Thus, each mechanical VT is created by the brief interruption and restoration of CPAP.

Airway pressure release ventilation can be delivered successfully only with equipment that meets stringent requirements. The continuous gas flow must meet the patient's peak inspiratory flow needs to allow unrestricted spontaneous ventilation. Flows of 90 to 100 L/min obviate the need for a demand valve or a reservoir bag in the inspiratory limb of the circuit. Currently marketed demand valves should not be used because they increase the work of breathing significantly. The high gas flow and rapid changes in airway pressure are necessary for successful CO_2 elimination; thus the humidifier, circuit, tubing, and connections must offer minimal flow resistance—less than 2 cm H_2O/100 L/min.

The release valve in the expiratory limb of the circuit must attain the fully open or closed position in 10 ms so that airway pressure can rise and fall rapidly. A switch controls the release valve and should allow it to stay completely open for 1.5 to 2 seconds so as to result in a short expiratory phase. This switch determines ventilatory cycle length and, therefore, the mechanical ventilatory rate.

The expiratory valve that creates CPAP must be a threshold resistor so that widely varying gas flows do not influence the level of CPAP. If a CPAP valve or other ventilator components create resistance to flow, airway pressure will vary with the gas flow in the circuit. If circuit flow varies markedly throughout the ventilatory cycle, the fluctuating airway pressure increases ventilatory work.[37] Further, if the patient coughs and greatly increases expiratory flow, exceptionally high peak airway pressures (in excess of 200 to 300 mm Hg) will result and may cause barotrauma.

TABLE 5–4.

Dogs With Acute Lung Injury That Were Ventilated With APRV and With Conventional Ventilation Plus PEEP ($\bar{x}$ + SD)

Variable	APRV	IPPV* + PEEP
Mean Paw* (cm H_2O)	12 ± 2	11 ± 3
Peak Paw (cm H_2O)	17 ± 5	23 ± 9[†]
V_E* (L/min)	6.2 ± 1.8	5.9 ± 2.2
$Paco_2$ (mm Hg)	34 ± 4	39 ± 3[†]
Pao_2 (mm Hg)	57 ± 14	50 ± 9[†]

*IPPV = conventional ventilation; Paw = airway pressure; V_E = minute ventilation.
[†]P < .04 when compared with APRV.

Clinical Application

The development of APRV is in its infancy. Initial animal studies published in 1987[36] demonstrated that APRV successfully ventilated the lungs and oxygenated the arterial blood of dogs with normal lungs. Cardiac function during APRV was similar to that during conventional ventilation. When the dog lungs were acutely injured, APRV and conventional ventilation with PEEP were compared. Mean airway pressures were kept constant for both modes of ventilation so that hemodynamic variables and arterial oxygenation could be compared. Compared with conventional ventilation with PEEP, APRV promoted improved arterial oxygenation, decreased physiologic dead-space ventilation, and lower peak airway pressures (Table 5–4). The peak airway pressure during APRV never exceeded the level of CPAP.

The first demonstration of APRV's efficacy in humans was in patients following cardiac operations. The primary purpose of this study was to demonstrate that APRV could oxygenate the arterial blood and eliminate CO_2 in humans. Cardiopulmonary bypass slightly increases lung water and mildly injures the lungs. To these patients with mild pulmonary impairment, APRV was delivered with CPAP levels of 10 to 12 cm H_2O; airway pressure was released to 2 cm H_2O. While apneic, patients received both APRV and conventional ventilation shortly after they arrived in the ICU. Compared with conventional ventilation with 5 cm H_2O PEEP, APRV produced lower peak airway pressures, similar hemodynamics, and similar gas exchange (Table 5–5).[38] Then patients received APRV until they no longer needed ventilatory support. Mechanical ventilation was discontinued by gradually decreasing the number of APRV breaths per minute as the patient increased his spontaneous minute ventilation. This APRV weaning method, which is similar to that with IMV, resulted in successful discontinuation of ventilatory support for all patients. Subsequently, CPAP was decreased from 10 to 5 cm H_2O, and patients were extubated without complication.

Currently, a multi-institutional investigation to examine the efficacy of APRV in patients with moderate to severe acute lung injury and concomitant ventilatory failure is in progress. Preliminary data from this study confirmed that APRV is effective in providing ventilatory support to patients with mild[39] and severe[40] acute respiratory failure.

TABLE 5–5.

Apneic Humans Ventilated With APRV and Conventional Ventilation After Cardiac Operations ($\bar{x}$ + SD)

Variable	APRV	Conventional Ventilation
Peak Paw (cm H_2O)	11 ± 1	32 ± 4
pHa	7.38 ± 0.04	7.39 ± 0.04
$Paco_2$ (mm Hg)	38 ± 4	36 ± 3
Pao_2/Fio_2 (mm Hg)	281 ± 45	263 ± 40
HR* (beats/min)	79 ± 16	79 ± 16
CO* (L/min)	5.2 ± 1.2	5.3 ± 0.9
$S\bar{v}o_2$* (%)	67 ± 4	63 ± 10

*HR = heart rate; CO = cardiac output; $S\bar{v}o_2$ = mixed-venous oxyhemoglobin saturation.

Further animal investigation demonstrated that instituting full ventilatory support with APRV did not disturb hemodynamic function when compared with spontaneous ventilation at a similar level of CPAP.[41] However, when conventional ventilation with PEEP (equal to the CPAP level during spontaneous ventilation) assumed full ventilatory support, stroke volume, cardiac output, and oxygen delivery significantly decreased (Table 5–6). In addition, conventional ventilatory support significantly increased oxygen extraction, whereas ventilatory support with APRV resulted in O_2 extraction and delivery similar to that during spontaneous ventilation with CPAP. Thus, APRV can assume full ventilatory support with no significant change in cardiac function. In contrast, assuming full ventilatory support with conventional ventilation and PEEP significantly impedes cardiac function.

Airway pressure release ventilation may support ventilation without hemodynamic embarrassment because of similarities in the intrapleural pressure pattern created by spontaneous ventilation and by APRV. Necessarily, the intrapleural pressure pattern reflects the airway pressure pattern. Thus, the dips in airway and intrapleural pressures during APRV correspond with lung emptying (mechanical exhalation). However, the brief dips in airway and intrapleural pressures that occur during spontaneous ventilation represent inspiration. Although the intrapleural pressure

TABLE 5–6.

Data Obtained During Spontaneous Ventilation With CPAP, APRV, and Conventional Ventilation With PEEP From Dogs With Acute Lung Injury ($\bar{x}$ + SD)

Variable*	CPAP	APRV	IPPV* + PEEP
SV (mL)	19 ± 5	18 ± 4	11 ± 3†
O_2 del (mL/min)	367 ± 97	394 ± 73	251 ± 54†
O_2 ex (%)	24 ± 6	22 ± 4	32 ± 12†

*SV = stroke volume; O_2 del = O_2 delivery; O_2 ex = O_2 extraction; IPPV = conventional ventilation.
†$P < .05$ when compared with CPAP and APRV.

patterns during APRV and spontaneous ventilation are similar, the direction of gas flow in or out of the lungs is opposite. Whether these notions maintain cardiac output during APRV require further testing.

In summary, APRV is a new ventilatory mode designed to deliver CPAP and to ventilate the lungs of patients with stiff lungs. Ventilation is accomplished by briefly interrupting CPAP and allowing airway pressure to fall and the lungs to passively empty. It ventilates humans with normal and mildly impaired lungs without disturbing hemodynamic function. Although initial results in humans with moderate to severe acute lung injury and ventilatory failure are promising, further investigation continues. Most APRV study has been directed toward efficacy. Studies to demonstrate the best airway pressure changes, best rates of ventilation, and limitations are either underway or waiting to be done.

CASE STUDY 1

A 27-year-old, 83-kg white man involved in a motor vehicle accident sustained a crushed chest, severe right pulmonary contusion, and a cardiac contusion. He also had a fracture of the left femur and left humerus. On initial examination the patient was noted to be tachypneic (42 bpm) with a blood pressure (BP) of 130/60 mm Hg and a pulse rate of 128/min. Arterial blood gas analysis revealed a pH of 7.26, a Pco_2 of 57 mm Hg, and a Po_2 of 44 mm Hg on room air. The patient was alert and oriented and complained of shortness of breath and chest pain. He was given 10 mg of morphine sulfate intravenously in increments and nasotracheally intubated. Conventional ventilatory support using the IMV mode was instituted with Vts of 1,200 mL at 10 breaths per minute, an Fio_2 of 0.35, and PEEP of 5 cm H_2O. Shortly after initiation of ventilatory support the patient's arterial BP started to fall, and the peak airway pressure was rising progressively with each mechanical breath. Examination of the chest revealed an asymmetrical chest wall excursion with hyperresonant percussion over the right side of the chest. A tension pneumothorax was diagnosed and a right thoracostomy tube inserted. The administration of 500 mL of normal saline restored his BP to 115/60 mm Hg. A persistent air leak was noted from the chest tube. Fiber-optic bronchoscopy did not identify any obvious tear in the major airways, and a diagnosis of traumatic bronchopleural fistula was made. Arterial blood gas analysis at this time showed persistent ventilatory failure with fair arterial oxygenation (Table 5–7). Despite a delivered Vt of 1,200 mL the exhaled Vt was only 700 mL, the other 500 mL escaping through the chest tube. The patient's spontaneous respiratory rate was 24 bpm. The peak airway pressure with each mechanical breath was 40 to 45 cm H_2O.

TABLE 5–7.

Case Study 1

Ventilatory Mode	Fio_2	Driving Pressure	T_{insp} (%)	PEEP (cm H_2O)	pHa	$Paco_2$ (mm Hg)	Pao_2 (mm Hg)
IMV	0.35	—	—	5	7.28	57	65
HFJV	0.35	20	25	5	7.33	49	64
HFJV	0.35	25	25	15	7.37	43	78
HFJV	0.35	12	25	15	7.41	39	84
Spont*	0.35	—	—	15	7.39	42	81
Spont*	0.35	—	—	5	7.38	42	79

*Spontaneous ventilation.

Discussion

The presence of a large bronchopleural fistula and markedly decreased lung compliance made conventional positive-pressure ventilation ineffective. The following are important questions that one must ask:

1. What do I want to accomplish?
2. What do I want to avoid?
3. What are my choices?

The patient exhibited two distinct pulmonary processes that together prevented conventional ventilation from being effective: a bronchopleural fistula and a pulmonary contusion that decreased lung compliance. Although PEEP may improve lung compliance, the peak airway pressures during conventional ventilation still exceeded 40 cm H_2O, which reflected persistant low pulmonary compliance. The goal of mechanical ventilatory support in patients with bronchopleural fistulas is to ventilate the lungs and eliminate CO_2 without increasing the pressure gradient across the fistula. An increased gradient encourages gas to escape through the path of least resistance, i.e., via the fistula and chest tube rather than into intact alveoli.

Similarly, the goals of ventilatory support with low lung compliance include maintenance of low peak airway pressures, delivery of supportive PEEP, and no decrease in cardiac function. Forms of ventilatory support that may satisfy these needs are HFJV, APRV, continuous-flow apneic ventilation,[42] and extracorporeal CO_2 removal.[43] Because extracorporeal CO_2 removal requires systemic anticoagulation, it was contraindicated in this patient with multiple trauma. Continuous-flow apneic ventilation has been used in animals with decreased lung compliance,[44] but in humans the success of this ventilatory mode depends, in part, on maintenance of arterial oxygenation with low FIO_2s.[45] There are insufficient human data to support the use of continuous-flow apneic ventilation in a critically ill man with decreased lung compliance.

Of the two remaining choices, APRV and HFJV, either are suitable ventilatory modes for patients with low lung compliance. No study yet has compared the two modes, and at this time there are insufficient clinical data on APRV to provide guidelines for its use in a patient with a bronchopleural fistula. However, the patient's bronchopleural fistula would probably benefit from as small an airway pressure change as possible; thus, HFJV appears to be the best choice for this patient.

CASE STUDY 1 CONTINUED

The goal of HFJV was to achieve ventilation with a mean airway pressure sufficient to support arterial oxygenation and maintain reasonable lung compliance. The FIO_2 was kept constant, and an initial jet driving pressure of 20 psi at 90 breaths per minute and a T_{insp} of 25% were instituted. Subjective evaluation and blood gas analysis revealed improved gas exchange and relief of ventilatory failure (see Table 5–7). However, slight respiratory acidemia persisted. The jet driving pressure was increased to 25 psi, which resulted in a normalization of $PaCO_2$ and pHa. Arterial oxygenation remained only marginally acceptable at 64 mm Hg. Mean airway pressure was increased by the application of PEEP in increments of 5 cm H_2O from 5 to 15 cm H_2O with resultant improvement in Pao_2 to 78 mm Hg. There were no adverse hemodynamic effects following institution of ventilatory support with HFJV and PEEP.

Discussion

A bronchopleural fistula is an alternate gas pathway with low resistance and high compliance relative to and in parallel with the natural airways and alveoli. Thus, the fistula significantly decreases downstream impedance to gas flow, thereby increasing entrainment at the jet source.[46] Loss of "ventilating" gas through the pathologic hole will be compensated by enhanced entrainment. During conventional ventilation, gas under pressure exits through the fistula, but little alveolar gas exchange occurs. However, during HFJV, gas may exit through the fistula, but not at the expense of alveolar gas exchange.[47-49] In an animal model of bronchopleural fistula, adequate CO_2 elimination could be achieved even when the fistula was as large as the cross-sectional area of the trachea.[50] Further, the low peak airway pressures probably prevent further enlargement of the pathologic opening. Therefore, although this patient's air leak persisted, adequate alveolar ventilation was achieved with HFJV, and arterial oxygenation and lung compliance were supported by ensuring an elevated mean airway pressure by the application of PEEP in conjunction with HFJV. Although the mean airway pressure could have been raised by continuing to increase the jet driving pressure, this would have increased minute ventilation and caused respiratory alkalemia. Instead, the jet driving pressure necessary to achieve normocarbia and normal pHa was used, and the mean airway pressure was raised by introducing a threshold resistor valve to the expiratory limbs of the circuit.

CASE STUDY 1 CONTINUED

Three days after admission following reduction of long-bone fractures, the patient's spontaneous ventilatory reserve had improved to a vital capacity of 1.4 L. Cardiovascular function was stable, and he required very little analgesia. Thus he appeared ready to assume spontaneous ventilation. Because the patient's lung compliance remained depressed from the pulmonary contusion, ventilatory support was withdrawn while maintaining an elevated mean airway pressure with PEEP. The jet driving pressure was decreased gradually over the next 24 hours until it reached 12 psi (see Table 5–7). The patient had a spontaneous respiratory rate of 24 breaths per minute and a Pao_2 of 84 mm Hg at an Fio_2 of 0.35. The HFJV was turned off, and the patient breathed through a continuous-flow CPAP system that delivered 15 cm H_2O airway pressure. During the next 48 hours, the CPAP level was decreased gradually to 5 cm H_2O without the need for increased Fio_2 and with an unchanged spontaneous respiratory rate and arterial oxygenation. The patient's trachea was extubated, and he was discharged from the hospital 3 weeks later.

CASE STUDY 2

A 69-year-old white man with severe chronic obstructive pulmonary disease was admitted to the ICU with a diagnosis of bacterial pneumonia. On examination he was febrile with a BP of 145/90 mm Hg and a pulse rate of 118/min. He was breathing 36 bpm with small V_T

on 32% O_2 delivered by a Venturi mask with a pHa of 7.12, a $Paco_2$ of 85 mm Hg, and a Pao_2 of 45 mm Hg. Previous medical records demonstrated that the patient breathed with a $Paco_2$ of 45 mm Hg and a Pao_2 of 62 mm Hg on room air while he was in his best state of health. Aggressive bronchodilator therapy and pulmonary toilet did not reverse the ventilatory failure, and the patient's respiratory rate continued to increase from 36 to 48 bpm. After endotracheal intubation, the patient was ventilated with the IMV mode at a rate of 8 bpm, a V_T of 12 mL/kg, and an $F_{I}O_2$ of 0.50, which resulted in acceptable arterial blood values (Table 5–8). He continued to breathe 18 bpm in addition to the mandatory mechanical breaths, which created peak airway pressures of 55 cm H_2O.

The patient was switched to PSV with 20 cm H_2O pressure support. The spontaneous respiratory rate increased to 36 bpm, and tachycardia, systolic hypertension, and mild alveolar hypoventilation developed (Table 5–8). The pressure support level was increased to 30 cm H_2O, which resulted in a decrease in the respiratory rate to 16 bpm and arterial Pco_2 to 36 mm Hg (Table 5–8). The patient's heart rate declined to 84 beats per minute, and his BP was 125/75 mm Hg.

Discussion

Pressure support ventilation was instituted because of the high peak airway pressures during conventional ventilation, probably secondary to the increase in airway resistance related to the bronchospastic component of his chronic lung disease. A pressure-limited technique, PSV results in peak airway pressures that are approximately equal to the level of pressure support. MacIntyre's protocol for successful use of PSV as a ventilatory mode requires the initial PSV level to support the bulk of the work of breathing.[28] This goal was achieved by raising the pressure level to 30 cm H_2O, which reduced the patient's work of breathing and resulted in a pattern of spontaneous breathing and cardiovascular function that was satisfactory. (See Chapter 3 for a discussion of detrimental work of breathing.)

CASE STUDY 2 CONTINUED

After 3 days of antibiotics and bronchial hygiene therapy, the patient became afebrile, and sputum production decreased. During the course of those 3 days, F_{IO_2} was decreased to 0.35 with maintenance of adequate arterial oxygenation. The respiratory rate declined to 10 bpm and his vital capacity was 1.2 L. Because of clinical improvement, weaning from ventilatory support was attempted. Pressure support was decreased in 5 bpm cm H_2O increments. Initially the patient maintained a respiratory rate of 12 to 20 bpm with adequate alveolar ventilation and arterial oxygenation. However, when the pressure support was reduced from 15 to 10 cm H_2O, his respiratory rate increased to 38 bpm and he became tachycardic. Pressure support ventilation was increased to 15 cm H_2O, and the respiratory rate and heart rate returned to baseline values.

The following day the patient breathed 16 times a minute with good arterial oxygenation and alveolar ventilation while receiving 15 cm H_2O pressure support. Pressure support was then decreased to 10 cm H_2O and subsequently to 5 cm H_2O with no clinical signs of detrimental work of breathing (see Table 5–8). Discontinuance of pressure support resulted in an increase in the respiratory rate to 36 bpm.

Discussion

The respiratory rate is probably one of the most sensitive indices of excessive

TABLE 5–8.
Case Study 2

Hospital Day	Pressure Support (cm H_2O)	Peak Paw (cm H_2O)	Spontaneous Respiratory Rate (bpm)	FIO_2	pHa	$PaCO_2$ (mm Hg)	PaO_2 (mm Hg)
Admit	0	—	48	0.36	7.09	85	46
Admit	0 (IMV)	55	12	0.5	7.38	44	69
Admit	20	20	36	0.5	7.32	51	65
Admit	30	30	16	0.5	7.42	36	72
Day 3	30	30	10	0.35	7.44	34	74
Day 3	20	20	18	0.35	7.40	40	72
Day 3	15	15	20	0.35	7.38	41	69
Day 3	10	10	38	0.35	7.39	41	73
Day 3	15	15	22	0.35	7.37	42	70
Day 4	15	15	16	0.35	7.38	39	85
Day 4	5	5	20	0.3	7.39	40	74
Day 4	0	—	36	0.3	7.38	42	70
Day 4	5	5	22	0.3	7.38	40	72
Day 4	Extubated	—	24	0.3	7.40	39	68

work of breathing and may be the best predictor of weaning success. The increase in respiratory rate that occurred when pressure support was decreased from 15 to 10 cm H_2O suggests that the patient probably still required 15 cm H_2O pressure support to avoid detrimental increases in his work of breathing. Twenty-four hours later, further resolution of pneumonia enabled a reduction in PSV to 5 cm H_2O. The increase in respiratory rate seen on discontinuance of PSV probably reflected a lack of tolerance for the additional work of breathing imposed by the endotracheal tube in a patient with chronically impaired pulmonary mechanics.

CASE STUDY 2 CONTINUED

Pressure support was increased to 5 cm H_2O, which resulted in a decrease in the spontaneous respiratory rate to 22 bpm with stable cardiac function and good gas exchange. He was subsequently extubated 2 hours later and had good gas exchange and a respiratory rate of 28 bpm.

Discussion

Pressure support ventilation enabled mechanical ventilatory support with lower peak airway pressure and allowed the patient to resume his work of breathing on a breath-by-breath basis. Patients with chronic obstructive pulmonary disease (COPD) who have flattened diaphragms and poor ventilatory muscle mechanics may benefit from the breath-by-breath support afforded by PSV.

Theoretically, PSV may be beneficial for patients who require muscle reconditioning. Tachypnea may be caused by an inspiratory work load that exceeds a patient's ventilatory muscle fatigue threshold. In a bench lung model, PSV changed the lung-thorax pressure-volume relationships so that lesser change in airway pressure is required to achieve the same VT. Although this has not been confirmed in patients, these data suggest that PSV may delay the onset of ventilatory muscle fatigue in susceptible patients. Pressure support ventilation may allow the fatigued muscle to reassume the responsibility for generating the transpulmonary pressure gradient gradually and may be advantageous for reconditioning the diaphragm and endurance muscle training.[51, 52] Further work is needed to demonstrate whether this effect will be seen in patients.

REFERENCES

1. Henderson Y, Chillingsworth FP, Whitney JL: The respiratory dead space. Am J Physiol 1915; 38:1.
2. Briscoe WA, Forster RE, Comroe JH Jr: Alveolar ventilation at very low tidal volumes. J Appl Physiol 1954; 7:27.
3. Sjostrand U: Review of physiological rationale for and development of high frequency positive pressure ventilation. Acta Anaesthesiol Scand Suppl 1988; 64:7.
4. Slutsky AS, Brown R, Lehr J, et al: High frequency ventilation: A promising new approach to mechanical ventilation. Med Instrum 1981; 15:229–233.
5. Chang HK, Harf A: High frequency ventilation: A review. Respir Physiol 1984; 57:135.
6. Kolton M, Cattran CB, Kent G, et al: Oxygenation during high-frequency ventilation compared with conventional mechanical ventilation in two models of lung injury. Anesth Analg 1982; 61:323.

7. Saari AF, Rossing TH, Solway J, et al: Lung inflation during high-frequency ventilation. *Am Rev Respir Dis* 1984; 129:333.
8. Fredberg JJ, Keefe DH, Glass GM, et al: Alveolar pressure nonhomogeneity during small-amplitude high-frequency oscillation. *J Appl Physiol* 1984; 57:788.
9. Sutton JE, Glass D: Airway pressure gradient during high-frequency ventilation. *Crit Care Med* 1984; 12:774.
10. Bourgain JL, Mortimer AJ, Sykes MK: Carbon dioxide clearance during high frequency jet ventilation (HFJV), in *Perspectives in High Frequency Ventilation*. Boston, Martinus Nijhoff, 1983, p 98.
11. Carlon GC, Ray C Jr, Groeger JS, et al: Tidal volume and airway pressure on high frequency jet ventilation. *Crit Care Med* 1983; 1:83.
12. Carlon GC, Miodownik S, Ray C Jr, et al: Technical aspects and clinical implications of high frequency jet ventilation with a solenoid valve. *Crit Care Med* 1981; 9:47.
13. Groeger JS, Carlon GC, Howland WS, et al: Experimental evaluation of high-frequency jet ventilation. *Crit Care Med* 1981; 12:747.
14. Miodownik S: High-frequency jet ventilation: Technical implications. *Crit Care Med* 1984; 12:718.
15. Carlon GC, Ray C Jr, Miodownik S, et al: Physiologic implications of high frequency jet ventilation techniques. *Crit Care Med* 1983; 11:508.
16. Woo P, Eurenius S: Dynamics of Venturi jet ventilation through the operating laryngoscope. *Ann Otol Rhinol Laryngol* 1982; 91:615–621.
17. Babinski MF, Bunegin L, Smith RB, et al: Application of double lumen tracheal tubes for HFV. *Anesthesiology* 1981; 55:370.
18. Calkins JM, Waterson CK: Clinical factors influencing the selection of high-frequency jet ventilators. *Crit Care Med* 1984; 12:806.
19. McEvoy RD, Davies JH, Hedenstierna G, et al: Lung mucociliary transport during high-frequency ventilation. *Am Rev Respir Dis* 1982; 126:452.
20. Nordin U, Keszler H, Klain M: How does high frequency jet ventilation affect the mucociliary transport? *Crit Care Med* 1981; 9:160.
21. Armengol JA, Man SFP, Logus JW, et al: Effects of high frequency oscillatory ventilation on canine tracheal mucous transport. *Crit Care Med* 1981; 9:192.
22. Nordin ULF, Klain M, Keszler H: Electron microscopic studies of tracheal mucosa after high frequency jet ventilation. *Crit Care Med* 1982; 10:211.
23. Ophoven JP, Mammel MC, Gordon MJ, et al: Tracheobronchial histopathology associated with high-frequency jet ventilation. *Crit Care Med* 1984; 12:829.
24. Polora T, Bing D, Mammel M, et al: Neonatal high-frequency jet ventilation. *Pediatrics* 1983; 72:27.
25. Rock J, Pfaelle H, Smith RB, et al: High pressure jet insufflation used to prevent aspiration and its effects on the tracheal mucosal wall. *Crit Care Med* 1976; 4:135.
26. Rouby JJ, Fusciardi J, et al: High frequency ventilation in post operative ventilatory failure. *Anesthesiology* 1983; 59:281.
27. Franz I, Close R: Elevated lung volume and alveolar pressure during jet ventilation of rabbits. *Am Rev Respir Dis* 1985; 131:134.
28. MacIntyre NR: Respiratory function during pressure support ventilation. *Chest* 1986; 89:677–683.
29. MacIntyre NR: Weaning from mechanical ventilatory support: Volume-assisting intermittent breaths versus pressure-assisting every breath. *Respir Care* 1988; 33:121–125.
30. Gibney RTN, Wilson RS, Pontoppidan H: Comparison of work of breathing on high gas flow and demand valve continuous positive airway pressure breathing systems. *Chest* 1982; 82:692.
31. Banner MJ, Kirby RR: Similarities between pressure support ventilation and intermittent positive-pressure ventilation. *Crit Care Med* 1985; 13:997–998.
32. Downs JB, Stock MC: Airway pressure release ventilation: A new concept in ventilatory support. *Crit Care Med* 1987; 15:459–461.
33. Brichant JF, Rouby JJ, Viars P: Intermittent positive pressure ventilation with either positive end-expiratory pressure or high frequency jet ventilation (HFJV), or HFJV alone in human acute respiratory failure. *Anesth Analg* 1986; 65:1135–1142.
34. Schuster DP, Klain M, Snyder JV: Comparison of high frequency jet ventilation to conventional ventilation during severe acute respirtory failure in humans. *Crit Care Med* 1982; 10:625–630.
35. Carlon GC, Howland WS, Ray C, et al: High-frequency jet ventilation: A prospective randomized evaluation. *Chest* 1983; 84:551–559.
36. Stock MC, Downs JB, Frolicher DA: Airway pressure release ventilation. *Crit Care Med* 1987; 15:462–466.
37. Banner MJ, Lampotang S, Boysen PG, et al: Flow resistance of expiratory positive-pressure valve systems. *Chest* 1986; 90:212–217.
38. Garner W, Downs JB, Stock MC, et al: Airway pressure release ventilation (APRV): A human trial. *Chest* 1988; 94:779–781.

39. Banner MJ, Kirby RR, Banner T, et al: Airway pressure release ventilation in patients with acute respiratory failure. *Crit Care Med* 1989; 17(suppl):32.
40. Cane RD, Stock MC, Lefebvre DL, et al: Airway pressure release ventilation in severe acute respiratory failure. *Crit Care Med* 1989; 17(suppl):32.
41. Rasanen J, Downs JB, Stock MC: Cardiovascular effects of conventional positive pressure ventilation and airway pressure release ventilation. *Chest* 1988; 93:911–915.
42. Smith RB, Babinski M, Bunegin L, et al: Continuous flow apneic ventilation. *Acta Anaesthesiol Scand* 1984, 28:631–639.
43. Gattinoni L, Pesenti A, Pelizzola A, et al: Reversal of terminal acute respiratory failure by low-frequency positive-pressure ventilation with extracorporeal removal of CO_2 (LFPPV-ECCO$_2$R). *Trans Am Soc Artif Intern Organs* 1981; 27:289–293.
44. Tallman RD, Yang YL, Marcolin R: Gas exchange by constant flow ventilation following oleic acid lung injury (abstract). *Anesthesiology* 1985; 63:296.
45. Stone E, Gelineau J, Bunegin L, et al: The effect of TI_{O_2} on arterial Pa_{CO_2} during continuous flow apneic ventilation in dogs. *Crit Care Med* 1986; 14:372.
46. Ray C Jr, Miodownik S, Carlon GC, et al: Pneumatic-to-electric analog model of high frequency jet ventilation of disrupted airways. *Crit Care Med* 1984; 12:711.
47. Carlon GC, Ray C Jr, Klain M, et al: High frequency positive pressure ventilation in the management of a patient with bronchopleural fistula. *Anesthesiology* 1980; 52:160.
48. Turnbull AD, Carlon GC, Howland WS, et al: High frequency jet ventilation in major airway or pulmonary disruption. *Ann Thorac Surg* 1981; 32:468.
49. Carlon GC, Ray C Jr, Pierri MK, et al: High frequency jet ventilation: Theoretical considerations and clinical observations. *Chest* 1982; 81:350.
50. Carlon GC, Griffin J, Ray C Jr, et al: High frequency jet ventilation in experimental airway disruption. *Crit Care Med* 1983; 11:353.
51. Braun NMT, Faulkner J, Hughes RL, et al: When should respiratory muscles be exercised? *Chest* 1983; 84:76–84.
52. Leith DE, Bradley M: Ventilatory muscle strength and endurance training. *J Appl Physiol* 1976; 41:508–516.

6/ Arrhythmias and Cardiac Failure

RICHARD DAVISON, M.D.
KERRY KAPLAN, M.D.

ARRHYTHMIAS AND CONGESTIVE HEART FAILURE

Continuous monitoring of the heart rhythm is inseparably intertwined with the concept of critical care medicine. Any time that there is cardiac pathology, arrhythmias will occur and will need to be identified and dealt with. Furthermore, cardiac arrhythmias are to be anticipated whenever any of the following circumstances are present: (1) dysfunction of the central and/or autonomic nervous system, (2) organ failure resulting in significant alteration of the metabolic and/or electrolytic internal milieu, (3) use of a variety of vasoactive or membrane-active drugs, and (4) placement of indwelling intracardiac devices. Of course, the majority of seriously ill patients will exhibit several of the above conditions and therefore be prone to arrhythmias.

But the detection of a disturbance in cardiac rhythm should not reflexly lead to an attempt at its correction. There are three aspects of the management of arrhythmias to be considered in an intensive care unit setting. First, when should attempts be made to terminate an ongoing arrhythmia? With the obvious exceptions of ventricular asystole or fibrillation, the treatment—or nontreatment—of an arrhythmia will be dictated primarily by the impact that the rhythm disturbance has on the patient's physiology. More harm may be done by pharmacologic interventions than by the arrhythmia they are directed at.[1]

A second issue that is frequently neglected in the haste to initiate antiarrhythmic therapy is the possibility that the arrhythmia may not be an expression of primary cardiac pathology but rather secondary to "extracardiac" factors. Some of the more commonly encountered circumstances are hypokalemia producing ventricular ectopy, sinus bradycardia as an expression of severe hypoxemia, congestive heart failure (CHF) presenting as atrial tachyarrhythmias, and the wide spectrum of drug-induced arrhythmias.

The third question is not as easily settled. When is an arrhythmia a harbinger of more serious events and therefore an indication for the initiation of suppressive therapy? Unfortunately there are no hard and fast rules. In general the propensity for a rhythm disturbance to develop into a life-threatening arrhythmia is directly proportional to the magnitude of the underlying cardiac pathology. It is very difficult to induce ventricular fibrillation in a normal heart.[2] Another important consideration is the trend displayed by the arrhythmia. Corrective measures should be more promptly initiated to treat a rapidly worsening disturbance than for what may be a more alarming but stable rhythm. For example, ventricular premature beats that progress from rare and isolated to frequent and in couplets may require earlier and more aggressive treatment than would ventricular triplets that have not changed in frequency over several days.

Once therapy is started, what should its aim be? Total suppression, or is "better" good enough? If total eradication of the rhythm disturbance can be accomplished without inordinate side effects, then that should be the goal. It is often wiser to settle for partial improvement. There is good evidence that the administration of antiarrhythmic drugs in doses that only *reduce* ectopic activity still lessen the chance of a lethal tachyarrhythmia.[3]

Congestive heart failure is the consequence of a persistent impairment in left ventricular function, with or without associated right ventricular involvement. In order to be clinically evident, it must be of sufficient severity to activate compensatory mechanisms that in turn are responsible for the majority of symptoms. It is a condition that, because of its chronic, slowly progressive course and the predictability of manifestations, should rarely be the primary reason for admission to an intensive care unit. Yet, because of the high incidence of hypertensive and ischemic heart disease, CHF very commonly complicates the care of the critically ill patient. Furthermore, the previously stable clinical status of a patient with CHF may take a sudden and dramatic turn for the worse with the development of complications such as arrhythmias, pulmonary embolism, and transient myocardial ischemia. These are basically reversible events that usually respond well to advanced supportive measures.

The same rationale should not be applied to patients with end-stage CHF where the introduction of intensive care techniques results in an ephemeral improvement that only lasts for as long as the measures are continued. As with other chronic organ failures, the final phase of CHF is due to an irreversible loss of function, a problem that is not appropriately dealt with in an intensive care unit setting.

CASE STUDY

A 58-year-old white male is brought to the emergency room with a 3-hour history of rapidly progressive shortness of breath. Prior to the onset of the respiratory distress, he had noted a "fast heartbeat" for several hours. The patient gave a history of "heart failure" for the past 10 years for which he was receiving a "digitalis" pill and a diuretic. On admission to the emergency room, the patient was sitting up in marked respiratory distress. The skin was cool, pale, and sweaty. His respiratory rate (RR) was 40/min, respirations were labored with prominent wheezing and "gurgling" noises, his pulse rate was 160/min and regular, and his blood pressure (BP) by cuff measured 120/90 mm Hg. Neck veins were distended to the angle of the jaw and had prominent pulsations. Fine and coarse moist rales and wheezes were heard throughout both lungs. A sustained apical impulse was visible and palpable over the fifth and sixth intercostal spaces, 13 cm lateral to the midsternal line. On auscultation, heart tones were distant and difficult to identify, but a gallop rhythm was clearly present. Examination of the abdomen revealed an enlarged liver (spanning 13 cm) that was tender to palpation. Peripheral pulses were thready but symmetrical. There was 2+ pitting edema of both ankles.

Arterial blood gas analysis (room air) showed a Po_2 of 42 mm Hg, a Pco_2 of 45 mm Hg, and a pH of 7.12. Routine chemistry was normal except for mildly elevated blood urea nitrogen (BUN), serum glutamic oxaloacetic acid (SGOT), and lactic dehydrogenase (LDH).

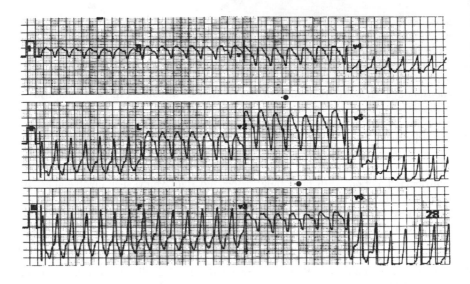

FIG 6–1.
"Wide-QRS" tachycardia: ventricular vs. supraventricular with aberrancy.

The chest x-ray film revealed bilateral alveolar infiltrates and pulmonary venous redistribution and congestion compatible with pulmonary edema. There was marked cardiomegaly. The electrocardiogram (ECG) is shown in Figure 6–1.

Oxygen was given by Venturi mask at an FIO_2 of 0.4, and the patient received 40 mg of furosemide and 4 mg of morphine sulfate intravenously (IV). His respiratory distress lessened and repeat blood gases were improved. The ECG was read as showing ventricular tachycardia. A bolus of 100 mg of IV lidocaine was given, but the bedside monitor showed persistence of the abnormal cardiac rhythm. Because of the lack of response to lidocaine, the original interpretation was questioned and a supraventricular tachycardia with aberrant intraventricular conduction postulated. Five milligrams of IV verapamil was given. The arrhythmia persisted, but the BP declined to 90/65 mm Hg. The patient was transferred to the intensive care unit.

Discussion

The patient presents to the emergency room with what appears to be an acute decompensation of chronic CHF that is precipitated by a tachyarrhythmia. Although the patient is in florid pulmonary edema, arterial BP and cerebral perfusion are adequate. Had either of them been seriously impaired, proper management would have required immediate electrical cardioversion. Therapy is initiated, including the administration of morphine sulphate, which is *not* contraindicated when CO_2 retention and respiratory acidosis are directly attributable to cardiac pulmonary edema.[4]

The ECG poses a dilemma that one faces often in acute cardiac crisis: the differential diagnosis of "wide-QRS" tachycardia. Wellens and colleagues[5] have identified those findings that suggest a ventricular origin for these tachyarrhythmias. They are summarized in Table 6–1. The ECG reproduced in Figure 6–1 does not

TABLE 6–1.

Findings Suggestive of Ventricular
Tachycardia

Heart rate, 130–170
Atrioventricular dissociation
QRS width >0.14 sec
Left-axis deviation
If RBBB*: Mono- or biphasic complexes in V1
If LBBB*: qR or QS complexes in V6

*RBBB = right bundle-branch block; LBBB = left bun-
dle-branch block.

fit several of the criteria listed, yet a ventricular origin for the tachycardia—later
confirmed by electrophysiologic testing—is strongly suggested by the very wide and
bizarre QRS.

Lidocaine (Xylocaine) has few deleterious effects on the cardiovascular system
and, therefore, is a wise choice as the initial agent for a therapeutic trial in a suspected
ventricular arrhythmia. Unfortunately, in the case under discussion effective blood
levels were probably never achieved because of an inadequate loading dose. A total
of 3 to 4 mg/kg of lidocaine, given in divided doses over a period of 10 minutes, will
usually result in therapeutic blood levels and is associated with a very low incidence
of toxicity. After the loading dose, a maintenance infusion must be initiated at a dose
as outlined in Table 6–2. Even with a continuous infusion of lidocaine, blood levels
will initially decline due to redistribution of the drug. When this occurs, it is common
to see a recrudescence of the original arrhythmia, and one or more small boluses
(12.5 to 25.0 mg) will be required to restore suppressive levels.[6]

In the event that lidocaine fails to control the ventricular arrhythmia, the next
parenteral drug of choice is procainamide (Pronestyl). Intravenous loading with this
agent is achieved by giving a 100-mg bolus (injected over a period of 2 minutes)
every 5 minutes until either the arrhythmia is suppressed, a total of up to 15 mg/kg
is given, or a side effect supervenes.[7] Close attention must be given to the development of hypotension and/or widening of the QRS. An increase in the duration of
the QRS of more than one third over control values should be construed as a warning
that toxic blood levels are being reached. Maintenance infusion rates will vary between 30 and 60 μg/kg/min and may initially require supplementation with small
50-mg boluses.

Bretylium tosylate (Bretylol), originally marketed for the treatment of ventricular
fibrillation, is now considered a second-line drug for the treatment of other ventricular
arrhythmias. The initial dose is 5 mg/kg given as an IV bolus that may be injected
rapidly if the patient is unresponsive. In the alert patient, unless it is given slowly,
vomiting will promptly follow. Up to 30 mg/kg can be administered as a loading dose
and followed with a maintenance infusion of 1 to 2 mg/min. The only common side
effect is postural hypotension. It is important to know that the antiarrhythmic effect
of bretylium may be delayed for 30 to 120 minutes.[8]

TABLE 6–2.
Intravenous Antiarrhythmics

Drug	Loading Dose	Maintenance Dose	Main Toxicity
Lidocaine	3–4 mg/kg	Normal: up to 55 µg/kg/min CHF*: up to 25 µg/kg/min Shock: up to 10 µg/kg/min	Dizziness Dysarthria Obtundation and/or agitation
Procainamide	Up to 15 mg/kg (100 mg q5 min)	30–60 µg/kg/min	Hypotension, IVCD*
Bretylium tosylate	5–30 mg/kg	1–2 mg/min	Postural hypotension, emesis

* CHF = congestive heart failure; IVCD = intraventricular conduction disturbances.

Following an apparent lidocaine failure, the alternate diagnosis of supraventricular tachycardia with aberrant intraventricular conduction was entertained and a therapeutic trial attempted with verapamil.[9] This substance, a calcium antagonist, has depressant effects on the atrioventricular and sinoatrial nodes, is a powerful arterial vasodilator, and exerts a considerable anti-inotropic effect. In a dose of 0.15 mg/kg divided into two IV boluses as needed, it is currently the agent of choice for the abolition of paroxysmal supraventricular tachycardia. Verapamil is also very effective when a prompt reduction of the ventricular response to atrial fibrillation or flutter is desired, although it will not commonly terminate these rhythms. On the other hand, our example illustrates a use of verapamil that is *not recommended*. In the setting of a patient who is hemodynamically impaired by an ill-defined tachyarrhythmia, the administration of verapamil—which has little effect on ventricular arrhythmias—may result in further cardiovascular deterioration. In comparison to other available antiarrhythmics, verapamil has myocardial and vascular depressant actions that are much too potent to allow its use as a safe "diagnostic" tool.

CASE STUDY CONTINUED

On arrival in the intensive care unit, the patient received another 150 mg of IV lidocaine in divided doses and reverted to a sinus tachycardia at a rate of 130/min. On auscultation moist rales were present over most of both lung fields, and a loud holosystolic murmur was heard at the apex with radiation to the axilla. The Foley catheter had yielded 30 cc of urine over the last hour. Repeat arterial blood gas analysis demonstrated a Po_2 of 58 mm Hg, a Pco_2 of 38 mm Hg, and a pH of 7.30 on an Fio_2 of 0.4. A repeat ECG showed nonspecific repolarization abnormalities suggestive of a digitalis effect and was compatible with left ventricular hypertrophy and left atrial disease. There were no changes suggestive of acute myocardial ischemia.

Eighty milligrams of furosemide was given IV. Shortly thereafter the monitor indicated the development of atrial fibrillation with a ventricular response of 145 beats per minute and frequent "aberrantly conducted" beats (Fig 6–2). With this there was little change in the clinical status. The BP was 110/85 mm Hg. Two doses of 0.125 mg of IV digoxin were given over the next 3 hours and the ventricular response slowed to 110 to 120/min. During this time, the urine output that had briefly risen to 120 cc/hr in response to the diuretic had again declined to 20 to 30 cc/hr. Furosemide was again administered, 120 mg by IV push. Within the next 15 minutes the pulse rate was noted to again rise to 140/min, the RR increased, and the patient was observed to become more agitated and diaphoretic. The BP was recorded at 90 mm Hg systolic by palpation, and preparations for the insertion of a pulmonary artery catheter were begun.

Discussion

The onset of atrial fibrillation poses several questions. First, could it be a manifestation of digitalis toxicity? Atrial fibrillation develops as a consequence of excess digitalis only exceptionally, and when it does, the ventricular response is *always slow* because of the associated atrioventricular block. In this instance, the atrial fibrillation is more likely related to dilatation of the atria secondary to the high filling pressures required by the failing ventricles.

The second question is whether synchronized electrical cardioversion should be used to terminate the atrial fibrillation. Although electrical cardioversion can be

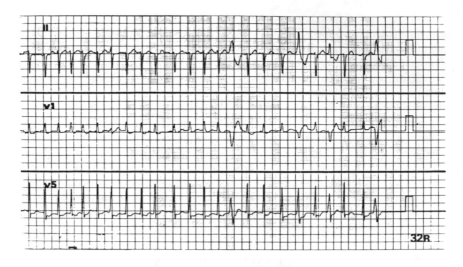

FIG 6–2.
Rhythm strip showing atrial fibrillation and frequent beats with a bizarre configuration. Intra-ventricular aberrant conduction (Aschman's) rather than ventricular premature beats is suggested by (1) the degree of aberrancy that is cycle dependent (i.e., it is greater with a long-short RR pattern); (2) lack of fixed coupling intervals; and (3) variable morphology.

performed safely in patients with no clinical evidence of digitalis toxicity,[10] the risk of inducing malignant ventricular arrhythmias may be heightened by concurrent hypoxemia and acidemia. But even more importantly, it serves no useful purpose to abolish a tachyarrhythmia unless the underlying precipitating factor(s) are also eliminated or at least modified. In the case under discussion, had cardioversion succeeded in restoring a sinus mechanism, it is highly probable that atrial fibrillation would have recurred promptly.

The final query is how to reduce the ventricular response to atrial fibrillation in a patient who is already "digitalized." Atrial fibrillation provides us with a unique end point to assess the degree of "digitalization": the ventricular response. Digitalis should be "pushed" gently in order to minimize the risk of toxicity. This is done by giving several small doses frequently since the effect of IV digoxin peaks at 2 to 4 hours. If the higher levels of digitalis are not well tolerated, the addition of small doses of a β-blocker (i.e., propranolol, 5 mg orally three or four times a day) or verapamil[11] may result in adequate slowing. Obviously these drugs are best avoided in patients with severe cardiovascular impairment, such as the case in discussion.

In fact, whenever a trial of β-blockade is entertained in a clinical setting where there is concern that such an intervention could make matters worse, esmolol becomes the drug of choice. Because of its elimination half-life of only 9 minutes, any untoward effects that it may precipitate will promptly subside on discontinuation. Treatment is initiated with a 1-minute loading dosage, an IV infusion of 500 μg/kg/min that is then reduced to a maintenance infusion of 50 μg/kg/min for 4 minutes.

TABLE 6–3.

Differential Between Ventricular Premature Beats and Aberrancy

Criterion	VPB	Aberrancy
Initial QRS deflection	Opposite to normal beat	Same as normal beat
Configuration in V1	Atypical RBBB (R or RS) or LBBB	Typical RBBB (RSR')
Fixed coupling	Diagnostic if present	Never present
"Long-short" pattern*	Not present	Present
Fusion beats	Diagnostic if present	Never present

*Long-short pattern refers to the tendency for the QRS that closes a short RR interval after a long RR interval to be aberrantly conducted. Figure 6–2 is a good example of this phenomenon.

If within 5 minutes a beneficial effect is not observed or is inadequate, the 1-minute loading dose is repeated, but now followed by a maintenance infusion of 100 μg/kg/min. This sequence is repeated as needed until a maintenance dose of 200 μg/kg/min is reached; exceeding this amount will not result in additional benefit.

One of the harder decisions that frequently comes up in acute cardiac care is whether wide and bizarre QRS complexes detected during atrial fibrillation are ventricular premature beats or aberrantly conducted inpulses, the so-called Aschman phenomenon. This dilemma is compounded by the fact that extra digitalis doses are usually being considered in an effort to slow the heart rate. Our first recommendation is that a 12-lead ECG be obtained before rendering an opinion. Monitor strips are good to document arrhythmias but not to diagnose them. Table 6–3 lists the criteria most commonly used in this differential diagnosis.

CASE STUDY CONTINUED

A Swan-Ganz catheter was inserted, and the initial hemodynamic information obtained is listed in Table 6–4 (column titled "Baseline"). The twice-normal arteriovenous O_2 difference reflects a marked desaturation of the central venous blood and confirms the accuracy of the measurement of a very low cardiac index (CI). Because the patient had received agents that dilate the veins (morphine and furosemide) as well as the arteries (verapamil), it was reasonable to assume that relative hypovolemia may have occurred. The filling pressures were indeed considerably lower than expected for an individual with long-standing CHF. Therefore, volume expansion with normal saline was initiated and 1,200 cc given over the next hour. This was attended by an improvement in the clinical status with slowing of the heart rate and decreased agitation and respiratory distress. A repeat set of hemodynamic parameters (Table 6–4, "After Volume Loading") demonstrated improvement, but the urine output remained depressed. Sodium nitroprusside (SN) therapy was started at an initial dose of 0.25 μg/kg/min. After 30 minutes, there was no significant change in the vital signs, and the dose was doubled. In the next hour, the urine output increased to 100 cc, and the final set of hemodynamic data were obtained (Table 6–4, "On Nitroprusside"). The patient's clinical status continued to improve over the next 24 hours. An angiotensin-converting enzyme inhibitor was administered and the SN gradually tapered and stopped. Lidocaine therapy was discontinued after several doses of oral procainamide, and good control of the ectopic activity was maintained. The patient was ambulated under monitored surveillance and sent home in good condition.

TABLE 6–4.

Hemodynamic Data*

Parameter	Baseline	After Volume Loading	On Nitroprusside
Mean right atrial pressure	10	13	8
Pulmonary artery pressures	50/16	65/22	45/14
Mean pulmonary artery pressure	27	36	24
Mean pulmonary artery occluded pressure	15	22	13
Mean arterial pressure	80	92	86
A/V O_2 diff† (vol %)	10.5	8.0	5.8
Cardiac output (L/min)	2.2	3.2	5.8
Cardiac index (L/min/m²)	1.3	1.9	2.8
Systemic vascular resistance (dynes·sec·cm^{-5})	2,545	1,728	1,075

*All pressures are expressed in mm Hg.
†A/V O_2 diff = arteriovenous oxygen content difference.

Discussion

If in the course of treating CHF the administration of IV furosemide is followed shortly by signs of deteriorating tissue perfusion, then it is very likely that the venodilating action of this drug has caused a critical reduction in the venous return to the heart.[12] The ensuing fall in preload adversely affects stroke volume (SV) and leads to reflex peripheral arterial constriction. As in the case under discussion, if measurements of the pulmonary artery occluded pressure are taken at this time, they are often found to be within the normal range. This finding in a chronically failing ventricle is evidence of relative hypovolemia. One is then placed in the apparently paradoxical situation of ordering volume expansion in a patient who up to that point was being vigorously treated for pulmonary edema and who, in fact, may still demonstrate moist rales on auscultation. This scenario results from a return of the ventricular function to baseline after the insult that precipitated pulmonary edema is overcome. A hypertrophied and dilated ventricle may then find that the same measures used to moderate the filling pressures at a time when they were acutely elevated are now responsible for suboptimal diastolic volumes.

The coexistence of physical findings compatible with the pulmonary venous hypertension with measurements that are within the normal range is simply due to a normal delay in the clearing of excessive interstitial fluid by the lymphatics of the lungs. Exemplified here is a circumstance where the clinical assessment of the patient's cardiovascular status has been obscured by therapeutic interventions, which makes the placement of a pulmonary artery catheter virtually mandatory.

As expected, improvement was brought on by the higher filling pressures achieved with fluid administration. However, further volume expansion was precluded by the risk of making the pulmonary congestion worse. At this point, additional circulatory support could be achieved in one of four ways: intra-aortic balloon counterpulsation, IV catecholamines, a phosphodiesterase inhibitor, or afterload reduction (AR). The primary indication for intra-aortic counterpulsation is an acute cardiovascular decompensation that is potentially amenable to surgical correction or amelioration. This is certainly not true in the case at hand. Catecholamines are a valid option, but a word of caution is timely. A patient who responds well to an IV agent may not always be successfully "weaned" from it, which may result in one being caught in the quandary of chronic support of the circulation with an IV preparation.

A similar limitation applies to the use of amrinone, the first member of a new family of drugs that produce their therapeutic effect via the inhibition of phosphodiesterase. The resulting increase in the concentration of intracellular cyclic adenosine monophosphate (AMP) exerts a positive inotropic action and induces peripheral arterial vasodilatation. Unfortunately, long-term administration of amrinone is associated with a high incidence of serious side effects such as thrombocytopenia and hepatic toxicity. "Second-generation" phosphodiesterase inhibitors, currently undergoing clinical testing, may allow for safer, long-term administration of these agents, but their ultimate contribution to the chronic treatment of CHF remains to be fully assessed.[13] For these and other reasons, an initial trial of AR is favored.

The purpose of this intervention is to reduce the peripheral arterial resistance with a vasodilator, enhance left ventricular emptying, and increase cardiac output.

For many years it was feared that hypotension would be a limiting factor. However, when AR is successful, the drop in resistance is associated with a compensatory increase in flow, and the BP changes little.[14] In short, AR attempts to transform a high-resistance, low-flow system into a low-resistance, high-flow system. The patient under discussion had evidence of a condition that makes AR an especially attractive alternative: mitral incompetence.[15] Reduction of the resistance in the outflow tract of the left ventricle will "redirect" flow and reduce the fraction of cardiac output that is regurgitated into the left atrium through the incompetent valve. For similar reasons, AR is also of special benefit in aortic valvular insufficiency and acute ventricular septal defects.

Therefore, AR should be entertained whenever low cardiac output is associated with any of the following: (1) cardiomegaly, (2) mitral regurgitation, (3) aortic insufficiency, and (4) acute ventricular septal defects. As a general rule, the higher the calculated systemic vascular resistance, the better the results.* However, because there is considerable overlap between responders and nonresponders, only a therapeutic trial provides the answer in an individual case.

SN is the drug most often used for AR.[16] It offers the following advantages: (1) it has a very brief duration of action that permits flexible titration; (2) it dilates both arteries and veins (a "balanced" vasodilator), thus reducing both afterload and preload; and (3) it has no effects other than those resulting from the vasodilation. Because it influences preload, the adequacy of filling pressures must be ascertained before it is administered for AR. The same limitation does not exist when SN is used in the management of hypertensive emergencies where BP is the main parameter monitored. Toxicity from SN is only observed in two circumstances: (1) when very large doses are given over a short period of time (such as with controlled hypotension techniques), the ability of the liver to detoxify cyanide into thiocyanate may be exceeded, and poisoning of the cellular respiratory enzymes occur; and (2) prolonged infusion in patients with severely limited renal function may lead to thiocyanate accumulation. The manifestations of thiocyanate intoxication are nausea, vomiting, psychosis, and convulsions; they are usually seen with serum levels of 10 μg/dL or more.

Nitroprusside is a very powerful drug that requires careful titration. The recommended starting dose for AR (0.25 μg/kg/min) is lower than that used in the treatment of hypertension. It should be escalated cautiously by increments of 50% until a change is noted in the circulatory parameters. These changes include a lowering of the pulmonary artery occluded or mean arterial pressures, a mild increase in the heart rate, or signs of clinical improvement such as an increase in the urine output. At that point, measurements of cardiac output and arterial and venous oxygen content should be done to document the beneficial effects. A successful application of AR should lead to (1) clinical improvement, (2) an increase in cardiac output, (3) only minor changes in mean arterial pressure and heart rate, and (4) a lowering of

---

*Systemic vascular resistance = (mean arterial pressure − mean right atrial pressure/cardiac output) × 80. Normal values are 1,200 ± 180 dynes·sec·cm^{-5}.

the pulmonary artery occluded pressure. Occasionally a disproportionate fall in pulmonary artery occluded pressure prevents infusion rates from becoming effective enough to reduce the afterload. In this setting, volume expansion will restore the filling pressures and permit further increases in the SN infusion.[17] In patients with pulmonary pathology and a significant ventilation-perfusion imbalance, SN may cause a worsening of intrapulmonary shunting. It does so by dilating pulmonary vessels and increasing perfusion to poorly ventilated areas.

As a safety measure it is wise to infuse the SN through a separate IV line that is not used for the administration of other IV medication. A bolus injection of another drug, given through tubing that is filled with an SN solution, can deliver enough of this agent to produce catastrophic hypotension.

IV nitroglycerin is now available as an alternative to SN, although its main action is exerted on the venous side of the circulation. Finally, there are several agents that permit an easy transition from parenteral to oral AR.

Both angiotensin-converting enzyme inhibitors[18] and the combination of hydralazine and oral nitrates[19] have improved the long-term survival of patients with CHF.

REFERENCES

1. Smith WM, Gallagher JJ: "Les Torsades de Pointes": An unusual ventricular arrhythmia. *Ann Intern Med* 1980; 93:578–584.
2. Josephson ME, Seides SF: *Clinical Cardiac Electrophysiology.* Philadelphia, Lea & Febiger, 1979, p 56.
3. Winkle RA, Alderman EL, Fitzgerald JW, et al: Treatment of recurrent symptomatic ventricular tachycardia. *Ann Intern Med* 1976; 85:1–7.
4. Aberman A, Fulop M: The metabolic and respiratory acidosis of acute pulmonary edema. *Ann Intern Med* 1972; 76:173–184.
5. Wellens HJJ, Bar FWHM, Lie KI: The value of the electrocardiogram in the differential diagnosis of a tachycardia with a widened QRS complex. *Am J Med* 1978; 64:27–33.
6. Collinsworth KA, Kalman S, Harrison DC: The clinical pharmacology of lidocaine as an antiarrhythmic drug. *Circulation* 1974; 50:1217–1230.
7. Giardina EGV, Heissenbuttel RH, Bigger JT Jr: Intermittent intravenous procaine amide to treat ventricular arrhythmias. Correlation of plasma concentration with effect on arrhythmia, electrocardiogram and blood pressure. *Ann Intern Med* 1973; 78:183–193.
8. Heissenbuttel RH, Bigger JT Jr: Bretylium tosylate: A newly available antiarrhythmic drug for ventricular arrhythmias. *Ann Intern Med* 1979; 91:229–238.
9. Stone PH, Antman EM, Muller JE, et al: Calcium channel blocking agents in the treatment of cardiovascular disorders. Part II. Hemodynamic effects and clinical applications. *Ann Intern Med* 1980; 93:886–904.
10. Ditchey RV, Karliner JS: Safety of electrical cardioversion in patients without digitalis toxicity. *Ann Intern Med* 1981; 95:676–679.
11. Klein HO, Kaplinsky E: Verapamil and digoxin: Their respective effects on atrial fibrillation and their interaction. *Am J Cardiol* 1982; 50:894–902.
12. Kiely J, Kelly DT, Taylor DR, et al: The role of furosemide in the treatment of left ventricular dysfunction associated with acute myocardial infarction. *Circulation* 1973; 58:581–587.
13. DiBianco R, Shabetai R, Kostuk W, et al: A comparison of oral milrinone, digoxin, and their combination in the treatment of patients with chronic heart failure. *N Engl J Med* 1989; 320:677–683.
14. Miller RR, Vismara LA, Williams DO, et al: Pharmacological mechanisms for left ventricular unloading in clinical congestive heart failure. Differential effects of nitroprusside, phentolamine, and nitroglycerin on cardiac function and peripheral circulation. *Circ Res* 1976; 39:127–133.
15. Goodman DJ, Rossen RM, Holloway EL, et al: Effect of nitroprusside on left ventricular dynamics in mitral regurgitation. *Circulation* 1974; 50:1025–1032.
16. Palmer RF, Lasseter KC: Sodium nitroprusside. *N Engl Med* 1975; 292:294–296.
17. Miller RR, Vismara LA, Zelis R, et al: Clinical use of sodium nitroprusside in chronic ischemic heart disease. Effects on peripheral vascular resistance and venous tone and on ventricular volume, pump and mechanical performance. *Circulation* 1975; 51:328–336.

18. The CONSENSUS Trial Study Group: Effects of enalapril on mortality in severe congestive heart failure: Results of the Cooperative North Scandinavian Enalapril Survival Study (CONSENSUS). *N Engl J Med* 1987; 316:1429–1435.
19. Cohn JN, Archibald DG, Ziesche S, et al: Effect of vasodilator therapy on mortality in chronic congestive heart failure: Results of a Veterans Administration Cooperative Study Group. *N Engl J Med* 1986; 314:1547–1552.

7 / Nutritional Support of the Critically Ill Patient

RICHARD M. VAZQUEZ M.D.

Malnutrition in the critically ill patient is extraordinarily common. Inadequate intake of nutrients as a result of both anorexia and dysfunction of the digestive system, increased demand for nutrients consequent on the hypermetabolism of critical illness, and malnutrition of chronic illness are the factors frequently associated with malnutrition in the critically ill patient. The impact of malnutrition on the ability of the critically ill patient to survive has been difficult to assess but appears to involve host immune defenses, wound healing, and muscular strength as well as many other physiologic processes.

METABOLIC RESPONSES TO STARVATION AND STRESS

The neuroendocrine response to stress or injury that occurs in the critically ill patient profoundly alters the protein and energy substrate utilization that may be observed in the unstressed individual. Adaptation to starvation characterized by a decrease in both protein and energy requirements fails to occur in the stressed individual. In simple starvation carbohydrate stores used to provide glucose to those organs that require this substrate as an energy source are exhausted within 12 hours. Glucose requirements are then met by gluconeogenesis from amino acids located in the largest pool of amino acids in the human body, the somatic musculature. The central nervous system (CNS), which is the largest obligate user of glucose, gradually shifts from glucose to fatty acid and ketone metabolism. By the tenth day of simple starvation, ketone bodies derived from adipose stores provide the majority of energy substrate required.[1]

This shift from glucose to fatty acid and ketone body metabolism then permits a decrease in gluconeogenesis from the glucogenic amino acids alanine and glutamine and thereby results in protein sparing. In early simple starvation a similar protein-sparing effect can be effected by parenteral infusion of 100 to 200 g of glucose per day.[2] This amount of glucose satisfies the needs of the CNS and obviates the majority of gluconeogenesis that would otherwise be required to supply the CNS with its primary fuel, glucose.

Concomitant with this shift in energy substrate is a decrease in resting metabolic expenditure. This is effected by several methods, but a good example is the decrease in protein synthesis afforded by a resting rather than active pancreas. Considerable energy is saved, since in the absence of digestible foodstuffs, the synthesis of proteolytic enzymes in the pancreas diminishes, thereby conserving the energy-consumptive process of proteolytic enzyme synthesis.[3] The preferential use of adipose tissue as energy substrate affords the best chance for survival of the organism by conserving the substrate necessary for the activity of the majority of physiologic functions, the proteins.

The neuroendocrine response to stress prevents the higher vertebrate organism from adapting to starvation. Therefore, the shift of energy substrate from glucose to fat does not occur. The consequence of this physiologic failure to shift fuel supplies is persistent protein catabolism to provide intermediates for the hepatic synthesis of glucose.[4]

In addition to continued glucose substrate requirement, the fasting, unadapted, but starved organism manifests a resistance to the glucose transport effect of insulin, the so-called diabetes of stress commonly observed in response to stress or sepsis. Even in fasting adapted starvation, certain tissues such as red blood cells and reparative tissues remain glucose obligate for their energy substrate, further adding to the burden of glucose provision in this starvation situation. Catabolism of 30% or more of lean tissue mass is associated with a negative impact on survival of the individual.[5]

Other changes in the endocrine milieu that accompany this response to stress are an increase in glucocorticoid, catechol, antidiuretic hormone (ADH), and aldosterone secretion. Increased secretion of ADH and aldosterone results in water and salt retention, a factor that complicates the nutritional support of the critically ill patient. In addition, the increased catechol and glucocorticoid secretion are partially responsible for the insulin resistance of stress (Fig 7–1). In the absence of these two adrenal hormones the usual response to hypovolemia that occurs with bloodshed does not occur, and significant but usually nonfatal hemorrhage results in death of the organism even if shed blood is promptly reinfused.[6] What this response to stress amounts to is preservation of the organism's ability to survive hemorrhagic shock at the expense of nutritional status. Such a situation has little consequence as pertains to survival of the host unless the exposure to shock, stress, and serious illness is prolonged or repetitive as it often is in the critically ill patient. The nutritional consequence of the neuroendocrine response to stress and sepsis is that the endocrinologic processes that are necessary for a homeostatic response to severe acute hypovolemia result in an embarrassment of the nutritional processes that are subsequently operational. Clearly then, the neuroendocrine response to injury benefits the organism in the immediate postinjury period; however, the chronic severe stress and reinjury process through which the critically ill individual is supported produces a prolongation of these usually transient neuroendocrine effects and their negative nutritional impact. Without critical care units this prolongation would have little meaning since most individuals would succumb after repeated but unsupported and untreated episodes of severe hemorrhage, sepsis, and other life-threatening illnesses.

NUTRITIONAL ASSESSMENT OF THE CRITICALLY ILL PATIENT

The nutritional assessment of the critically ill patient is made in the main by using common sense as pertains to the history and physical examination at the bedside with the aid of a diminutive value from laboratory investigations. Clearly the most

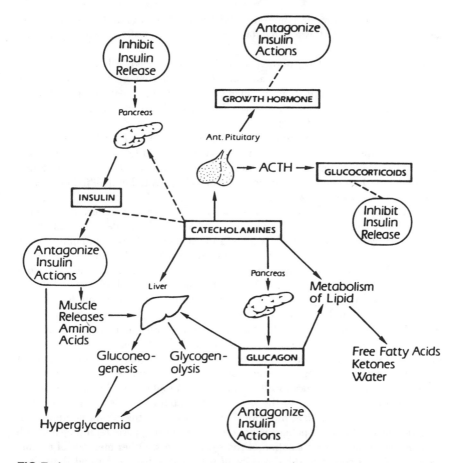

FIG 7–1.
The principal endocrine changes and their effects on energy substrate utilization following trauma. The *straight line* represents stimulation; *dotted line,* inhibition. (From Beal JM: *Critical Care for Surgical Patients.* Macmillan Publishing Co, Inc, 1982. Used by permission.)

important aspect of nutritional assessment is a past history of malnutrition antedating the critical illness or a history of illness known to interfere with normal nutritional processes. For example, patients with chronic respiratory illnesses are frequently malnourished in part because they have such difficulty maintaining adequate ventilation that proper oral intake of nutrients does not occur. Those patients with gastrointestinal (GI) diseases that interfere with nutrient absorption such as regional ileitis frequently experience additional nutritional insult secondary to the catabolic effect of steroid therapy.

The classical approach to nutritional assessment relies upon anthropometric measurements that include body weight and calculation of the skeletal muscle mass, or somatic protein compartment, and fat stores. These calculations are based upon measurement of the arm circumference and triceps skin fat fold. The results of the calculations are reported as a percentage of the normal expected muscle mass and body fat.

In the eumetabolic state, normal renal function assumed, a linear relationship exists between creatinine excretion and muscle mass.[7] Serum creatinine and 24-hour urinary creatinine determinations are made to calculate the creatinine height index as a method to estimate muscle mass while other laboratory studies are used to estimate the visceral protein stores.

The visceral protein measurement that may have retained value in the nutritional assessment of the critically ill patient is the serum albumin level. In the unstressed individual a serum albumin content less than 3.5 g/dL is considered to be indicative of depletion of the visceral protein pool. This level needs to be modified downward for elderly individuals to 3.2 g/dL.

The anthropometric measurements of body weight, arm circumference, and triceps skin fold thickness are altered by the all-too-common edematous condition experienced by many critically ill patients. Indeed, the fluid resuscitation necessary to guarantee proper cardiac function frequently results in dilution of the serum proteins. This is particularly true in the resuscitation of septic patients, who lose serum proteins by way of capillary leak or transudation into third-space compartments. The nonspecificity of the depression of serum albumin levels to reflect a purely nutritional etiology has been observed with many of the other readily measured serum proteins. The use of serum albumin levels for monitoring the efficacy of nutritional support is unrewarding; a low albumin level remains refractory to the provision of what is considered to be optimal nutritional support until the patient enters the convalescent stage of illness. Actually, hypoalbuminemia in the critically ill patient population correlates well with low survival rates. This has led the author and other investigators to favor the use of serum albumin levels as an indicator of severity of illness rather than nutritional state.[8] A rise in the serum albumin concentration of a critically ill patient may be observed during parenteral infusion with albumin, dehydration, or resolution of the severe illness. Other methods of making a nutritional assessment of the critically ill patient that have not stood the test of time are the measurement of the total lymphocyte count, the serum transferrin level, and the use of cell-mediated immunity.[9]

Clinical Nitrogen Balance

Measurement of the clinical nitrogen balance is useful for monitoring the adequacy of nutrient provision. Ninety percent of the nitrogenous products of protein catabolism are excreted in the urine as urea. A baseline 24-hour nitrogen excretion measurement correlates well with protein catabolism during the collection period. This baseline measurement provides a useful method to estimate anticipated protein requirements. The quantitative excretion of urine urea nitrogen (UUN), may be used during nutritional support to monitor the adequacy of the provision of protein.

An unstressed adult male usually excretes about 7 g of urea nitrogen each 24 hours. A 50% increase in the resting metabolic rate will usually increase the excretion of urea nitrogen to 10 or 11 g per 24 hours. For obvious reasons, the 24-hour UUN concentration has been called a poor man's method of calculating energy expenditure.

As the goal of nutritional support is to achieve nutritional repair through anabolism, a positive nitrogen balance is desirable. Nitrogen balance is calculated by subtracting the nitrogen output from the nitrogen input. The nitrogen input is calculated during nonvolitional feedings by multiplying the volume of the nitrogen-containing infusate times the concentration of nitrogen per unit volume of the infusate. The nitrogen content of parenteral amino acid preparations cannot be calculated by multiplying the weight of the amino acids present by 16% (the nitrogen content of high–biologic value intact proteins). The protein equivalence of these products is determined by the amount of available nitrogen present and must be obtained from the manufacturer's package insert literature.

The nitrogen output may be calculated by measuring UUN and adding to this determination 2 g for other nitrogenous waste not measured by urea analysis. In addition, 1 g of nitrogen is added to compensate for skin desquamation, and 1 g of nitrogen is added for fecal nitrogen loss. The 24-hour nitrogen balance is then calculated by subtracting the output from the input. A positive state (more nitrogen assimilated than lost) implies an anabolic state, providing the serum urea nitrogen remains stable over the collection period. A rising serum urea nitrogen signifies that the patient may be receiving an excessive amino acid load, is becoming dehydrated, or has compromised renal function.

Factors that may influence the nonurea nitrogen concentration in the calculation are (1) excessive stooling, (2) severe skin desquamation, and (3) protein loss from serum protein weeping from open wounds or burns. Nitrogen utilization can be optimized by provision of sufficient energy to permit protein synthesis. If insufficient nonprotein energy is provided, the amino acids will be used as fuel rather than as components for the synthesis of body proteins.

NUTRITIONAL SUPPORT

Nutritional support of the critically ill patient is based upon two major principles: removal of those factors inducing or prolonging the catabolic neuroendocrine response of the patient and the provision of adequate amounts of appropriate metabolic substrates in a suitable form to maintain and restore the normal composition of the body. Therefore, the basic principles of patient care such as treatment of pain, hemorrhage, tissue necrosis, and sepsis must be undertaken either before or concomitantly with the initiation of nutritional support. Also, nutritional support is never an emergency and should not be instituted until proper fluid and electrolyte resuscitation has been administered and cardiovascular stability secured. The addition of variables attributable to nutritional support to those exigencies demanding immediate correction during volume and electrolyte resuscitation cannot be justified by the negligible potential immediate benefit to the patient.

NUTRITIONAL REQUIREMENTS
Energy Supply

Energy needs to be supplied in sufficient amount to minimize catabolism or, if the clinical situation permits, to promote lean tissue synthesis. On occasion, an increase in body fat is desirable, but such a circumstance would rarely be present in the critical care unit. Sedentary adult surgical patients at liberty to move about in the hospital setting generally require 2,000 to 2,200 kcal/day. Those same patients when subjected to the stress of major operations required 1,800 to 2,200 kcal/day. This diminution in energy requirement may be explained by the minimal locomotion activity exhibited by the immediately postoperative patient at bed rest.

The optimal energy supply for those adult patients in critical care units is estimated to fall within the range of 2,400 ±200 kcal/day. A more precise determination of energy requirements may be obtained by using indirect calorimetry, a complicated process that has not been widely accepted. The frequency with which metabolic carts were successfully used by nutritional support teams possessing them has been reported to be 60%. Calibration difficulties and clinical factors greatly interfered with their use.

During the 1970s the tendency toward overfeeding was evident in the clinical practice of nutritional support. The deleterious effect of overfeeding was appreciated in 1980 by Askenazi et al.[10] Besides constituting a waste of expensive nutrient infusates, the excessive CO_2 production associated with overfeeding of those patients with marginal CO_2 excretory capacity became evident. The metabolism of carbohydrate energy sources produces a respiratory quotient (RQ) of 1, that is, for each mole of oxygen consumed, 1 mol of carbon dioxide is produced and needs to be excreted. Overfeeding sufficient to result in lipogenesis (RQ = 7.0) further increases carbon dioxide production. Metabolism of fat has an RQ of 0.7 mol of CO_2 per mole oxygen.[10] Supplying energy substrate in correct amounts to meet the patient's needs, with fat as 50% of the energy source, may be expected to decrease carbon dioxide production by less than 30% of the amount produced by a pure carbohydrate energy supply.[11]

For the subset of patients in critical care units with marginal CO_2 excretory capacity, a small increase in CO_2 production may perpetuate the need for mechanical ventilatory support. For this group of patients a more precise method of determining energy requirements should be considered. Indirect calorimetry measurement may be useful in this group of patients so that energy can be provided in more correct amounts than by simple predictive methods. In general, an energy supply of about 30 to 35 kcal/kg body weight is sufficient to maintain body mass. An additional 500 kcal/day is usually provided when weight gain as body fat and lean mass is desired.

The most abundant and inexpensive energy source for parenteral solutions is carbohydrate in the form of dextrose. Since hydrated glucose supplies 3.4 kcal/g, 500 mL of a 60% dextrose solution will contain 300 g of glucose or contain 1.02 nonprotein kilocalories per milliliter when diluted with 500 mL of an amino acid solution (300 g × 3.4 kcal/g = 1,020 calories per liter, or approximately 1 kcal/mL).

Parenteral fat emulsions are isotonic and supply more energy per unit volume than do isotonic carbohydrate solutions. A 10% emulsion provides 550 kcal in a volume of 500 mL of isotonic emulsion. Essential fats must be provided to prevent the occurrence of essential fatty acid deficiency. Provision of 8% of the calorie requirements as fat emulsion supplies the required 20 g of linoleic acid per day.[12] The provision of more than 60% of the daily energy requirement with fat is associated with serum lipemia and fat overload syndrome. The latter is associated with thrombocytopenia. These considerations provide the lower and upper limits of the percentage of fat to be parenterally infused, i.e., between 8% and 60% of the nonprotein energy requirement.[13] The provision of 25% to 40% of the nonprotein energy requirements as lipid minimizes the difficulties with both glucose metabolism and hypertriglyceridemia that are caused by insufficient utilization of infused lipid.

Protein Requirements

Provision of adequate protein substrate promotes a positive nitrogen balance, the synthesis of protein for tissue repair, and the synthesis of hormones necessary for the control of biochemical and physiologic activities and regulation of metabolic processes.

Adults at zero nitrogen balance require 50 g of protein or 8 g of nitrogen per day (0.8 to 1 g of protein per kilogram of body weight per day).[14] Requirements for critically ill patients are increased to 1.5 to 2 g of protein per kilogram of body weight per day. The relative amounts of protein and nonprotein energy supplied by parenteral or enteral diets is frequently expressed as a calorie-to-nitrogen ratio. For example, a person whose dietary intake provides 2,000 kcal/ day and 10 g of nitrogen may be referred to as having a diet with a calorie-to-nitrogen ratio of 200 kcal/1 g of nitrogen. The severely ill patient appears to require more nitrogen than do those patients with simple starvation and is therefore better supported by diets with a calorie-to-nitrogen ratio closer to 120 to 150 kcal/g nitrogen.

Patients with renal and/or hepatic failure are intolerant of protein. Some chronic renal failure patients fed special low-nitrogen diets with 1.5 to 4 g/day of nitrogen present as essential amino acids have achieved nitrogen equilibrium when sufficient nonprotein energy substrate was provided.[13]

The carbon skeleton of an essential amino acid cannot by synthesized by an organism in amounts adequate to provide for optimal growth and development. An absence of any one essential amino acid will result in growth failure. The amino acids known to be essential for healthy adults are listed in Table 7-1. In uremic chronic renal failure patients, histidine increases nitrogen retention following intravenous hyperalimentation (IVH). Premature infants require cysteine. Therefore histidine and cysteine, which are usually considered to be nonessential, may be considered essential in these situations (see Table 7-1).[5]

A particular protein will be synthesized only if all amino acids required for its synthesis are provided in sufficient amounts. A deficiency of any component amino acid may limit synthesis of the particular protein. In addition, sufficient cofactors such as vitamins, trace elements, and nonprotein energy must also be present. The weight of the essential amino acids divided by the total nitrogen content of any amino acid mixture has been termed the *E/T ratio*. It has been shown in humans that optimal nitrogen retention is associated with an E/T ratio of 1:2.22, i.e., approximately 30% of the amino acids administered are essential amino acids. The amino acid solution used should be sufficient to provide each of the amino acids necessary to meet requirements. Solutions containing <10% essential amino acids would probably not provide sufficient quantities of these amino acids. Diets containing more than

TABLE 7–1.

Essential and Nonessential Amino Acids

Amino Acid	Abbr	Essential
Alanine	Ala	No
Arginine	Arg	No
Asparagine	Asn	No
Aspartic acid	Asp	No
Cysteine	Cys	No
Glycine	Gly	No
Glutamic acid	Glu	No
Glutamine	Gin	No
Histidine	His	Semi
Isoleucine	Ile	Yes
Leucine	Leu	Yes
Lysine	Lys	Yes
Methionine	Met	Yes
Phenylalanine	Phe	Yes
Proline	Pro	No
Serine	Ser	No
Threonine	Thr	Yes
Tryptophan	Trp	Yes
Tyrosine	Tyr	No
Valine	Val	Yes

50% essential amino acids may produce adverse effects on the growth rate and result in amino acid imbalance, antagonism, or toxicity.[12]

Vitamin and Trace Element Requirements

The provision of vitamins and trace elements to patients receiving nutritional support needs specific attention, especially for those patients who have disease processes that are known to interfere with vitamin absorption or increase requirements. Biliary obstruction and jaundice as well as the hepatic dysfunction of cirrhosis are associated with vitamin K deficiency. Biliary tract obstruction decreases the bile salt concentration in the gut, which leads to decreased absorption of fat-soluble vitamins. Usually, the addition of 10 mg of vitamin K per week to the parenteral infusate is sufficient to prevent the development of vitamin K deficiency.[15]

Thiamin, riboflavin, and pyridoxine deficiencies are associated with alcoholism, as is vitamin A deficiency resulting from inadequate dietary intake and interference with absorption.[16] These potential deficiencies may necessitate adjustment of nutrient prescriptions.

Criticaly ill patients may be folate deficient, a condition that may be manifested by peripheral thrombocytopenia.[17] Burn patients have increased needs for ascorbic acid. Abnormal collagen synthesis associated with a deficiency of vitamin C may lead to poor wound healing or dehiscence of traumatically or surgically created wounds.[18]

Vitamin E, a known antioxidant, plays a protective role in retinal oxygen toxicity of the newborn and appears to require selenium as a permissive agent for its activity. The role of vitamin D as it pertains to calcium metabolism is well known but rarely becomes a cause for concern in the intensive care unit (ICU) nutritional support setting.

The nutrient prescription should contain 10 mL/day of a commercially available multivitamin preparation. Those currently on the market contain sufficient amounts of all of the fat- and water-soluble vitamins to repair mild deficiencies of all vitamin deficiencies except vitamin K deficiency. Vitamin K is not a component of the multivitamin infusions due to storage and compatibility considerations and therefore must be administered in addition to the multiple vitamin infusion.

Pharmacologic dosing of vitamin A in doses of 10,000 to 40,000 units/day has been reported to reduce the incidence of stress ulcers from 63% to 18% in patients with large surface area burns. High-dose vitamin A has also been used to counteract the adverse wound-healing effect of steroid therapy.[19]

Overwhelming sepsis may result in a marked increase of all vitamin requirements. The metabolic rate and nutrient requirements of the patient are increased, and bacteria compete with the infected host for the same vitamins to maintain their own metabolic functions.

Trace Elements in Parenteral Nutrition

Those trace elements noted to be essential for humans include copper, chromium, cobalt, iron, iodine, zinc, manganese, fluorine, molybdenum, and selenium. In the short-term parenteral nutrition critical care patient, zinc, copper, chromium, manganese, and selenium should be added to the nutritional prescription.

Zinc is required for normal wound healing. Zinc deficiency is usually unmasked during the recovery phase from severe illness. The symptoms include diarrhea, depression, and dermatitis at the nasolabial fold. The provision of 5 mg of zinc to parenteral nutritional prescriptions usually prevents such a deficiency from occurring.[20]

Copper should be infused in a dose of 0.4 to 0.5 mg/day. Because copper is excreted through the biliary tract, its use should be restricted in the presence of obstructive jaundice. The deficiency state is characterized by neutropenia and anemia due to the involvement of copper in hematopoiesis.

The role of chromium and its relationship to carbohydrate metabolism have been described by Mertz and Schroeder.[21] Insulin resistance may be observed in the chromium-deficient patient without apparent explanation such as the coexistence of sepsis. Ten micrograms per day is the recommended dosage.[22]

Like copper, manganese is excreted primarily in bile, and therefore its parenteral use should be discontinued during biliary tract obstruction. Otherwise, 0.5 mg/day as a parenteral additive is sufficient. Approximately 100 to 150 μg of selenium should be given each day in parenteral nutritional infusions. Selenium is required for normal hematopoiesis and for cardiac muscle function.

METHODS OF NUTRITIONAL SUPPORT

To provide complete or total nutritional support, nutrients must be administered into either the gut or vascular system. The enteral route requires a functional intestinal tract, whereas nutrient infusion of glutamine into the gut promotes integrity of the gut mucosal barrier to bacterial invasion.[23] The expense and potential complications of the parenteral route may be avoided if enteral feeding suffices. Ileus, GI hemorrhage, and GI intolerance manifested by emesis or diarrhea limit the usefulness of the enteral route. Pulmonary aspiration of emesis may occur in those unable to protect the airway. The enteral nutrients may be delivered into the intestinal tract through small-caliber enteral feeding tubes of silicone rubber or polyurethane. These tubes are usually placed with relative ease at the bedside; however, placement of these feeding tubes with the aid of a stiffening stylet has been associated with penetration of the esophagus as well as unintentional tracheobronchial positioning of the devices.

The proper method of placement of a nasoenteral feeding tube in a patient who cannot or will not cooperate with tube insertion requires gentle passage of a well-lubricated feeding tube followed by radiographic confirmation of the location of the tip of the feeding tube. Injection of air into the tube with concomitant auscultation of the left upper quadrant for bubbling of air is sometimes misleading with regard to the location of the tip of the feeding tube.

Continuous feeding appears to be tolerated by the critically ill surgical patient better than bolus feedings. The continuous mode of feeding permits gradual adjustment of the osmolarity of the nutrient and better emptying of the gut which results in better patient tolerance and less morbidity. In addition, duodenal or jejunal feeding past the pylorus may be preferable to gastric feeding and less likely to result in pulmonary aspiration.

Surgical access by gastrostomy or jejunostomy are alternate means of providing enteral feedings and are probably best reserved for those patients undergoing abdominal operations for problems other than malnutrition only. Gastric feedings are not well tolerated by the critically ill patient, but jejunal feeding, especially when combined with proximal gastric decompression by nasogastric tube or gastrostomy, is well tolerated. The technique of needle-catheter feeding jejunostomy has a low complication rate and may be performed rapidly. Continuous infusion of low-viscosity tube feedings can be given by this needle-catheter method even in the immediate postoperative period.

Parenteral feedings may be combined with enteral feedings for those patients who are being weaned from parenteral feeding or who cannot tolerate the entire nutrient prescription by the enteral route.

Parenteral Nutrition

Intravenous hyperalimentation (IVH) infused by the central venous route has developed to a degree of safety such that reports of technical and septic complications of less than 3% are common.[24]

Central venous access by supraclavicular or infraclavicular subclavian venipuncture is the preferred route for acute IVH. Placement of a catheter in the superior vena cava by cephalic or external jugular vein cutdown, median basilic vein puncture, as well as other methods of catheter placement, are acceptable. Because sepsis is to be avoided, the catheters must be placed and cared for after insertion using strict asepsis. If possible, the catheter should be dedicated to IVH administration. The preferred material for central venous catheterization in decreasing stiffness and thrombogenicity is silicone, followed by polyurethane, and then polyvinylchloride catheters. Upper extremity thrombosis has been reported at frequencies of 4% to 25% and is occasionally the cause of pulmonary embolism or serious morbidity.[25] Because of its stiffness, Teflon should not be used for superior vena caval catheterization. The use of a transparent, water vapor–permeable, bacteria-impermeable dressing is associated with less than a 1% incidence of catheter-induced sepsis.[26]

Parenteral Infusates

Intravenous hyperalimentation solutions composed of a mixture of 500 mL of 8.5% to 10% amino acids mixed with an equivalent volume of hypertonic glucose (40% to 70%) are commonly used basic nutrient prescriptions (see Table 7–2).

Fat emulsions may also be given by the central route or by a peripheral vein, may be mixed with the amino acid and glucose solution, or may be administered by piggyback or a "y" connector into the central venous catheter. The provision of sufficient electrolytes, trace elements, and vitamins needs consideration as well.

It is convenient to consider a standard solution not only for the purposes of discussion but also since many patients outside the ICU with essentially normal major organ system function can be safely and adequately nourished with a standard solution or prescription. Modification of such a prescription to suit the particular requirements of the ICU patient may be made by reference to departure from some of the components. For those patients with profound major organ system dysfunction the approach of designing the prescription without reference to any type of standard solution is easier and not contrived. For example, the standard solution currently in use at Northwestern Memorial Hospital (NMH) uses 500 mL of 60% glucose mixed with 500 mL of an 8.5% amino acid solution. As previously discussed, such a mixture results in a solution that provides about 1 kcal/mL, or 1,000 calories per liter. The particular amino acid solution used by NMH (Aminosyn) provides 6.5 g of nitrogen or a protein equivalent of 39 g/L (6.5 g N per liter × 6 g protein per g N = grams of protein per liter).

For the remainder of this discussion please refer to Table 7–2.

The energy and fluid requirements of many patients can be provided at infusion rates of 60 to 75 mL of infusate per hour, assuming that an additional 500 mL of 10% fat emulsion will also be infused each day. At an infusion rate of 60 mL/hr, or 1 mL/min, the volume of amino acid/glucose solution delivered each day equals 1,440 mL/day. As each milliliter of this infusate provides about 1 kcal/mL, the infusion provides 1,440 kcal of carbohydrate energy per day. If 500 mL of 10% fat emulsion is also infused, an additional 550 kcal of lipid is provided for a total of 1,990 nonprotein kilocalories administered per day. By increasing the infusion rate of the glucose

TABLE 7–2.

Guidelines for Parenteral Feeding and Suggested Parenteral Infusates

Protein:

                Adult baseline: 1 g protein/kg/day ideal body weight

                Daily requirement: 11–16 g N/day (1 g N/6 g protein)*

                    7% Aminosyn = 5.5 g N/500 cc

                    8.5% Aminosyn = 6.5 g N/500 cc

                    10% Aminosyn = 7.8 g N/500 cc

Fats:

Minimum requirement: 8% of caloric intake given daily or weekly as supplements

Maximum daily dose for adults = 2.5–4.0 g/kg or 50%–60% of nonprotein calorie requirements for adults

                10% Liposyn = 550 calories/500 cc

                20% Liposyn = 1,000 calories/500 cc

Electrolytes:

Hyperlyte is a multiple electrolyte additive with a concentrated vol of 20 mL†

Ingredient	mEq/L TPN‡
Na	25
K	40.5
Mg	8
Ca	5
Cl	33.5
Acetate	40.6
Gluconate	5

Sample regimen:

  500 cc Aminosyn (protein source)

  20 cc Hyperlyte

  10 cc MVI-12 (multivitamin)

Caloric needs: 35 calories/kg IBW‡/Day (2,450 calories/Day for 70-kg Person)

	Calories/L TPN	Calories/mL	Calories/Day at Various Infusions (mL/hr)					
			50	60	75	83	100	125
D40	680	0.7	840	1,000	1,260	1,400	1,680	2,100
D50	850	0.85	1,020	1,220	1,500	1,700	2,040	2,550
D60‖	1,020	1.0	1,200	1,440	1,800	2,000	2,400	3,000
D70	1,200	1.2	1,440	1,700	2,160	2,400	2,900	3,600

Vitamins—MVI-12§ ingredients:

Ascorbate:	100 mg	Niacinamide:	40 mg
Vitamin A:	3,300 IU	Pantothenic acid:	15 mg
Vitamin D:	200 IU	Vitamin E:	10 IU
Thiamine:	3 mg	Biotin:	60 µg
Pyridoxine:	4 mg	Folate:	400 µg
		Vitamin B_{12}:	5 µg

Trace elements can also be added to the bottle each day:

Zinc:	4 mg	Maganese:	0.5 mg	Selenous acid: 100–150 mg
Copper:	0.4 mg	Chromium:	10 µg	

*Severely ill people may require 1.5–2 times more.
†Phosphate is not included, so 15 mmol/L will need to be added.
‡TPN = total parenteral nutrition; IBW = ideal body weight.
§MVI-12 does not supply vitamin K (10 mg/wk).
‖Standard solution.

amino acid component to 75 mL/hr, or 1,800 mL/day, the CHO energy infusion is increased to 1,800 calories per day, and the nonprotein energy infusion is increased to a total of 2,350 kcal/day.

If we consider the protein content of an infusion of 1,800 mL of this reference solution, 1.8 L that contains 6.54 g of nitrogen per liter supplies 11.8 g of nitrogen or 71 g of protein daily. This amount of protein may not be sufficient to satisfy the protein requirement of a critically ill patient, because severely ill patients frequently require 1.5 g of protein per kilogram of body weight.[27] Depending on other issues such as water requirements, potential remedies for this problem include (1) increasing the amino acid concentration to 10% i.e., 7.8 g N per liter; (2) mixing the glucose and amino acid solution with 600 mL amino acid and 400 mL glucose per liter (70% glucose may be substituted for 60% so as not to lessen the CHO energy component significantly); (3) increasing the infusion rate; and (4) using any combination of these remedies to suit the patient's needs.

Regardless of which infusate rate is selected each day, the patient should be given at least 10 mL of a multiple vitamin infusion, trace elements in the amounts indicated in Table 7–2, and vitamin K at 10 mg/wk unless contraindicated for medical reasons.

Management of Electrolyte Balance

The nutrient prescription usually contains sufficient fluid and electrolyte components to meet the patient's individual requirements. In addition to the anticipated need for sodium and chloride replacement, patients receiving parenteral nutrition have increased requirements for those electrolytes that occur in the intracellular fluid. These requirements may reflect not only the addition of new cellular mass but may also be related to depletion during the pretreatment phase of illness. Other factors that need be considered are organ dysfunction, medications that cause wasting of certain electrolytes such as steroids or diuretics, and so forth. Phosphate depletion is particualrly dangerous, and its occurrence may be insidious since multiphase electrolyte panels do not include serum phosphate levels and serum phosphate levels are not routinely frequently tested. A serum phosphate level <1.0 mg/dL may be associated with muscular dysfunction severe enough to result in ventilatory failure or cardiac arrest.[28] Refer to Table 7–2 for a list of the electrolytes contained in a commonly used multiple electrolyte additive. Notice the absence of phosphate, which must be added separately.

COMPLICATIONS OF NUTRITIONAL SUPPORT

Complications of nutritional support may be divided into technical, metabolic, or septic categories. Parenteral feedings are specifically associated with technical and septic complications related to the intravenous (IV) catheter. Metabolic complications may occur with either route and are usually related to insufficiently frequent monitoring of fluid and electrolyte status or excessive or inadequate intake of specific components of the diet. Enteral feedings are associated with the technical problems secondary to the delivery of large volumes of hyperosmolar solutions into the GI tract and also a significant risk of pulmonary aspiration.

A previously unrecognized complication of parenteral infusions is the inadequate provision of nutrient to the mucosa of the gut with consequent loss of mucosal barrier function. Loss of the gut mucosal barrier results in chronic septicemia and bacteremia with enteric organisms.

Metabolic Complications

Frequent evaluation of the metabolic, fluid and electrolyte, and acid-base status of the patient is of fundamental importance. The frequency of such determinations is dependent upon the rapidity and severity of changes in the patient's response to the infusate. Volume replacement and cardiovascular resuscitation should be accomplished prior to initiating nutritional support. Correction of fluid and electrolyte as well as acid-base abnormalities may take place concomitantly with hyperalimentation.

Electrolyte Problems

Critically ill patients with normal renal function commonly have depletion of potassium, chloride, and magnesium stores secondary to the widespread use of diuretics and loss of GI secretions. In addition, loss of fixed acid or base in GI secretions may cause acid-base abnormalities. Other common causes of potassium depletion other than the loss of potassium associated with malnutrition are caused in the main by medications. For example, steroids commonly used for the treatment of nonspecific inflammatory bowel disease cause large losses of potassium in the urine. Similarly, amphotericin antifungal therapy is associated with nephrotoxicity and urinary potassium loss.

Magnesium deficiency accompanies diuretic use as well as GI secretion loss. Depletion of total body stores of the intracellular electrolytes magnesium, phosphate, and potassium is associated with malnutrition. Measurement of serum levels of these electrolytes frequently does not reflect their depletion, a depletion that is frequently unmasked by the initiation of total parenteral nutrition. Hence comes the recommendation that serum electrolyte determinations be made frequently at the inception of hyperalimentation therapy.

For further discussion concerning disorders of extracellular and intracelluar electrolytes see Chapter 14 of this text.

The swiftness and intensity of the correction of these fluid and electrolyte abnormalities should be tempered by several considerations. Overzealous correction usually embraced by the novice all too frequently results in wide swings in serum electrolyte levels, confuses and frustrates the nursing staff, and results in wastage of large amounts of ill-prescribed hyperalimentation fluid. Critical to their proper management is the anticipation of possible changes in serum electrolyte levels and the measurement of serum samples frequently enough to prevent surprises to the physician and staff.

Acid-Base Imbalance

In addition to correction of pulmonary and renal dysfunction the health care team has the option of manipulating changes in acid-base balance through the hyperalimentation prescription. Bicarbonate cannot be added to the IVH formula because the resultant change in the pH of the solution causes precipitation of calcium carbonate. Addition of fixed base to the solution is achieved by the addition of sodium or potassium as acetate salts. The acetate is metabolized to bicarbonate, thereby achieving the goal. Conversely, the subtraction or replacement of acetate salts with chloride salts results in a diminution in the amount of substrate that can be metabolized to bicarbonate, and the fixed acid concentration in the blood increases.

The advisability of making these manipulations requires consideration of the etiology of the change and whether metabolic treatment of the abnormalities would be of benefit or detriment to the patient.

Other Metabolic Complications

Volume overload.—Volume overload can be a problem, particularly in those patients with cardiac disease and those requiring mechanical ventilatory support. Positive-pressure ventilation results in changes in ADH secretion, renal perfusion, and water balance such that these patients tend to retain water. In addition, some patients, such as those with head or spinal cord injury, are predisposed to the syndrome of inappropriate antidiuretic hormone (SIADH).

Glucose intolerance.—The critically ill patient frequently manifests glucose intolerance. Persistent glycosuria produces an osmotic diuresis and often leads to nonketotic hyperosmolar dehydration and coma in nondiabetic patients and a ketoacidotic state in the diabetic patient. If prompt control of the serum glucose level cannot be obtained, the following treatment may be required: (1) the discontinuation of IVH infusion and (2) volume resuscitation to correct the volume depletion consequent on persistent osmotic diuresis. Avoidance of this complication is achieved by frequent monitoring of the patient for glycosuria, the addition of small amounts of insulin to the IVH infusion, and a shift away from glucose as the major nonprotein energy substrate. Effective control of the blood sugar concentration by the addition of insulin to the infusate occurs despite the adherence of much of the insulin to the delivery apparatus.[29]

Chromium deficiency has been reported as an uncommon cause of glucose intolerance. Chromium trichloride may be added to the IV solutions in a dose of 10 μg/day to maintain normal serum chromium levels.[22]

Technical Complications

The most frequently occurring complications of central venous catheterization are pneumothorax and unintentional arterial puncture. Pneumothorax may require treatment with chest tube insertion. Unsuccessful venipuncture on one side should not be followed by attempted catheterization of the other side until a chest radiograph for possible complication of catheterization has been obtained. Arterial puncture leads to morbid complication in those patients with coagulopathies. Hemothorax or chest wall hematoma may occur in these patients with hemorrhagic disorders.

By far the most serious technical complications of central vein catheterization result from penetration of major vascular structures or the heart. Hydrothorax, hydromediastinum, or even cardiac tamponade may result.[30] Penetration of these anatomic structures appears to be related to overzealous passage of devices into the central circulation and to the stiffness of the catheter material. The conscious patient will experience visceral thoracic pain or substernal chest pain during catheter placement or during infusion through the malpositioned device. If any doubt about the proper intravascular location of the catheter exists, the catheter may be studied under fluoroscopy with injection of radiographic contrast material or removal of the catheter and replacement with a new device.

Nutrient infusion should not be started until these catheters are demonstrated to be in proper location, usually by an upright anteroposterior (AP) chest radiograph. Infusion of these hyperosmolar substances into veins with insufficient flow may result in thrombosis of the great veins or superior vena cava. Those patients with protein C, protein S, or antithrombin III deficiencies are at increased risk—greater than the 4% to 8% rate of venous occlusion reported. Pulmonary embolism can occur as a result of upper extremity vein thrombosis, as may septic pulmonary embolism.

Septic Complications

Because sepsis is prone to develop in critically ill patients, the differential diagnosis of sepsis after the introduction of a central venous catheter and initiation of hyperalimentation is important. The search for a septic focus includes evaluation of other potential causes for infection by cultures of blood, sputum, and urine; examination of the patient; and culture of any removed intravascular devices for bacteria or fungi. The single most important factor in identifying the central venous catheter as the source of sepsis is resolution of the septic focus upon removal of the device. The decision to remove and replace catheters suspected to be contaminated or to exchange them over guide wires is controversial. The author recommends exchange of the catheter over a guidewire if (1) the catheter was originally placed under sterile conditions, (2) there is no purulent discharge from the catheter skin puncture site, and (3) the patient is not in bacteremic shock. However, if a patient being evaluated for catheter-induced sepsis actually goes into septic shock, all intravascular devices should be removed and replaced at a new site if at all possible. When any serious doubt exists regarding the sterility of a central venous catheter, the catheter should be removed and replaced at a new clean site.[31]

The mainstay of treatment of catheter-induced sepsis is prevention. Attention to the details of technique both anatomic and aseptic during catheter insertion and frequent inspection of the properly dressed catheter insertion site later are necessary. Catheter colonization seems to occur more frequently when these devices are used for multiple purposes, if the devices have multiple rather than single lumina, or if the patient has a remote site of invasive infection.

CASE STUDY

A 64-year-old man with an 8-year history of chronic obstructive pulmonary disease was seen in the emergency room with a complaint of increasing shortness of breath and coughing of 2 days' duration. The patient had two previous admissions in the past 18 months for pneumonia. He normally produced small quantities of whitish sputum but had been producing approximately half a cup per day of thick yellow sputum for the last 2 days. Further questioning revealed a loss of appetite and a weight loss of 30 lb over the last 6 months associated with severe depression after the death of his wife.

On examination he was noted to be markedly cachectic and weighed 55 kg. His heart rate was 115/min with occasional ventricular ectopic beats, and his blood pressure (BP) was 160/90 mm Hg. His extremities were cyanotic, and the fingernails were clubbed. There was no evidence of jugular venous distention or peripheral edema. Auscultation of the heart revealed a marked P2 component to the second heart sound, and no murmurs were heard. His respiratory rate (RR) was 35/min with a tidal volume (VT) of 300 mL, and the patient was using accessory ventilatory muscles. The AP diameter of his chest was enlarged, and the chest was hyperresonant to percussion. Diaphragmatic excursion was minimal, and rhonchi and fremitus were noted in the right middle and lower lobe regions. The rest of the physical examination was unremarkable.

Initial laboratory investigations revealed the following values: serum sodium, 143 mEq/L; potassium, 4.8 mEq/L; chloride, 90 mEq/L; bicarbonate, 36 mEq/L; serum glucose, 270 mg/dL; and blood urea nitrogen (BUN), 28 mg/dL. The patient's hemoglobin concentration was 17 mg/dL; and the white blood cell (WBC) count was 18,000 mm^{-3} with a leftward shift. Arterial blood gas analysis on room air revealed a pH of 7.51, a Pco_2 of 45 mm Hg, and a Po_2 of 40 mm Hg. Gram staining of the sputum showed the presence of many WBCs and gram-positive diplococci. A sputum sample was sent for a culture and sensitivity determination. Urinalysis was within normal limits. The electrocardiogram (ECG) showed sinus tachycardia with occasional ventricular premature beats. Chest x-ray films revealed infiltrates in the right, middle, and lower lobe; flattened diaphragms; and hyperinflation. A preliminary diagnosis of acute bacterial pneumonia superimposed on chronic obstructive pulmonary disease was made and the patient's poor nutritional status noted.

The patient was administered penicillin for his presumed pneumococcal pneumonia and given 24% oxygen via an air entrainment mask, which resulted in arterial blood gases with a pH of 7.50, a Pco_2 of 45 mm Hg, and a Po_2 of 44 mm Hg. The F_IO_2 was increased to 0.28 with resultant improvement in the arterial oxygenation, a decrease in heart rate and BP, and a change in respiratory pattern to a rate of 28/min with a VT of 350 mL and a vital capacity (VC) of 1.1 L. Arterial blood gas analysis on 28% oxygen showed a pH of 7.46, a Pco_2 of 50 mm Hg, and a Po_2 of 52 mm Hg. Chest physical therapy was ordered to help the patient mobilize secretions, and the nutritional support service was requested to review the patient's nutritional status. Three hours later the patient was noted to have increasing RR, heart rate, and systemic BP. Repeat on arterial blood gas analysis on 28% oxygen revealed a pH of 7.32, a Pco_2 of 68 mm Hg, and a Po_2 of 43 mm Hg. The patient was deemed to be developing acute ventilatory failure and was ventilated with a manual resuscitator and face mask in preparation for nasotracheal intubation to facilitate mechanical ventilatory support. Following uneventful placement of a nasotracheal tube, the patient was put on a mechanical ventilator at a rate of 8 breaths per minute, mechanical VT of 1,000 mL, and 40% oxygen with +5 of positive end-expiratory pressure (PEEP), which resulted in a pHa of 7.42, a $Paco_2$ of 53 mm Hg, and a Po_2 of 71 mm Hg. At this time the patient was noted to have no spontaneous respiratory efforts at all and was resting quietly. Sputum cultures confirmed the diagnosis of pneumococcal pneumonia.

Assessment of the patient's nutritional status revealed the following:

Anthropometric Measurements

- Mid-upper-arm circumference, 15.2 cm (60% of standard)

- Triceps skin fold thickness, 7.5 mm (60% of standard)
- Arm muscle circumference, 0.0314 × TSF = 15.0 cm (60% of standard)

Laboratory Measurements

- Serum albumin, 2.9 gm/dL
- WBC, 18,000 mm^{-3} with 6% lymphocytes
- Serum magnesium, 1.5 mg/dL
- Serum calcium, 7.0 mg/dL
- Serum phosphorus, 2.5 mg/dL
- 24-hour UUN, 2 g
- Liver and renal function, normal

On the basis of these measurements, the patient was deemed to have severe depletion of somatic protein compartments and a mixed marasmus and kwashiorkor-like state of malnutrition.

The patient's ideal body weight was 70 kg, and therefore it was determined that he required 2,450 kcal/day (35 kcal/kg) and 105 g of protein (1.5 g protein per kilogram per day). The patient was started on enteral feedings administered via a nasogastric tube because the patient had no evidence of abnormal GI function. Fifty cubic centimeters of full-strength Isocal was administered per hour via the nasogastric tube. Gastric residual volumes, urine glucose, and acetone were checked every 4 hours. This diet gave the patient 1,200 calories per day with 41 g of protein in a volume of 1.2 L/day.

The patient was tolerating mechanical ventilatory support and required 2 mg of IV morphine every 2 to 4 hours for sedation. The 50-cc/hr nasogastric feedings were well tolerated in the first 24 hours, with no sugar or acetone noted in the urine. The following day the feedings were increased to 75 cc/hr, and 4 hours later the gastric residual was noted to be 150 cc. Examination of the patient revealed decreased bowel sounds and slight abdominal distention. Feedings were cut back to 50 cc/hr, and the patient was started on 10 mg of IV metaclopramide every 6 hours. On day 4, feedings were again increased to 75 cc/hr, which resulted in marked abdominal distention, nausea, vomiting, and a gastric residual of 200 cc after 4 hours. A flat-plate x-ray film of the abdomen was taken and was consistent with an ileus.

Discussion

The initial premise that the patient's GI function was adequate to enable enteral feedings was clearly incorrect. The probable causes for this ileus include the morphine sedation and the initiation of mechanical ventilatory support. Metaclopramide enhances GI motility and has an antiemetic action. Although it often helps increase tolerance for enteral feedings, metaclopramide was ineffective for this patient. Fifty cubic centimeters per hour of Isocal feedings are insufficient to provide the patient's caloric and protein requirements. Therefore, it is necessary to either stop the feedings until the factors producing the ileus can be corrected or switch the patient to a regimen of IV alimentation. In view of the severe degree of the patient's nutritional depletion and the probability that this nutritional depletion will adversely impact on the patient's response to infection and the ability to resume spontaneous ventilation, it was decided to switch to IV alimentation.

CASE STUDY CONTINUED

A right subclavian silicone catheter was inserted under aseptic technique to enable IVH. A chest x-ray film taken after placement of the line confirmed the position of the line and revealed no evidence of pneumothorax or hemothorax. The patients WBC count at this time had decreased to 11,000 mm^{-3}, and the patient was normothermic with a normal temperature curve. Intravenous alimentation was started with a mixture of 60% dextrose and an 8.5% amino acid solution with additional electrolytes, trace elements, and vitamins. The infusion was started at a rate of 50 mL/hr, with the goal of increasing it over time to 100 cc/hr, which would provide the patient with 2,448 calories and 102 g of protein per day. To prevent the development of essential fatty acid deficiencies, 500 mL of a 10% lipid emulsion was administered twice a week to provide an additional 1,100 calories per week. The patient tolerated the IV alimentation at 50 cc/hr with no acetone or glucose in the urine. After 24 hours of IV alimentation, the rate was increased to 75 cc/hr, which resulted in 0.1% glucose detected in the urine by Clinitest, no acetone, and a serum glucose level of 180 mg/dL. On the third day of IV alimentation, the infusion rate was increased to 100 mL/hr, which resulted in a 1% urinary glucose and a serum glucose of 325 mg/dL. Fifteen units of regular insulin were added to each liter of hyperalimentation solution and resulted in a lowering of the serum glucose concentration to 120 mg/dL with no glucose or acetone detected in the urine.

Over the next 48 hours the patient continued to tolerate IV feedings and a routine monitoring of arterial blood gases on 40% oxygen revealed a pH of 7.52, a P_{CO_2} of 53 mm Hg, and a P_{O_2} of 71 mm Hg.

The chest x-ray findings showed no significant changes in the infiltrates at this time. The patient remained afebrile. The serum potassium level was noted to have decreased to 3.6 mEq/L with a serum chloride content of 90 mEq/L. Additional potassium chloride was added to the patient's IV fluids to bring it to a total of 40 mEq/L. On the eighth day of IV alimentation (12th hospital day), the serum potassium was 4.3 mEq/L, and arterial blood gases on full ventilatory support with an F_{IO_2} of 0.4 showed a pH of 7.43, a P_{CO_2} of 54 mm Hg, and a P_{O_2} of 83 mm Hg. The UUN was 7 g/day, and a calculated nitrogen balance was $+5.3$ g.

Discussion

Metabolic disturbances are common during hyperalimentation. Close attention must be paid to monitoring serum electrolyte and glucose concentrations because most of these problems are easily corrected.

The following formulas are used to calculate nitrogen balances:

$$\text{Nitrogen balance} = \text{nitrogen in} - \text{nitrogen out}$$

$$\text{Nitrogen balance} = \frac{\text{protein intake}}{\text{grams usable N}_2} - (\text{UUN} + 4)$$

The usable nitrogen per gram of protein is 6.25, and the factor of 4 added to the UUN represents 2 g for nonurea urinary nitrogen, 1 g for fecal nitrogen, and 1 g for nitrogen lost from desquamation of skin and epithelial surfaces. A nitrogen balance of 0 to $+4$ g/day is indicative of anabolism equal to catabolism. Nitrogen balances of $+4$ to $+6$ indicate anabolism occurring at a rate sufficient to restore nutritional status and promote growth.

This patient had now been in the hospital for 12 days and had received a full course of antibiotics and 8 days of appropriate nutritional support. He had a positive nitrogen balance, although only for a short period of time. It would be reasonable to assess the patient with the objective of attempting to wean him from mechanical ventilatory support. Before attempting to wean, it is essential to first determine that the primary reason for the development of ventilatory failure has been corrected and second that there are no other acutely correctable factors that may limit the patient's ability to ventilate spontaneously. These factors would include electrolyte disturbances, hemodynamic imbalances, acid-base imbalances, and inadequate hemoglobin concentration. Because this patient was a known CO_2 retainer, he may in part depend on a hypoxic drive to maintain spontaneous ventilation. Therefore, the inspired oxygen concentration should be decreased to return the arterial oxygenation to a level closer to what is normal for this patient with chronic lung disease.

CASE STUDY CONTINUED

Assessment of the patient revealed marked improvement on the chest x-ray film and clinical findings implying resolution of pneumonia. His electrolyte status was within normal limits. The patient was afebrile and had a positive nitrogen balance. The F_iO_2 was decreased to 0.25, which resulted in the following arterial blood gas values: a pH of 7.42, a Pco_2 of 51 mm Hg, and a Po_2 of 55 mm Hg. The patient was noted to have some spontaneous ventilation at a rate of 20 breaths per minute with a V_T of 250 cc. His measured VC was 900 mL. The patient was placed on a free-flowing continuous positive airway pressure (CPAP) system at +5 cm of water and an F_iO_2 of 0.25. He had a heart rate of 115 beats per minute and a BP of 130/90 mm Hg. The patient felt comfortable. Over the next 4 hours his heart rate increased steadily to 130 beats per minute, and his BP rose to 170/100 mm Hg. The patient complained of shortness of breath, and repeat arterial blood gas analysis revealed a pH of 7.33, a Pco_2 of 64 mm Hg, and a Po_2 of 49 mm Hg on F_iO_2 of 0.25. Mechanical ventilatory support was reinstituted, and the patient's condition stabilized on the ventilator at 8 breaths per minute with a V_T of 1,000 mL.

Repeat measurement of serum albumin revealed a concentration of 3 g/dL, and the serum phosphorus concentration was 2.2 mg/dL. The patient was given IV potassium phosphate, and on the following day the serum phosphorus concentration had risen to 3.8 mg/dL. Carbon dioxide production was measured and found to be 302 mL/min.

Discussion

Hypophosphatemia is associated with ventilatory failure, although the onset of ventilatory failure is usually seen only with levels of phosphorus below 1.8 mg/dL. It is not clear whether the low phosphorus content measured in this patient was a significant factor in his failure to be weaned from mechanical ventilatory support. However, it was deemed wise to correct this deficiency because it may have played a part in the failure to wean.

The high carbon dioxide production measured in this patient probably reflects the high caloric intake of a carbohydrate source. Carbohydrate energy substrates are metabolized with a respiratory quotient of 1 and are associated with marked increase in CO_2 production and minute ventilatory requirements.[10] The metabolic demand on the ventilatory system can be decreased by reducing the total number of calories given to a patient or by reducing the carbohydrate source of those calories and replacing it with fat. Fats are metabolized with a lower respiratory quotient of 0.7

and a lower CO_2 production. In addition, if patients are overfed with carbohydrates, excess carbohydrate will be converted to fats. This process of lipogenesis has a respiratory quotient of 7.0 and is therefore associated with a high CO_2 production.[32]

CASE STUDY CONTINUED

The patient's IV alimentation was changed to a mixture of 40% dextrose and 8.5% amino acid solution, with 25 cc of a 20% lipid emulsion added per hour to provide the appropriate number of calories. This change gave the patient a total of 2,506 calories, of which 1,200 were derived from lipids and 1,306 from carbohydrate sources with 102 g of protein per day. The patient was maintained on mechanical ventilatory support and the new alimentation regimen for 2 days. Carbon dioxide production was remeasured. At this time carbon dioxide production had decreased to 210 cc/min, and the nitrogen balance was found to be +4.3. Once again the patient was removed from mechanical ventilatory support and allowed to breathe spontaneously on a free flowing CPAP system with essentially the same result of a rising arterial PCO_2 and a falling pH. No immediately correctable reason for the patient's inability to ventilate spontaneously could be identified, and it was felt that he required further nutritional repletion. A tracheostomy was performed. The patient was maintained on mechanical ventilatory support with the intention of providing 2 weeks more of IV alimentation before further attempts at weaning would be undertaken.

Twenty-four hours later the patient spiked a fever to 70°C rectally. He had been afebrile for the preceding 7 days.

Discussion

Acceptance of the need for strict aseptic technique in catheter placement and maintenance has led to a fall in catheter-related sepsis to 3% from 7%.[33] Alimentation catheters must be placed under conditions of surgical sterility and dedicated solely to the infusion of alimentation solutions. When a patient receiving IV alimentation develops a fever, a full fever workup should be performed. In addition, the alimentation catheter tip and fluids must be cultured. Inspection of the catheter site often provides useful information. If the catheter grows organisms, then another catheter must be inserted in a new site. If the catheter is found to be uninfected, then alimentation can be reinstituted via the existing site.[34]

CASE STUDY CONTINUED

Blood, urine, and sputum samples were collected and sent for culture and sensitivity studies. A WBC count was measured. Blood was drawn through the alimentation catheter and sent for culture and sensitivity determination, and the IV alimentation solution was returned to the pharmacy for culture and sensitivity tests. The skin site of the subclavian catheter was inspected and looked clean. The subclavian catheter was removed after a guide wire had been inserted through it and the catheter tip sent for culture and sensitivity studies. A fresh catheter was introduced over the guide wire and hyperalimentation fluids discontinued while the patient received 10% dextrose and water through the new catheter. All the cultures were negative, and 24 hours later the patient's fever had subsided. IV alimentation was recommenced at this time. Because the patient's ileus had resolved, it was decided to attempt to reinstitute enteral feedings. A Dobhoff nasoenteral tube was inserted. Once the position of the Dobhoff tube had been verified by x-ray to be in the duodenum, enteral feedings of Isocal were instituted. Over a period of several days, the rate of enteral feedings was increased while the IV alimentation was decreased. During this period the relative volumes and concentrations of enteral and parenteral feedings were adjusted to maintain the same daily delivery of protein, calories, and volume that the patient had been receiving when on full parenteral alimentation. After 4 days the patient was tolerating 125 mL/hr of enteral feedings, and the IV alimentation was discontinued. The patient was maintained on this regimen for 12 more days and remained afebrile during this period. The chest x-ray film was clear, and the WBC count was 7,000 mm^{-3}. Electrolytes were appropriate for a patient with chronic obstructive pulmonary disease, and arterial blood gas analysis on 30% oxygen showed a pH of 7.41, a Pco_2 of 52 mm Hg, and a Po_2 of 72 mm Hg. Remeasured carbon dioxide production was 190 mL/min, and the patient had been in positive nitrogen balance for 3 weeks. His serum albumin concentration was 3.8 g/dL, and serum magnesium, calcium, and phosphorus levels were all within normal limits. Skin antigen testing revealed an appropriate response.

Once again the Fio_2 was reduced to 0.24, and the patient's Pao_2 at this inspired oxygen concentration was 53 mm Hg. Ventilatory support was discontinued, and the patient was maintained on a free-flowing CPAP system with +5 cm of water pressure. His spontaneous ventilatory rate was 22/min with a VT of 280 mL. Vital capacity was 1.1 L. The patient was comfortable and maintained this level of ventilation. His heart rate was 95/min with a BP of 130/90 mm Hg. The extremities remained warm, and the patient continued to pass urine. After 24 hours off mechanical ventilatory support, the tracheostomy tube was replaced with a fenestrated tracheostomy tube that was subsequently corked to enable the patient to breathe through the upper airway. The patient did not develop any further problems, and 2 days later the trachea was decannulated without event.

REFERENCES

1. Keys A, Brozek J, Henschel A: *The Biology of Human Starvation*. Minneapolis, University of Minnesota Press, 1970.
2. O'Connell RC, et al: Nitrogen conservation in starvation: Graded response to intravenous glucose. *J Clin Endocrinol Metab* 1974; 39:555.
3. Addis T, Poo LJ, Lew W: The quantities of protein lost by various organs and tissues of the body during a fast. *J Biol Chem* 1936; 115:111–116.
4. Cahill GF Jr: Starvation in man. *N Engl J Med* 1970; 282:668–675.
5. Moore FD, Brennan MF: Surgical injury: Body composition, protein metabolism and neuroendocrinology, in Ballinger WF, Collins JA, Drucker WR, et al (eds): *Manual of Surgical Nutrition*. Philadelphia, WB Saunders Co, 1975, pp 169–222.
6. Gann DS, Amari JF: Endocrine and metabolic responses to injury, in Schwartz SI, Shires GT, Spencer FC, et al (eds): *Principles of Surgery*, ed 5. New York, McGraw-Hill International Book Co, Inc, 1989, pp 17–19.
7. Bistrian BR, Blackburn GL, Sherman M, et al: Therapeutic index of nutritional depletion of hospitalized patients. *Surg Gynecol Obstet* 1975; 141:512–516.
8. Furst P, Bergstrom J, Liljedahl SO, et al: Nutritional assessment in severe trauma, in *Nutritional Assessment—Present Status, Future Directions and Prospects, Report of the 2nd Ross Conference on Medical Research*. Columbus, Ohio, Ross Laboratories, Columbus, 1986, pp 26–29.
9. Murray MJ, Marsh HM, Wochos DN, et al: Nutritional assessment of intensive care unit patients. *Mayo Clin Proc* 1988; 63:1106–1115.
10. Askanazi J, Rosenbaum SH, Hyman AL, et al: Effects of parenteral nutrition on ventilatory drive. *Anesthesiology* 1980; 53:5185.
11. Dowling RJ, Alexander MA, Mullen JL: Use of fat emulsions, in Deitel M (ed): *Nutrition in Clinical Surgery*, ed 2. Baltimore, Williams & Wilkins, 1985, pp 142–143.
12. Jeejeebhoy KN: Total parenteral nutrition. *Ann R Coll Phys Surg Can* 1976; 9:287–300.
13. Meng HC: Parenteral nutrition: Principles, nutrient requirements, techniques and clinical applications, in Schneider HA, Anderson CE, Coursin DB, (eds): *Nutritional Support of Medical Practice*. New York, Harper & Row Publishers, Inc, 1977, pp 152–183.
14. Recommended Dietary Allowances. A Report of the Food and Nutrition Board, National Research Council, National Academy of Science, ed 8, 1974.
15. Vazquez RM: Vitamin requirements in total parenteral nutrition, in Deitel M (ed): *Nutrition in Clinical Surgery*. Baltimore, Williams & Wilkins, 1985, pp 148–159.

16. Mant MJ, Connolly T, Gordon PA, et al: Severe thrombocytopenia probably due to acute folic acid deficiency. *Crit Care Med* 1979; 7:297–300.
17. Dreyfus PM, Victor M: Effects of thiamin deficiency on the central nervous system. *Am J Clin Nutr* 1961; 9:414–425.
18. Levenson SM, Green RW, Taylor FH, et al: Ascorbic acid, riboflavin, thiamin and nicotinic acid in relation to injury, hemorrhage, and infection in humans. *Ann Surg* 1946; 124:840–856.
19. Chernov MS, Cook FB, Wood M, et al: Stress ulcer: A preventable disease. *J Trauma* 1972; 12:831–833.
20. Shils ME: Guidelines for total parenteral nutrition. *JAMA* 1972; 22:1721–1729.
21. Mertz W, Schroeder HA: Some aspects of glucose metabolism of chromium-deficient rats raised in a strictly controlled environment. *J Nutr* 1965; 86:107–112.
22. Freund H, Atamian S, Fischer JE: Chromium deficiency during total parenteral nutrition. *JAMA* 1979; 241:496–498.
23. Deitch EA, Winterton J, Berg R: The gut as the portal for entry for bacteremia: The role of protein malnutrition. *Ann Surg* 1987; 205:681–692.
24. Nehme AE: Nutritional support of the hospitalized patient: The team concept. *JAMA* 1980; 243:1906–1908.
25. Bozzetti F, Scarpa D, Terno G, et al: Subclavian venous thrombosis due to indwelling catheters: A prospective study on 52 patients. *J Parenter Enteral Nutr* 1983; 7:560–562.
26. Vazquez RM, Jarrard MM: Care of the central venous catheterization site: The use of a transparent polyurethane film. *J Parenter Enteral Nutr* 1982; 8:181–186.
27. Elwyn DH: Repletion of the malnourished patient, in Blackburn GL, Grant JP, Young (eds): *Amino Acids, Metabolism and Medical Applications*. London, John Wright, PSG, Inc, 1983, p 359.
28. Varsano S, Shapiro M, Taragan R, et al: Hypophosphatemia as a reversible cause of refractory ventilatory failure. *Crit Care Med* 1983; 11:908–909.
29. Oh TE, Dyer H, Wall BP, et al: Insulin loss in parenteral nutrition systems. *Anaesth Intens Care* 1976; 4:342–346.
30. Brandt RL, Foley WJ, Fink GH, et al: Mechanism of perforation of the heart with production of hydropericardium by a venous catheter and its prevention. *Am J Surg* 1970; 119:311–316.
31. Bozzetti F, Terno G, Bonfanti G, et al: Prevention and treatment of central venous catheter sepsis by exchange via a guidewire. *Ann Surg* 1983; 198:48–52.
32. Saltarauh A, Salyano JV: Effect of carbohydrate metabolism upon respiratory gas exchange in normal man. *J Appl Physiol* 1971; 30:228.
33. Copeland EM, MacFayden BV, McGowan C, et al: The use of hyperalimentation in patients with potential sepsis. *Surg Gynecol Obstet* 1974; 138:377–380.
34. Blackburn GL: Hyperalimentation in the critically ill patient. *Heart Lung* 1979; 8:67–70.

8/Pain Control and Symptom Management in Critically Ill Patients

DONALD M. SINCLAIR, M.B.B.CH.
ANTHONY GIAMBERDINO, M.D.

Two major symptom complexes of concern in the intensive care unit (ICU) are pain and anxiety. The two complexes are mutually interactive, and each is capable of potentiating the other. Admission to a critical care unit is frequently unplanned and precipitate, and one's attention is naturally given first to control of respiratory, cardiovascular, and other variables. One should remember when the dust of admission settles to spare a thought for symptoms that the patient may have and that he may not be able to communicate. Pain and anxiety are the most common of these. Where admission is planned, the most frequent reason is postoperative care. All patients who have had surgery will have some degree of pain. In a preplanned admission full explanation of the reason for admission, the anticipated treatment and monitoring, a description or even visit to the unit, and where possible, meeting some of the personnel who would be caring for that particular patient will go a long way in allaying fear and anxiety.

Pain is defined as "an unpleasant sensory and emotional experience associated with actual or potential tissue damage, or described in terms of such damage."[1] Anxiety is a psychophysiologic response to real or anticipated danger.

PAIN CONTROL

Pain is the most common symptom of patients seeking medical help. Most often pain is ephemeral and its cause self-limiting. Most headaches and lower back pains, for example, pass either with self-treatment or minor symptomatic treatment by the physician. The pain may, however, be a warning symptom pointing to more sinister underlying pathology that must be diagnosed and treated. **All pain should first be considered a pointer to pathology. Only after this should one consider symptomatic treatment of the pain.** To quote Francis Bacon, "I esteem it the office of a physician not only to restore health but to mitigate pain and dolors." Once it has served its warning and diagnostic functions, pain is both purposeless and unnecessary. When pain has been present for a long time—a matter of months or more—a chronic pain state develops in which the pain is a disease in itself, limiting and crippling the sufferer.

Pain relief is offered primarily for humanitarian reasons. It is probably the oldest function of the physician and the shaman or witch doctor before him to offer comfort and to assuage pain. Prayers and exorcisms for the removal of pain are found in humanity's earliest documents, the clay tablets and papyri of Babylon and Egypt. Even more compelling today is the evidence that apart from its warning value, pain is in itself detrimental to the patient and relief of pain may significantly improve the prognosis.

EFFECTS OF PAIN ON THE BODY

Acute pain is a warning of malfunction. It enforces rest and protection of injured tissue through reflex muscle spasm and splinting. But it also has detrimental effects, especially in the postoperative setting.[2-4]

Many patients with good underlying health are able to tolerate the physiologic "side effects" of pain without apparent adverse effects but, nonetheless, find the pain emotionally disturbing. Some patients are unable to complain of their pain. Adequate pain control can provide a calmer, more rational patient who is better able to comprehend his situation, participate in the decision-making process, and cooperate more actively with treatments such as physical therapy.

Ventilatory Effects

Pain and anxiety lead to hyperventilation with a low P_{CO_2} and high pH.[2, 5, 6] The patient will be breathing rapidly and shallowly and will be reluctant to cough lest this exacerbate the pain. With such splinted respiratory patterns there is a tendency to atelectasis of the dependent portions of the lung and resultant hypoxemia and ultimately to possible pulmonary infection. A markedly reduced functional residual capacity aggravates these changes. Thoracic and upper abdominal surgery have the most marked effects on ventilatory function, but even such relatively periperal surgery as hip replacement significantly changes ventilatory patterns.

Cardiovascular Effects

Pain and anxiety lead to marked changes in the cardiovascular system.[2, 3] These changes are mediated largely through increased sympathetic tone. Increased heart rate, contractility, stroke volume, total peripheral resistance, and blood pressure all lead to additive increases in myocardial oxygen consumption. This can obviously threaten the myocardium in patients with compromised myocardial reserves and, even more critically, those with acute myocardial infarction. It can also be a limiting factor in other patients such as those with burns, infections, or major trauma who already have elevated metabolic rates and oxygen consumptions (V_{O_2}). The V_{O_2} is also markedly raised by circulating catecholamines, and it has been shown that this in itself can be a determining factor in survival. Adequate control of pain that results in a peaceful resting patient minimizes strains on oxygen homeostasis. Regional blood flow is also altered by catecholamines, with especially decreased flow to the periphery and to the splanchnic region. This shunting can have an untoward effect on the outcome in patients with illness in these regions, especially intra-abdominal and peripheral vascular pathologies.

Hematologic Effects

The blood is greatly altered in function by cortisol and catecholamine changes secondary to pain.[2, 7] Blood viscosity and platelet aggregation are increased and fibrinolysis and clotting time altered. Increased viscosity combined with decreased regional blood flow can further threaten homeostasis. There is a definite increase in the incidence of deep-vein thrombosis in those with pain that limits leg movement.

THE NEUROPHYSIOLOGIC BASIS OF PAIN AND THERAPY

For a noxious stimulus to give rise to a perception of pain four processes are involved—transduction, transmission, modulation, and perception.[8] Recall of these processes in an orderly fashion whenever a plan for pain management is being evolved will ensure that all possible sites and methods of pain control are considered.

Transduction

Nerve endings that are sensitive to noxious stimuli are simple, free nerve endings connected to either unmyelinated C fibers or small myelinated A-delta fibers. The process of transduction is the activation of the nerve endings by a stimulus. The stimulus may be tissue trauma, e.g., from sharp instruments, heat, or cold, or it may be pain-producing substances including those released within the tissues such as potassium, serotonin, substance P, histamine, and prostaglandins. These may either directly stimulate the nerve ending, as in the case of potassium, or may sensitize the nerve ending and lower the threshold for painful stimuli, as in the case of prostaglandins. Treatment at the level of transduction is frequently forgottten. Removing the cause in the form of drainage, the use of nonsteroidal anti-inflammatory drugs (NSAID), and the use of local anesthetics topically applied can stop the process of transduction or raise the threshold of transduction. Topical anesthetics on sensitive mucous membranes before interventions such as urinary catheterization and dermal application before large-bore needle interventions, even in the noncommunicative patient, may prevent unnecessary pain. The use of local anesthetic-containing dress-ings at skin graft donor sites greatly reduces pain from the region. Immunosuppressed patients such as those with the acquired immunodeficiency syndrome (AIDS), pa-tients who have had courses of chemotherapy, and older patients in general may develop shingles. This condition is painful in the acute stage, but there is also a tendency to develop post-herpetic neuralgia. This is an exquisitely painful disorder, and the longer treatment is delayed, the harder it is to eliminate the pain. It should be treated in the ICU right along with the patient's other problems. It would be ironic for the patient to be successfully discharged only to find that quality of life is minimal because of resistant neuralgia. A very successful therapy is transdermal capsaicin, which selectively blocks free nerve endings on a long-term basis. While still at the surface as it were, there are recent developments in the transdermal administration of narcotics, especially fentanyl, the transmucosal administration of buprenorphine; and the rectal administration of morphine. These nonstandard routes of administration may occasionally meet the special needs of a patient and offer advantages where fluid load restriction is necessary.

Transmission

Transmission is via the spinothalamic and reticulothalamic pathways (Fig 8–1). The rate of transmission is slow because the fibers involved are small. They are more sensitive than the larger fibers are to local anesthetics, so it is possible to block nerves differentially to remove pain and leave other sensory modalities and motor function at least partially functional. This is done by adjusting the concentration of the local anesthetic used. It is possible to interrupt transmission via these pathways at the six points marked by the methods listed (Fig 8–1).

Modulation

In recent years it has become increasingly apparent that the transmission pathway for pain is amenable to considerable modification. The modulation pathways have their origin in the frontal cortex and the supraoptic hypothalamic nuclei (Fig 8–2). This means that the pain pathways can be powerfully modulated by psychogenic factors. Beecher's observation that soldiers wounded in the heat and excitement of battle require considerably less analgesic than do civilians with similar injuries[9] shows how powerful this modulation can be. Patients who have been prepared for pain deal with it far better than the unprepared.[10] Most available for modification to us is the synaptic region in the dorsal spinal cord where modulating influences act on the incoming signals (the asterisk in Fig 8–2). Some of the modulating synapses here have opioid receptors. Melzack and Wall[11] also postulated a gate mechanism at this site in which a balance of types of input modulates transmission (Fig 8–3). A preponderance of signals via thicker-diameter fibers tends to close the gate to pain transmission, and a preponderance of finer-fiber signals tends to open the gate to pain transmission, thus allowing transmission through to the cortex. Thick-fiber actions ranging from the soothing stroke of a caring hand through warm packs to the use of transcutaneous electrical nerve stimulation (TENS) units all act, at least partially, via this gating mechanism. The application of narcotics to the area of the dorsal route has been a recent major advance.

Perception

This is the most complex part of the pain pathway. Loss of consciousness leads

Transmission

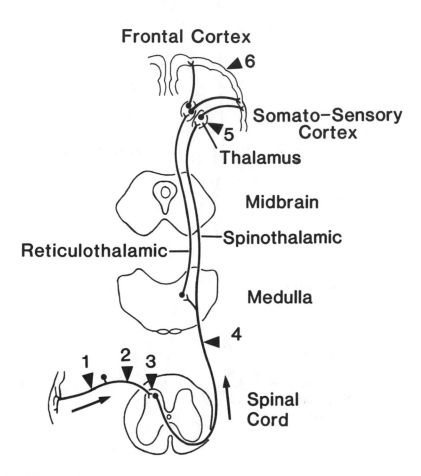

FIG 8–1.
Pain transmission pathway from periphery to cortex. The numbers *1* to *6* represent levels
at which one may modify or block the transmission. (Modified from Fields H: *Pain.* New York,
McGraw-Hill Book Co, 1987, pp 1–131.)

Modulation

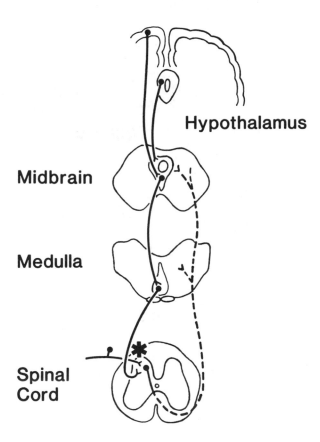

Hypothalamus

Midbrain

Medulla

Spinal Cord

FIG 8–2.
Pain modulation pathways. These are shown as arising at all levels of the neuraxis and acting on the substantia galatinosa (*). Knowledge of these modulating pathways is growing exponentially and this is the site of future pain control growth. (Modified from Fields H: *Pain.* New York, McGraw-Hill Book Co, 1987, pp 1–131.)

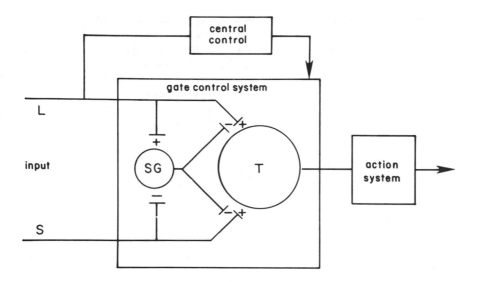

FIG 8–3.
Schematic diagram of the gate control theory of pain. L = large-diameter afferents; S = small-diameter afferents; SG = substantia gelatinosa; T = first transmission cells; + = excitation; − = inhibition. An inhibitory effect is exerted by the SG on the afferent axonal terminals when activated by impulses in the large afferents; this inhibitory effect is decreased by activity in the small afferents. The central control trigger is represented by a line running from the large afferent system to the central control mechanisms; the latter, in turn, project back to the gate control system.

obviously to a loss of perception, and anesthesiologists use the route to conquer pain every day. More complex is modifying perception in the conscious patient. There is a strong cultural component in the interpretation of pain, with some societies being more resistant to pain, this frequently being coupled with a lack of fear of death. There is also an enormous individual variation from the stoical to the near hysterical. Calm explanation of what to expect and of what has happened are very helpful in optimizing perception. Anxiety must be minimized—see below. Other techniques such as biofeedback and hypnosis are very helpful in modifying chronic pain behavior and pain perception but have little place in the critical care setting.

OPIOID RECEPTORS

In the pain pathways discussed there are many synapses where a whole host of peptides and other chemicals act as synaptic transmitters.[12, 13] Of special interest are the opioids. Opium and its derivatives have been a blessing and a curse to humanity as far back as the earliest Mediterranean civilizations. It is only in the 1970s that opium-like substances and their receptors were demonstrated in mammalian nervous systems. These receptors have been classified into μ, κ, and σ opioid receptors and subserve differing functions. The main function of interest, analgesia, is subserved by κ receptors at the spinal level and μ-receptors at a supraspinal level. The other well-known effects of narcotics are ventilatory depression, euphoria or depression, addiction, miosis, skin itching, and urinary difficulty (increased detrussor tone). There is a search for a drug that provides analgesia without respiratory depression or an addictive tendency. Because these actions are from common receptors, this search has so far been unavailing. The demonstration of opioid receptors in the spinal cord has given us a very potent analgesic tool in the form of spinally or epidurally applied narcotics.

TREATMENT OF PAIN

General Approach

Anticipation

Pain should first be anticipated and prevented wherever possible. The use of local anesthetics, regional anesthesia, and intravenous (IV) sedation and analgesics or the administration of general anesthesia where indicated for painful and invasive procedures should always be encouraged. The desirability of these administrations must be weighed against the physiologic state of the patient at the time and the danger to the patient of the administration. It is also possible to prevent pain by the timely performance of a nerve block. For example, a cryoprobe can be used at the time of a thoracotomy to temporarily stop conduction in intercostal nerves. The appropriate use of local anesthesia to skin and mucous membranes has already been mentioned.

Seeking the Cause

A cause for pain must always be sought and the cause removed or treated wherever possible. This is particularly important when a new pain arises. Patients in ICUs frequently develop other problems—often complications of their primary disease or their therapy. Appendicitis, strangulated hernias, infarction of the bowel, expanding aneurysms, kidney stones, carcinomas, and fractures, particularly in the fragile old bedridden patient, are all sources of "unrelated" pain. They may indeed be unrelated to the immediate pathology responsible for admission, but they are most certainly related in that they belong to the patient at hand. They should never be unsuspected.

Therapy

Keep the treatment as simple and safe as possible. This is the therapeutic Occam's razor. If oral therapy with a well-tried drug gives adequate relief, use it in preference to a more exotic "high-tech" method that is certain to be far more expensive and more likely to have graver complications. For example, a patient recovering from plating of a pathologic fracture of the hip and awaiting radiotherapy to the region complained of severe lower back and rib cage pain. The pains were due to other new pathologic fractures. A suggestion had been made to insert a long-term epidural catheter for giving narcotics and/or local anesthetics. Further consideration suggested that there were no contraindications to oral medications or to the use of aspirin. Adequate dosing with oral aspirin combined with judicious later radiotherapy for the bone metastases led to very adequate pain control. On the other hand, what at first thought seems to be the simplest method may turn out to be tedious and complicated on further consideration. Take the time-honored standard hospital regimen of intramuscular (IM) meperidine (Demerol) every 6 hours as needed. The patient develops pain and decides to ride it out because medication is bad for you and, besides, he does not want to disturb the busy nurse. The pain worsens. He has to have relief right now. He calls for the nurse, who takes some time in responding, then frequently continues other more urgent duties, and eventually gives a scaled-down IM dose that takes an hour to peak at an inadequate level. Such a chain of need and response is complex and time-consuming and leads to a poor result. A patient-controlled analgesia (PCA) system may seem a complex solution but is in fact a labor-saving, cheap, and effective answer to this patient's need.

It is important to remember that you cannot measure the patient's pain. In an intensive care setting one is particularly used to dealing in hard ordinal data. But pain is a subjective experience. You may infer pain when a stimulus that you expect to have caused pain leads to an appropriate response—a cry, withdrawal of a limb, tachycardia, or raised blood pressure. But only the patient can measure the pain and tell you about it, either by describing it or marking an analogue pain scale. A problem arises when you feel that the patient has inappropriate pain and is asking for too much medication. You must still accept that the patient, not you the clinician, is the measurer of the pain. Recheck for other causes of pain that may explain why the patient has what you consider to be an inappropriate pain response: Maybe an abscess is forming, a bowel obstruction is developing, or bleeding into a closed space is occuring and leading to more severe pain. Also consider that your patient may be a narcotics addict, that the dose you have given may thus be inadequate, and that you have the problem of narcotic withdrawal to deal with as well. This problem is dealt with later in this chapter. Other pain measurement problems such as exaggerated patient response in the hope of boosting medicolegal or Workmens' Compensation claims are far less likely to give problems in the intensive care setting.

Lastly, individualize your treatment of this very variable and difficult-to-measure symptom. Tailor your plan to the patient, judge the response to the best of your ability, and then modify your plan as needed.

ANALGESICS

Nonsteroidal Anti-inflammatory Drugs and Other Nonnarcotic Analgesics

All these medications offer analgesic, antipyretic, and anti-inflammatory actions. There are a large number available. The possible routes of administration, doses, durations, and side effects vary. Useful lists are available.[14, 15]

Indomethacin, 50 mg, given by rectal suppository has been found to be particularly useful in helping to control visceral pain, especially pain at the site of an intercostal drain, and helps reduce the amount of narcotic required. IV NSAIDs are frequently used to help control temperature. If aspirin is used, its effect of prolonging bleeding time should be remembered, and it should not be used in children.

Ketamine, a phencyclidine, acts on σ-receptors and is a powerful analgesic and anesthetic agent. It also may cause unpleasant disorientation and hallucination. Its use is largely confined to dressing changes and other short painful procedures in intensive care settings. An anesthesiologist with suitable equipment should be present. It has been tried as an analgesic via epidural catheters but not found to be very reliable or efficacious.

Narcotics/Opioid Analgesics

Narcotics are the most commonly used analgesics in the intensive care setting.[16, 17] Many are available, and many new ones are being introduced, especially into anesthetic practice. The term *narcotic* is slipping from pharmacologic fashion, and it is used so widely in the law enforcement field where it refers to a wide number of drugs that may have no narcotic analgesic action, e.g., cocaine. The term *opioid* is replacing it and refers to all drugs, natural, synthetic, or semisynthetic, that act at the opioid receptor sites in the body. Because the term opioid includes the pure antagonists such as naloxone, the term *opioid analgesics* is useful in serving to include only the agonists and mixed agonist-antagonist drugs.

Morphine

Morphine, the main active ingredient of the juice from the seedpod of the poppy, *Papaver somniferum*, remains the mainstay of analgesia in the ICU. There are a host of other synthetic or semisynthetic opiates available, but their advertised advantages do not warrant a change. Morphine is also by far the cheapest of the opiates available. When a patient is allergic or has idiosyncratic reactions to morphine, meperidine (Demerol) may be used.

Morphine acts primarily at the μ-receptors but also at other opioid receptor sites. In the nervous system it is a powerful analgesic that acts on the μ-receptors in the substantia gelatinosa. It probably acts at other sites as well to modify nociceptive impulses. Morphine also acts within the nervous system to depress respiration in a dose-dependent fashion and acts on the oculomotor nerve nucleus to cause pupil constriction—miosis. More variable is its action on higher centers to produce mood changes ranging from euphoria to dysphoria with a peaceful state somewhere between. This variability of response is wide and is both individual and dependent on the presence of pain (less likely to become dysphoric) and emotional state at the time of administration. Action on the chemoreceptor trigger zone is also variable and may cause nausea and vomiting. Addiction is a last and complex central nervous system (CNS) action. In the ICU setting and in a narcotic-naive patient, addiction is very rarely a problem. Substance abuse is far more likely to be a problem in staff and family than in the patient, unless the patient is already a substance abuser.

Morphine causes constipation by its actions on the small and large bowel and may lead to itching of the skin that may be very unpleasant.

Morphine may lead to histamine release in patients, and this may be associated with troublesome hypotension or bronchospasm. The hypotension may be particularly marked in patients where other causes for hypotension are also present, most notably relative hypovolemia. Morphine administration should thus be started cautiously with small incremental dosing.

For all its side effects, morphine is a most satisfactory drug when tailored in dose, frequency, and route of administration to each patient's needs.

Meperidine

Meperidine (Demerol) is a synthetic opioid introduced into medicine in 1939. It has similar side effects to morphine, and in equianalgesic doses it causes equal respiratory depression. It is about ten times less potent. Its pharmacokinetics have been widely studied, and it has been shown that satisfactory analgesia is best obtained by the use of some system to avoid excessive swings in plasma concentration. There is a high incidence of dizziness in mobile patients, and excessively high concentrations may lead to convulsions that are caused by an accumulation of a metabolite.

Other Opiates

Fentanyl

Patients may arrive in the ICU already heavily narcotized with other opiates. The most common example is patients who have had high-dose narcotic anesthetics, especially high-dose fentanyl for open heart surgery. Fentanyl is a synthetic phenylpiperidine 800 to 1,000 times more potent than meperidine. It has a major advantage over morphine and meperidine in that it does not release histamine from mast cells and so may be given at a relatively high rate to rapidly achieve very high serum levels. This has made it popular in anesthesia. Fentanyl serum levels decrease very sharply, 98% having disappeared in the first hour after administration, largely due to equilibration with (1) the vessel-rich organs and (2) fat. It is eliminated from the body by the liver, and because there is virtually 100% extraction by the liver, the rate of elimination is hepatic blood flow dependent. Hepatic blood flow may be markedly altered in sick patients. In effect, if "industrial doses" have been used, the patient is heavily sedated at arrival in the ICU and requires ventilation for at least some hours, usually until the next morning. As the fentanyl wears off, these patients may become agitated, but their respiratory drive may still be inadequate for weaning. In this case they need adequate sedation.

Sufentanil

This drug is ten times more potent than fentanyl is and is the most potent opioid currently available for human use. Sufentanil enjoys especial popularity in some circles in achieving "stress-free" anesthesia, especially for major vessel surgery. It's pharmacokinetics are midway between those of fentanyl and alfentanil, and those who use this drug find that the patients are often ready for extubation about 6 hours after the loading dose. Because major vascular surgery may often outlast this period, many of these patients reach the recovery room or the ICU extubated. The danger in these patients is that they may either spontaneously develop respiratory depression or may react very sensitively to any further narcotic given in response to pain. They should be watched very carefully.

Alfentanil

This drug is only one quarter as potent as fentanyl. It has a very short elimination half-life and has found special application in the field of neuroanesthesia. General anesthesia usually depresses many CNS actions along with its depression of consciousness. In some circumstances it is desirable to maintain some of these neurologic functions at a normal or near-normal level. This is so that one is able to monitor the integrity of the neuraxis during surgery. Stimuli are fed into the neuraxis below the site that may be disrupted, and consequent evoked signals are monitored above this site—evoked-potential monitoring. Alfentanil by continuous infusion in combination with infused benzodiazepines or more commonly with a low dose of forane, an inhalation anesthetic agent, allows for both satisfactory anesthesia and evoked-potential monitoring. Patients receiving this type of anesthesia are characteristically awake and breathing spontaneously very soon after its use has been discontinued—even after anesthesias lasting half a day or more. They frequently arrive in the recovery area breathing spontaneously and even extubated. They require even more meticulous watching than do patients administered sufentanil because their remarkable state of consciousness lulls one into a false sense of security while they may in fact develop inadequate ventilation in the following hours, and the onset of this failure may not be gradual.

Reversal of Narcotic Effect

If the patient is already extubated, one must weigh reintubation against reversal of the respiratory depression by administration of either naloxone or naltrexone. These are pure opioid antagonists. Before using them, remember that you will reverse not only the respiratory depressive effects of the narcotic but also the analgesic effects and you may change from having an unduly depressed patient to having a restless, anxious patient in pain. This change may lead to trading a ventilatory problem for cardiovascular instability (tachycardia, hypertension, arrhythmias, and pulmonary edema may all follow the use of naloxone, especially if given rapidly or in large dose) or raised intracranial pressure now not due to a rising pCO_2 but to the straining of the patient. Any reversal should be carefully titrated to effect, and one should remember that the antagonist's effect may wear off before the underlying narcotic problem has adequately waned. Naloxone in increments of 40 μg (i.e., 1 cc of a 1-in-10 dilution of naloxone) may be given IV at 2-minute intervals, and with patience a state will be reached in which ventilation is adequate but the patient is still comfortable. Until this state is reached, the patient may be told to breathe more, or the ventilation may be assisted by a manual ventilator and mask.

Other Opioids

Mixed agonist-antagonists are used for analgesia. Their use in the ICU is limited at this time. Pentazocine, for instance, has a ceiling effect for analgesia that may be too low for satisfactory pain relief, and there is a high incidence of dysphoria and hallucinations. It also causes undesirable cardiovascular side effects, most especially increases in both systemic and pulmonary vascular resistances. Finally, when administered to a patient already loaded with a pure agonist, the mixed effect of this drug along with its low potency may in fact lead to a decrease rather than an increase in analgesia. More recent mixed agonist-antagonists such as butorphanol show more promise and may provide adequate analgesia with fewer respiratory depressant effects and an acceptable incidence of other side effects. We have no experience with these drugs in the ICU setting, where morphine still reigns supreme.

ROUTES OF ADMINISTRATION
Intramuscular Injection

Narcotics have traditionally been given to patients by IM injection. This has a series of major disadvantages. There is a time delay from the patient requesting analgesia to its administration. There is a further time delay with absorption of the drug, and its peak effect is only reached at 45 minutes to 1 hour in the physiologically sound. In patients with vasoconstriction and impaired circulation, the delay is unknown. In fact, placement of any drug into muscle tissue in such a patient is like lighting a fuse of unknown delay. Drugs administered may remain in the vasoconstricted muscle until the circulation is improved, at which time the drug, perhaps long forgotten, is absorbed. In an ICU such a route is inappropriate. Subcutaneous injection is even more inappropriate.

Intravenous Injection

The replacement of IM injection by IV bolus injection of opioids represented a quantum leap forward. There is a certainty of the fate of the drug, the peak effect is seen in minutes, the desired end point is reached rapidly, and the dose may be repeated to effect as needed. The problem with this is that it is labor intensive for personnel involved because dosing is repeated more often than with IM injections. With morphine, typical boluses for an adult would be 2 mg. With meperidine this would be 20 to 25 mg. This bolus would be repeated every 5 minutes until adequate analgesia was reached. As understanding of pharmacokinetics has improved along with changing technology of small pumps suitable for continuous administration, it has become possible to load the patient with boluses as described and then to maintain analgesia with a continuous infusion. This spares labor and ensures a more even and, we hope, a more satisfactory blood level of the drug. The disadvantages are that the technique adds a level of complexity to the care and also makes it easier to not monitor the patient as closely. Without careful observation, overdosage is a danger.

A dosage with morphine may well begin at 10 μg/kg lean body mass per hour and be adjusted as needed. As long as the dangers and limitations are understood, this is an elegant and effective method of obtaining analgesia in the ICU. The meperidine dosage would be 75 to 100 μg/kg/hr. There would be little sense in the ICU setting in using the shorter-acting and more expensive newer narcotics to achieve long-term results.

Patient-Controlled Analgesia

In patients who are conscious and able to understand and move, there is the option of using PCA, a system in which the patient controls his own analgesia by pressing a button whenever he feels that he needs more pain relief.[18-20] This releases an IV bolus of preselected amount. The patient may trigger the system as often as he needs. A safety lockout is built in that prevents more than a physician has selected as the maximum amount per hour. As the patient becomes pain free and sedate, he ceases activating the apparatus, and so the blood levels start to wane with concomitant waxing of the pain. This arouses the patient, who presses the button once more, thus relieving the pain and lapsing into rest again. While this may seem to be degrading the patient to the Pavlovian level of a trained reflex responder, it is in fact a very satisfactory method of pain control. The patient does not perceive himself as an automated link in a feedback loop, but rather as master of some small part of his destiny and well-being in what from the patient's viewpoint is otherwise a threatening and dependent-making environment. Patients require less opioid, experience better pain relief, and express more overall satisfaction with this method than with the more traditional methods. In the postoperative setting, this has also been shown to lead to fewer postoperative complications, shorter ICU stays, and earlier hospital discharge.

The PCA systems range from sophisticated pumps with complex programming possibilities and the ability to track the dosage given and how often the patient has requested medication to a simple disposable system in which there is a fixed volume delivered per bolus and a fixed maximum per hour. Here the dosage is changed by changing the concentration of the dose delivered. Morphine is again the most common opioid used, and typical boluses would be 1 mg in the adult with a maximum of 6 mg/hr. Patient size, physiologic status, other drugs, previous drug experience, and wide variation of need will mean that the bolus may be in the range of 0.5 to 3 mg and the hourly maximum from 2 to 20 mg. The maximum dose per hour may also be expressed as a lockout period. If the bolus is 1 mg and the maximum allowed per hour is 6 mg, the lockout period is 10 minutes. Doses for meperidine would again be seven to ten times the morphine dose.

Epidural Administration

Insertion of an epidural catheter allows profound analgesia to be achieved.[21] If the patient is to have surgery, this may be done preoperatively. The catheter is placed at an appropriate vertebral level—usually lumbar, but occasionally thoracic.

TABLE 8–1.

Analgesic Dose Averages*

	Morphine	Meperidine	Fentanyl
Bolus dose†	0.025 mg/kg	0.1 mg/kg	0.001 mg/kg
Infusion			
Concentration	0.1 mg/cc saline	5 mg/cc saline	0.01 mg/cc saline‡
Rate	5 cc/hr	5 cc/hr	5 cc/hr
Dose/hr	0.5 mg	25 mg	0.05 mg

*These doses are guidelines only. Dosages may vary widely.
†All in 10 cc normal saline.
‡Mix 20 cc of fentanyl (0.05 mg/cc) in 80 cc saline to give a concentration of 0.01 mg/cc.

The accuracy of placement is checked by giving a test dose of local anesthetic through the catheter after aspirating for blood or cerebrospinal fluid (CSF). If aspiration is positive, no test dose is given, and the catheter is removed and reinserted. The test dose may be 3 cc of 1% lidocaine with 1-in-100,000 epinephrine. If the pulse is monitored, an increased rate and strength of the pulse should be felt if the dose has been given IV and a noticeable spinal level obtained with leg weakness if the catheter is intrathecal. Again, in either case the catheter must be removed and reinserted. It is very important to ritualistically check for catheter misplacement to avoid unwanted surprises and complications. A further 3 cc of plain 1% lidocaine should give a pronounced band of analgesia on the trunk if the catheter is correctly inserted.

After surgery the catheter may be used to supply analgesia. Morphine and fentanyl are the most common drugs used. If using morphine, a special preservative-free formulation should be used to avoid possible nerve damage. Morphine is less lipid soluble than fentanyl is and therefore binds less with the spinal cord and is more likely to reach CSF concentrations that may depress respiration when the morphine reaches the fourth ventricle region. CSF circulation is slow, and it may take as long as 8 hours for it to circulate from the lumbar region to the ventricle. This means that careful monitoring of respiration is essential if the patient is breathing spontaneously.

A bolus of the drug selected should be given and is usually diluted in 10 cc of preservative-free saline. This volume is required to achieve wide-enough anatomic spread to involve the necessary dermatomes. This bolus takes about half an hour to work and so should be given in advance of anticipated awakening. In the awake patient the pain should be controlled by IV opiates until the epidural drugs become effective. A continuous-infusion pump is then started, where again the dose and the volume used should be sufficient to achieve a density of analgesia over the involved dermatomes.

Table 8–1 lists average doses and infusion rates as guides that must be adjusted to the individual patient's needs. It is usual to alter the volume first to achieve more or less analgesia as needed and only to alter the concentration if it is felt that spread is sufficient but the density of analgesia is insufficient. In changing concentrations, it is normal to double the concentration and then to cut back on the volume given per hour. Local anesthetic agents may be infused along with or in lieu of the opioids.

Bupivicaine, 0.125%, is the usual drug chosen for length of action and adequate analgesia. This strength may have to be increased to 0.25% in some patients. The local anesthetic blocks not only the thin pain-conducting fibers but also the sympathetic efferents and may lead to hypotension, especially if there is hypovolemia. The heavy limbs that result from motor nerve block are also a problem. The patient must be assisted when moving and not allowed to stay in a fixed position for too long lest he develop venous stasis or pressure effects.

Side effects of the opioids are nausea and vomiting, pruritus, and urinary retention. All of these effects may be reversed by the administration of naloxone. If it is titrated carefully in the minimal necessary dosage, the analgesia may remain satisfactory. Migration of the catheter into the CSF or the blood stream is always a possibility that should be borne in mind. Infection may occur at the site of the catheter, and unexplained tenderness in the area or unexplained pyrexia should lead one to review this possibility.

Epidural catheters are contraindicated in the face of systemic infection or where blood coagulation is not adequate. If the catheter is to be used for longer than 3 days or so, it should be tunneled in the same manner as a central line placed for long-term use. These catheters have been used for longer than 6 months. Such long-term use is usually in patients with malignancy. The cost of preservative-free morphine is very high, and ordinary morphine has been used for long periods of time with no apparent neurologic sequelae in these long-term patients.

NONPHARMACOLOGIC METHODS OF PAIN CONTROL

There are some nonpharmacologic methods of pain control that may be used alone or more frequently in combination with other methods.

Transcutaneous Electrical Nerve Stimulation

TENS is the most common nonpharmacologic method of pain control.[22] A small electrical current is applied in the area of the source of the pain. The device is organized so that the strength, frequency, and pulse width can all be altered. The stimulus is designed to stimulate large myelinated fibers so as to alter the "balance" in the spinal gating mechanism and thus help block small-fiber pain transmission. Sterile electrodes are available for placement parallel to the sound site at surgery. It is seldom that TENS will offer adequate pain relief alone in the acute situation, but it has been shown to decrease the need for opioids significantly.

Psychological Coping Strategies

Various cognitive coping strategies using distraction, attention, or both can modify patient response to noxious stimuli.[23, 24] To an extent, PCA may work by allowing the patient to cope and control one small aspect of their being in the busy and dominant ICU environment. Learned techniques may also be added and include deep breathing, relaxation, self-hypnosis, and the use of imagery.

While all of these techniques are useful, they require instruction of the patient before admission to the ICU. This limits them at this time to postoperative patients. However, counseling and the application of psychological techniques in appropriate patients and for families in the ICU setting should always be considered.

CONTROL OF ANXIETY

Anxiety and agitation may have similar detrimental physiologic effects to pain.[25, 26] A restless, agitated patient is also difficult to manage, and vital IV and other lines may be threatened by the patient thrashing about. So prompt and adequate treatment of anxiety is an important part of intensive care medicine. Treatment varies with the severity of symptoms. For purposes of discussion it will be assumed that adequate analgesia has already been provided and we are faced with a patient who remains anxious.

Anxiety can arise from two different sources. First, the illness itself or its treatment may have a direct effect on CNS function. Table 8–2 lists common medical causes of anxiety that need to be considered. Second, the illness may have an effect on the patient's mind. Although CNS function is normal, the psychological reaction to being ill may cause fear, depression, agitation, paranoia, or hostility. These psychological processes are frequently the result of disorientation, fear of death or disability, loss of autonomy, disturbances in sleep patterns, stress of procedures, voicelessness from intubation, and poor interactions with staff. The role of communication and good rapport cannot be overemphasized. Repeated orientation and a discussion of the pathophysiology, treatment plan, and prognosis on a layman level with patient and family can often reduce the need for medication. If these measures prove ineffective, anxiolytic therapy should be started. The ideal drug would possess no hemodynamic or respiratory side effects, have a short elimination half-life, and would not depend on normal renal or hepatic function for clearance. The ideal drug does not exist at this time.

Narcotics have been discussed under analgesic therapy above. Morphine is useful as a sedative, especially if there is a component of pain. Advantages include staff familiarity with dosing and side effects and the ability to reverse its action if necessary. However, morphine is only a mild anxiolytic, and large doses may be required to

TABLE 8–2.

Common Medical Causes of Anxiety

Drug side effect/toxicity/withdrawal	Meningitis/encephalitis
Electrolyte imbalance	Seizures
Hepatic failure	Sepsis
Hypertensive encephalopathy	Shock
Hypoglycemia	Thyroid dysfunction
Hypoxemia/hypercarbia	Uremia
Intracranial pathology	Wernicke's disease

calm more agitated patients. This may lead to undesired respiratory depression and venodilation. Narcotics may also produce dysphoria.

Benzodiazepines

The drugs of choice for treating anxiety are the benzodiazepines. Because drugs in this group possess similar anxiolytic properties, the choice of a particular agent is based on elimination half-life, duration of action, and personal familiarity. Like narcotics, benzodiazepines are metabolized in the liver with subsequent renal excretion. Prolonged effects can be expected in patients with impaired hepatic function. Many of the benzodiazepines are converted to active metabolites that themselves have long half-lives. Examples include diazepam, chlordiazepoxide, and clorazepate. Continued use of these drugs can lead to an accumulation of active metabolites and excessive sedation, especially in the elderly. Examples of benzodiazepines with weakly active or inactive metabolites include lorazepam, oxazepam, temazepam, and the newest agent, midazolam. In addition to their anxiolytic (low dose) and hypnotic (higher dose) effects, benzodiazepines possess anticonvulsant and muscle relaxant activity. These drugs have a very useful amnesic property as well, which can be most desirable in the ICU setting.

Athough the benzodiazepines are generally considered to have a high therapeutic index, even in critically ill patients, they do have the potential to produce undesirable side effects. Respiratory effects are reductions in tidal volume with a compensatory increase in respiratory rate. The net effect is minimal in usual doses. Subanesthetic doses decrease the hypoxic respiratory drive. In large IV doses they can cause apnea, especially when used in combination with narcotics (which blunt the compensatory increase in respiratory rate). This risk is increased in patients with preexisting respiratory disease. Therefore, smaller doses and greater caution should be used when combining benzodiazepines with narcotics or other CNS depressants.

Hemodynamic effects are usually minimal in sedative doses. Small decreases in peripheral resistance and cardiac output are common. This can lead to hypotension in patients with unstable cardiovascular function. It is best to administer these drugs in small IV increments with adequate bedside monitoring and titrate them to effect. CNS effects increase with age and include light-headedness, psychomotor impairment, anterograde amnesia, and lassitude. The onset of slurred speech has been suggested as a useful end point for therapy. There is great individual variation in dose requirements. Paradoxical excitation can occur and is thought to result from disinhibition of arousal centers. Although there are numerous benzodiazepines available, we will limit the discussion to the commonly used IV agents.

Diazepam is the most commonly used benzodiazepine in the intensive care setting. Its initial dose is typically 2 to 5 mg IV or orally, with less given to elderly or more compromised patients. Larger doses may be required for more agitated patients. Its peak effect is reached in to 2 to 20 minutes when given IV and 30 to 180 minutes after oral doses. Nordiazepam is the primary metabolite and is active with a half-life of 100 to 200 minutes. Repeat doses may lead to prolonged sedation. Once the patient is calmed, IV dosing should be as needed (2 to 4 mg every 4 hours).

Alternatively, the patient can be administered two or three oral doses daily. Diazepam should not be administered IM because absorption is unpredictable. Diazepam is not water soluble and is manufactured in 40% propylene glycol. It can cause pain and phlebitis at the injection site. The manufacturer recommends 5 mg/min to be the maximum injection rate.

Lorazepam is advocated for use in intensive care because it produces fewer adverse effects on cardiopulmonary function when compared with diazepam. Furthermore, it has a shorter elimination half-life (1.5 hour) and inactive metabolites. It can be given IM and sublingually (SL) in addition to oral and IV administration. The initial IV or IM dose is 1 to 2 mg. The oral or SL dose is 0.5 to 1 mg. The time to peak effect is somewhat slower than with diazepam, 60 to 120 minutes for IM and oral administration and 20 to 60 minutes for SL and IV dosing. Once the patient is calmed, three-times-daily (TID) oral or as-needed IV dosing may proceed. As with diazepam, lorazepam can cause pain and phlebitis at the injection site. The manufacturer recommends a 2-mg/min maximum injection rate.

Midazolam is a newer benzodiazepine. It has the advantages of rapid onset and short elimination half-life. It is also water soluble and does not cause tissue reactions at the injection site. The initial IV dose is 1 to 2 mg (a quarter to half of the diazepam dose). Its peak effect is reached in 3 to 5 minutes. This rapid onset makes midazolam easier to titrate. The elimination half-life is 2 to 4 hours. After the patient is calmed, subsequent doses can be given as needed every 1 to 2 hours, or an infusion can be started at 0.1 to 0.4 μg/kg/min. Continuous infusion of midazolam regimens is becoming increasingly popular in the ICU setting. The initial IM dose is 2 to 4 mg, with a peak effect in 30 to 60 minutes. There is no oral preparation.

The initial doses stated above are conservative starting points for stable adults. Adequate time should be allowed for the peak effect before administering subsequent doses. If the initial dose has minimal or no effect, subsequent doses should be increased until the desired effect is seen. Maintenance doses should start at 25% of the initial sedating dose. Rebound anxiety or insomnia is more frequently associated with drugs with a shorter half-life. A benzodiazepine antagonist is under investigation but is not yet available.

Miscellaneous Drugs

Other drugs have been used for sedation in intensive care. Etomidate infusions offer the advantage of better hemodynamic stability and more rapid onset. However, etomidate has been shown to inhibit adrenal steroidogenesis and has been largely abandoned. Barbiturates have the disadvantages of myocardial depression and long elimination half-lives. Although they are still used in neurointensive care for brain protection, they have been largely replaced by the benzodiazepines for sedation. Nitrous oxide/oxygen mixtures are effective for sedation and analgesia but are in limited use because of resultant bone marrow suppression, neurotoxicity, and the need for specialized equipment and scavenging systems. Ketamine offers the advantages of respiratory and hemodynamic stimulation as well as intense analgesia. It can be used as an infusion for sedation but is more commonly used for sedation and analgesia during short, stimulating procedures such as dressing changes. It has the disadvantages of occasional dysphoric reactions and increased airway secretions.

TREATMENT OF DELIRIUM

Delirium is defined as "a condition of extreme mental, and usually motor excitement, marked by a rapid succession of confused and unconnected ideas, often with illusions and hallucinations." As anxiety increases, a combination of personality, environment, and disease can decrease the meaningfulness of sensory input and detaches the patient from his surroundings. As with anxiety and milder agitation it is important to pursue organic etiologies. However, treatment must often be initiated before a full workup can be completed because delirious patients often jeopardize their own safety. Anxiolytics and narcotics are usually ineffective, as are psychosocial measures.

Intensive care unit psychosis is a transient psychotic reaction to the stress of the intensive care environment. It has become a popular catchall term for all agitated patients in intensive care without demonstrated organic etiology. However, true psychosis is uncommon in intensive care. Delirium is more commonly a manifestation of panic, fear, disorientation, depression, or hostility. Therefore, patients with true ICU psychosis account for a small subset of delirious patients.

Treatment goals in delirium are protection of the patient (and staff) from injurious behavior, control of agitation, and resolution of any organic etiology.[25-27] The use of restraints is the quickest way to protect the patient from self-injury. This is a temporizing measure while pharmacologic therapy and organic workup is begun. Restraints may increase agitation, especially in paranoid patients, and should be cautiously discontinued after agitation has been adequately controlled. Commonly, patients have already been treated with an anxiolytic or a narcotic by the time their agitation has progressed to delirium. Attempts to increase the dosage of these agents to control delirium may lead to deleterious respiratory depression or circulatory instability. This will complicate delirium by adding hypoxemia, hypercarbia, or hypotension to the problem. For this reason a neuroleptic agent should be used once "reasonable" doses of anxiolytics or narcotics have failed. In contrast to benzodiazepines and narcotics, neuroleptics have little or no potential for exacerbating delirium.

At this time there are no clear data demonstrating advantages of one neuroleptic over another. Therefore, it seems prudent to become familiar with the use of one drug. Haloperidol is the most common neuroleptic used in the intensive care setting. IV administration is recommended for acute situations because IM dosing can increase discomfort and agitation and has been associated with a high incidence of extrapyramidal side effects. Intravenous haloperidol does not have Food and Drug Administration (FDA) approval at this time, so documentation of risks and benefits is recommended. Haloperidol has trivial effects on respiratory and hemodynamic function when compared with the benzodiazepines and narcotics. It possesses mild α-antagonistic properties. Hypotension is rare and is usually seen where low systemic vascular resistance or hypovolemia already exists. Concurrent administration of haloperidol and propranolol has been associated with hypotension and cardiopulmonary arrest. Laryngeal dystonia is a rare complication, but airway support equipment should be readily available. QT prolongation may be seen after extremely high doses. Haloperidol has a slower onset of action (11 minutes) when compared with benzodiazepines and narcotics. Therefore, dosing intervals of 20 to 30 minutes are recommended. Its peak effect is reached in 45 minutes. The initial IV dose is 2 mg for mild and 5 to 10 mg for moderate to severe agitation. Subsequent doses should be doubled until the desired effect is observed. The addition of 1 mg lorazepam to haloperidol doses over 20 mg may reduce the required haloperidol dose through a synergistic effect. Once the patient is calmed, smaller doses can be administered two to three times daily, with a larger dose given at night when delirium is more common. As the patient's condition improves, therapy can be tapered to a single nightly dose. The oral dose is two times the IV dose. Haloperidol precipitates in solution with heparin or phenytoin.

Nondepolarizing Muscle Relaxants

In the event that all attempts at sedation fail, it may be necessary to pharmacologically paralyze the patient. This should be considered a last resort in patients with life-threatening agitation or incapacitating side effects from sedative therapy (respiratory depression, laryngeal dystonia, hypotension). Nondepolarizing muscle relaxants are used. Pancuronium in doses of 0.05 to 0.1 mg/kg work within 5 minutes with a duration of 1 to 2 hours. Subsequent doses of 1 to 2 mg can be given every 1 to 2 hours. Side effects include antimuscarinic actions and block of norepinephrine reuptake, both of which can elevate the heart rate, blood pressure, and cardiac output. Vecuronium in an identical loading dose has minimal hemodynamic effects. However, its short duration of action makes a maintenance infusion more practical than intermittent bolus dosing.

Neuromuscular blocking agents can be used only in patients who are intubated and ventilated. It must be remembered that these drugs possess no amnestic or sedative properties and that paralysis can be a terrifying experience. Provisions must be made for adequate sedation, analgesia, and amnesia even though the patient appears calm. Explanation and reassurance are also essential. The use of neuromuscular blocking agents and mechanical ventilation increases the risk of pulmonary complications and deep venous thrombosis. Meticulous attention to positioning is necessary to prevent traction and pressure injuries. It is sometimes necessary to paralyze an agitated patient to enable placement of lines and monitors and for initiation of supportive therapy. Once these goals have been achieved, more conventional sedation can be used. If paralysis is to be used, rapid sequence intubation is mandatory if the possibility exists that the stomach may be full. This protects against aspiration.

WITHDRAWAL FROM NARCOTICS AND OTHER ABUSED SUBSTANCES

A subset of patients manifesting anxiety or agitation are those experiencing substance withdrawal.[28, 29] Substance abuse is seen most commonly in multiple trauma victims. By their life-styles, these patients are especially prone to trauma. In general, withdrawal syndromes consist of rebound activity in the physiologic systems that are modified by the abused drug. In most withdrawal syndromes, sympathetic hyperactivity is a dominant manifestation. Unfortunately, it is also a dominant manifestation of agitation from other etiologies. This point emphasizes the importance of taking a thorough history and developing a strong clinical suspicion. The cornerstone of withdrawal therapy is substituting a cross-tolerant drug for the abused substance. Using the appropriate drug obviates the need for large doses of a drug that is not cross-tolerant to gain control of the situation.

Alcohol Withdrawal

Alcohol depresses neuronal excitability, conduction, and transmitter release. Chronic ingestion leads to neurophysiologic compensation for this state of continuing depression in an attempt to normalize function. In abrupt withdrawal, these compensatory changes become maladaptive and give rise to neural hyperexcitability within 6 to 8 hours. The intensity of withdrawal is related to the intensity and duration of previous alcohol consumption. In mild withdrawal, symptoms include tremor, insomnia, and irritability. These usually resolve within 48 hours. In severe withdrawal these symptoms progress to tremulousness, confusion, hallucinosis, hyperpyrexia, and lowering of the seizure threshold. These more severe symptoms are usually manifested 48 to 72 hours after the last alcohol consumption. Severe alcohol withdrawal is also referred to as delirium tremens and occurs in approximately 5% of hospitalized alcoholics. Mortality from delirium tremens can be as high as 15% but is probably much lower because of improvements in supportive care. The second component of alcohol withdrawal is a stress response to the hyperexcitability phenomenon that is characterized by elevated levels of circulating catecholamines. Their effect is potentiated by preexisting upregulation of β-adrenergic receptors induced by chronic alcohol ingestion. The net result is an increase in cardiac output (by increasing both heart rate and contractility), blood pressure, and the potential for dysrhythmias. Other abnormalities frequently encountered in alcohol withdrawal are listed in Table 8–3.

Treatment goals include control of subjective symptoms, treatment of coexisting medical pathology, control and prevention of seizures and dysrhythmias, and prep-

TABLE 8–3.

Pathologic Abnormalities Frequently Associated With Alcohol Withdrawal

Hepatic dysfunction	Malnutrition
Hypoglycemia	Pneumonia
Hypokalemia	Respiratory alkalosis
Hypomagnesemia	Upper GI hemorrhage

aration for rehabilitation. Many drugs have been used successfully in the treatment of alcohol withdrawal, including barbiturates, antihistamines, chloral hydrate, and the major tranquilizers. However, these drugs have been largely replaced by the benzodiazepines because they offer the advantages of familiarity, a high therapeutic index, and anticonvulsant activity. There is currently no evidence supporting the use of one benzodiazepine over another. Diazepam, chlordiazepoxide, and clorazepate are commonly used. Again, it seems wise to become familiar with the use of one drug and use it consistently. Treatment is begun with diazepam, 10 mg IV slowly, followed by 5 mg every 5 to 10 minutes until the patient is completely calm. Typical loading doses range from 30 to 60 mg. The patient can then receive oral therapy, 5 to 20 mg every 6 hours. The daily dose is then tapered by 25% every day. These are just guidelines because therapy must be individualized. Some advocate switching to a short–half-life drug for oral therapy to avoid the possibility of accumulating active metabolites with subsequent oversedation. Oxazepam or lorazepam would be appropriate choices. Midazolam infusions have also been used successfully. Seizures are treated with IV diazepam and suitable airway maintenance and protection. There is no need for prolonged phenytoin therapy unless the patient has a preexisting seizure disorder. Small doses of haloperidol (0.5 to 2 mg) may be helpful in controlling hallucinosis. All patients suspected of having alcohol withdrawal should be given 100 mg of thiamine on admission to prevent Wernicke's syndrome. Propranolol can be used to treat adrenergic hyperactivity.

Opiate Withdrawal

Opiate withdrawal has features in common with alcohol withdrawal. The syndrome is variable and depends on the drug, dose, interval, duration of use, and personality of the abuser. Typically, symptoms begin 8 to 15 hours after the last dose and consist of anxiety, depression, restlessness, and irritability. These progress over a period of 24 hours to the constellation of symptoms and signs listed in Table 8–4.

Very rarely the syndrome may progress to convulsions and cardiovascular collapse. Symptoms usually subside in 5 to 10 days. The syndrome is more gradual in onset, less intense, and longer in duration when withdrawal is from longer-duration drugs such as methadone.

Withdrawal can be precipitated within seconds by the administration of opioid antagonists or mixed agonist/antagonists to patients with unsuspected opiate addic-

TABLE 8–4.

Signs and Symptoms of Opiate Withdrawal

Abdominal cramps	Dilated pupils	Sneezing
Anorexia	Gooseflesh*	Tachycardia
Coryzia	Hypertension	Tremors
Diaphoresis	Nausea	Weakness
Diarrhea		

*hence the term *cold turkey*

tion. Treatment of withdrawal consists of titration of a parenteral narcotic in incremental doses until symptoms subside. The patient can then receive oral methadone, usually 20 to 40 mg/day, which is then gradually tapered. Clonidine replaces opiate depression with α_2-mediated CNS depression and has been used to control withdrawal symptoms. In the ICU setting, it would probably be best to maintain the patient on a narcotics regimen and institute weaning and counseling during a later recovery phase.

TREATMENT OF MECHANICALLY VENTILATED PATIENTS WHO ARE AGITATED

A final subgroup of agitated ptients deserving special attention are those receiving mechanical ventilation.[30, 31] As with spontaneously breathing patients, goals for sedation include analgesia, relief of anxiety, safety, and simplicity. However, in contrast to spontaneously breathing patients, reduction of the respiratory drive may be desirable and will promote more efficient interaction between patient and ventilator. This decreases the work of breathing and allows a more favorable distribution of cardiac output to the critical organs (brain, heart, kidneys). Opiates are the most appropriate choice for this purpose. Morphine is commonly used and titrated in 1- to 2-mg increments until the patient is adequately sedated. Subsequent doses can be given in bolus form as needed, typically 1 to 4 mg/hr.

Morphine may also be administered as an infusion. The patient is given 0.1 mg/kg over a 30-minute period, and the infusion is started at 0.025 mg/kg/hr. This is just a guideline—individual doses must be tailored to patient needs. The potential for morphine to cause hypotension through venodilation must be kept in mind. Infusions have the advantages of minimizing the periods of oversedation and undersedation commonly seen with bolus dosing. The achievement of stable plasma concentrations with infusions frequently leads to a smaller cumulative dose. The newer narcotics fentanyl and alfentanil have the advantages of more rapid onset and shorter duration of action, which makes them more suitable for infusion. They also possess fewer cardiovascular side effects. Tolerance to the effects of fentanyl given as an infusion has been described. As with haloperidol, a small dose of benzodiazepine added to the narcotic may decrease dose requirements. Nondepolarizing muscle relaxants may be required for those patients too unstable to tolerate adequate doses of sedatives.

CASE STUDY 1

The patient was a 52-year-old man admitted for a left nephrectomy. The metastatic workup was negative. His past medical history was significant for asthma treated with oral theophylline and albuterol inhaler. He had dyspnea on exertion after walking three blocks.

The physical examination was remarkable for occasional expiratory wheezes. Chest x-ray films showed some pulmonary hyperinflation. Pulmonary function tests (PFTs) showed moderate obstructive disease. The pain control service (PCS) was consulted preoperatively for evaluation.

Discussion

Goals for postoperative management include maximization of pulmonary function. Upper abdominal surgery is associated with a 60% reduction in vital capacity and a 30% reduction in FRC. These changes compromise a patient's ability to cough, deep breathe, and clear secretions. Postoperative pain with splinting and lack of deep breathing contributes to the problem. Aggressive bronchial hygiene combined with good analgesia can minimize these changes. Parenteral opioids can be effective, but they lead to significant respiratory depression. Intercostal blocks provide excellent analgesia but are limited by their relatively short duration. Epidural analgesia with opioids offers the advantages of being continuous while causing minimal hemodynamic side effects and no motor blockade. This promotes deep breathing and early ambulation. Epidural local anesthetics also provide excellent analgesia but have the potential to cause hypotension and motor blockade. A last option is insertion of an intrapleural catheter for infusion of local anesthesia.

CASE STUDY 1 CONTINUED

After a discussion of available options with the patient, an epidural opioid infusion was chosen to provide the postoperative analgesia. An epidural catheter was placed preoperatively at T11–12. Its function was confirmed by injecting 6 cc of 1% lidocaine and observing a band of analgesia from T10 to T12 bilaterally. The patient was then brought to the operating room (OR) where surgery proceeded uneventfully under general anesthesia. Thirty minutes before the end of anesthesia the patient was given 10 cc of a solution containing 10 μg/cc of fentanyl in preservative-free saline via the epidural catheter. He was then taken to the recovery room, at which time PCS was called for further management. They decided to continue with the fentanyl and use an infusion of 10 μg/cc at the rate of 5 cc/hr. One hour after the infusion was begun, the patient complained of pain. A bolus of 5 cc of the fentanyl mixture was administered. The pain was not any less after half an hour.

Discussion

The pain was mild at rest and severe when the patient coughed. The inadequate pain relief may have resulted from either a still-insufficient dose of fentanyl or misplacement of the catheter. At this point it was decided to confirm that the catheter was in position. This can be done by administering 3 to 5 cc of 1% lidocaine and again looking for a band of analgesia. If this does not give a band of anesthesia, it must be presumed that the catheter is no longer in the epidural space, and a new catheter should be placed if one planned to continue with this form of analgesia. If the band of anesthesia were found, a decision would have to be made between continuing with epidural opioids in increased dose, switching to an epidural infusion of local anesthetic, or using a combination of the two.

CASE STUDY 1 CONTINUED

The test dose of 5 cc of 1% lidocaine showed a good band of anesthesia on the right half of the body but no anesthesia on the left. This suggested that the catheter was in the epidural space but was to the right of a midline band that is sometimes present and this band was preventing the medication from reaching the left half of the epidural space. To correct this the catheter was pulled back 1 cm and a further bolus given. The pain improved somewhat but was still not satisfactory, so a mixture of fentanyl and local anesthetic was substituted for the fentanyl. The mixture consisted of fentanyl, 10 μg/cc, and bupivacaine, 0.125%. This gave excellent pain relief. The patient became hypotensive.

Discussion

The hypotension should not be unexpected because the patient had significant sympathetic blockade from the local anesthetic. Relative hypovolemia after surgery exacerbates the hypotension. Continuous monitoring of the blood pressure is essential when initiating therapy with local anesthetics. The hypotension should respond to IV fluids. The Trendelenburg position may also be used as well as a short-acting vasopressor such as ephedrine in 5-mg boluses to support the blood pressure temporarily while fluids are given. Because of the potential for hypotension and motor blockade the patient should be monitored closely and assisted during position changes.

CASE STUDY 1 CONTINUED

The hypotension was resolved after infusion of 500 cc of normal saline, and analgesia was excellent. Nevertheless, the patient remained restless and anxious. He was alert and oriented. Physical examination and blood gas values were within normal limits, as were serum electrolytes and glucose. Although the patient was reassured that he was doing well and was given 2 mg of diazepam IV, he spent a restless night. As the service made rounds the next morning, they found the patient to be more anxious and restless. Upon questioning, he denied pain but stated that he felt shaky. He was somewhat disoriented and easily distracted. Physical examination revealed moderate tachycardia and hypertension as well as hyperreflexia. Blood gas, serum electrolyte and blood glucose values remained within normal limits.

Discussion

At this point, the appropriate workup had been done to rule out the most common medical causes of agitation. Other considerations at this time included hypothyroidism, substance withdrawal, and CNS infections. Based on the tremor and hyperreflexia, substance withdrawal seemed likely, and the history may clarify the situation.

CASE STUDY 1 CONTINUED

Upon questioning, the patient admitted to heavy alcohol intake for the past 10 years. His last drink was on the night of admission, approximately 36 hours previously. He denied ever experiencing major withdrawal but was frequently tremulous in the morning and steadied up after a drink. At this point the patient was given 100 mg of thiamine and 10 mg of diazepam IV slowly. Further IV diazepam was given in 5-mg increments every 10 minutes until the patient was mildly sedated and no longer exhibited tremor or hyperreflexia. This required a total of 40 mg of diazepam. He then received 10 mg every 6 hours for the next day. This dose was decreased 25% each day thereafter. The social work service was involved for counseling and alcohol rehabilitation. He received magnesium supplementation after his serum level was found to be low. Use of the epidural catheter was discontinued on the third postoperative day and the patient switched to oral analgesic use. The remainder of his hospital stay was unremarkable.

CASE STUDY 2

The patient was a 68-year-old woman about to undergo laparotomy for a presumptive ruptured diverticulum. The PCS was consulted about a possible epidural catheter for postoperative analgesia. The past medical history was significant for chronic stable angina and congestive heart failure. The physical examination elicited a temperature of 39.2°C and right lower quadrant pain and guarding. Laboratory results showed a white blood cell count of 24,000 mm^{-3} with a left shift.

Discussion

One of the important goals in the management of this patient was adequate analgesia. Acute pain with subsequent sympathetic activation leading to tachycardia and vasoconstriction has adverse effects on myocardial oxygenation and function. This could aggravate both the heart failure and angina. Options for providing analgesia are the same as in case 1. The requested epidural catheter was relatively contraindicated in this patient, who has signs of active systemic infection.

CASE STUDY 2 CONTINUED

It was decided to provide PCA for postoperative analgesia. A demand dose of morphine at 0.5 mg with a lockout interval of 6 minutes was ordered. The PCA unit was demonstrated and explained to the patient before surgery, the surgery done, and the patient brought to the recovery room extubated. The PCA was plugged into the patient's IV. The patient soon complained of incisional pain. The recovery room nurse asked whether she could use the PCA unit to treat the pain.

Discussion

The principle of PCA is to have the patient self-administer small IV doses of opioid at relatively frequent intervals in order to maintain analgesic blood levels. Used in this manner PCA roughly resembles an infusion. As with most infusions it is desirable to start with an initial larger bolus of drug to rapidly achieve therapeutic levels. Given the small doses ordered for PCA, one would predict that it would take some considerable time to achieve symptom relief. Therefore, the recovery room staff should be instructed to administer morphine IV over a 15- to 20-minute period to a threshold dose sufficient to achieve analgesia. The PCA unit may be used by the patient once this bolusing has achieved adequate relief.

CASE STUDY 2 CONTINUED

The patient required 6 mg of morphine to achieve adequate analgesia. The patient was then instructed to use the PCA unit as needed. She was transferred to the ICU to continue postoperative management. Two hours later the patient complained of moderate incisional pain. The ICU nurse called the PCS to request that the PCA demand dose be increased.

Discussion

When faced with a patient on PCA complaining of pain, one first needs to make sure that there is no new cause for pain and that the patient is in fact using the unit. Ask the patient how often she is using the unit and inspect the unit to determine how many doses have in fact been given. The most common cause for inadequate analgesia is failure of the patient to use the unit properly. Frequently, the explanation of PCA was inadequate or was given at a time for which the patient was amnestic. Many patients are hesitant to give themselves doses for fear of overdosing. For these reasons it is necessary to frequently re-explain the unit to the patient, encourage her to use it, and reassure her that it is not dangerous. If the patient has been demanding doses frequently but still has pain, one must inspect the unit for proper setup and function. One should also check that the IV line is working. Only after ruling out these explanations for inadequate analgesia should one consider increasing the demand dose.

CASE STUDY 2 CONTINUED

Upon questioning, the patient stated that she had pushed the button only once or twice in the past 2 hours. Inspection of the unit confirmed this. The unit and the concept of PCA were reexplained, and she was urged to use it as frequently as needed. Two milligrams of IV morphine was given to reestablish an analgesic morphine level. She then used the PCA unit appropriately and remained comfortable thereafter. On the second postoperative day the service was called to the ICU because the patient had become severely agitated. She had become progressively more disoriented over the previous night despite reassurance and reorientation by the nursing staff. She had become agitated and combative over a 45-minute period and pulled out her arterial cannula while trying to get out of bed. She had been given 4 mg of IV diazepam, which seemed to increase her agitation. She began speaking incoherently and was held in bed by two nurses. She was hypertensive and tachycardiac. Physical examination was difficult to perform under the circumstances, but the results were grossly unchanged from the previous day. She had no neurologic deficits. She had received only 3 mg of morphine in the preceding 6 hours. There had been no recent change in drug therapy. Serum electrolyte levels, glucose concentration, and a complete blood cell count (CBC) measured 3 hours before were within normal limits.

Discussion

At this point the patient was delirious. Workup for an organic cause should be promptly undertaken. Appropriate first steps include arterial blood gas analysis, electrocardiogram (ECG), and measurement of serum electrolytes and blood glucose.

However, the immediate concern is protection of the patient from self-injury and control of agitation. An increased sympathetic tone is highly undesirable in a patient with ischemic heart disease. Such a patient should be restrained and pharmacologic therapy begun to rapidly control agitation while the workup is under way. Supplemental oxygen should be provided. Because the agitation increased after benzodiazepine administration, a neuroleptic was indicated.

CASE STUDY 2 CONTINUED

The patient was placed in restraints and given 40% O_2 by face mask and 5 mg of haloperidol IV. An arterial sample was obtained and sent for gas analysis and electrolyte and glucose determination. An ECG was not able to be obtained at this point because of the patient's struggling. Ten minutes later the agitation was improved, but she was still pulling against the restraints and disoriented. The blood results were within normal limits. An ECG was now able to be obtained and revealed T-wave inversions in the lateral precordial leads. A nitroglycerin infusion was begun and arterial cannulation reestablished. An additional 10 mg of haloperidol was administered, and the patient calmed down over the next 15 minutes. The T-wave inversions resolved. Thorough neurologic examination revealed no deficits. The patient gradually became oriented. Upon questioning, she was amnestic for the entire event. She was given haloperidol IV three times daily over the next 2 days. This was then tapered to a single nightly dose and eventually discontinued. Myocardial infarction was ruled out by serial cardiac isoenzyme determinations.

Discussion

The only abnormality found in the workup for this delirium was the T-wave inversion. It is possible that an anginal episode in this disoriented patient could have precipitated her delirium, and it is equally possible that the delirium preceded the ischemia, which was then secondary to the combative behavior and the associated increase in myocardial oxygen consumption. Regardless, rapid control of agitation was necessary to prevent self-injury, allow a thorough evaluation, and reduce sympathetic overactivity.

CASE STUDY 3

A 25-year-old man was admitted to the ICU after thoracotomy for a bullet wound to the chest. A bronchopleural fistula developed and the patient required prolonged ventilation. Within days he was more difficult to control on the ventilator and complained of pain in notes written to the staff. His morphine doses were increased, and he became temporarily manageable. He soon required 20 mg of morphine IV per hour.

Discussion

The patient was developing a tolerance to morphine. Tolerance may develop with prolonged use of opioids and may become a problem as ever-higher doses of opioid are required to achieve the same end point. This will not occur to a problematic extent in most patients, although there is evidence that all patients receiving opioids do develop a tolerance to some extent. If tolerance becomes a problem, it is best to switch to another opioid because cross-tolerance is not complete.

CASE STUDY 3 CONTINUED

The patient received oral methadone via a nasogastric tube that was not being used for feeding. A dose of 20 mg every 4 hours for 2 days followed by a dose of 20 mg every 8 hours controlled him adequately. During the changeover it was necessary to give some IV morphine as needed until the absorbtion of the methadone was sufficient to take over.

Discussion

Because tolerance had developed to the morphine, a dose that would give about half the analgesic equivalent of the morphine was chosen. Ten milligrams of oral methadone is approximately equianalgesic to 5 mg IV morphine, hence 20 mg was the appropriate dose. Consideration of the pharmacokinetics of methadone led to the appropriate timing of the doses.

CASE STUDY 3 CONTINUED

The patient remained satisfactory for the next week. The fistula closed, and the methadone was reduced to 5 mg every 12 hours in anticipation of weaning. The patient was found to be diaphoretic, shaking, pyrexial, and restless late the next day.

Discussion

The causes of the clinical picture are many, and one must rapidly ensure that hypoxemia and infection are not responsible. These urgent causes excluded, withdrawal symptoms should be suspected. It has been shown that even short exposures to opioids may lead to physical dependence with consequent withdrawal symptoms upon rapid weaning from the drugs.

CASE STUDY 3 CONTINUED

Withdrawal was managed by giving more opioid until the symptoms abated. In this case cautious use of IV morphine was used, and the patient felt much better when 8 mg had been given in 2 mg increments. The methadone dose was increased, and weaning was taken more slowly.

REFERENCES

1. Mersky H: Classification of chronic pain: Descriptions of chronic pain syndromes and definitions of pain terms. *Pain Suppl* 1986; 3:217.
2. Bonica J: Past and current status of pain research and therapy. *Semin Anesthesiol* 1986; 5:82–99.
3. Kehlet H: Pain relief and modification of the stress response, in Cousins M, Phillips G (eds): *Acute Pain Management*. New York, Churchill Livingstone, Inc, 1986, pp 49–75.

4. Moore R, McQuay H: Neuroendocrinology of the postoperative state, in Smith G, Covino B (eds): *Acute Pain.* Woburn, Mass, Butterworths, 1985, pp 133–154.
5. Harman E, Lillington G: Pulmonary risk factors in surgery. *Med Clin North Am* 1979; 63:1289–1295.
6. Craig D: Postoperative recovery of pulmonary function. *Anesth Analg* 1981; 60:46–52.
7. Ogston D, McDonald G, Fullerton H: The influence of anxiety in tests of blood coagulability and fibrinolytic activity. *Lancet* 1962; 2:521–523.
8. Fields H: *Pain.* New York, McGraw-Hill International Book Co, 1987, pp 1–131.
9. Beecher H: Relationship of significance of wound to pain experienced. *JAMA* 1956; 161:1609–1613.
10. Chapman C: Psychological factors in postoperative pain, in Smith G, Covino B (eds): *Acute Pain.* Woburn, Mass, Butterworths, 1985, pp 22–41.
11. Melzack R, Wall, P: Pain mechanisms: A new theory. *Science* 1965; 150:971–978.
12. Levinthal C: *Messengers of Paradise: Opiates and the Brain.* New York, Anchor Press, 1988, pp 11–54.
13. Yaksh T: Neurologic mechanisms of pain, in Cousins M, Bridenbaugh P (eds): *Neural Blockade in Clinical Anesthesia and Management of Pain,* ed 2. Philadelphia, JB Lippincott, 1988, pp 791–844.
14. Tollison J: Special considerations in pharmacologic pain management, in Tollison C (ed): *Handbook of Chronic Pain Management.* Baltimore, Williams & Wilkins, 1989, p 108.
15. Di Gregorio G, et al: *Handbook of Pain Management.* Westchester, Pa, Medical Surveillance, Inc, 1986, pp 30–34.
16. Stanley T: Sleep, pain and sedation, in Schoemaker W, et al (eds): *Textbook of Critical Care,* ed 2. Philadelphia, WB Saunders Co, 1989, pp 1155–1169.
17. Twycross R, McQuay H: Opioids, in Wall, P, Melzack R (eds): *Textbook of Pain,* ed 2. New York, Churchill Livingstone, Inc, 1989, pp 686–701.
18. White P: Patient-controlled analgesia, in Brown D (ed): *Problems in Anesthesia 2, Perioperative Analgesia.* Philadelphia, JB Lippincott, 1988, pp 339–350.
19. White P: Use of patient-controlled analgesia for management of acute pain. *JAMA* 1988; 259:243–247.
20. White P: Patient-controlled analgesia: An update on its use in the treatment of postoperative pain. *Management of Postoperative Pain. Anesthesiol Clin North Am* 1989; 7:63–78.
21. Cousins M, Bromage P: Epidural neural blockade, in Cousins M, Bridenbaugh P (eds): *Neural Blockade in Clinical Anesthesia and Management of Pain,* ed 2. Philadelphia, JB Lippincott, 1988, pp 253–361.
22. McMeeken J, Stillman B: Transcutaneous nerve stimulation, in Burrows G, et al (eds): *Handbook of Chronic Pain Management.* New York, Elsevier Science Publishing Co, Inc, 1987, pp 259–270.
23. VanDalfsen P, Syrjala K: Psychological strategies in acute pain management. *Anesthesiol Clin North Am* 1989; 7:63–78.
24. Hendler N: *Diagnosis and Management of Chronic Pain.* New York, Raven Press, 1981.
25. Cassem H: Psychiatric problems of the critically ill patient, in Schoemaker W, et al (eds): *Textbook of Critical Care,* ed 2. Philadelphia, WB Saunders Co, 1989, pp 1404–1414.
26. Egan K: Psychological issues in postoperative pain. *Anesthesiol Clin North Am* 1989; 7:183–192.
27. Tesar G, Stern T: Rapid tranquilization of the agitated intensive care unit patient. *J Intens Care Med* 1988; 3:195–201.
28. Schuckit M: Alcohol and alcoholism, in Braunwald E, et al (eds): *Harrison's Principles of Internal Medicine,* ed 11. New York, McGraw-Hill International Book Co, 1987, pp 2106–2111.
29. Schuckit M, Segal D: Opioid drug use, in Braunwald E, et al (eds): *Harrison's Principles of Internal Medicine,* ed 11. New York, McGraw-Hill International Book Co, 1987, pp 2111–2115.
30. Merriman H: The techniques used to sedate ventilated patients. *Intens Care Med* 1981; 7:212–224.
31. Bird T, et al: Intravenous sedation for the intubated and spontaneously breathing patient in the intensive care unit. *Acta Anaesthesiol Scand* 1984; 28:640–643.

9/Drug Overdose

ROY D. CANE, M.B.B.CH.

DRUG OVERDOSE

The definition of a poison is as imprecise as are the statistics on the incidence of both accidental and deliberate poisoning. Poisoning may be defined as exposure to a substance in sufficient quantity that it will produce untoward effects on the majority of individuals thus exposed. This chapter will deal with poisoning due to drug overdose, with particular reference to sedatives, narcotics, and common household chemical agents. The reader is referred to other texts for more general information regarding the wider range of poisons.[1-3]

EPIDEMIOLOGY OF DRUG OVERDOSE

The American Association of Poison Control Centers National Data Collection System reported 1,098,894 cases of poisoning from 57 centers in 1986[4] and 1,166,940 cases from 63 centers in 1987.[5] Table 9–1 shows the nature and frequency of substances most frequently involved in poisonings for 1986 and 1987. Individuals under the age of 17 years were involved in 72.1% of poisonings in 1986[4] and 72% of poisonings in 1987.[5] Male-female involvement was 50%:48.3% in 1986 and 50.1%:48.5% in 1987.[4, 5] More than 90% of poisonings occur in the home.[5] The majority of poisonings occur accidentally (89%), while about 9% are the result of suicidal intent.[4, 5] Accidental poisonings are most common in individuals under the age of 12 years, whereas intentional poisonings are most common in individuals over the age of 13 years.[5] Poisoning with more than one substance occurs in about 6% of cases.[4, 5] In 1986, 406 of 1,098,894 cases of poisoning were fatal, and in 1987, 397 of 1,166,940 cases were fatal.[4, 5]

Table 9–2 shows the patterns of poisonings for the 5-year period 1983 to 1987.[5] The causes of death from drug overdose are due primarily to depression of vital functions with consequent respiratory and circulatory failure. Aspiration of gastric contents is a significant cause of morbidity and may produce death. Aspiration pneumonia may be the most common preventable complication in acute drug overdose (see Chapter 13).

TABLE 9–1.

Substances Most Frequently Involved in Human Poison Exposures*

Substance	1986 (%)[†]	1987 (%)[†]
Cleaning substances	9.2	9.4
Analgesics	9.0	9.1
Cosmetics	7.1	7.7
Plants	7.4	7.2
Cough and cold preparations	4.9	5.1
Hydrocarbons	4.1	3.8
Bites/envenomations	3.2	3.6
Topicals	3.8	3.4
Foreign bodies	3.7	3.3
Pesticides	4.0	3.1
Food poisoning	3.4	3.1
Sedative/hypnotics/antipsychotics	3.3	3.0
Antimicrobials	2.9	2.9
Chemicals	3.0	2.9
Alcohols	2.8	2.6
Vitamins	2.9	2.6

*Modified from Litovitz TL, Martin TG, and Schmitz B: 1986 Annual Report of the American Association of Poison Control Centers National Data Collection Systems. Am J Emerg Med 1987; 5:405; and Litovitz TL, Schmitz BF, Matyunas N, et al: 1987 Annual Report of the American Association of Poison Control Centers National Data Collection Systems. Am J Emerg Med 1988; 6:479.
[†]% based on total number of ingested substances, not on number of cases.

DIAGNOSIS OF DRUG OVERDOSE

The diagnosis of drug overdose will depend on the history, physical examination, and laboratory evaluation. The signs and symptoms of overdose will vary depending on both the nature of the agent that has been ingested and also the quantity and timing of such ingestion.

History

Valuable information can be obtained from careful questioning of the patient and the patient's family, friends, neighbors, and physician. Frequently the patient will be admitted to the hospital comatose, and a history can only be obtained from secondary sources. A detailed family history and psychological assessment of the patient can be invaluable because preexistent psychosocial problems are common in poisoning victims.[6–9] Knowledge of medications prescribed for other family members may help identify a putative drug. Certain substances require immediate specific therapy. Therefore, direct questioning concerning possible exposure to substances such as acetaminophen, ethylene glycol, lead, lithium, methanol, or salicylates is mandatory.[2]

TABLE 9–2.
Five-Year Patterns of Poisonings and Fatalities*

	1983	1984	1985	1986	1987
No. of reported poison exposures	251,012	730,224	900,513	1,098,894	1,116,940
Exposures involving children aged <6 yr (%)	64.1	64.9	63.9	63.0	66.6
No. of deaths	95	293	328	406	397
Annual exposures that are deaths (%)	0.038	0.040	0.036	0.037	0.034
No. of suicides	60	165	178	223	226
Annual deaths that are suicides (%)	63.2	56.3	54.3	55.0	57.0

*Modified from Litovitz TL, Schmitz BF, Matyunas N, et al: 1987 Annual Report of the American Association of Poison Control Centers National Data Collection System. Am J Emerg Med 1988; 6:479.

Physical Examination

It is imperative when dealing with the comatose patient suspected of drug overdose that immediate assessment of the adequacy of cardiopulmonary function be undertaken prior to any further examination or therapy. In addition to clinical observation of peripheral perfusion, skin temperature, color, urine output, and blood pressure (BP), this assessment should always include arterial blood gas analysis. Alveolar hypoventilation cannot readily be documented on clinical observation alone.

When examining a patient examine the skin and the mucosa to look for bullae at pressure points, which may occur in overdose with barbiturates, opioids, and other sedatives.[2] The patient may have stigmata of drug abuse that can be identified by careful physical examination of the extremities. A detailed neurologic examination is essential. It is important to check for evidence of cervical injuries before attempting to move the head. Practically any neurological finding can occur in drug overdoses,[10] and furthermore, the clinical picture can be obscured because of head injury, intracranial bleeding, and generalized or localized central nervous system (CNS) ischemia superimposed on drug overdose.

The differential diagnosis of coma[10] is very extensive and beyond the scope of this text. However, the two important conditions to rule out immediately are an intracranial lesion and meningitis. If an intracranial lesion is suspected, computed tomography will invariably help make a diagnosis. Meningitis can be detected by an evaluation of intracranial pressure and cerebrospinal fluid analysis.

Laboratory Tests

Laboratory investigations can be of value in identifying a specific drug and may be of use in guiding therapy. The laboratory can undertake screening in suspected drug overdoses for common agents, but it is important to remember that the range of potential drugs that could have been abused is very large. The presence of drugs can be sought in gastric contents, blood, urine, or feces. Laboratories commonly employ chromatographic and mass spectrometric techniques to identify substances in bodily fluids. The routine use of a laboratory for toxicology screening is difficult to justify because of the enormous cost and the relatively low yield. Furthermore, the laboratory may detect the presence of substances routinely prescribed to patients for therapeutic reasons, not because of ingestion of excessive quantities.

Serum Electrolytes

Use of the clinical laboratory for measurement of serum electrolytes may help confirm the suspicion of a drug overdose. Estimation of serum osmolality from measured serum electrolytes when compared with a measured osmolality may identify the presence of a significant concentration of occult osmoles, which would suggest the possibility of poisoning with an alcohol. This discrepancy in estimated and measured osmolality can be misleading in patients given glycerol, mannitol, or isosorbide and in the face of a significant lipemia.[2] Assessment of the anion gap may be useful because occult anions may result from tissue hypoxia secondary to poisoning with cyanides or sulfides, from the formation of acid metabolites of methanol and ethylene glycol, or from the lactic acidosis produced by substances that inhibit oxidative cellular metabolism.

Serum Drug Concentration

Laboratory measurement of specific drug serum concentrations is of limited value because serum levels will rise following ingestion of a drug and then subsequently decline with time. A particular level on the upswing is far more significant than the identical level on the downswing of that particular drug serum concentration curve. When evaluating any particular drug serum level, it is important to consider the timing at which the blood sample was taken relative to ingestion of the drug, history of prior drug exposure, interactions among detected drugs, and the influence of age and disease. Serum drug concentrations are of little prognostic value because with appropriate care and support almost all patients will survive poisoning with therapeutic drugs. Trends in serum drug concentrations can be of qualitative value in assessing and managing an acute overdose.

The laboratory was shown to be useful in identifying toxins in 58% of 235 patients with a clinical diagnosis of drug overdose.[11] The correlation between drug level and clinical state was poor. Of these 235 patients, only 21 required active therapy, and in no instance was this therapy influenced by the toxicologic analyses. Similar results have been reported by other workers.[12, 13]

MANAGEMENT OF DRUG OVERDOSE

The management of drug overdose involves supportive therapy and specific measures aimed at decreasing the absorbance of the ingested drug, enhancing removal of the ingested drug, or antagonizing the specific effects of an ingested drug.

Supportive therapy should be aimed at guaranteeing airway maintenance and protection, tissue perfusion, and ventilation. Consideration must be given to the correction of any significant disturbances of arterial oxygenation and acid-base balance.

Decreasing Drug Absorbance

Most drug overdoses result from oral ingestion of the substance, and therefore, most measures are aimed at removal of the drug from the gastrointestinal (GI) tract. Parenteral self-administration of drugs is less common. Most ingested drugs will have left the stomach within the first 4 hours[14]; however, some drugs may in themselves directly decrease or inhibit gastric and intestinal motility, thereby vastly prolonging the period of time in which there is potential access to the drug in the stomach. This is particularly true for glutethimide and salicylates and, in fact, may account for the fluctuating levels of consciousness observed with glutethimide. Because there is no specific interval after drug ingestion that makes recovery of drug from the stomach unlikely,[15] it is wise to give serious consideration to lavage or emesis in all suspected drug overdoses.

Lavage

Lavage and emesis can be effective in removing drugs contained in the stomach; however, both are associated with significant risks of pulmonary aspiration and esophageal rupture. It is of vital importance to assess patients' airway and their ability to protect their airway before undertaking lavage or inducing emesis. If there is any doubt as to patients' ability to protect their airway, it is imperative that a cuffed endotracheal tube be inserted prior to attempting lavage or induction of emesis. In patients with adequate airway protection reflexes, it is important to continually reassess these reflexes during the period of lavage or emesis. Patients may lose this ability to protect their airway with time if the drug concentration in the brain is still rising. Introduction of large volumes of fluid to the stomach will promote emptying of the stomach into the intestine and, therefore, should be avoided.[16] Lavage should be undertaken with small volumes or via double-lumen tubes that allow continuous drainage while fluid is being introduced into the stomach. Lavaging should be continued until such time as the fluid returned is clear of any drug or food particles. Lavaging with tap water can lead to water intoxication, but there is only a minimal risk of increasing gastric emptying, which occurs more readily with large volumes of isotonic fluids. If large volumes of lavage fluid are required, body-temperature saline is probably the wisest fluid to use. Gastroscopy offers an additional means of identifying and removing tablets and drug masses from the stomach.

Emesis

Many emetics have been described, although most are associated with toxicity of their own and probably should be avoided.[17] Syrup of ipecac and apomorphine are effective in emptying the stomach and are the agents of choice for the induction of emesis.[18, 19] Apomorphine may be associated with hypoventilation and sedation due to central depression. The effects of central depression can be antagonized with naloxone. A common misconception in relation to the use of emetics is that large volumes of fluid should be given to the patient to enhance emesis. The administration of fluid does not enhance vomiting[20] and may in itself promote emptying of the stomach; therefore, it should be avoided.[16] Emetics are safer to use in children than adults and are generally more effective than lavage because of the technical difficulties of lavage in small children.

Adsorbents

The administration of an adsorbent to a patient is probably safer and is at least as effective as emetics.[21-23] Charcoal is the principal adsorbent used and will effectively decrease absorption of most drugs from the gut with the exception of organic solvents and inorganic salts.[24] It may be necessary to repeat the administration of adsorbent in patients who have taken drugs excreted in bile and returned to the gut or in patients who have active metabolites excreted in bile. Cathartics such as castor oil or osmotic cathartics are less effective than adsorbents are in preventing the absorption of drugs from the gut and will decrease the efficacy of activated charcoal.[25, 26]

Enhancing the Removal of Drugs

Specific measures aimed at hastening elimination of the drug include forced diuresis, dialysis, hemoperfusion, exchange transfusion, and the use of antibodies.

Many drugs are excreted in the urine, and forced diuresis may facilitate drug removal. It is important to remember, however, that the efficacy of diuresis is limited by renal perfusion and it may be necessary to enhance renal perfusion with a dopamine infusion. Osmotic diuretics are effective in increasing the excretion of barbiturates, salicylates, and phencyclidine, whereas the efficacy of furosemide and thiazides have not yet been established.[2] The degree of drug ionization is in some instances a function of urinary pH. Alkalinization of the urine can enhance renal clearance of some drugs, particularly barbiturates and salicylic acid. Acidification of the urine generally enhances excretion of basic substances such as phencyclidine, amphetamine, and quinidine.

Peritoneal dialysis is generally ineffective in clearing drugs because the rate of exchange of dialysis fluid is slow and peritoneal blood flow and diffusion of drug across the peritoneum is not great. Hypertonic dialysis and alkaline dialysis can enhance peritoneal removal of some drugs but have associated risks.[27]

Hemodialysis is considerably more effective than peritoneal dialysis. Provided the patient's BP is adequate, the preferred method for removing drugs is by dialysis. Drugs with high lipid solubility may be more effectively dialyzed out by employing a lipid dialysate; however, the data to substantiate this claim are not strong.[27–29]

Hemoperfusion against an adsorbent is usually more effective than hemodialysis. Hemoperfusion employing oil, hydrocarbons, charcoal, and other resins has the advantage of increasing the surface area of contact between blood and the sorbent. For most drugs charcoal hemoperfusion is approximately twice as effective as aqueous hemodialysis and half as effective as XAD-4 resin hemoperfusion.[27, 30, 31] Charcoal and resin hemoperfusion cartridges will also adsorb platelets and white cells, an undesirable effect that may be controlled with the administration of thromboxane and prostacyclin. Anuria constitutes an important indication for hemoperfusion because it may represent the only possible means of eliminating the drug.

An exchange transfusion may be useful in clearing drugs in small children but is of little value in adults. Specific antibodies to individual drugs administered intravenously (IV) bind the drug, and the antibody-drug complex is then excreted, thereby greatly enhancing removal of a drug from the blood.[2] Unfortunately, there are very few specific drug antibodies presently available.

Techniques to enhance removal of the drug from the blood are probably most effective if implemented early during the phase of rising blood concentration secondary to absorption of drug from the gut. The more aggressive forms of management such as hemodialysis or hemoperfusion probaby should be used in patients who have taken very large doses of drugs or who have high blood concentrations of drug.

Antagonizing Drug Effects

Specific antidotes can be given in cases of overdose with certain agents. These

TABLE 9–3.
Commonly Encountered Toxic Substances and Antidotes

Agent	Antidote
Acetaminophen	Sulfates, dimercaprol, methionine, N-acetyl cysteine
Acid, corrosive	Weak alkali
Alkali, caustic	Weak alkali
Alkaloids	Potassium permanganate
Amphetamine	Phenothiazine
Anticoagulants, oral	Phytonadione
Atropine	Physostigmine, pilocarpine
Cholinesterase inhibitors	Atropine sulfate, pralidoxime
Cocaine	Propranolol
Codeine	Naloxone
Coumadin derivatives	Phytonadione
Cyanide	Sodium thiosulfate, hydroxycobalamin
Diazepam	Physostigmine
Ethylene glycol	Ethyl alcohol
Heparin	Protamine sulfate
Heroin	Naloxone
Meperidine	Naloxone
Methadone	Naloxone
Methyl alcohol	Ethyl alcohol
Morphine	Naloxone
Opium alkaloids	Naloxone
Phenothiazine tranquilizers	Diphenhydramine
Physostigmine	Potassium permanganate
Scopolamine	Physostigmine
Tricyclic antidepressants	Physostigmine

antidotes are given to (1) modify drug metabolism; (2) antagonize drug actions, e.g., opioids, cholinergic agents; or (3) bind or chelate drugs and their metabolites, e.g., cyanide, heavy metals. Some of the more commonly encountered toxic substances and their antidotes are listed in Table 9–3.

For a more comprehensive list of drug and toxin antidotes, the reader is referred to the work of Arena.[1, 3] Modifications of drug metabolism may prevent the formation of toxic metabolites, hasten the production of harmless metabolites, or bind and inactivate toxic metabolites.

PROGNOSIS

With appropriate supportive and specific therapy and good general nursing care, the prognosis in most instances of drug overdose is good. Almost all patients will survive poisoning with therapeutic drugs if they reach the hospital alive. Measurement of serum drug concentrations or electroencephalographic (EEG) studies have little or no prognostic value.[32] Elderly patients or those with significant cardiorespiratory disease will not tolerate a period of coma as well as a younger, healthier individual and therefore warrant greater consideration for more aggressive therapy.

Because drug overdose is frequently a result of suicidal intent, the long-term outlook for these patients is poor. Adults who have previously attempted to kill themselves have a 4 to 20-fold increase in their predicted death rates as a result of further suicide attempts.[2, 33] Psychiatric care will reduce the incidence of repeated suicide attempts, and it has been shown that such care can be as effectively delivered by general physicians as by psychiatrists.[33]

DIAGNOSIS AND MANAGEMENT OF SPECIFIC POISONINGS

Lithium

An acute overdose of lithium usually presents a paucity of clinical signs despite a high serum level. Chronic overdose results in tissue accumulation with presenting signs of progressive CNS depression, cardiac arrhythmias, polydipsia, and polyuria secondary to nephrogenic diabetes insipidus.[34] Permanent encephalopathy may result.

Treatment involves hemodialysis for severe poisonings and correction of the associated sodium and water deficiencies.

Cholinesterase Inhibitors

Organophosphate insecticides bind and inactivate the anticholinesterase found in myoneural junctions to produce a cholinergic syndrome characterized by salivation, lacrimation, urination, defecation, GI cramping, emesis, diaphoresis, miosis, muscle fasciculations, bronchorrhea and bradycardia. Severe cases may develop seizures and coma. The administration of atropine reverses the signs and symptoms but does not directly affect the binding of the enzyme. A favorable response to a test dose of 2 mg of atropine should lead to repeated doses until pulmonary secretions are diminished. Very large doses of atropine may be necessary in severe cases and will not produce signs of atropinization.[35]

Pralidoxime hydrochloride can be administered to displace the bound inhibitor in doses of 1 g as a 30-minute IV infusion in 250 mL of saline repeated every 6 to 12 hours for 24 hours. Greatest efficacy is seen when the drug is administered as soon as possible after the poisoning.[35]

Tricyclic Antidepressants

Tricyclic antidepressants produce cardiac arrhythmias, conduction disturbances, and CNS depression including respiratory depression and seizures.[36] Patients not uncommonly appear stable for several hours following admission and then show rapid deterioration. Serum levels are not of value, and the best way to monitor the patients is the electrocardiogram (ECG). Widening of the QRS interval to >0.12 seconds is associated with an increased incidence of arryhthmias and seizures.[37]

No specific antidotes are available. Close ECG monitoring of the patient for at least 6 to 8 hours with general supportive therapy and measures aimed at reducing drug absorption are recommended.

Glycol and Methanol

Although these two substances are of low toxicity themselves, they are metabolized by alcohol dehydrogenase to substances of much greater toxicity.[38] They produce signs of behavioral alteration, metabolic acidosis, and widening of the anion gap. CNS and respiratory depression may result. Because these substances are osmotically active, patients will usually show a disparity between measured and calculated serum osmolality.

General supportive therapy in conjunction with correction of the metabolic acidosis with sodium bicarbonate and fluid and electrolyte replacement are essential. Determination of serum levels is useful for prognostication and to guide therapy. Levels <10 mg/dL in otherwise asymptomatic patients do not require any specific therapy. Patients with levels between 20 and 50 mg/dL require the administration of ethyl alcohol to block the alcohol dehydrogenase mediated conversion to toxic metabolites. Serum ethanol levels of 100 to 130 mg/dL should be maintained.[39] Blood sugar monitoring for hypoglycemia during ethanol administration is recommended, especially in pediatric patients. Patients with serum levels >50 mg/dL or those with severe symptoms and acidosis are best managed with hemodialysis.[38, 40, 41]

CASE STUDY 1

A 38-year-old white man was admitted to the emergency room after he had been found unresponsive and cyanotic on the floor of his apartment following a call from his estranged wife. She had not been able to contact him for 24 hours after he had threatened to take an overdose of glutethimide. He had a past history of chronic sedative abuse and two previous episodes of deliberate sedative drug overdose. On examination he was well developed and well nourished but unresponsive to deep pain. His pulse rate was 120/min, BP was 140/60 mm Hg, and his respiratory rate (RR) was 50/min and shallow. His pupils were at midpoint and sluggishly reactive to light. No nystagmus was noted. Examination of the chest revealed coarse rhonchi bilaterally, although it was more marked on the right than the left. His heart rate was regular, heart sounds normal, and no S_3 S_4, or murmurs were heard. The abdomen was scaphoid and had hypoactive bowel sounds. Peripheral perfusion was adequate.

Examination of the skin revealed multiple areas of pressure necrosis over the ankles and elbows. Evaluation of the airway demonstrated obtunded protective reflexes. The initial arterial blood gas analysis obtained in the emergency room on room air revealed a pH of 7.40, a P_{CO_2} of 36 mm Hg, and a P_{O_2} of 41 mm Hg.

Discussion

Two immediate problems were identified by the initial evaluation: (1) lack of airway protection and (2) severe hypoxemia. Airway protection must be provided by intubation with a cuffed endotracheal tube prior to the initiation of any specific therapy. The most likely explanation of the hypoxemia is pulmonary aspiration. The patient should receive oxygen therapy and further pulmonary evaluation concomitantly with specific therapy for the drug overdose.

CASE STUDY 1 CONTINUED

A cuffed endotracheal tube was passed nasally, 50% oxygen given, and gastric lavage with activated charcoal initiated. Lavage returned greenish material consistent with glute-thimide tablets. A chest x-ray film was obtained that showed a right basilar infiltrate. The patient was admitted to the intensive care unit and received 5 cm H_2O continuous positive airway pressure (CPAP) with an FIO_2 of 0.5. Arterial blood gas analysis revealed a pH of 7.41, a PCO_2 of 36 mm Hg, and a PO_2 of 60 mm Hg. Routine laboratory tests revealed normal serum electrolyte and hemoglobin concentrations and a white blood cell (WBC) count of 18,000 mm.$^{-3}$ Fiber-optic bronchoscopy was performed, and copious yellow-green secretions were observed in the right lower and middle portions of the lobes. No particulate matter was identified. Secretions were suctioned during the bronchoscopy, and following bronchoscopy a chest physical therapy treatment was given to the patient. Repeat arterial blood gas analysis following these interventions revealed a pH of 7.44, a PCO_2 of 32 mm Hg, and a PO_2 of 73 mm Hg with an FIO_2 of 0.5.

Discussion

Aspiration is a frequently encountered cause of morbidity in patients following sedative drug overdose. Not all aspirations are associated with an infective pneumonitis (see Chapter 13); however, the nature of the secretions seen on bronchoscopy in conjunction with an elevated WBC count strongly suggests a pneumonia. A sputum culture and sensitivity should be performed prior to commencing antibiotic therapy. The patient may have developed a pneumonia due to secondary bacterial infection superimposed on either the chemically induced lung injury of aspiration or because of hypostasis and retention of pulmonary secretions.

A bronchoscopy was performed to determine whether the patient had aspirated drug masses. If aspirated particles of large size are found, consideration needs to be given to repeat the bronchoscopy with a rigid bronchoscope to remove these particles. Chest physical therapy is indicated to facilitate the suctioning and removal of retained secretions.

CASE STUDY 1 CONTINUED

Gram staining and a culture of the aspirated sputum revealed a *Pseudomonas* organism, and appropriate antibiotic therapy was started. The patient's condition stabilized. He maintained good urine output and was maintained on 5 cm H_2O CPAP with an FIO_2 of 0.5 and continued to receive antibiotic and chest physical therapy. His arterial oxygenation steadily improved, and the FIO_2 was decreased to 0.4. Fourteen hours later arterial blood gas analysis revealed a pH of 7.43, a PCO_2 of 36 mm Hg, and a PO_2 of 78 mm Hg with an FIO_2 of 0.4. Eight hours later the patient was still unconscious but now responded to noxious stimuli. Twelve hours later the patient regained consciousness.

Discussion

Glutethimide intoxication may be associated with the clinical phenomenon of waxing and waning levels of consciousness. This phenomenon may be due to one of several mechanisms. First, glutethimide prolongs gastric emptying time, and drug masses in the GI tract may break down and release more drug for absorption. This can cause a consequent secondary rise in serum and subsequently in brain drug concentration. Second, the drug may be metabolized to a pharmacologically active metabolite that in itself will depress CNS function. Third, the primary drug or an active metabolite may be excreted in the bile and, hence, be returned to the GI tract and reabsorbed, a process termed enterohepatic recirculation. Finally, highly lipid soluble drugs will accumulate in fatty tissues in large concentrations. They will be released into the serum following an acute reduction in serum concentration secondary to dialysis or hemoperfusion and result in a secondary rise in serum concentration. Therefore, consideration has to be given to the possibility that this patient may relapse into unconsciousness with a possible loss of the ability to protect his airway. If the patient is tolerating the endotracheal tube, the wisest course of action is to leave the patient intubated for a further 4 to 8 hours. In the event that the endotracheal tube is not being tolerated, the patient can be extubated, maintained on nil per mouth, and frequently reevaluated with respect to level of consciousness and ability to protect his airway.

CASE STUDY 1 CONTINUED

The patient was not tolerating the endotracheal tube and was extubated. Following extubation while receiving 40% oxygen via face mask, arterial blood gas analysis revealed a pH of 7.42, a P_{CO_2} of 34 mm Hg, and a P_{O_2} of 77 mm Hg.

The patient did not lose consciousness again, and his pneumonia resolved over the next 2 days. He was subsequently transferred from the intensive care unit to the psychiatric ward for long-term management of his drug abuse problem and suicidal tendencies.

CASE STUDY 2

A 24-year-old woman was brought to the emergency room by her roommate after she had been found confused and barely rousable. An empty medication vial marked codeine was found by the patient's bedside. The patient's friend volunteered the information that the patient had recently broken off her engagement with her boyfriend. She was not aware of any previous suicide attempts on the part of her friend.

On examination the patient was noted to be a well-nourished female of approximately 55kg weight who was obtunded but could be aroused with difficulty. Her RR and tidal volume (VT) were 8/min and 300 mL, respectively. Her heart rate was 60/min and regular, and BP was 90/60 mm Hg. An arterial blood sample was sent for blood gas analysis and the patient given 40% oxygen to breathe via an air entrainment mask. While awaiting the results of blood gas analysis, further examination showed pinpoint pupils that reacted sluggishly to light. Tendon reflexes were symmetrically depressed. The patient showed none of the stigmata of IV drug abuse. The rest of the examination revealed a sluggish gag reflex and hypoactive bowel sounds but no other demonstrable abnormalities. Arterial blood gas analysis revealed a pH of 7.28, a P_{CO_2} of 55 mm Hg, and a P_{O_2} of 65 mm Hg ($F_{IO_2} = 0.21$). An IV line was established and 0.4 mg of naloxone administered by slow IV injection. The patient's level of consciousness improved, and her RR increased to 18/min with a VT of 420 mL. Her pulse rate was 85/min and regular and BP was 110/60 mm Hg. The patient was hostile and refused to answer questions. Repeat arterial blood gas analysis at this time on 40% oxygen revealed a pH of 7.38, a P_{CO_2} of 45 mm Hg, and a P_{O_2} of 170 mm Hg. The oxygen mask was bothering the patient and was replaced with a nasal cannula with an oxygen flow of 2 L/min. Routine laboratory investigations revealed a normal serum chemistry and blood count. The chest x-ray findings were normal. The patient was now adequately protecting her airway. A nasogastric tube was inserted, and the aspirate contained white material consistent with codeine tablets. Gastric lavage with saline was performed and activated charcoal administered. The patient was transferred to the intensive care unit for observation and further evaluation.

Discussion

The single most important aspect of management in acute narcotic overdose is cardiopulmonary support. Direct respiratory center depression will result in hypoventilation and acute ventilatory failure. It is imperative that blood gas analysis be performed to assess the adequacy of alveolar ventilation and that ventilatory support be provided when indicated until the respiratory depression can be reversed with a narcotic antagonist. The cardiovascular effects of narcotic overdose include bradycardia and hypotension. The hypotension is secondary to venodilatation and will respond to the administration of IV fluids and usually will reverse following the administration of a narcotic antagonist. In this patient the degree of hypoventilation and hypotension were such that it was appropriate to administer an antagonist as a primary step. If the degree of CNS obtundation had been greater, then mechanical ventilatory support would have to have been initiated as a primary step. The safest way to provide this is by endotracheal intubation with a cuffed endotracheal tube and ventilation with a manual resuscitation bag or a mechanical ventilator.

Naloxone is the narcotic antagonist of choice because it has little intrinsic narcotic activity. It is important to remember that the duration of action of the narcotic may exceed that of the antagonist and that repeat doses of antagonist may be required. For this reason, patients should be closely monitored for evidence of renarcotization for at least 12 hours. The other problem that may be encountered with the administration of narcotic antagonist is acute narcotic withdrawal. This is usually seen in individuals who habitually take narcotics. This patient showed none of the stigmata associated with chronic narcotic abuse, and hence, withdrawal phenomena were not anticipated. Lavage is helpful only in removing unabsorbed drug, thereby limiting any further rise in serum and brain drug concentration.

CASE STUDY 2 CONTINUED

The patient's friend, who had returned to their apartment, telephoned to report finding an empty container of a proprietary preparation of acetaminophen in the bathroom. She did not know how many tablets had been in the bottle. Repeat questioning of the patient confirmed that she had taken these tablets in addition to the codeine. She denied taking any other medications, substances, or alcohol. Blood was immediately sent to the toxicology laboratory for measurement of the acetaminophen concentration. Two grams of methionine was immediately administered to the patient orally, and orders were written to repeat this every 4 hours for a total of four doses. The patient's serum acetaminophen concentration was 120 mg/L. Blood was sent for measurement of serum bilirubin, enzymes, albumin, methemoglobin, and a coagulation profile. Urine was sent for measurement of hemoglobin. Serum bilirubin, enzymes, albumin, and coagulation studies were all normal. The urine contained no hemoglobin, and the serum methemoglobin concentration was 1.5% of the total hemoglobin.

Discussion

Acetaminophen is a commonly used analgesic marketed as a safe alternative to aspirin. Unfortunately, it is anything but safe when used in larger doses. Five grams will produce liver damage, and 10 gm may be lethal.[2] The toxicity of the drug is related to its metabolites. Normal metabolism of acetaminophen by mixed-function oxidase systems results in the formation of a highly reactive compound that binds to liver cell proteins, thereby disrupting hepatic function. These metabolites are normally bound to the sulfhydral group of glutathione, which renders them harmless. An overdose of acetaminophen, induction of the oxidase enzymes, or depletion of glutathione may all result in the formation of larger amounts of these toxic metabolites and produce liver damage.

Other than nausea, there are no early signs or symptoms of acetaminophen intoxication. This is one circumstance where the toxicology laboratory is of paramount importance because hepatotoxicity is accurately predicted by the serum concentration of acetaminophen. Concentrations >200 mg/L 4 hours after ingestion or 80 mg/L 12 hours after ingestion will be associated with hepatotoxicity.[2] The half-life of acetaminophen is approximately $2\frac{1}{2}$ hours, although this can be prolonged by liver damage to 7 to 8 hours.

Active therapy aimed at reducing the concentration of toxic metabolites will effectively prevent liver damage if initiated promptly. The administration of sulfate will enhance conjugation of acetaminophen. The preferred and more effective approach is to increase the availability of sulfhydral groups to bind these metabolites. Methionine, N-acetylcysteine, or cysteamine are useful. Untreated acetaminophen poisoning will result in liver damage in 70% of patients, while prompt administration of methionine will reduce the incidence to 10%.[2] There may be slight toxicity due to the antidote, including nausea and vomiting or rashes. Administration of an antidote is the cornerstone of therapy; however, activated charcoals and lavage are indicated to reduce further absorption of drug.

Other problems that may be encountered in acetaminophen overdose include hemolysis and rarely the formation of methemoglobin. Hemolysis is more frequently encountered in chronic abuse of the drug but may occur in an acute overdose in individuals with red blood cell glucose-6-phosphate dehydrogenase deficiency.

CASE STUDY 2 CONTINUED

Three hours after the initial dose of naloxone, the patient was noted to be more somnolent, and a second dose of 0.2 mg naloxone was given IV, which resulted in a prompt improvement in the level of consciousness. The serum acetaminophen concentration measured 4 hours after the initial measurement was 50 mg/L. Treatment with methionine was completed as originally ordered. No further problems developed, and the patient was transferred from the intensive care unit to the psychiatric unit 24 hours later.

REFERENCES

1. Arena JM: The treatment of poisoning. *Clin Symp* 1978; 3:38.
2. Thompson WL: Poisoning: The twentieth century black death, in Shoemaker WC, Thompson L (eds): *Critical Care State of the Art*. Chapter N, Society of Critical Care Medicine, Fullerton, Calif, 1980.
3. Arena AM: *Poisoning: Toxicology-Symptoms-Treatment*, ed 4. Springfield, Ill. Charles C Thomas Publishers, 1978.
4. Litovitz TL, Martin TG, Schmitz BF: 1986 Annual Report of the American Association of Poison Control Centers National Data Collection System. *Am J Emerg Med* 1987; 5:405.
5. Litovitz TL, Schmitz BF, Matyunas N, et al: 1987 Annual Report of the American Association of Poison Control Centers National Data Collection System. *Am J Emerg Med* 1988; 6:479.
6. McIntire MS, Angle CR: The taxonomy of suicide as seen in poison control centers. *Pediatr Clin North Am* 1970; 17:597–706.
7. White HC: Self-poisoning in adolescents. *Br J Psychiatry* 1974; 124:24–35.
8. McIntire MS, Angle CR: Psychological "biopsy" in self-poisoning of children and adolescents. *Am J Dis Child* 1973; 126:42–46.
9. Bancroft J, Skrimshire A, Casson J, et al: People who deliberately poison or injure themselves: Their problems and their contacts with helping agencies. *Psychol Med* 1977; 7:289–303.
10. Plum F, Posner JB: *The Diagnosis of Stupor and Coma*, ed 2. Philadelphia, FA Davis Co Publishers, 1972.
11. Qirbi AA, Poznanski WJ: Emergency toxicology in a general hospital. *Can Med Assoc J* 1977; 116:884–888.
12. Bobik A, McLean AJ: Drug analysis in the overdosed patient: Its application to clinical toxicology. *Med J Aust* 1977; 1:367–369.
13. Wiltbank TB, Sine HE, Brody BB: Are emergency toxicology measurements really used? *Clin Chem* 1974; 20:116–118.
14. Nimmo WS: Drugs, diseases and altered gastric emptying. *Clin Pharmacokinet* 1976; 1:189–203.
15. Blake DR, Bramble MG, Evans JG: Is there excessive use of gastric lavage in the treatment of self-poisoning? *Ann Intern Med* 1977; 87:721–722.
16. Henderson ML, Piccioni AL, Chin L: Evaluation of oral dilution as a first aid measure in poisoning. *J Pharm Sci* 1966; 55:1311–1313.
17. Manno BR, Manno JE: Toxicology of ipecac: A review. *Clin Toxicol* 1977; 10:221–242.
18. Corby DG, Decker WJ, Moran MJ, et al: Clinical comparison of pharmacologic emetics in children. *Pediatrics* 1968; 42:361–364.
19. MacLean WC, Jr: A comparison of ipecac syrup and apomorphine in the immediate treatment of ingestion of poisons. *J Pediatr* 1973; 82:121–124.
20. Friday KL, Powell SH, Thompson WL, et al: Emetics in poisoned dogs: Efficacy independent of ingested volume. *Crit Care Med* 1980; 8:233.
21. Lipscomb DJ, Widdop B: Studies with activated charcoal in the treatment of drug overdosage using the pig as an animal model. *Arch Toxicol* 1975; 34:37–46.
22. Decker WJ: In quest of emesis: Fact, fable and fancy. *Clin Toxicol* 1971; 4:383–387.
23. Chin L: Induced emesis—a questionable procedure for the treatment of acute poisoning. *Ariz Med* 1973; 30:28–30.
24. Greensher J, Mofenson HC, Piccioni AL, et al: Activated charcoal updated. *JACEP* 1979; 8:261–263.
25. Powell SH, Van deGraaff WB, Thompson WL, et al: Charcoals, emetics and cathartics in care of poisoned patients. *Crit Care Med* 1980; 8:233.
26. Scholtz EC, Jaffe JM, Colaizzi JL: Evaluation of five activated charcoal formations for inhibition of aspirin absorption and palatability in man. *Am J Hosp Pharm* 1978; 35:1355–1359.
27. Winchester JF, Gelfand MC, Knepshield JH, et al: Dialysis and hemoperfusion of poisons and drugs—update. *Trans Am Soc Artif Intern Organs* 1977; 23:762–842.
28. von Hartitzch B, Pinto MH, Mauer SM, et al: Treatment of glutethimide intoxication: An in vitro comparison of lipid aqueous and peritoneal dialysis with albumin. *Proc Clin Dial Transplant Forum* 1973; 3:102.
29. Kopelman R, Miller S, Kelly R, et al: Camphor intoxication treated by resin hemoperfusion. *JAMA* 1979; 241:727–728.
30. Winchester JF, Gelfand MC, Knepshield JH, et al: Present and future uses of hemoperfusion with sorbents. *Artif Organs* 1978; 2:353–358.
31. Winchester JF, Gelfand MC, Tilstone WJ: Hemoperfusion in drug intoxication: Clinical and laboratory aspects. *Drug Metab Rev* 1978; 8:69–104.
32. Bird TD, Plum F: Recovery from barbiturate overdose coma with a prolonged isoelectric electroencephalogram. *Neurology* 1968; 18:456–460.

33. Lonnqvist J, Niskanen P, Achte KA, et al: Self-poisoning with follow-up considerations. *Suicide* 1975; 5:39–46.
34. Hansen HE, Amidsen A: Lithium intoxication. *Q J Med* 1978; 186:123.
35. Hayes WJ: Phosphorus pesticides, treatment of poisoning in man, in Hayes WJ (ed): *Pesticides in Man* Baltimore, Williams & Wilkins, 1982, p 312.
36. Callaham M: Tricyclic antidepressant overdose. *JACEP* 1979; 8:413.
37. Boehnert MT, Lovejoy FH: Value of the QRS duration versus the serum drug level in predicting seizures and ventricular arrhythmias after an acute overdose of tricyclic antidepressants. *N Engl J Med* 1985; 313:474.
38. Kulig K, Duffy JP, Linden CH, et al: Toxic effects of methanol, ethylene glycol and isopropyl alcohol. *Curr Top Emerg Med* 1984; 6:14.
39. Jacobsen D, Jansen H, Wijk-Larsen E, et al: Studies on methanol poisoning. *Acta Med Scand* 1982; 212:5.
40. Gordon HL, Hunter JM: Ethylene glycol poisoning. *Anesthesia* 1982; 37:332.
41. Ekins BR, Rollins DE, Duffy DP, et al: Standardized treatment of severe methanol poisoning with ethanol and hemodialysis. *West J Med* 1985; 142:337.

10 / Smoke Inhalation

PAUL S. MESNICK, M.D.

SMOKE INHALATION

Injury to the pulmonary system by inhalation of thermal gaseous or particulate products of combustion is generically referred to as *smoke inhalation*. The United States has the highest rate of fire deaths among the industrialized nations that record fire statistics. The majority of these deaths are attributed to asphyxia and the inhaled products of combustion.[1] The synergistic lethal relationship between body surface area burn and pulmonary injury secondary to smoke inhalation is well documented. The chemical and particulate nature of a specific fire produces a potential complexity of direct and indirect effects on the pulmonary system that frequently makes it impossible to determine the specific nature of an airway or pulmonary injury.[2] Smoke inhalation may be considered in terms of immediate manifestations (carbon monoxide poisoning, airway injury, and lung burn) occurring within minutes to hours and the delayed effects occurring within days to weeks.

EARLY MANIFESTATIONS OF SMOKE INHALATION

Carbon monoxide poisoning and the onset of upper airway obstruction are the earliest and most life-threatening problems associated with smoke inhalation. The toxic, gaseous products of combustion include numerous pulmonary irritants that may produce bronchoconstriction and various degrees of noncardiogenic pulmonary edema, which may occur hours after the initial exposure.

Carbon Monoxide Poisoning

Smoke inhalation may be considered a form of carbon monoxide poisoning complicated by the addition of gaseous and particulate materials of combustion superimposing their direct and indirect chemical effects upon the pulmonary system. Carbon monoxide gas is a product of incomplete hydrocarbon combustion that lacks a characteristic odor. It is tasteless and nonirritating. Clinical and experimental data indicate that carboxyhemoglobin (HbCO) levels measured shortly after injury are proportional to an inhaled dose of smoke.[3–5]

Inhaled carbon monoxide combines readily with hemoglobin to form HbCO, a compound 210 times more stable than normal oxyhemoglobin (HbO$_2$). Not only does

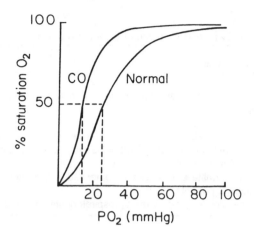

FIG 10–1.
Hemoglobin:oxygen dissociation curve showing a leftward shift of the curve for Hbco. *CO* = carbon monoxide.

Hbco diminish the blood's oxygen-carrying capacity, it also shifts the oxygen dissociation curve (Fig 10–1) to the left, which means the "unloading" of oxygen at the tissue level is impaired. It is important to realize that in the presence of an arterial Po_2 above 80 mm Hg, the available hemoglobin moieties (those not saturated with carbon monoxide) will be fully saturated with oxygen. Tissue hypoxia may occur because the hemoglobin is less capable of "giving up" oxygen to the tissues.

The peripheral chemoreceptors (aortic and carotid bodies) respond chiefly to deficits in arterial oxygen tensions rather than to the arterial oxygen content. A patient suffering from carbon monoxide poisoning usually has an adequate arterial Po_2 and therefore may not have a cardiopulmonary response to tissue hypoxia until lactic acidemia occurs.[6, 7]

In addition to the well-documented effects of carbon monoxide on oxygen transport and delivery, a number of studies suggest that carbon monoxide may have a disrupting effect on cellular oxidative metabolism by interfering with the function of intracellular cytochrome oxidase systems.[8, 9] This may account for occasional discrepancies between the severity of the patient's clinical status and the measured level of blood Hbco.[10]

DIAGNOSIS OF CO POISONING

The clinical diagnosis of carbon monoxide poisoning is usually based on a history of exposure to smoke or exhaust fumes. The classical textbook description of "cherry red" facial coloration is rarely seen in clinical practice. The milder symptoms of carbon monoxide poisoning, e.g., headache, nausea, fatigue, and occasional breathlessness (Table 10–1) are rarely seen below Hbco levels of 15%. Symptoms of

TABLE 10–1.

CO Poisoning Signs and Symptoms at Various Percentages of Hbco

Hbco (%)	Signs and Symptoms
0–10	None
10–20	Tightness across forehead; slight headache; dilatation of cutaneous blood vessels
20–30	Throbbing headache
40–50	As above with possibility of syncope; increased respiratory and pulse rates
50–60	Syncope; increased respiratory and pulse rates; coma with intermittent convulsions; Cheyne-Stokes respiration
60–70	Coma with intermittent convulsions; depressed cardiovascular and respiratory function; possible death
70–80	Weak pulse, slow respiratory rates; respiratory failure and death

confusion, disorientation, and dizziness are seen in patients who remain in contaminated atmospheres after initial symptoms develop.

Carbon monoxide manifests its effects primarily on the central nervous system (CNS) by producing a stupor that leads to an eventual loss of consciousness and death. Various phases of disorientation, athetosis, and paresis have all been reported.[11-13] Of course, tissue hypoxia secondary to carbon monoxide poisoning may cause irreversible damage and further aggravate preexisting cardiovascular or cerebrovascular disease.

The definitive diagnosis of carbon monoxide poisoning is accomplished by measurement of the percentage of total hemoglobin that is saturated with carbon monoxide, i.e., Hbco. These levels are readily determined by a multiple-band spectrophotometer such as the IL 232 Co-Oximeter, an instrument that should be available in any appropriately equipped laboratory providing blood gas measurements. An Hbco >20% is usually considered carbon monoxide poisoning. Because most smoke inhalation victims are receiving oxygen therapy prior to their arrival at the hospital, an Hbco level >40% assumes the patient has had a severe exposure. It is at these levels, >40% Hbco, that the more severe neurologic sequelae of ataxia, cortical blindness, and behavioral disturbances manifest themselves. Levels in excess of 50% Hbco may produce irreversible CNS damage.

The use of a pH-Po_2 nomogram to calculate an assumed Hbo_2 saturation will be totally misleading in the presence of significant Hbco because the nomogram assumes all hemoglobin is either reduced or saturated with oxygen. When the Hbo_2 is measured, the diagnosis of carbon monoxide poisoning may be suggested by the presence of a significantly lower Hbo_2 saturation than would be predicted from the arterial Po_2 level. In other words, a discrepancy between expected Hbo_2 and measured Hbo_2 may be due to the presence of Hbco.

Arterial Pco_2 may be normal, decreased, or elevated in carbon monoxide poisoning, depending on the patient's CNS, pulmonary, and acid-base status. Severely poisoned patients frequently exhibit a lactic acidemia secondary to tissue hypoxia. The resulting metabolic acidemia frequently stimulates minute ventilation, and a lower-than-normal $Paco_2$ is then produced.

TREATMENT OF CO POISONING

The definitive treatment of carbon monoxide poisoning is to facilitate elimination of the gas via the lungs. Because the hemoglobin affinity for carbon monoxide is so great, less than 2 mm Hg P_{CO} will result in greater than 50% Hb_{CO}. This means that even after the victim is removed from the carbon monoxide source and the alveolar P_{CO} approaches zero there is an extremely small carbon monoxide tension gradient from blood to alveolar gas. The elimination of carbon monoxide results in an exponentially decreasing Hb_{CO} level that is most commonly referred to as the "Hb_{CO} half-life." The Hb_{CO} half-life when breathing room air is approximately 5 hours, i.e., 30% Hb_{CO} will be reduced to approximately 15% in 5 hours and approximately 7% in another 5 hours when breathing room air at 1 atm.

Since oxygen competes with carbon monoxide for the same sites on the hemoglobin molecule, increased arterial oxygen tensions mean that increased numbers of dissolved oxygen molecules are competing for the hemoglobin sites occupied by carbon monoxide. This competitive factor of an increased arterial P_{O_2} is so significant that breathing 100% oxygen at 1 atm will change the Hb_{CO} half-life to approximately 1 hour. Thus, *increasing the arterial P_{O_2} is the single most important factor in carbon monoxide elimination.* Severe cases of carbon monoxide poisoning, especially in the obtunded, unconscious, or chronic lung disease patient, may require endotracheal intubation and mechanical ventilation to safely increase the arterial P_{O_2} maximally.

The use of the hyperbaric oxygen chamber is a useful therapeutic tool in the rapid elimination of carbon monoxide since an arterial P_{O_2} greater than 1,500 mm Hg can be achieved.[14, 15] Its use remains controversial in circumstances that require hospital transfer or ambulance bypass of closer emergency medical care facilities. The use of a hyperbaric facility may be considered for the more severe cases of carbon monoxide poisoning or those patients who fail to respond appropriately to treatment; however, definitive evidence of an improved prognosis following the use of hyperbaric oxygenation is lacking.[16]

Airway Injury

The efficient heat exchange and cooling mechanisms of the upper airway are highly protective of subglottic structures under most circumstances. An exception is the inhalation of hot steam, which contains 4,000 times the heat capacity of air.[17] However, there is little or no protection for the glottis and supraglottic structures, which explains why the most immediate threat to life from thermal injury is typically tissue edema in the region of the hypopharynx. The presence of progressive hoarseness or stridor, especially when it appears in the first 2 hours, must be carefully evaluated and followed. Tissue edema may be further aggravated by the infusion of large volumes of resuscitative fluids required with large surface area burns. Burns of the tongue are particularly hazardous.

Early endotracheal intubation may be required to prevent a significant compromise of an obstructing airway. This should be accomplished as expeditiously and atraumatically as possible. It is important to contemplate the intervention well in

TABLE 10–2.

Toxic Products of Combustion

Substance Burned	Toxic Products
Wood, cotton, paper	Acrolein, acetaldehyde, formaldehyde, acetic acid, formic acid
Petroleum products	Acrolein, acetic acid, formic acid
Melamine resins	Ammonia, hydrogen cyanide
Nitrocellulose film	Oxides of nitrogen, acetic acid, formic acid
Polyvinyl chloride	Hydrogen chloride, phosgene, chlorine
Polyurethane (nitrogen-containing compounds)	Isocyanate, hydrogen cyanide
Polyfluorocarbons	Octafluoroisobutylene

advance before a life-threatening obstruction occurs. Emergency cricothyroidotomy or tracheostomy is best reserved for cases in which intubation is not possible because of hypopharyngeal edema or other factors.[18] Tracheostomy is best performed electively once control of the airway has been gained by placement of an endotracheal tube. In addition to thermal injury, the various gaseous and particulate products of combustion produce a wide range of chemical components that either separately or in combination cause airway irritability and obstructive symptoms (Table 10–2). Tissue reaction of the pulmonary mucosa results in impaired mucociliary action and cellular sloughing, and this creates an accumulation of epithelial debris and secretions. Inflammation, retained secretions, bronchospasm, and hemorrhage may combine and interact to compromise both central and peripheral airways.[19, 20]

Lung Tissue Injury

The toxic constituents of smoke create a complex and still poorly understood series of interactions leading to profound tissue damage at the alveolar level. Modern office furnishings and construction materials include compounds capable of producing a wide range of toxic chemicals and gases upon combustion.[19, 21] A few of the various gases produced from combustion of modern synthetic polymers are hydrogen cyanide; hydrochloric, sulfuric, acetic, and formic acids; phosgene; acrolein; and oxides of nitrogen and sulfur. These substances may directly destroy alveolar epithelium and indirectly damage capillary endothelium. Furthermore, the burn patient is susceptible to factors resulting in acute lung injury (see Chapter 18). The vigorous administration of resuscitative fluids required by the burn patient will increase water and colloid conductance across the capillaries due to increased permeability of the endothelium.[21, 22]

Fire-retardant materials are slow to ignite and burn, but they readily decompose in fires and release gases of fluorides, bromides, and iodides. These substances may actually produce sedative effects (bromides) and have anesthetic qualities that diminish the cough reflex and further allow corrosive acids and alkalis to invade the tracheobronchial tree.

LATE MANIFESTATIONS OF SMOKE INHALATION

The neurologic and behavioral complications of carbon monoxide poisoning are quite variable. A latent period of 1 to 9 days after apparent complete recovery may ensue before symptoms develop. Late sequelae of carbon monoxide poisoning are extensive and include mental retardation, personality changes, ataxia, parkinsonism, apraxia, dysphagia, and temporal-spatial forms of disorientation.

Bedside forced expiratory spirograms are useful as diagnostic aids in assessing obstructive and restrictive functions following smoke inhalation injury.[23, 24] Fiberoptic bronchoscopy affords a good evaluation of the cord structures, trachea, and large bronchi for erythema, hemorrhage, edema, soot, and ulceration, but it must be used with caution in the face of significant upper airway inflammation and edema.[24, 25] Xenon perfusion-ventilation scanning may be useful in detecting early pulmonary damage subsequent to smoke inhalation several days before positive findings become apparent on the chest roentgenogram. False-positive scans, especially in the face of preexisting lung disease, must be appreciated.[26, 27]

Pneumonias in the burn patient are usually secondary to nosocomial gram-negative bacteria and are often polymicrobial. Aspiration, hematogenous spread of bacteria from infected wounds, disruption of the normal tracheal muscosal protective barrier by the introduction of endotracheal tubes or tracheostomy all provide portals of entry for opportunistic organisms. The compromised nutritional status and depression of the autoimmune system in the burn patient further aids the development of pneumonia and sepsis. The use of prophylactic antibiotics has not been shown to be beneficial in preventing bacterial pneumonias and may well "select out" drug-resistant bacterial flora.[28]

Functional residual capacity may be increasingly compromised in burn patients by circumferential eschar formation and edema fluid about the thoracic and abdominal regions. Decompression by escharotomy will help improve functional residual capacity in these patients and guard against further restrictive pulmonary compromise. Some decompression may also be required because of chest wall edema developing within several days of the burn injury.

CASE STUDY

A 52-year-old building superintendent was brought to the emergency room at 10:45 A.M. as a result of a flash basement fire, that involved electrical insulating materials. He had been trapped in the basement for approximately 15 minutes prior to being rescued by the fire department. He was given oxygen on the scene and while being transferred to the hospital. He had a general history of good health except for occasional mild bronchitis. He smoked two packs of cigarettes a day for approximately 30 years.

Physical examination revealed a well-developed, slightly obese, middle-aged white male. The patient appeared anxious and confused. His skin color was normal, but his face was covered with a sooty material. Vital signs showed a blood pressure (BP) of 160/100 mm Hg, a pulse of 110/min, respirations of 24/min, and tidal volume (VT) of 400 mL. Auscultation of the patient's lungs demonstrated scattered rhonchi and occasional wheezes. His voice exhibited a mild degree of hoarseness, and no stridor was noted. Carbonaceous material was noted about his nasal passages and in his sputum. Superficial burns were present about the facial region. Indirect laryngoscopy revealed the pharyngeal mucosa to be erythematous and slightly edematous. The cords were not clearly visualized, and no further attempts at instrumentation by other endoscopic techniques were carried out.

Laboratory data revealed normal serum electrolytes, a hemoglobin of 14.5 gm/dL, a hematocrit of 45%, and a white blood cell (WBC) count of 10,000 mm^{-3}. Arterial blood gas analysis on 4 L/min of nasal oxygen showed a pH of 7.50, a P_{CO_2} of 22 mm Hg, a Pa_{O_2} of 90 mm Hg, an HCO_3 of 16.5 mEq/L, and a base deficit of -5 mEq/L. The Hb_{CO} level was 32% with an Hb_{O_2} of 66%. A "stat" chest x-ray film was read as essentially normal with evidence of increased lung markings and some discoid atelectasis in the lower lobes. The electrocardiogram (ECG) showed ST depression in leads II and V4–6.

Discussion

A careful history to ascertain the nature and extent of the patient's exposure to smoke inhalation was appropriately attempted. Information as to the nature of confinement, intensity of exposure, and loss of consciousness is a useful indicator of the extent of pulmonary injury. Unfortunately, initial accurate information is usually difficult to obtain owing to both the confusing nature of rescue activities and the often confused, obtunded, and otherwise impaired mental state of the victim.

Inspection of the facial area for evidence of burns or carbonaceous material about the nares, mouth, or oropharynx was carried out. The ventilatory pattern should be observed for regularity and ease of air movement and the chest ausculated for wheezes, rales, and rhonchi. Hoarseness of speech was noted and requires further scrutiny. This may be accomplished by repeated observation of airway status, indirect laryngoscopy, or direct laryngoscopy via a fiber-optic laryngoscope or bronchoscope. A strong case may be made to avoid unnecessary instrumentation so that further tissue trauma is avoided.

The use of indirect laryngoscopy as carried out in this case may represent a reasonable compromise. Although it is difficult to clearly visualize the glottic structures with this technique, the hypopharynx can usually be well visualized with little risk of trauma. The decision not to proceed with further efforts to visualize the cords seems reasonable since significant oropharyngeal and posterior pharyngeal edema and mucosal damage are already present. The patient should be frequently examined for progressive airway compromise.

The Hb_{CO} of 32% confirms carbon monoxide poisoning. The arterial P_{O_2} of 90 mm Hg is inadequate treatment.

CASE STUDY CONTINUED

A no. 18 intravenous (IV) catheter was established in the left forearm, and lactated Ringer's solution was administered. The patient was placed on a high-flow oxygen system with an F_{IO_2} of 1.0.

An arterial blood gas sample was obtained approximately 1 hour later and showed a pH of 7.46, a P_{CO_2} of 30 mm Hg, a P_{O_2} of 228 mm Hg, and a Hb_{CO} of 19%. The patient was more alert and better able to answer questions. He denied having lost consciousness at any time in the course of the fire.

Closer assessment of his upper airway demonstrated burned nasal hairs and slight oropharyngeal edema. The patient was transferred to the intensive care unit where an arterial line was established. A course of high-dose steroids (methylprednisolone [Solu-Medrol], 1 g every 6 hours for 24 hours) was initiated. Respiratory therapy was begun and consisted of tapering oxygen therapy when the Hbco fell below 10% and using incentive spirometry and aerosolization therapy with racemic epinephrine every 4 hours. A Gram stain of the sputum showed small carbon particles and polymorphonuclear leukocytes but no predominant organisms.

Throughout the first 24 hours the patient continued to cough up thin watery secretions. He complained of a sore throat and continued to exhibit hoarseness without evidence of stridor or shortness of breath.

Discussion

The Hbco level responded as expected. The absence of progressive stridor and dyspnea is encouraging. Bronchodilators in parenteral or aerosolized form may prove useful in reducing bronchospasm. The use of agents such as racemic epinephrine in addition to bronchodilation may prove useful and effective as a mucosal decongestant and thereby relieve glottic edema early in the course of patient management. It should be realized that most commercially available inhalation bronchodilators do not contain decongestants. Humidification of inspired air by aerosol techniques such as ultrasonic nebulization may aid the patient by thinning inspissated mucoid secretions so he can cough them up.

The presence of a PaO_2 of 228 mm Hg on a high-flow oxygen system with an FIO_2 of 1.0 may indicate the preexistence of pulmonary disease. This is certainly compatible with his history of heavy cigarette smoking. This must increase the concern for secondary complications such as bronchospasm, bronchitis, and pneumonia. However, it must always be kept in mind that patients suffering from smoke inhalation often have a lowered arterial PaO_2 secondary to pulmonary injury and irritation due to the inhaled toxic constituents of smoke. This effect alone may account for or contribute to any and all of the above findings.

The use of prophylactic corticosteroids is controversial and is best reserved for specific indications such as glottic edema. Prophylactic antibiotics are not indicated (see Chapter 13 for further information on these topics).

CASE STUDY CONTINUED

After 24 hours in the intensive care unit, he still complained of throat soreness and difficulty in swallowing. He was specifically examined for stridor on an hourly basis. Serial arterial blood gas measurements allowed for an initial reduction in his high-flow oxygen therapy to an FIO_2 of 0.5. At 24 hours post admission on an FIO_2 of 0.5, he showed a pHa of 7.44, a $PaCO_2$ of 33 mm Hg, a PaO_2 of 140 mm Hg, and an Hbco of 3%. The FIO_2 was reduced to 0.3 with an arterial PO_2 of 80 mm Hg. Bedside spirometry was performed with his respiratory therapy treatments and showed a VT of 400 mL and a vital capacity (VC) of 2.0 L. His mental status remained alert and oriented. His temperature was 97.3°F; pulse 82/min and regular; respirations, 18/min; and BP, 155/70 mm Hg.

Laboratory data showed his serum electrolytes to be within normal limits. His hematocrit was 46% and his WBC count measured 12,700 mm^{-3}. Recorded fluids for the first 24 hours was 1,330 cc of fluid intake and 845 cc of output. His latest ECG showed resolution of the ST depression noted on admission.

The patient was discharged from the intensive care unit after 2 days and made an uneventful recovery.

REFERENCES

1. Gaston SF, Schumann LL: Inhalation injury. *Am J Nurs* 1980; 80:94–97.
2. Fein A, Leff A, Hopewell PC: Pathophysiology and management of the complications resulting from fire and the inhaled products of combustion: Review of the literature. *Crit Care Med* 1980; 8:94.
3. Kindwall EP: Carbon monoxide and cyanide poisoning, in Davis JC, Hunt TH (eds): *Hyperbaric Oxygen Therapy*. Bethesda, Md, Undersea Medical Soc, 1977, pp 177–190.
4. Zawacki BE, Jung RC, Joyce J, et al: Smoke, burns, and the natural history of inhalation injury in fire victims. *Ann Surg* 1977; 185:100–109.
5. Chu C: New concepts of pulmonary burn injury. *J Trauma* 1981; 21:958–961.
6. Chiodi H, Dill DB, Consolagio F, et al: Respiratory and circulatory responses to acute carbon monoxide poisoning. *Am J Physiol* 1941; 134:683.
7. Beuhler JH, et al: Lactic acidosis from carboxyhemoglobinemia after smoke inhalation. *Ann Intern Med* 1975; 82:803.
8. Goldbaum LR, Ramirez RG, Absalom KB: What is the mechanism of carbon monoxide toxicity? *Aviat Space Environ Med* 1975; 46:1289–1291.
9. Chance B, Ericinisha M, Wagner M: Mitochondrial responses to carbon monoxide toxicity. *Ann NY Acad Sci* 1970; 174:193.
10. Norkool DM, Kilpatrick JM: Treatment of acute carbon monoxide poisoning with hyperbaric oxygen: A review of 115 cases. *Ann Emerg Med* 1985; 14:1168–1171.
11. Garland H, Pearce J: Neurological complications of carbon monoxide poisoning. *Q J Med* 1967; 144:445–455.
12. Meigs JW, Hughes JPW: Acute carbon monoxide poisoning—an analysis of one hundred five cases. *Arch Indust Hyg Occup Med* 1952; 6:344.
13. Plum F, Posner JB, Hain RF: Delayed neurological deterioration after anoxia. *Arch Intern Med* 1962; 110:18.
14. Myers RA, Snyder SK, Linberg S, et al: Volume of hyperbaric oxygen in suspected carbon monoxide poisoning. *JAMA* 1981; 246:2448–2480.
15. Smith G, Sharp GR: Treatment of carbon monoxide poisoning with oxygen under pressure. *Lancet* 1960; 1:905–906.
16. Olson KR: Carbon monoxide poisoning: Mechanisms, prevention and controversies in management. *J Emerg Med* 1984; 1:233–243.
17. Phillips AW, Tanner JW, Cope O: Burn therapy. IV. Respiratory tract damage (an account of the clinical x-ray and postmortem findings) and the meaning of restlessness. *Ann Surg* 1963; 158:799.
18. Echauser FE, Billote J, Burke JF, et al: Tracheostomy complicating massive burn injury: A plea for conservatism. *Am J Surg* 1974; 126:418.
19. Summer W, Haponik E: Inhalation of irritant gases. *Clin Chest Med* 1981; 2:273–285.
20. Harrel L, Walker MS, Charles G, et al: Experimental inhalation injury in the goat. *J Trauma* 1981; 21:962–964.
21. Eckhardt RE, Hindin R: The health hazards of plastics. *J Med* 1973; 15:803–817.
22. Moncrief JA: Burns, in Schwartz SI (ed): *Principles of Surgery*, ed 2. New York, McGraw-Hill International Book Co, 1974, pp 253–274.
23. Whitener DR, Whitener LM, Robertson KJ, et al: Pulmonary function measurements in patients with thermal injury and smoke inhalation. *Am Rev Respir Dis* 1980; 122:731–739.
24. Hunt JL, Ager RN, Pruitt BA Jr: Fiberoptic bronchoscopy in acute inhalation injury. *J Trauma* 1975; 15:641.
25. Robinson L, Miller RH: Smoke inhalation injuries. *Ann J Otolaryngol* 1986; 7:375–380.
26. Petroff PA, Hander EW, Clayton WH, et al: Pulmonary function studies after smoke inhalation. *Am J Surg* 1976; 132:346–351.
27. Schall GL, McDonald HD, Carr LB, et al: Xenon ventilation—perfusion lung scars. *JAMA* 1978; 240:2241–2445.
28. Achauer BM, Allyn PA, Furmes DW, et al: Pulmonary complications of burns: The major threat to the burn patient. *Ann Surg* 1973; 177:311.

11/Critical Care of Neurosurgical Patients

WILLIAM T. PERUZZI, M.D.
TOD B. SLOAN, M.D., PH.D.

The care of the neurologically injured patient encompasses several aspects of critical care medicine. Among the most common reasons for admission to a neurosurgical intensive care unit (NSICU) are traumatic head injury, cerebral edema, and intracranial hemorrhage due to aneurysms or hypertension. The primary central nervous system (CNS) disorders frequently result in intracranial hypertension, reduction of cerebral blood flow, respiratory abnormalities, cardiovascular instability, and metabolic derangements. These secondary disorders can result in further neurologic injury. In order to avoid the sequelae of these pathophysiologic processes, intervention by the critical care physician must be rapid and effective.

HEAD INJURY

Recent studies have indicated that the incidence of head injury ranges between 200 and 610 individuals per 100,000 members of the general population.[1, 2] These injuries account for greater than half of the mortality associated with overall accidental injury.[1, 3] The survivors of head injury often suffer severe and debilitating sequelae including motor and sensory deficits, speech impairments, epilepsy, and personality disorders.[1] As stated previously, neurologic dysfunction results not only from the primary injury to neural structures but also from secondary pathophysiologic processes as well. Given appropriate supportive care during the acute episode, the neurologic sequelae can be minimized, and many of these patients can recover to highly functional and even normal levels.

INTRACRANIAL HYPERTENSION

One of the most frequent problems one must face in treating the neurologically injured patient is that of intracranial hypertension. There are several causes of increased intracranial pressure (ICP), such as widespread cerebral edema, hydrocephalus, and mass lesions. Increased intracranial volume in the face of a nondistensible container (cranium) and relatively noncompressible contents (brain, cerebrospinal fluid [CSF], blood) is the common underlying pathophysiologic problem in these causes of intracranial hypertension. The CSF compartment is normally maintained at a pressure of 7 to 10 mm Hg.[4] CSF absorption has been shown to cease below an ICP of 5 mm Hg and to increase linearly at values between 5 and 18 mm Hg.[4, 5] As ICP rises, up to 40 mL of CSF can be acutely translocated to the dural sleeves of the spinal cord. In addition, approximately 40 mL of venous blood can be shifted outside the calvarium. In children with open fontanelles and cranial sutures, the cranium remains distensible, and the head circumference can increase. Although these compensatory mechanisms can ameliorate rises in ICP during times of increased intracranial volume, they are rather limited and can be rapidly overwhelmed.

Intracranial Compliance

Intracranial volume expansion is well tolerated to a point (Fig 11–1) but is then followed by exponential rises in pressure with further volume increases. Absolute ICP measurements can be helpful in determining the patient's intracranial volume status if they are elevated; however, ICP values in the normal range are less informative. Intracranial compliance testing can yield much more information about the patient's location on the curve (Fig 11–1).[6] Compliance testing can only be

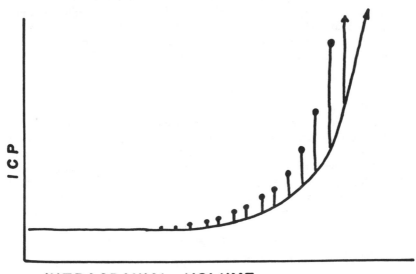

INTRACRANIAL VOLUME

FIG 11–1.
Intracranial compliance curve. As volume is acutely added to the intracranial vault, the pressure remains relatively unchanged until the compensatory mechanisms are exhausted. From this point, the pressure begins an exponentially increasing climb. If small volumes are intermittently added to the curve, the small pressure rise also exponentially increases (the response to a small-volume injection is shown by the *vertical lines* on the basic curve). Thus, both the absolute ICP value and the compliance response to a small injected volume can be used to assess the placement of the patient on the curve.

accomplished when ICP monitors are in place. Small volumes of saline (0.5 to 2.0 mL) are injected into the intracranial vault and the pressure response noted. Greater than a 2.0–mm Hg rise in ICP is considered abnormal. Testing is most safely accomplished via an intraventricular catheter because fluid can be drained should the ICP increase to dangerous levels; however, such testing has been done with an intracranial bolt in place by using smaller volumes of fluid (0.1 mL).[6, 7]

Cerebral Perfusion

Brain perfusion (cerebral perfusion pressure [CPP]) is determined by the difference between the mean arterial pressure (MAP) entering the skull and the venous outflow pressure.[8] Since ICP effectively represents the cerebral outflow pressure,[9] CPP = MAP − ICP. Normally, a CPP above 50 mm Hg ensures adequate intracranial blood flow. However, an injured brain may require 90 mm Hg for adequate perfusion.[10] As the ICP approaches MAP, blood flow will be compromised, and ischemia will result. The overall consequences of brain ischemia are several. Medullary ischemia may promote systemic hypertension and a reflex bradycardia. Brain stem ischemia or injury may also result in abnormal ventilatory patterns.[11] The combination of raised ICP, hypertension, and bradycardia is known as Cushing's triad. An irregular ventilatory pattern associated with Cushing's triad is known as Cushing's syndrome. These are severe and late signs of increased ICP and are not always present. The classical "Kocher-Cushing signs" are mainly associated with posterior fossa lesions unless there has been a sudden increase in supratentorial and intraventricular pressures, with transmission of these pressures to the infratentorial region.[12] It should be noted that patients with cervical or high thoracic spinal cord trauma may not show the Cushing response due to a loss of autonomic tone.[13] Also, since bradycardia is a reflex phenomenon, it occurs less commonly than isolated hypertension does in patients with increased ICP.

Mechanism of Brain Injury

The mechanism of injury to the brain in closed head trauma is rather complex. The bony skull forcefully collides with the brain substance at impact because each is accelerated and decelerated at different rates. These mechanical forces produce neuronal injury by several mechanisms (Table 11–1). Impact pressures as high as 4,000 mm Hg have been demonstrated in an animal model.[14–18] Pressure waves of 1,000 to 2,000 mm Hg cause a transient loss of consciousness with apnea, although no neuronal damage may be demonstrated. Pressure waves greater than 2,000 mm Hg may produce disruption of larger blood vessels and subarachnoid hemorrhage (SAH). Acceleration-deceleration within the brain tissue may lead to neuronal disruption with small vascular hemorrhages (brain contusion). In rapid deceleration, it appears that the shift of the surface of the cortex is relatively greater than is the shift of the deeper structures.[19–21] These shear forces often create the greatest damage on the side opposite the site of impact (contracoup lesion). A transient loss of consciousness and amnesia (concussion) is most commonly due to such cortical-level damage,

TABLE 11–1.

Mechanisms of Neuronal Injury

Primary factors
  Direct mechanical axonal injury
  Neurotransmitter failure
  Toxins
Secondary factors
  Ischemia
  Hemorrhage
  Edema

whereas brain stem injury or more severe cortical injury results in longer periods of unconsciousness.

Preexisting metabolic disease such as diabetes mellitus or alcohol intoxication are known to worsen the neuronal injury secondary to trauma. Alcohol is present in up to 40% of head trauma victims, and this complicates the clinical evaluation as well as potentially worsens the brain injury.[26-30]

Secondary causes of neuronal damage must be considered as soon as possible (Table 11–1). Ischemia is the common denominator of these secondary insults and may be due to hypotension, hypercarbia, hypoxia, or intracranial hypertension with compromised cerebral perfusion. The loss of airway patency and/or airway protective reflexes must be constantly evaluated. Ensuring adequate ventilation and oxygenation is crucial.[11] Since aspiration, atelectasis, and hypoventilation are common concomitants of head injury, hypoxemia is present in 30% to 50% of victims.[11, 13, 31] Abnormal ventilatory patterns are also common in patients with CNS injuries, but they do not usually cause hypoventilation.[11] However, oxygen therapy should be delivered with a system that will provide an appropriate and consistent FIO_2 despite the presence of an abnormal or unstable pattern of ventilation.

Neurologic Evaluation

Early assessment of the extent of head injury is crucial in determining appropriate therapy. The most widely accepted method for the classification of head injury is the Glasgow Coma Scale (GCS), which is outlined in Table 11–2.[22] It must be noted that the GCS does not evaluate brain stem function. This is best evaluated by testing for oculocephalic ("doll's eyes") and oculovestibular reflexes. A dysconjugate gaze is suggestive of a brain stem lesion. A normal oculovestibular response will result in tonic deviation of the eyes away from the side of cold water infusions in the ear canal. Intact oculocephalic reflexes are demonstrated by deviation of the eyes in a direction opposite to that of head motion. Testing of the oculocephalic reflex is contraindicated when cervical spine injury is suspected. Oculovestibular testing is contraindicated when inner ear damage is suspected.

Pontine damage is suggested when pinpoint pupils are observed in the absence of drug effects or in the presence of ocular bobbing (fast downward gaze followed by a slow upward gaze).[23] Irregular, ataxic ventilation may also result from pontine

TABLE 11–2.

The Glasgow Coma Scale*

Response	Points
Eye opening	
Spontaneously	4
To speech	3
To pain	2
Never	1
Best verbal response	
Oriented	5
Confused	4
Inappropriate	3
Garbled	2
None	1
Best motor response	
Obeys commands	6
Localizes pain	5
Withdrawal	4
Abnormal flexion	3
Extension	2
None	1

After evaluation of the patient, the points are summed. Severe head injury is often defined as a score below 8 for more than 6 hours.

damage.[11] Medullary damage is suggested by a loss of the gag and cough response, bradycardia, and hypotension.[24] Hypotension in the patient with head trauma is a preterminal event when due to the brain injury.[25] However, shock in a traumatized patient is usually due to other causes, such as abdominal bleeding, and must be aggressively evaluated and treated.

Increased Intracranial Pressure and Herniation Syndromes

The consequences of uncontrolled intracranial hypertension are several. As ICP approaches MAP, the CPP falls, and ischemia and cell death result. As pressure increases from focal areas of intracranial pathology, pressure gradients can develop between the various intracranial compartments, and brain tissue may be forced from its native intracranial compartment to other areas within or outside of the cranial vault. This phenomenon is known as herniation, the signs of which are dependent upon the neurologic structures that are compressed in the process. There are essentially five major herniation syndromes that have been described[32]: (1) cingulate herniation, (2) transtentorial (central) herniation, (3) uncal herniation, (4) upward transtentorial herniation, and (5) cerebellar tonsilar herniation into the foramen magnum (Fig 11–2).

Cingulate herniation occurs when the increase in supratentorial pressure forces the cingulate gyrus across the midline and under the falx cerebri (Fig 11–2,A). The most significant problems occurring directly from this process are compression of the ipsilateral anterior cerebral artery and/or the internal cerebral vein posteriorly.[33] This results in cerebral ischemia, vascular congestion, worsening cerebral edema, and exacerbation of intracranial hypertension. This pattern is usually due to a unilateral enlarging lesion and is followed by transtentorial herniation if the process is allowed to progress. The physical signs and symptoms of this type of herniation are rather nonspecific and primarily related to the injuries caused by vascular compromise.

Transtentorial herniation may occur in two forms: (1) central herniation (Fig 11–2,B) and (2) uncal herniation (Fig 11–2,C). Both of these syndromes involve displacement of brain parenchyma through the tentorial notch; however, they differ in the sequence of signs and symptoms.

The central syndrome, most frequently associated with subacute or chronic neu-

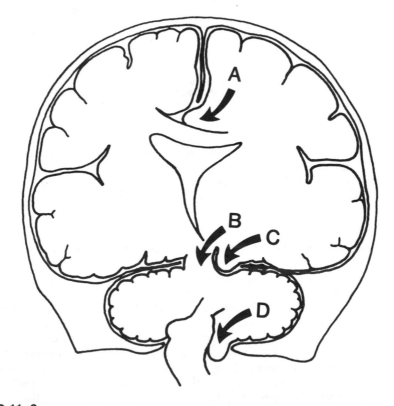

FIG 11–2.
Herniation syndromes. A = cingulate gyrus herniation; B = central transtentorial herniation; C = uncal herniation; D = cerebellar tonsillar herniation. Upward transtentorial herniation is not indicated but is essentially the opposite direction of B.

ropathology, usually results from space-occupying parenchymal lesions in the frontal, parietal, or occipital lobes or from extraparenchymal lesions at the vertex, the frontal, or the occipital poles. Anatomically, there is caudal displacement of the cerebral hemispheres and basal nuclei that results in compression and displacement of the diencephalon (thalamus, hypothalamus, epithalamus, and subthalamus) and the midbrain through the tentorial notch. This process occurs in stages. The early compression of diencephalic structures causes a general change in consciousness. The patients may find it difficult to concentrate and may become agitated or somnolent. Unfortunately, these are rather nonspecific findings that can be secondary to other factors. There are other helpful signs, however. The ventilatory pattern may be essentially normal, but with frequent sighs or yawns, or the patient may demonstrate Cheyne-Stokes (periodic) breathing. In this early stage, the pupils are small and have a narrow range of contraction. Depending upon the degree of diencephalic compression, the oculocephalic and oculovestibular responses may remain intact, or there may be roving eye movements with resistance to interruption during the "doll's head maneuver" and loss of the fast component of the oculovestibular response to cold water irrigation. Also, pressure on the superior colliculi and diencephalic pretectum may impair upward conjugate gaze in response to neck flexion. The motor response to noxious stimuli is appropriate early in the syndrome. During progression, however, preexisting contralateral hemiparesis may worsen, paratonic resistance on the side ipsilateral to the lesion may develop, and the plantar responses may become extensor bilaterally (more so on the side contralateral to the underlying lesion), thus indicating corticospinal and extrapyramidal dysfunction. Further injury to the diencephalon results in the emergence of grasp reflexes followed by decorticate (arms flex and legs stiffen) posturing. As the midbrain and upper portion of the pons are damaged, the respiratory pattern changes from Cheyne-Stokes breathing to persistent tachypnea. The pupils dilate irregularly to the midposition (3 to 5 mm) and remain fixed. Oculocephalic and oculovestibular reflexes become grossly abnormal and dysconjugate. The motor response to noxious stimuli becomes decerebrate (upper and lower extremity extension and pronation). Progression of injury to the lower part of the pons and upper portion of the medulla results in a rapid and shalow respiratory pattern, fixed pupils that remain in the midposition, no response to maneuvers testing oculocephalic or oculovestibular reflexes, and flaccid extremities with little or no response to noxious stimuli. Further medullary compromise results in irregular or agonal ventilatory patterns followed by apnea and death.

Uncal herniation is more commonly the result of acute or rapidly expanding supratentorial lesions (i.e., hematomas, severe cerebral edema), especially those arising in the lateral middle fossa or the temporal lobe.[32] In contrast to the central herniation syndrome, the pressure differential first forces the medial-basal portion of the uncus and the hippocampal gyrus over the tentorial edge. Initially, this tissue shift compresses the third cranial nerve and the posterior cerebral artery on the side of the mass lesion. Therefore, the earliest sign of uncal herniation is unilateral pupillary dilatation on the same side of the mass causing the herniation (94% of cases).[32, 34] During the early phases of this process the patient's consciousness, respiratory pattern, oculocephalic and oculovestibular reflexes, and motor response to noxious stimuli are often no more abnormal than would be expected on the basis of their underlying CNS lesion.[32] Although the pupillary abnormality may persist for hours without signs of brain stem compression, treatment should not be delayed. This syndrome tends to proceed quickly to irreversible midbrain compromise, without preceding evidence of diencephalic involvement. This results in rapid progression to loss of consciousness, loss of oculocephalic and oculovestibular reflexes, hemiplegia on the side ipsilateral to the lesion (due to compression of the contralateral cerebral peduncle), and evolution of decorticate posturing in response to painful stimuli. As the medulla is compressed, the opposite pupil will dilate, and eventually both pupils will become fixed at the midposition. The remainder of the progression is the same as that for the central syndrome.

During the early portion of the diencephalic stage the vascular supply has not been compromised sufficiently to cause infarction; therefore, the process remains reversible. As evidence of midbrain involvement emerges, the presence of infarction becomes more likely, and the chance of reversibility decreases accordingly. Plum and Posner[12] have noted that no adult subject displaying fully developed signs of midbrain injury due to a supratentorial lesion has ever recovered full neurologic function, thus mandating early recognition and rapid intervention if neurologic function is to be preserved.

Upward transtentorial herniation involves displacement of the cerebellum and mesencephalon rostrally through the tentorial notch, and this results in the rapid onset of coma due to midbrain compression, interruption of CSF drainage, and compromise of both the arterial supply to and venous drainage from various critical areas of the brain.

Downward herniation of the cerebellar tonsils through the foramen magnum is essentially a terminal event producing brain stem compression with resultant respiratory arrest and cardiovascular collapse. Should the patients survive the acute event, infarction of the cerebellar tonsils, the medulla, and the upper cervical spinal cord will occur due to compromise of the vascular supply.

CASE STUDY 1

A 33-year-old man was brought to the emergency department at 10:00 P.M. following a motor vehicle accident. He was previously in good health with no known allergies. According to witnesses, he lost consciousness for about 5 minutes after striking his head on the windshield.

Paramedical personnel stated that when they arrived on the scene the patient was slightly confused and recalled none of the accident. On initial evaluation he complained of a headache and neck pain. He was slightly confused as to time and place. On physical examination he was slightly restless and had several scalp lacerations over the left parietal region in addition to bilateral bloody nostrils. No other physical or neurologic abnormalities were noted. Vital signs were as follows: blood pressure (BP), 170/85 mm Hg; pulse, 55 beats per minute and regular; and respiratory rate (RR), 15/min and regular.

A preliminary diagnosis of mild intracranial injury with a possible basilar skull fracture or nasal injury was made. An intravenous (IV) line was started, and blood specimens were obtained for a complete blood cell count, electrolyte level determination, blood typing and crossmatching, and blood alcohol level determination. Skull, chest, and cervical spine radiologic studies were also ordered.

At 10:50 P.M., while in the radiology department, the patient developed mild right arm weakness that was followed by progressive obtundation over the next 15 minutes. By 11:20 P.M. he responded only to pain with incomprehensible utterances and normal flexor withdrawal of the left arm. The eyes opened in response to painful stimuli, but the right arm and leg appeared paretic. The left pupil was dilated and slowly responsive to light. The vital signs were BP, 180/90 mm Hg; pulse, 48 beats per minute; and RR, 24/min and irregular.

The chest x-ray findings were normal. Skull films revealed a linear skull fracture over the left parietal region. Cervical spine films revealed no abnormality. Blood studies had normal values.

Discussion

The patient's rapid deterioration suggests significant intracranial injury with rapidly increasing ICP. The physical findings are consistent with uncal and early transtentorial herniation. Approximately 50% of deaths from head injury occur within 2 hours of injury, often before hospital arrival.[35] Initial evaluation and resuscitation are of great importance. Many believe it is safest to assume that increased ICP exists when the GCS is 7 or less, thus necessitating intubation and hyperventilation.[36] The justification for this approach is that the nervous system has limited reserves and aggressive early therapy is the best way to avoid irreversible damage. Intubation in this setting provides airway protection from aspiration; allows hyperventilation to acutely lower the ICP; and prevents airway obstruction, thus avoiding increased intrathoracic pressure, hypercarbia, and worsening of the intracranial hypertension.

CASE STUDY 1 CONTINUED

The trachea was orally intubated following the application of 70% oxygen by mask and the IV administration of 5 mg/kg of sodium pentothal, 1.5 mg/kg of lidocaine, and 1 mg/kg of succinylcholine. The patient was placed on mechanical ventilatory support designed to provide hyperventilation (rate, 10 breaths per minute; tidal volume (V_T 1,200 cc) and adequate oxygenation (F_iO_2, 0.5; positive end-expiratory pressure [PEEP], 0). Arterial blood gas (ABG) analysis revealed a pH of 7.52, a P_{CO_2} of 28 mm Hg, and a P_{O_2} of 250 mm Hg. The BP was 135/70 mm Hg with a regular pulse of 73 beats per minute. Mannitol (0.25 to 0.5 g/kg) was administered IV preceded by furosemide (0.5 mg/kg). A Foley catheter was inserted, and arrangements were made for an emergency craniotomy.

Discussion

Airway Management in Intracranial Hypertension

The intubation was accomplished orally to avoid intracerebral intubation through a possible basilar skull fracture and to allow appropriate measures to minimize increases in ICP during the procedure. Care was taken to avoid neck movement, despite the apparently normal cervical spine films. Up to a 10% incidence of cervical spine injury has been reported with head trauma, and emergency department radiographs may not be of sufficient quality to allow detection of all abnormalities, especially those in the lower cervical vertebra.[30, 37, 38]

Succinylcholine was chosen for prompt and short-term neuromuscular blockade to facilitate intubation and to allow rapid neurologic reevaluation. In patients with denervation injuries (i.e., paraplegia or hemiplegia) present for greater than 5 days, depolarizing neuromuscular blocking agents such as succinylcholine should be avoided in favor of nondepolarizing drugs (i.e., pancuronium, vecuronium, atracurium).[39] Denervation results in significant proliferation of acetylcholine receptors on the sarcoplasmic membrane. Simultaneous depolarization of all of the receptors can result in a massive extracellular potassium flux and cardiac arrest due to hyperkalemia.[40] The period of maximal susceptibility for this occurrence has been reported to be within the first 6 months and longer in patients with progressive muscle degener- ation.[41, 42] This effect has also been reported in a patient with a closed head injury and no evidence of peripheral paralysis.[43] Caution must be exercised when admin- istering depolarizing agents to patients with significant CNS injuries.

Sodium pentothal and lidocaine were used to minimize the autonomic and ICP response to tracheal manipulation, to decrease ICP by direct vasoconstriction, and to decrease the cerebral metabolic rate.[44–47] Sodium pentothal is a rapidly acting (10 to 15 seconds) and predictable sedative that allows neurologic examination within 5 to 10 minutes of administration.[46] The choice and dosage of drugs will depend on the cardiovascular status of the patient. Whenever possible, drugs with a short duration of action should be utilized to rapidly allow reevaluation of the patient's neurologic status.

Management of Increased Intracranial Pressure

Hyperventilation and oxygenation.—The management of increased ICP rests on the principle of decreasing intracranial volume. This is readily accomplished by diminishing the venous and capillary blood volume. Elevation of the head to 30 to 40 degrees in the neutral position promotes venous drainage. Airway obstruction or Valsalva maneuvers increase intrathoracic pressure and impede venous drainage. Maintaining a clear airway, including endotracheal intubation when indicated, can obviate this problem.

The cerebral vasculature and, hence, cerebral blood volume (CBV) is responsive to an arterial P_{CO_2} between 20 and 80 mm Hg (Fig 11–3). A reduction in arterial P_{CO_2} results in vasoconstriction and a decrease in CBV and ICP within minutes (Fig 11–4). The effect will be sustained for approximately 1 hour.[48] Once established, hyperventilation should be continued until the underlying problem has begun to resolve in order to avoid a decrease in CSF pH and an increase in cerebral blood flow (CBF). Ongoing cerebral ischemia may also result in continued CSF acidosis, cerebral vasodilatation, and the continued need for hyperventilation to maintain control of ICP. There is experimental evidence to suggest that extreme levels of hyperventilation (Pa_{CO_2} <20 mm Hg) can compromise blood flow and oxygen delivery to normal areas of brain because it is the normal cerebral blood vessels that are affected by the induced CSF alkalosis.[49] This may lead to local tissue hypoxia, in- creased tissue lactate formation, and a compensatory increase in CBF due to de- creased tissue and CSF pH. Profound hypoglycemia will abolish this hypoxia-induced increase in CBF, presumably due to a lack of the substrate needed to produce lactic acid.[50] The initial goal of hyperventilation should be to achieve a Pa_{CO_2} of 28 to 30 mm Hg. This will decrease ICP rapidly and allow for further hyperventilation in the event of an acute worsening of the intracranial hypertension.

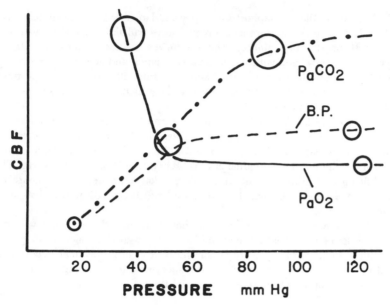

FIG 11–3.
Physiologic variables and CBF. Arterial oxygen, carbon dioxide, and BP cause alterations by causing vasoconstriction or vasodilation (depicted on the curves, *open circles* represent the degree of vessel dilation). Vessel dilation with rising flow will cause a proportionate rise in CBV and, therefore, will also cause a corresponding rise in ICP.

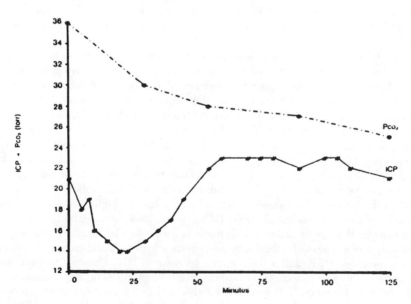

FIG 11–4.
Change in ICP with hyperventilation.

Mechanical ventilatory support for hyperventilation is best accomplished with high VTs (15 to 20 cc/kg or more if airway pressures will allow) and a low ventilatory rate (8 to 10 breaths per minute). This minimizes the rise in mean intrathoracic pressure that is associated with mechanical ventilation and achieves a minimal impairment of venous return to the heart.[51] Many patients with intracranial hypertension who are capable of maintaining their airway and ventilation without assistance demonstrate spontaneous hyperventilation.

Because an arterial Pao$_2$ below 50 mm Hg promotes cerebral vasodilation (see Fig 11–3), it is essential that significant hypoxemia be immediately corrected in patients with increased ICP. Fig 11–3 also indicates that autoregulation of blood flow occurs in the normal individual at a MAP between 50 and 150 mm Hg. These limits shift upward in the patient with hypertension of greater than 1 month's duration. Rapid changes in BP may have profound effects on CBF in the head-injured patient.

Osmolar therapy.—The use of osmotic therapy to alter the pressures within the CNS was described in 1919 by Weed and McKibben[52] and has since developed into one of the most important modalities for the control of intracranial hypertension. Several agents have been used to increase serum osmolarity including dextrose, urea, glycerol, and mannitol. Of these agents, mannitol has become the most frequently employed.

Traditional theory has been that osmolar agents exert their influence on ICP by inducing osmotic gradients between the intravascular and the extravascular space, thereby resulting in reduction of brain edema. Experimental evidence has indicated that the effects of mannitol may be due to decreases in blood viscosity, increased CBF, and compensatory cerebral artery vasoconstriction.[53, 54] However, studies using magnetic resonance imaging (MRI) to estimate brain water content have shown that mannitol therapy indeed results in a decrease in the water content of abnormal brain tissue.[55]

Mannitol is commercially available in a 20% solution (20 g/100 cc) for IV infusion. A dose of 0.25 g/kg of mannitol has been shown to be as effective as 0.5 or 1.0 g/kg.[56] However, the dose required to decrease ICP may vary significantly among patients. Treatment must be individually determined depending upon the clinical situation and response to therapy. A serum osmolarity of 295 to 305 mOsm/L is a reasonable therapeutic range.[48] If this does not reduce ICP, the serum osmolarity can be increased to as high as 320 mOsm/L. Beyond this point, hemodynamic instability and renal dysfunction may result. Since the hemodynamic instability associated with mannitol therapy is usually secondary to hypovolemia, the fluid status may need to be monitored invasively. Normal saline is the crystalloid of choice to maintain the intravascular volume status because it has the highest osmolarity (310 mOsm/L) of the most commonly used IV solutions. Caution must be exercised in using osmotic therapy in patients with tenuous cardiovascular function. The initial mobilization of extravascular fluid may precipitate a hypervolemic state, pulmonary edema, increased CBF, and a concomitant increase in ICP. Osmolar therapy can also cause an increase in sodium, potassium, magnesium, phosphorus, calcium, uric acid, and urea excretion.[57] The reason for this is that the osmotic agents cause a decrease in the renal tubular concentration gradients that favor reabsorption of these substances and an increase in distal renal tubular flow rates, thus favoring excretion of the various substances, especially potassium.[57] This may require electrolyte supplementation as therapy continues.

Of concern during the discontinuation of osmolar therapy is the so called "rebound phenomenon." This is thought to result from equilibration of mannitol across cell membranes (and an abnormal blood-brain barrier) with the development of an osmotic gradient that favors intracellular fluid transfer.[58] The incidence of this has been reported to be as high as 30%; however, several workers report this occurring in fewer than 5% of the patients treated with mannitol.[48, 59, 60] In an event, discontinuation of mannitol administration should be gradual if treatment has been maintained for any significant period of time.

The effects of dextrose are transient because of the intracellular metabolism that it undergoes.[61] This ultimately results in the administration of a significant quantity of free water, which is a situation to be avoided in these patients. Also, there is experimental evidence and some limited clinical evidence that hyperglycemia at the time of neurologic injury may promote intracellular acidosis in the areas of ischemia and worsen the neurologic outcome.[62, 63]

The use of urea as an osmotic diuretic has essentially been abandoned in most centers because of several unfavorable effects, including a significant rebound phenomenon, nausea, anorexia, vomiting, seizures, and others.

Glycerol has also been shown to be efficacious in ICP control. It undergoes intracellular metabolism and thus can act as an energy source as well.[64, 65] Glycerol can be administered orally (every 4 to 6 hours), or it can be administered IV (every 2 hours) as a 10% solution in 0.45% or 0.9% saline. Preparation of glycerol in appropriate concentrations of saline will prevent the hemolysis that is noted with IV administration in water.[64] Unfortunately, because of the lack of commercial availability, IV glycerol solutions must be prepared on site. Various dosage regimens ranging from 0.5 to 1.75 g/kg IV every 2 hours have been described.[64, 66, 67] The fluid and electrolyte disturbances noted with glycerol administration are similar to that of mannitol; however, the incidence and severity of renal failure seem to be less.[64]

Diuretic therapy.—The loop diuretics (i.e., furosemide, ethacrynic acid, etc.) decrease ICP by (1) creating a water concentration gradient between serum and brain that results in mobilization of brain water and (2) decreasing the rate of CSF production.[48] These agents are very useful in the management of patients with increased ICP who are at risk for congestive heart failure. When diuretics and osmolar agents are used in conjunction, care must be taken to avoid dehydration to the point of cardiovascular compromise and a resultant fall in cardiac output (CO), MAP, CPP, and tissue oxygen delivery.

Steroid therapy.—Steroid treatment of cerebral edema resulting from brain tumors was proved to be effective nearly 30 years ago.[68] Data from MRI studies indicate that dexamethasone treatment, while improving the clinical situation, does not result in a decrease in brain water content as does osmotic therapy.[55] Several studies of the efficacy of steroid therapy in head injury patients have failed to demonstrate a beneficial effect on neurologic outcome or on ICP control.[69–72]

CASE STUDY 1 CONTINUED

An emergency computed tomographic (CT) scan was conducted at 11:50 P.M. During the scan the patient became restless and required sedation with morphine sulfate (20 mg) and neuromuscular blockade with IV pancuronium bromide (0.1 mg/kg). The scan revealed a 7-mm midline shift to the right with a radiodense mass adjacent to the skull fracture over the left hemisphere.

Discussion

Intracranial Bleeding

The neurologic deterioration in this patient was consistent with the CT findings of an expanding intracranial mass because the deterioration was too rapid to be attributed to cerebral edema. Increased ICP secondary to cerebral edema usually develops over a 12- to 24-hour period.

The patient exhibited hypertension on admission and had a consistently slow heart rate. All trauma patients with hypertension should be evaluated for increased ICP before treatment, especially before the administration of vasodilators that might further raise the ICP.

Approximately 3% of patients with major head trauma have intracranial bleeding, and 40% of these are comatose on arrival at a hospital.[73, 74] There are four major types of bleeding: extradural, subdural, infratentorial (posterior fossa), and intracerebral.

The primary injury may either tear extradural veins (middle meningeal veins or venous sinuses), or the middle meningeal artery may be torn by fractures of the temporal or parietal bones. Skull fractures are associated with a 20-fold increased incidence of extradural hematomas.[75] These hematomas can be manifested by otorrhagia (blood in the ear canal) or hematotympanum (blood behind the tympanic membrane). In the classical presentation of an epidural hemorrhage or hematoma, the patient has a lucid interval followed by deterioration; however, one third of patients follow this pattern, another one third never lose consciousness, and the remaining are never conscious following the injury.[76]

Acute subdural hematomas are 2 to 3 times as common as epidural hematomas and have twice the mortality.[77] These are frequently due to injury to the bridging veins or arterial rupture on the cortical surface caused by rapid acceleration/deceleration. Acute subdural hematomas can also be due to small-vessel hemorrhage in a cortical contusion.[78] Patients with subdural hematomas may also have a lucid interval (15%); however, the majority are never conscious (55%).[78] Mortality is markedly increased (60% to 100%) if bilateral or multiple lesions occur.[78–81]

Subdural hematomas can develop gradually (more than 24 hours) by slow leakage from venous structures (subacute hematoma), or they may develop at a later time (chronic subdural hematoma), as is often seen in elderly or alcoholic patients. Posterior fossa hematomas are quite uncommon (2.5% of the masses) and are highly lethal due to brain stem compression and upward herniation.[34] However, with rapid diagnosis and surgical intervention, these patients can have a good recovery.

Supratentorial mass lesions are common in patients with severe head injury and can be rapidly diagnosed by a shift of the midline structures in the cerebrum. In one study of 200 head-injured patients with a GCS less than 8, 62% had a midline shift in excess of 1 cm.[82] Midline shifts can be detected easily with CT scanning, but arteriograms and other tests that assess midline structures are acceptable alternatives.

When increased ICP is caused by a mass lesion, the survival and morbidity depend on immediate operative intervention. The percentage of patients surviving mass lesions with functional recovery has been reported at 60% to 70% when surgery was conducted within 4 hours, but only 10% (with 3 to 4 times the total morbidity) when surgery was delayed beyond 4 hours.[77]

CASE STUDY 1 CONTINUED

The patient was rushed to the operating room at 1:00 A.M. for evacuation of the hematoma and insertion of an intraventricular pressure monitor. Anesthesia was maintained with narcotics (fentanyl citrate) supplemented with small concentrations of isoflurane and oxygen. Paralysis was maintained with additional pancuronium bromide. A moderate-sized epidural hematoma was evacuated and the fractured bone flap realigned.

Following surgery the patient was transferred to the intensive care unit (ICU) where a central venous catheter and orogastric tube were inserted. His pupillary responses returned to normal. He was positioned with his head up 30 degrees and remained on full ventilatory support with a $Paco_2$ ranging between 30 and 35 mm Hg. The inspired oxygen concentration was gradually tapered to 30% with a Pao_2 ranging between 70 and 80 mm Hg. Regular doses of phenytoin (Dilantin) and nafcillin and sedation with phenobarbital were begun.

Discussion

Intracranial Pressure Monitoring

More than 50% to 88% of patients who require operative treatment of head injuries have postoperative ICP rises greater than 20 mm Hg.[74, 83–85] Elevations in ICP were found in 30% of head-injured patients who were unable to follow simple commands and in 69% when a cerebral contusion was present.[74, 83, 84] ICP monitoring is particularly valuable when the patient's mental status cannot be assessed due to coma or pharmacologic therapy. Clinical experience suggests that neurologic abnormalities are consistently observed with an ICP above 40 mm Hg and in some patients with an ICP above 25 to 30 mm Hg.[86] For this reason, most clinicians aggressively treat ICP rises over 15 to 20 mm Hg. The importance of ICP in outcome is emphasized by the correlation of mortality with raised ICP. If the ICP is sustained over 60 mm Hg, the result is uniformly fatal in adults (children are generally more tolerant of higher pressures). Elevations from 40 to 60 mm Hg correlate with a 40% to 62% mortality, whereas levels from 20 to 40 mm Hg correlate with a 26% mortality. The mortality falls to 14% when the ICP remains below 20 mm Hg.[83, 85] In general, intracranial hypertension is thought to be the principal cause of half of the deaths due to head trauma.[84]

The ventricular catheter is among the most commonly used and reliable methods of ICP monitoring. In addition to accuracy and reliability, it allows for the drainage of CSF as needed to help control ICP. Unfortunately, this method is the most invasive and carries with it a higher risk of infection.[87-90] Daily CSF samples should be sent for a cell count, protein and glucose determinations, culture and sensitivity, and Gram staining while the device is in place. The use of prophylactic antibiotics is controversial; however, many advocate the use of an antistaphylococcal penicillin while the catheter is in place and for a period of time after it is removed (24 hours).

A subarachnoid screw or bolt is also commonly used. It carries with it less risk of infection and is more easily inserted; however, it carries a greater chance of malfunction, which has prompted many centers to abandon its use. Another disadvantage of this device is that it does not usually allow for removal of CSF in order to decrease ICP.

There are other monitoring devices that are placed either epidurally or subdurally and that utilize counterpressure techniques to determine ICP. These devices carry a lower risk of CSF infection but do not necessarily provide for continuous pressure monitoring.[91] Also, errors in pressure measurement due to malfunctions in the system are not always readily detected. Most recently a fiber-optic ICP measuring device has been developed that utilizes membrane-mounted mirrors to reflect light through fiber-optic channels. The mirrors undergo pressure-dependent position changes and reflect a quantity of light that is proportional to the ICP. The system cannot be zeroed in vivo, and fracture of the fiber-optic strands may cause a failure of the device. Breakage and failure, however, are easily detectable.

While ICP monitoring can be very helpful, a conventionally placed ICP monitor may not accurately reflect the intracranial pathophysiology in situations where there are focal areas of brain compression or lesions in the temporal lobe and/or posterior fossa.[7]

Lundberg was among the first to report a technique for safe long-term monitoring of ICP via ventriculostomy.[92] He reported three different wave forms. B and C waves are associated with changes in the respiratory cycle and BP, respectively. These waves were felt to be of limited clinical significance except for their association with a decreased level of consciousness. A waves or plateau waves represent abrupt and profound increases in ICP lasting 5 to 20 minutes and are thought to be abnormal autoregulatory responses to cerebral ischemia.[92-94] They are often associated with a deterioration in neurologic status, especially when they occur very frequently.

CASE STUDY 1 CONTINUED

The ICP gradually rose to 20 mm Hg over the next 12 hours. By 4:00 P.M. on the day following admission (18 hours after injury), the ICP continually rose above 20 mm Hg. Concomitant with the ICP rise was a return of hypertension (160 to 180 mm Hg systolic) and restlessness. Upper and lower extremity motion was bilaterally symmetrical in response to pain. Additional doses of mannitol (0.25 g/kg) were given IV, which kept the ICP below 20 mm Hg except for transient rises during stimulation. Due to the progressive deterioration, the patient underwent a repeat CT scan at 6:00 P.M. that revealed edema in the region of the cortex adjacent to the site of the hematoma. Neurologic examination revealed eye opening and appropriate motor withdrawal from pain but no verbal response. The electroencephalogram (EEG) showed generalized slowing with no spike activity. Evoked-potential studies revealed a slightly delayed right median nerve response but normal brain stem auditory evoked responses.

Discussion

Cerebral Edema

Cerebral edema is a major problem in the head-injured patient. There are three general patterns of swelling: swelling adjacent to a contusion or hematoma, swelling of the ipsilateral hemisphere in association with a mass lesion, and diffuse bilateral swelling due to global ischemia.[95, 96]

The formation of edema is postulated to occur by several mechanisms, but the most important is related to a transient blood-brain barrier malfunction that occurs at the time of injury.[97, 98] This is termed vasogenic edema and is due to focal disruption of vascular integrity with leakage of water through the vessel walls and can be exacerbated by hypertension.[99] The peak level of edema occurs at 24 to 72 hours after injury.[99, 100] Other mechanisms of edema formation include dysfunction of membrane transport mechanisms, cytotoxic injury with cellular water uptake, and interstitial fluid accumulation. Also postulated but poorly substantiated is edema formation by neurogenic mechanisms or the production of edemagenic factors (i.e., free radicals, serotonin, prostaglandins, etc.).[101–105] Electrolyte disturbances (i.e., hyponatremia) can promote cerebral edema; thus fluid and electrolyte regulation is crucial in these patients.

Electrophysiologic Monitoring in the Intensive Care Unit

In the patient who is obtunded or pharmacologically blunted, an assessment of neurologic function and damage can be difficult. Although radiologic studies are valuable in defining anatomic abnormalities, the electrophysiologic assessment of neurologic function can localize more subtle degrees of injury.

The EEG is produced by the postsynaptic potentials of the pyramidal cells in the granular layer of the cerebral cortex.[106] As such, it can be used to assess the overall state of health of the cortex. EEG findings will become abnormal when regional blood flow falls below 16 to 18 cc/min/100 g of brain tissue and absent below 12 cc/min/100 g of brain tissue.[107]

There are two types of signal-processed EEG monitors commercially available at present. The first is the compressed spectral array (CSA) monitor, which takes the voltage-vs.-time signals of the unprocessed EEG and presents them as three-dimensional "power spectra" that are graphic representations of power vs. frequency for a given time period. This results in a 1,000-fold decrease in the amount of information presented, provides an easily interpreted "peaks-and-valleys" display, and allows for rapid trend analysis at a glance. Unfortunately, the processing that allows for the above also eliminates the ability to identify certain EEG patterns and discrete events.[108] However, this technique has shown good correlation with the prediction of outcome in comatose patients. In patients with ischemic infarctions, the assessment of background activity via the processed EEG also proved to be a good predictor of outcome and was better at predicting the side of the lesion than the raw EEG was.[106]

The second is the cerebral function monitor (CFM), which uses a single-channel EEG designed to provide trending of EEG amplitude and amplitude variability. This device processes the EEG signal by filtering out certain EEG frequencies, amplifying others, and compressing the amplitude logarithmically.[108] The tracing is presented as a single line of variable thickness and height, which correlate with amplitude and frequency, respectively.[108] Because this instrument displays a single channel representing activity throughout the entire cortex, injury cannot be localized to a specific region unless multiple units are applied to different areas of the head.[108] This modality has been shown to be useful in predicting outcome in various coma states and following cardiac arrests.[106] Also, it has been found helpful in the pediatric ICU for seizure observation.[106]

The EEG, while a potentially useful monitor in the ICU, is not routinely used in this setting. The reasons for this are several. The provision of good and reliable tracings requires a degree of technical skill and knowledge that is not commonly available in ICU personnel. Interpretation of the signals, especially for those who are unfamiliar with EEG analysis, can be difficult. The expense of a system to provide continuous EEG monitoring can be considerable and prohibitive. Finally, the EEG provides information concerning the function of the cerebral cortex but provides no information concerning the function of the deeper brain structures.

Whereas EEG only examines the 20% of the cerebral cortex that is near the surface of the brain, evoked potentials can detect injury in deeper structures and peripheral nerve pathways. In these studies, a stimulus applied to the nervous system evokes an electrical response in a select neural pathway where the health of the nervous system can be selectively evaluated. The traditional pathways evaluated include the visual pathway, the auditory pathway (notably the brain stem), and the somatosensory system (from stimulation of the major peripheral nerves). Evoked-potential responses correlate well with CBF, CPP, tissue hypoxia, ischemia, and compression of neural structures.[106] Short-latency auditory evoked potentials are essentially unaffected by barbiturate coma and hypothermia; therefore they are useful in monitoring brain stem function in such patients.[108] The use of these techniques to assess the function of peripheral nerves, the spinal cord, the brain stem, and cortical structures in patients with head injury and coma is well accepted. Again, because of the need for personnel with advanced skills, difficulty with interpretation, and expense, these techniques have not met with widespread continuous use in the ICU setting.

CASE STUDY 1 CONTINUED

The ICP continued to rise to more than 30 mm Hg despite mannitol administration, hyperventilation, and sedation. A pulmonary artery catheter was inserted to allow optimization of the patient's hemodynamic status during the institution and maintenance of barbiturate coma. The initial hemodynamic profile was as follows: MAP, 123 mm Hg (180/95); central venous pressure (CVP), 4 mm Hg; pulmonary artery occluded pressure (PAOP), 3 mm Hg; CO, 4.6 L/min; systemic vascular resistance (SVR), 2,070 dynes-sec-cm^{-5}; ICP, 32 mm Hg; and CPP, 91 mm Hg. The patient was fluid loaded with 1,000 cc of 0.9% NaCl in 250-cc increments. The PAOP was checked and the lungs examined for rales after each fluid bolus. The hemodynamic profile after fluid loading was as follows: MAP, 115 mm Hg (170/88); CVP, 10 mm Hg; PAOP, 12 mm Hg; CO, 5.8 L/min; SVR, 1,448 dynes-sec-cm^{-5}; ICP, 28 mm Hg; and CPP, 87 mm Hg. The patient was then placed in a barbiturate coma with 15 mg/kg of pentobarbital IV push over a period of 10 minutes. The patient's BP decreased significantly at the completion of the loading dose. The hemodynamic profile at that time was as follows: MAP, 77 mm Hg (102/65); CVP, 6 mm Hg; PAOP, 7 mm Hg; CO, 4.4 L/min; SVR, 1,291 dynes-sec-cm^{-5}; ICP, 18 mm Hg; and CPP, 59 mm Hg. The patient was given an additional 500 cc of 0.9% NaCl over a 15-minute period, also in 250-cc increments and with close monitoring of fluid status, with the following results: MAP, 82 mm Hg (110/68); CVP, 13 mm Hg; PAOP, 14 mm Hg; CO, 5.1 L/min; SVR, 1,082 dynes-sec-cm^{-5}; ICP, 19 mm Hg; and CPP, 63 mm Hg. An infusion of dopamine was started at 4 µg/kg/min to stimulate CO and allow maintenance of the barbiturate infusion without compromising the CPP. The hemodynamic profile with inotropic support was as follows: MAP, 91 mm Hg (123/75); CVP, 12 mm Hg; PAOP, 12 mm Hg; CO, 5.8 L/min; SVR, 1,089 dynes-sec-cm^{-5}; ICP, 17 mm Hg; and CPP, 74 mm Hg. A continuous infusion of pentobarbital was begun at a rate of 15 mg/kg/hr for 2 hours to maintain serum concentrations during drug redistribution. This was followed by a maintenance infusion of 0.8 mg/kg/hr. The serum pentobarbital level was measured every 12 hours and the infusion adjusted to maintain the level within a range of 25 to 40 µg/mL. The patient's hemodynamic status was maintained with fluid infusion and titration of inotropic support in the manner outlined above.

Discussion

Barbiturate Coma

It is known that barbiturates can significantly decrease the cerebral metabolic rate for oxygen (CMRO$_2$) and can decrease ICP by increasing cerebral vascular resistance and decreasing CBF.[109] The decrease in CMRO$_2$ exceeds the decrease in CBF; thus the net effect is to improve the overall metabolic balance by maintaining energy supply above energy demand. Since cerebral vessels supplying focal areas of brain ischemia are maximally vasodilated due to the local tissue milieu (vasomotor paralysis), barbiturate-induced cerebral vasoconstriction will theoretically affect only the vessels supplying adequately perfused brain and shunt blood to the areas of greater need. Barbiturates have also been shown to decrease free radical activity, which would provide a theoretical advantage when dealing with cerebral edema due to hypoxia. The anticonvulsant properties of barbiturates make them useful in the dealing with the significant increase in CMRO$_2$ secondary to unchecked seizure activity. Unfortunately, the theoretical advantages of barbiturate therapy have not been consistently borne out in the clinical situation. Many of the human studies concerning the use of barbiturates in various types of CNS pathology (trauma, Reye's syndrome, anoxic injury) have been poorly structured and controlled, thus making firm conclusions impossible. Several animal experiments have shown good results with the use of barbiturates to lessen or prevent the injuries associated with various neurologic insults; however, extrapolation of animal data to humans is often problematic. Recent controlled, randomized studies in situations after cardiac arrest and head trauma have failed to demonstrate a difference in outcome between the barbiturate-treated groups and the control groups.[110, 111] Because of the complex nature of brain function and injury, this topic is difficult to study and remains controversial.[112–114]

Barbiturates can cause venodilatation, myocardial depression (in a dose-dependent fashion), and hemodynamic instability. Therefore, when barbiturate coma is instituted, invasive hemodynamic monitoring (pulmonary artery catheter) is necessary to guide fluid and inotropic therapy and ensure that an adequate CPP can be maintained.

CASE STUDY 1 CONTINUED

The ICP decreased to 18 to 20 mm Hg with initiation of barbiturate coma, and the patient remained hemodynamically stable with inotropic support. On the second day of barbiturate coma, the patient began to develop progressive hypoxemia (ABG analysis: pH, 7.51; $Paco_2$, 29 mm Hg; Pao_2, 52 mm Hg; mechanical ventilator settings: RR, 10 breaths per minute; V_T, 1,400 cc; F_iO_2, 0.4; PEEP, 0 cm H_2O. Chest x-ray examinations revealed bilateral patchy infiltrates in the dependent portions of the lungs. The patient's effective static lung compliance decreased from 55 cc/cm H_2O to 28 cc/cm H_2O. The ICP increased to values consistently greater than 20 mm Hg. This was attributed to the arterial hypoxemia. Simultaneous arterial and mixed venous blood gas samples were obtained and the shunt fraction (QspQt) and arterial-venous oxygen content difference calculated. QspQt and the $Ca-Vo_2$ were determined to be 38% and 3.8 vol%, respectively. Positive end-expiratory pressure was added to the ventilator therapy at an initial level of 5 cm H_2O. Repeat arterial and mixed venous blood samples yielded the following ABG results: pH, 7.49; $Paco_2$, 30; Pao_2 60; QspQt, 30%; and $Ca-Vo_2$, 3.6 vols%. The hemodynamic profile and ICP remained stable: CO, 5.9 L/min; MAP, 93 mm Hg; PAOP, 13 mm Hg; ICP, 20 mm Hg; and CPP, 73 mm Hg. Positive end-expiratory pressure was increased to a level of 15 cm H_2O in 5 cm H_2O increments. Determinations of QspQt, $Ca-Vo_2$, the hemodynamic profile, ICP, and CPP were made at each incremental change in PEEP. At 15 cm H_2O PEEP with an F_iO_2 of 0.4 and mechanical ventilator settings as listed above, the following information was obtained: QspQt, 17%; $Ca-Vo_2$, 3.9 vols%; CO, 5.7 L/min; MAP, 89 mm Hg; ICP, 19 mm Hg; CPP 70 mm Hg; pH, 7.48; $Paco_2$, 31 mm Hg; and Pao_2, 85 mm Hg.

Discussion

Neurogenic Pulmonary Edema

Neurogenic pulmonary edema (NPE) is a form of acute lung injury (ALI). The pathophysiology and treatment of ALI is discussed in Chapter 18. The etiology of NPE appears to be related to an imbalance in autonomic nervous system activity. Portions of the medullary reticular formation have been found to mediate the hypertensive response and the development of NPE when inhibitory influences from the nucleus solitarius are removed.[115] The caudal hypothalamus can produce a similar syndrome when the inhibitory influence of the lateral preoptic region is removed.[116] There is experimental evidence that lesions in other portions of the brain will produce pulmonary edema mediated by mechanisms other than sympathetic discharge.[117, 118]

The precise mechanism by which this sympathetic activity results in NPE is unclear, but there are several theories. Left atrial hypertension has been postulated to be a factor; however, sustained left atrial hypertension to a level sufficient to cause significant ongoing pulmonary edema has not been reported in cases of pure neurologic injury. Profound pulmonary vasoconstriction might play a role, especially if the vasoconstriction were nonuniform and resulted in focal areas of increased pulmonary capillary hydrostatic pressures. Pulmonary capillary endothelial cells may be innervated by sympathetic nerve fibers that, when massively discharged, could result in the activation of contractile elements in endothelial cells, opening of endothelial tight junctions, and leakage of protein-rich fluid into the lung interstitium.[117, 119] Alternatively, there may be a constriction of pulmonary lymphatic vessels and an accumulation of edema fluid due to impaired removal. Of course, any combination of these theories may play a role in NPE.

As is discussed in Chapter 18, the mainstay of supportive therapy for ALI/NPE is the application of PEEP to the airway. While some of the data are conflicting, the studies done in humans have indicated that the application of PEEP in patients with decreased intracranial compliance (increased elastance) and normal lung compliance resulted in a significant increase in ICP.[120, 121] However, in patients with decreased lung compliance, increased QspQt, and arterial hypoxemia in addition to decreased intracranial compliance, PEEP therapy did not appear to adversely affect ICP.[122–125] Additionally, the improvement in arterial oxygenation with PEEP therapy has been associated with a rapid (within 24 hours) improvement in intracranial compliance.[125] Thus, the application of appropriate levels of PEEP therapy, when clinically indicated on the basis of lung pathology, does not appear to adversely affect ICP and should not be avoided on that basis. In situations where intracranial compliance is significantly decreased, ICP monitoring should be instituted so that therapy can be guided by direct measurements.

CASE STUDY 1 CONTINUED

During the next 24 hours the patient continued to require mechanical ventilatory support and PEEP levels of 15 cm H_2O to maintain a Pao_2 of more than 60 mm Hg. The ICP remained near 20 mm Hg, with periodic and prolonged increases to greater than 40 mm Hg despite the continuation of barbiturate coma, osmolar therapy, and hyperventilation. In the morning of his third day of hospitalization the patient developed a urine output of 250 cc/hr that increased rapidly to 400 cc/hr over the next 4 hours. Initial serum and urine electrolyte determinations revealed a serum osmolarity of 308 mOsm/L and a urine osmolarity of 112 mOsm/L. The serum Na concentration was 148 mEq/L, and the urine Na concentration was 78 mEq/L. As the urine output continued to increase, the serum osmolarity increased to 319 mOsm/L, and the serum Na increased to 163 mEq/L. This was felt to be consistent with diabetes insipidus (DI). The IV infusion rate was increased to maintain an equal fluid balance and the IV solution changed to 5% dextrose/0.2% NaCl in order to compensate for the free water that was being lost in the urine. Over the next 2 hours the urine output increased to 600 cc/hr, and vasopressin therapy was begun (5 mg subcutaneously every 4 to 6 hours).

Discussion

Endocrinologic Disorders

Acute endocrinologic disorders resulting from hypothalamic and pituitary dysfunction are often associated with CNS trauma, brain tumors, CNS infections, and intracranial birth defects.[126–128] DI and the syndrome of inappropriate antidiuretic hormone (SIADH) secretion are two of the more frequently encountered hormonal abnormalities. In those patients suffering from head trauma, SIADH (20% to 36%) is significantly more common than DI is (2% to 26%).

Diabetes insipidus.—Traumatically induced DI has been reported to occur primarily in severe head injury associated with skull or facial fractures, cranial nerve dysfunction, or prolonged periods of amnesia; however, it has also been reported following relatively minor head injury and in association with brain death from nontraumatic causes.[129] In the case of head trauma, the onset of symptoms can occur within hours or may be delayed for months, but they will usually appear within 10 days from the time of injury.[129] Autopsy studies of patients who developed DI after head trauma have indicated that the disorder appears to result from a stretch injury to the pituitary stalk that is induced by the shear forces of the precipitating trauma rather than actual hypothalalamic or neurohypophyséal damage.[129–132] Conversely, autopsies of patients who developed DI following anoxic episodes revealed hypothalamic injury characterized by perineuronal edema and nerve cell destruction.[133] Production of experimental DI in animals supports this finding.[134] The onset of DI in patients with nontraumatic brain injury has been heralded as a poor prognostic indicator and evidence of brain death.[134, 135] In this situation, DI may be caused by transtentorial herniation with migration of the diencephalon caudally through the tentorial notch, stretching of the infundibular stalk, and interruption of antidiuretic hormone (ADH) transport.[136]

The diagnosis of DI is based on the findings of polyuria, increased serum osmolarity, and decreased urinary osmolarity. Profound hypernatremia may occur if free water is not replaced at a rate adequate to compensate for the amount of renal water excretion. Postsurgical or traumatic DI may follow one of several patterns.[137] First, the polyuria may develop within 1 to 2 days and be only transient, with normal urine production returning within 4 to 7 days. Second, the polyuria may develop within the same time course and continue permanently. Third, the polyuria may occur and then resolve transiently, only to be followed by permanent DI. In the last category, the interval of improvement may represent the death and degeneration of neurosecretory cells with a final release of stored endogenous vasopressin.[137]

The treatment of DI consists of the maintenance of physiologic fluid and electrolyte balance and supplementation of the deficient hormone if necessary. Often the patient will be able to maintain adequate fluid intake during the transient episodes of DI following surgical manipulations. If this is not possible, IV fluids containing the proper proportion of free water and sodium should be administered. In the event of permanent or severe DI where proper fluid and electrolyte balance cannot be maintained, the deficient hormone should be supplemented pharmacologically. There are several hormone preparations available.[137] In the past, pitressin tannate in oil was administered intramuscularly in doses of 5 to 10 *United States Pharmacopeia (USP)* units every 2 to 3 days. This treatment was largely replaced with aqueous pitressin, which has a duration of action of only a few hours. This was followed by the development of a synthetic lysine vasopressin nasal spray with a duration of action of 4 to 6 hours. Most recently, desamino-8-D-arginine vasopressin (DDAVP, desmopressin), a synthetic hormone with approximately twice the antidiuretic potency of the native molecule, essentially no pressor properties, and an increased resistance to metabolic degradation, has been developed. Desmopressin is administered either intranasally (10 to 25 µg, twice daily) or parenterally (1 to 2 µg daily). Other drugs such as chlorpropamide (Diabinese) and clofibrate (Atromid-S) have also been effective in decreasing the polyuria of DI. The above agents are effective only in neurogenic DI. There is little or no response when they are used in the face of nephrogenic DI.

Syndrome of inappropriate antidiuretic hormone secretion.—This syndrome has been associated with meningitis, cerebral abscesses, cavernous sinus thrombosis, hydrocephalus, brain tumors, SAH, head trauma, and other neurologic pathology.[126, 137] The incidence of SIADH in patients with neurologic lesions has been reported to be from less than 5% to greater than 40%, depending upon the time frame of the study period. There is evidence that there may be two peak time periods for the development of SIADH.[126] It may occur "early," within the first 4 days, or "late," between the 7th and 19th days following injury. It is crucial that individuals caring for these patients realize that the risk of developing this syndrome is present for a period of time that extends well beyond the normal period of ICU confinement. Of concern is that the hyponatremia that results can bring about or exacerbate various neurologic abnormalities such as confusion, agitation, seizures, and coma. If the process is not appropriately addressed, it can eventually lead to severe and permanent neurologic injury or death.

The syndrome is present if the serum sodium content is less than 135 mEq/L, the urine sodium concentration is greater than 25 mEq/L, the serum osmolarity is less than 280 mOsm/L, and the urine osmolarity is greater than that of plasma.[126] Plasma vasopressin and renin levels can also be obtained in order to confirm the diagnosis. The diagnosis must be made in the absence of other causes of hyponatremia such as hyperglycemia, mannitol therapy, alcohol ingestion, elevated plasma protein or lipid levels, hypovolemia, thiazide diuretic therapy, hypotension, liver disease, congestive heart failure, adrenal insufficiency, hypothyroidism, or renal disease.[126, 137, 138]

Inappropriate antidiuretic hormone secretion can be managed in several different ways depending upon the degree of hyponatremia and the symptoms manifested by the patient. Fluid restriction is the mainstay of therapy for asymptomatic hyponatremia associated with SIADH. To be effective in the reduction of excess body water, however, the total daily fluid intake must be at least 500 cc less than urine output.[137] This degree of fluid restriction is sometimes difficult to achieve and results in a very gradual increase in serum osmolarity (1% to 2% per day).[137] Demeclocycline (up to 1.2 g/day) has been used to inhibit the antidiuretic effects of vasopressin on the kidney.[138] Again, this form of therapy will take an extended period of time to work and probably should be used only for the mildly symptomatic or asymptomatic patient. Furosemide has been used in conjunction with IV or oral NaCl administration in order to facilitate free water excretion and restoration of the serum sodium concentration.[137, 138] This method will help correct moderate to severe hyponatremia in a reasonable time frame (24 hours) and is useful in symptomatic patients in danger of developing seizure activity. Hypertonic saline (3% NaCl) can also be used in the patient who is demonstrating neurologic symptoms due to hyponatremia. When the 3% saline solution is administered IV at a rate of 0.1 cc/kg/min, the plasma sodium concentration and osmolarity will increase by approximately 2% per hour.[137] Since there have been reports of central pontine myelinolysis in association with rapid correction of the hyponatremia associated with SIADH and the primary concern when correcting the hyponatremia is to avoid exacerbation or precipitation of neurologic injuries, appropriate caution must be exercised when treating this disorder.[137, 139, 140]

Subarachnoid Hemorrhage, Cerebral Aneurysms, and Cerebral Vasospasm

Subarachnoid hemorrhage is estimated to occur in 10 to 28 individuals per 100,000 members of the population per year (approximately 25,000 cases per year in the United States).[32, 139, 141, 142] Most SAH is secondary to ruptured intracranial aneurysms, 4% to 5% are due to arteriovenous malformations (AVMs), and 13% to 22% of those with SAH have an unidentified source of bleeding.[141, 143] Several studies have been undertaken to identify significant risk factors for SAH in order to increase the potential for prevention since the available treatments have done little to improve overall survival or outcome over the last 20 to 30 years.[124] The data tend to be rather controversial; however, the major risk factors that have been identified include age, tobacco abuse, and hypertension, with the latter being the most significant.[124, 144] Although hypertension may predispose to SAH, intracranial hemorrhage directly related to hypertension or a hypertensive crisis often results in intracerebral hemorrhage, especially in the area of the basal ganglia.[145, 146] Other possible factors in question include sex, oral contraceptive use, collagen-vascular disease, and hereditary predisposition.[124]

Approximately 70% of those with SAH caused by an intracranial aneurysm rupture die or are severely disabled.[32, 147] Even those patients admitted with minimal neurologic injury show significant morbidity and mortality. A study by Ropper and Zervas[148] during which they followed over 100 patients for 1 year post-hemorrhage revealed that only 46% recovered fully, there was an 11% mortality, 17% had persistent neurologic injury (primarily due to vasospasm), and 25% suffered from emotional or psychological problems that interfered significantly with their lives (1% were lost to follow-up). Those patients with SAH and an unidentifiable source of bleeding following a thorough radiologic evaluation have a lower incidence of rebleeding and a better prognosis for long-term survival and recovery of function.[124, 143, 149]

The classification of SAH is based upon clinical signs and symptoms. A modification of the Hunt-Hess classification is outlined in Table 11–3.[150] Although mortality rates may vary among different institutions, in general, mortality increases significantly with the clinical grade.

TABLE 11–3.

Classification of Patients With Subarachnoid Hemorrhage According to Signs, Symptoms, and Perioperative Risk

Grade	Criteria	Mortality (%)
0	Unruptured aneurysm	
I	Asymptomatic or minimal headache and slight nuchal rigidity	0–5
Ia	Stable, residual neurologic deficit past the period of acute cerebral reaction	
II	Moderate to severe headache, nuchal rigidity, no neurologic deficit other than cranial nerve palsy	2–10
III	Drowsiness, confusion, or mild focal deficit	10–15
IV	Stupor, moderate to severe hemiparesis, possibly early decerebrate rigidity and vegetative disturbances	60–70
V	Deep coma, decerebrate rigidity, moribund appearance	70–100

Management of these patients includes stabilization of their respiratory and cardiovascular status, manipulation of cerebral perfusion in an attempt to avoid the risk of cerebral ischemia and infarction due to vasospasm, and surgical correction of the underlying problem when appropriate. The timing of surgical intervention is a controversial topic and is based on several factors including clinical grade, the presence or absence of vasospasm or mass effect from an intracerebral hematoma, the location of the aneurysm, and the patient's overall medical status. One philosophy is to operate on patients in grade I or II SAH and evacuate the subarachnoid clot as soon as possible (within 72 hours) following hemorrhage. The rationale for this is to avoid the risk of rebleeding, eliminate any mass effect that may increase ICP, and decrease the risk of cerebral artery vasospasm.[151] Patients admitted with grade III hemorrhage have evidence of clinical vasospasm. Some studies have indicated that early surgery in this situation will improve outcome, while others have provided evidence to the contrary.[147, 151] When patients present several days after hemorrhage or if they have grades IV or V SAH without space-occupying hemorrhagic lesions causing increased ICP, surgical intervention is often delayed until their neurologic status improves. Many would agree that, because of the overall poor prognosis, grade IV and V patients should not be surgically manipulated; however, surgical intervention in all grades of SAH must be considered on an individual basis.

CASE STUDY 2

The patient was a 58-year-old white woman who noted the sudden onset of an intense right-sided headache while working at home. She was brought to the emergency room by her husband. She complained of a persistent moderate headache and neck stiffness but denied any chest discomfort. Her past medical history was unremarkable except for three normal pregnancies, a 38 pack-per-year history of tobacco abuse, and an allergy to pencillin. She had a history of good exercise tolerance without dyspnea on exertion. Physical examination revealed her vital signs as follows: BP, 145/88 mm Hg; pulse, 88 beats per minute; RR, 26 breaths per min; and temperature, 37.2°C. The patient was alert and oriented to person, place, time, and situation. All cranial nerves were intact. Motor and sensory function were intact and bilaterally symmetrical. The remainder of her physical examination was normal. Laboratory studies in the emergency department were as follows: hemoglobin, 12.8 g/dL; Na, 138 mEq/L; K, 4.1 mEq/L; Cl, 108 mEq/L; CO_2, 24 mEq/L; ABG pH, 7.48; $Paco_2$, 32 mm Hg; and Pao_2, 84 mm Hg on room air. Coagulation studies were within normal limits. Chest radiographic findings were normal, but the electrocardiogram (ECG) revealed diffuse T-wave inversions most prominent in the anterolateral leads. A CT scan of the head revealed subarachnoid blood in the basal cisterns. The patient was admitted to the NSICU where an arterial line was inserted and arrangements made for an emergency cerebral angiogram.

Discussion

Neurogenic Electrocardiographic Changes

The changes noted on the admission ECG are not unusual in patients with neurologic injuries. This is most commonly seen in patients with SAH but can also occur with head trauma, brain tumors, strokes, seizure disorders, and other neurologic pathology.[117] Patients may present with T-wave changes varying from peaking to deep inversions, prolonged QT intervals, and U waves unrelated to electrolyte imbalances.[152, 153] It is believed that the sympathetic discharge associated with insults to various parts of the brain is responsible for the ECG changes noted.[117] Gross postmortem examination of the heart in several patients has failed to reveal significant injury associated with these ECG changes; however, electron microscopy has provided evidence of widespread myofibrillar necrosis that is virtually identical to "catecholamine cardiomyopathy."[117, 154] Many patients who present with SAH are within the age group at risk for primary cardiac disease. Thus, neurogenic ECG changes must be a diagnosis of exclusion, and patients with such changes should be observed carefully, evaluated thoroughly, and treated for myocardial ischemia as clinically indicated.

Cardiac dysrhythmias are also very common in patients with neurologic insults.[155] Bradycardia and varying degrees of heart block related to high vagal tone are frequently encountered. In addition, malignant ventricular ectopy can be precipitated by an asymmetrical sympathetic discharge.[156]

CASE STUDY 2 CONTINUED

Cerebral angiography revealed a right anterior communicating artery aneurysm. The patient underwent emergency craniotomy, successful aneurysmal clipping, and subarachnoid clot evacuation. She gradually awoke from surgery without evidence of a significant focal neurologic deficit. On the fifth day following SAH evacuation she became progressively more somnolent and developed a mild left hemiparesis.

Discussion

Cerebral Artery Vasospasm

Cerebral artery vasospasm is the most common (30%) and one of the most devastating consequences of SAH.[32] Vasospasm is classified in terms of angiographic and clinical findings. Angiographic vasospasm is the observation of cerebral arterial narrowing during diagnostic angiographic procedures. This may or may not be accompanied by clinical vasospasm, which is the compendium of clinical signs and symptoms associated with cerebral ischemia due to a compromise of CBF. Progressive arterial narrowing can lead to cerebral infarction and permanent neurologic deficits.

Retrospective and prospective studies have indicated that the volume and distribution of subarachnoid blood is important in determining the risk of vasospasm.[157, 158] Those factors associated with increased risk of vasospasm are (1) clots larger than 5 × 3 mm in length or width, (2) vertical layers of blood clot greater than 1 mm thick as shown by CT sections, and/or (3) clotted blood in the basal cisterns.[157] Diffusely distributed subarachnoid blood, clotted blood located other than in the basal cisterns, and no blood on CT scan appear to be associated with a diminished chance of severe vasospasm.[157]

While there is a strong correlation between the amount and distribution of blood in the subarachnoid space and the development of vasospasm, the mechanism by which the presence of blood evokes this response is unclear. Several theories have been advanced including (1) direct vascular smooth muscle constriction in response to the liberation of vasoactive substances; (2) inhibition of normal vasodilatory responses due to prostacycline–thromboxane A_2 imbalance, hemoglobin in the CSF, or hypoxia of arterial smooth muscle cells; (3) mechanical distortion of the cerebral arteries by a periarterial clot; (4) deposition of circulating immune complexes in the media of the cerebral arteries; (5) leukocyte invasion of the arterial walls and adhesion to the endothelial surfaces; (6) smooth muscle cell and fibroblast proliferation; and (7) abnormal ionic conductance across the cerebrovascular smooth muscle membranes. [32, 147, 159, 160]

The time course for the development of cerebral artery vasospasm appears somewhat different in experimental animals than in humans. [160] In dogs there appears to be a biphasic response with an immediate vasospasm that peaks in 30 minutes and reverses within 2 days. This is followed by late or chronic vasospasm that begins within 48 hours of SAH and persists from days to weeks. The early spasm has not been well demonstrated in humans. Although vasospasm in humans has been reported to occur any time between the first day and several weeks following SAH, chronic vasospasm has been shown to reach its maximal intensity within 5 to 7 days after the hemorrhagic event. [32, 160] As in the patient presented here, vasospasm usually begins with the gradual onset of signs of decreased global CBF such as somnolence, confusion, semicoma, or stupor. This is often followed by the development of focal neurologic deficits such as speech abnormalities and/or weakness in various muscle groups. It is unusual for focal neurologic deficits to occur without a more generalized change in consciousness. [160] While it has been shown that there is a decrease in global CBF in association with SAH and that this worsens with the clinical grade of the patient, it does not seem to be clearly related to angiographic vasospasm. [160–166] Studies of regional cerebral blood flow (rCBF) have produced conflicting results; however, many authors have shown decreases in rCBF in the distribution of spastic cerebral arteries. [160, 162, 167–169]

Although the standard method for the evaluation of vasospasm is cerebral angiography, transcranial Doppler measurement of cerebral blood velocity is generating interest. It has been demonstrated that the velocity of blood flow through middle cerebral arteries classified as spastic by angiography is related in an inverse fashion to the diameter of the arteries as measured from the angiograms. [170] The relationship is less clear when applied to the anterior cerebral arteries, most likely due to collateral blood flow channels. [170] Abnormal flow velocities in cerebral arteries have been related to the occurrence and severity of clinical vasospasm. [171, 172]

CASE STUDY 2 CONTINUED

Because the patient's changing neurologic status was thought to be due to cerebral vasospasm, a pulmonary artery catheter was inserted to aid in optimization of the patient's hemodynamic status. The initial hemodynamic profile was as follows: CVP, 7 mm Hg; right ventricular pressure (RP), 22/0 mm Hg; pulmonary artery pressure (PAP), 22/8 mm Hg; PAOP, 7 mm Hg; CO, 4.6 L/min; MAP, 98 mm Hg; and SVR, 1,582 dynes·sec·cm^{-5}. The pertinent laboratory values at that time were hemoglobin, 12.8 g/dL; Na, 139 mEq/L; and K, 4.1 mEq/L. The patient was given fluid boluses with 0.9% NaCl and 5% albumin until the PAOP was raised to 15 mm Hg. At this point the other hemodynamic parameters were CVP, 14 mm Hg; PAP, 28/17 mm Hg; CO, 6.9 L/min; MAP, 105 mm Hg; and SVR, 1,055 dynes-sec-cm^{-5}. The patient appeared to be more responsive and began to regain strength in her left side. Repeat laboratory studies revealed the following: hemoglobin, 11.2 g/dL; Na, 144 mEq/L; and K, 3.8 mEq/L.

Discussion

Therapy for Cerebral Artery Vasospasm

Therapy for cerebral artery vasospasm is only marginally effective. Attempts at biochemical manipulation have included prostaglandins with vasodilatory activity and inhibitory effects on platelet aggregation (prostacyclin, carbacyclin) and thromboxane synthetase inhibitors.[173] Steroids in various doses, nonsteroidal anti-inflammatory agents, and calcium channel blockers have been investigated in various animal models of cerebral vasospasm.[32, 174–177] While these therapies show promise, some of them carry risks of significant adverse side effects.[32, 175] Nimodipine, a calcium channel blocker, has been heavily studied, and evidence has been produced that neurologic outcome in patients with cerebral artery vasospasm is improved with this treatment.[178, 179]

The mainstay of therapy in humans has been the manipulation of the patient's hemodynamic status in order to maximize cardiac output with the goal of preservation of perfusion to the area of brain at risk for infarction.[180–182] The first step in this "hyperperfusion protocol" is to optimize the filling pressures.[183] These patients are often relatively hypovolemic and may benefit significantly from fluid loading. However, even those who are euvolemic may benefit from the maximizing of filling pressures in order to increase cardiac output and blood flow as much as possible. If this is done with the appropriate hemodynamic monitors (i.e., pulmonary artery catheter), it can be done safely with the avoidance of fluid overload and pulmonary edema. If such patients improve neurologically, they are maintained at the hemodynamic level at which improvement is maximal.

CASE STUDY 2 CONTINUED

The patient responded to fluid loading for approximately 36 hours, at which point she again appeared to become more somnolent and developed more weakness in her left upper extremity. At that time her hemodynamic profile was as follows: CVP, 15 mm Hg; PAP, 28/18 mm Hg; PAOP, 17 mm Hg; CO, 5.2 L/min; MAP, 98 mm Hg; and SVR, 1,277 dynes-sec-cm^{-5}. Dobutamine therapy was started at a rate of 3 μg/kg/min. After approximately 30 minutes, a repeat hemodynamic profile revealed the following: CVP, 14 mm Hg; PAP, 27/16 mm Hg; PAOP 15 mm Hg; CO, 6.1 L/min; MAP, 103 mm Hg; and SVR, 1,167 dynes-sec-cm^{-5}. There was no significant neurologic improvement. The PAOP was raised to 18 mm Hg with 500 cc of 0.9% NaCl, and a new hemodynamic profile was obtained, the results of which are as follows: CV P, 17 mm Hg; PAP, 30/19 mm Hg; PAOP, 18 mm Hg; CO, 6.8 L/min; MAP, 106 mm Hg; and SVR, 1,047 dynes-sec-cm^{-5}. The patient appeared to awaken significantly and to regain some strength in her left arm. She was maintained at this level of support and observed for further neurologic changes.

Discussion

If the patient does not improve neurologically or if the patient improves initially and then deteriorates, CO is further augmented with inotropic and sometimes chronotropic support.[32, 183] This is probably best done while maintaining arterial BP and SVR within normal limits (SVR of 800 to 1,200 dynes-sec-cm^{-5}). Close attention must be paid to the patient's myocardial status during these manipulations, especially if these patients are within the age group where coronary artery disease must be considered. The addition of inotropic and chronotropic agents (i.e., dobutamine, dopamine, isoproterenol) have the potential to significantly increase myocardial oxygen consumption and precipitate ischemia. Serial ECG tracings may be helpful when the patient is unable to communicate symptoms of myocardial ischemia.

CASE STUDY 2 CONTINUED

The hyperperfusion protocol was continued for 3 more days, at which point the patient had evidence of a mild residual left upper extremity weakness. Inotropic agents were withdrawn and fluid loading discontinued without a deterioration in the patient's neurologic status. The patient was transferred from the NSICU to the floor and eventually to a rehabilitation unit for treatment of her residual neurologic deficit.

DISCUSSION

The final outcome for the patient with CNS injury rests on the ability of the critical care physician to manage the acute sequelae of the initial insult and produce a favorable milieu for neuronal recovery. As is demonstrated by the cases presented here, the physiologic derangements that can accompany a primary neurologic injury can be significant. Since the major portion of the neurologic damage is often fixed at the time of the initial event, the true challenge for the physician caring for these patients is to minimize secondary injury caused by the pathophysiologic sequelae brought about by the primary CNS disorder.

REFERENCES

1. Jagger J, Levine JI, Jane JA, et al: Epidemiologic features of head injury in a predominantly rural population. *J Trauma* 1984; 24:40–44.
2. Kalsbeek WD, McLaurin RL, Harris BSH III, et al: The national head and spinal cord injury survey: Major findings. *J Neurosurg* 1980; 55(suppl):19–31.
3. Baker CC, Oppenheimer L, Stephens B, et al: Epidemiology of trauma deaths. *Am J Surg* 1980; 140:144–150.
4. Allen R: Intracranial pressure: A review of clinical problems, measurement techniques and monitoring methods. *J Med Eng Technol* 1986; 10:299–320.
5. Cutler RWP, Page L, Galicich J, Watters GV: Formation and absorption of cerebrospinal fluid in man. *Brain* 1968; 91:707–720.
6. Miller JD, Garibi J, Pickard JD: Induced changes of cerebrospinal fluid volume: Effects during continuous monitoring of ventricular fluid pressure. *Arch Neurol* 1973; 28:265–269.
7. Rockoff MA, Kennedy SK: Physiology and clinical aspects of raised intracranial pressure, in Ropper AH, Kennedy SF (eds): *Neurological and Neurosurgical Intensive Care*, ed 2. Rockville, Md, Aspen Publishers, Inc, 1988, pp 9–21.
8. Rockoff MA, Kennedy SK: Physiology and clinical aspects of raised intracranial pressure, in Ropper AH, Kennedy (eds): *Neurological and Neurosurgical Intensive Care*, ed 2. Rockville, Md, Aspen Publishers, Inc, 1988, pp 11–12.

9. Johnston IH, Rowan JO: Raised intracranial pressure and cerebral blood flow: 3. Venous outflow tract pressures and vascular resistances in experimental intracranial hypertension. *J Neurol Neurosurg Psychiatry* 1974; 37:392–402.

10. Miller JD: Physiology of trauma. *Clin Neurosurg* 1982; 29:103–130.

11. North JB, Jennett S: Abnormal breathing patterns associated with acute brain damage. *Arch Neurol* 1974; 31:338–344.

12. Plum F, Posner JB: Supratentorial lesions causing coma: Diagnosis of coma from supratentorial mass lesions, in *The Diagnosis of Stupor and Coma*, ed 3. Philadelphia, FA Davis Co Publishers. 1980, pp 101–102.

13. Sinha RP, Ducker TB, Perot PL: Arterial oxygenation: Findings and its significance in central nervous system trauma patients. *JAMA* 1973; 224:1258–1260.

14. Lindgren S, Rinder L: Experimental studies in head injury. *Biophysik* 1965; 2:320–329.

15. Sullivan HG, Nartubexm AJ, Becker DP, et al: Fluid percussion model of mechanical brain injury in the cat. *J Neurosurg* 1976; 45:520–534.

16. Bremer AM, Yamada K, West CR: Ischemic cerebral edema in primates: Effects of acetazolamide, phenytoin, sorbitol, dexamethasone and methylprednisone on brain water and electrolytes. *Neurosurgery* 1980; 6:149–154.

17. Saunders ML, Miller JD, Stablein D, et al: The effects of graded experimental trauma on cerebral blood flow and responsiveness to CO_2. *J Neurosurg* 1979; 51:18–26.

18. Wei EP, Dietrich DW, Povlishock JT, et al: Functional morphologic and metabolic abnormalities of the cerebral microcirculation after concussive brain injury in cats. *Circ Res* 1981; 48:95–103.

19. Holbourn AHS: Mechanisms of head injuries. *Lancet* 1943; 2:438–441.

20. Pudenz RH, Shelden CH: Lucite calvarium: Method for direct observation of the brain, cerebral trauma and brain movement. *J Neurosurg* 1946; 3:487–505.

21. Strich SJ: Shearing of nerve fibers as a cause of brain damage due to head injury: A pathological study of twenty cases. *Lancet* 1961; 2:443–448.

22. Teasdale G, Jennett B: Assessment of coma and impaired consciousness: A practical scale. *Lancet* 1974; 2:81–84.

23. Fisher CM: Ocular bobbing. *Arch Neurol* 1964; 11:543–546.

24. Sevitt S: Fatal road accidents in Birmingham: Times of death and their course. *Injury* 1973; 4:281–293.

25. Illingworth G, Jennett WB: The shocked head injury. *Lancet* 1965; 2:511–514.

26. Jennett B: Some medicolegal aspects of the management of acute head injury. *Br Med J* 1976; 1:1383–1385.

27. Patel AR, Jennett B, Galbraith SL: Alcohol and head injury. *Lancet* 1977; 1:1369–1370.

28. Flamm ES, Demopoulos HB, Seligman ML; et al: Ethanol potentiation of central nervous system trauma. *J Neurosurg* 1977; 46:328–335.

29. Galbraith SL: Misdiagnosis and delayed diagnosis in traumatic intracranial hematoma. *Br Med J* 1976; 1:1438–1439.

30. Trowbridge A, Giesecke AH: Multiple injuries. *Clin Anesthesiol* 1976; 11:79–84.

31. Katsuada K, Yamada R, Sugimoto R: Respiratory insufficiency in patients with severe head injury. *Surgery* 1973; 73:191–199.

32. Kassell NF, Sasaki T, Colohan ART, et al: Cerebral vasospasm following aneurysmal subarachnoid hemorrhage (review). *Stroke* 1985; 16:562–572.

33. Sohn D, Levine S: Frontal lobe infarctions caused by brain herniation: Compression of anterior cerebral artery branches. *Arch Pathol* 1967; 84:509–512.

34. Pitts L: Neurologic evaluation of the head injury patient. *Clin Neurosug* 1982; 29:203–224.

35. Gobb CP, Schwartz DJ, Wynne JW, et al: Antacid pulmonary aspiration in the dog. *Anesthesiology* 1979; 51:380–385.

36. Cooper PR: Resuscitation of the multiply injured patient. *Clin Neurosurg* 1982; 29:225–239.

37. Beck GP, Nwill LW: Anesthesia for associated trauma in patients with head injuries. *Anesth Analg* 1963; 42:687–695.

38. Crighton HC, Giesecke AH: One year's experience in the anesthetic management of trauma. *Anesth Analg* 1966; 45:835–842.

39. Gronert GA, Theye RA: Pathophysiology of hyperkalemia induced by succinylcholine. *Anesthesiology* 1975; 43:89–99.

40. Miller RD, Savarese JJ: Pharmacology of muscle relaxants and their antagonists, in Miller RD (ed): *Anesthesia*, ed 2, vol 2. New York, Churchill Livingstone, Inc, 1986, pp 889–943.

41. Cooperman LH: Succinylcholine-induced hyperkalemia in neuromuscular disease. *JAMA* 1970; 213:1867–1871.

42. Cooperman LH, Strobel GE Jr, Kennell EM: Massive hyperkalemia after administration of succinylcholine. *Anesthesiology* 1970; 32:161–164.

43. Stevenson PH, Birch AA: Succinylcholine-induced hyperkalemia in a patient with a closed head injury. *Anesthesiology* 1979; 51:89–90.

44. Donegan MF, Bedford RF: Intravenously administered lidocaine prevents intracranial hypertension during endotrachial suctioning. *Anesthesiology* 1980; 52:516–518.
45. McKay RD: Head trauma: Anesthesia, in Newfield P, Cottrell JE (eds): *Handbook of Neuroanesthesia: Clinical and Physiologic Essentials.* Boston, Little Brown & Co, Inc, 1983, pp 314–336.
46. Way WL, Trevor AJ: Pharmacology of intravenous nonnarcotic anesthetics, in Miller RD (ed): *Anesthesia,* ed, vol 2. New York, Churchill Livingstone, Inc, 1986, pp 799–833.
47. Bedford RF, Persing JA, Pobereskin L, et al: Lidocaine or thiopental for rapid control of intracranial hypertension. *Anesth Analg* 1980; 59:435–437.
48. Ropper AH, Rockoff MA: Treatment of intracranial hypertension, in Ropper AH, Kennedy SF (eds): *Neurological and Neurosurgical Intensive Care,* ed 2. Rockville, Md, Aspen Publishers, Inc, 1988, pp 23–41.
49. Plum F, Posner JB: Blood and cerebrospinal fluid lactate during hyperventilation. *Am J Physiol* 1967; 212:864–870.
50. Miller JD, Bell BA: Cerebral blood flow variations with perfusion pressure and metabolism, in Wood JH (ed): *Cerebral Blood Flow: Physiologic and Clinical Aspects.* New York, McGraw-Hill International Book Co, 1987; pp 119–130.
51. Cane RD, Shapiro BA: Clinical principles of positive pressure ventilation. *Anesthesiol Clin North Am* 1987; 5:717–747.
52. Weed L, McKibben P: Pressure changes in the cerebrospinal fluid following intravenous injections of solutions of various concentrations. *Am J Physiol* 1919; 48:512–530.
53. Muizelaar JP, Wei EP, Kontos HA, et al: Mannitol causes compensatory cerebral vasoconstriction and vasodilation in response to blood viscosity changes. *J Neurosurg* 1983; 59:822–828.
54. Muizelaar JP, Lutz HA, Becker DP: Effect of mannitol on ICP and CBF and correlation with pressure autoregulation in severely head-injured patients. *J Neurosurg* 1984; 61:700–706.
55. Bell BA, Kean DM, MacDonald HL, et al: Brain water measured by magnetic resonance imaging: Correlation with direct estimation and changes after mannitol and dexamethasone. *Lancet* 1987; 1:66–69.
56. Marshall LF, Smith RW, Rausher LA, et al: Mannitol dose requirements in brain injured patients. *J Neurosurg* 1978; 48:169–172.
57. Gennari FJ, Kassirer JP: Osmotic diuresis. *N Engl J Med* 1974; 291:714–720.
58. Marshall LF, Smith RW, Rauscher LA, et al: Mannitol dose requirements in brain injured patients. *J Neurosurg* 1978; 48:169–172.
59. Goluboff B, Shankin A, Haft H: The effects of mannitol and urea on cerebral hemodynamics and cerebrospinal fluid pressure. *Neurology* 1964; 14:891–898.
60. James HE, Langfitt TW, Kumar V, et al: Treatment of intracranial hypertension; analysis of 105 consecutive continuous recordings of intracranial pressure. *Acta Neurochir* 1977; 36:189–200.
61. Shenkin HA, Spitz EB, Grant FC, et al: The acute effects on the cerebral circulation of the reduction of increased intracranial pressure by means of intravenous glucose or ventricular drainage. *J Neurosurg* 1948; 5:466–470.
62. Lanier WL, Stanglnad KJ, Scheithauer BW, et al: The effects of dextrose infusion and head position on neurologic outcome after complete cerebral ischemia in primates: Examination of a model. *Anesthesiology* 1987; 66:39–48.
63. Stewart DJ, DaSilva CA, Flegel T: Elevated blood glucose levels may increase the danger of neurological deficit following profoundly hypothermic cardiac arrest. *Anesthesiology* 1988; 68:653.
64. Swedlow DB, Schreiner MS: Management of Reye's syndrome. *Crit Care Clin* 1985; 1:285–311.
65. Solviter HA, Shimkin P, Suhara K: Glycerol as a substrate for brain metabolism. *Nature* 1970; 210:1334.
66. MacDonald JT, Uden DL: Intravenous glycerol and mannitol therapy in children with intracranial hypertension. *Neurology* 1982; 32:437–440.
67. Nahata MC, Kerzner B, McClung HJ, et al: Variations in glycerol kinetics in Reye's syndrome. *Clin Pharmacol Ther* 1981; 29:782–787.
68. Galicich JH, French LA: Use of dexamethasone in the treatment of cerebral edema resulting from brain tumors and brain surgery. *Am Pract Dig Treat* 1961; 12:169–174.
69. Saul TG, Ducker TB, Salcman M, et al: Steroids in severe head injury: A prospective randomized clinical trial. *J Neurosurg* 1981; 54:596–600.
70. Braakman R, Schouten HJA, Blaauw–van Dishoeck M, Minderhoud JM: Megadose steroids in severe head injury; results of a prospective double-blind clinical trial. *J Neurosurg* 1983; 58:326–330.
71. Cooper PR, Moody S, Clark WK, et al: Dexamethasone and severe head injury: A prospective double-blind study. *J Neurosurg* 1979; 51:307–316.
72. Dearden NM, Gibson JS, McDowall DG, et al: Effect of high-dose dexamethasone on outcome from severe head injury. *J Neurosurg* 1986; 64:81–88.
73. Kalsbeek WD, McLaurin RL, Harris BSH, et al: The national head and spinal cord injury survey: Major findings. *J Neurosurg* 1980; 53(suppl):19–31.

74. Becker DP, Miller JD, Ward JD, et al: The outcome from severe head injury with early diagnosis and intensive management. *J Neurosurg* 1977; 47:491–502.
75. Jennett B, Teasdale G: *Management of Head Injuries. Contemporary Neurology Series*, no. 20. Philadelphia, FA Davis Co Publishers, 1981.
76. Jamieson KG, Yelland JDN: Extradural hematoma: Report of 167 cases. *J Neurosurg* 1968; 29:13–23.
77. Seelig JM, Becker DP, Miller JD, et al: Traumatic acute subdural hematoma: Major mortality reduction in comatose patients treated within four hours. *N Engl J Med* 1981; 304:1511–1518.
78. Jamieson KG, Yelland JDN: Surgically treated traumatic subdural hematomas. *J Neurosurg* 1972; 37:137–149.
79. Fell DA, Fitzgerald S, Moiel RH, et al: Acute subdural hematomas: Review of 144 cases. *J Neurosurg* 1975; 42:37–42.
80. Moiel RH, Caram PC: Acute subdural hematoma: A review of 84 cases. A six year evaluation. *J Trauma* 7:660–666.
81. Talalla A, Morin MA: Acute traumatic subdural hematoma: A review of 100 consecutive cases. *J Trauma* 1971; 11:771–777.
82. Frost EAM, Arancibia CU, Shullman K: Pulmonary shunt as a prognostic indicator in head injury. *J Neurosurg* 1979; 50:768–772.
83. Miller JD: Disorders of cerebral blood flow and intracranial pressure after head injury. *Clin Neurosurg* 1982; 29:162–173.
84. Miller JD, Becker DP, Ward JD, et al: Significance of intracranial hypertension in severe head injury. *J Neurosurg* 1977; 47:503–516.
85. Miller JD, Butterworth JF, Gudman SK, et al: Further experience in the management of severe head injury. *J Neurosurg* 1981; 54:289–299.
86. Greenberg RP, Mayer DJ, Becker DP: Correlation in man on intracranial pressure and neuroelectric activity determined by multimodality evoked potentials, in Beks JFW, Bosch DA, Brock M (eds): *Intracerebral Pressure*, vol 3. Berlin, Springer-Verlag, 1976.
87. Mayhill CG, Archer NH, Lamb VA, et al: Ventrulostomy-related infections. *N Engl J Med* 1984; 310:553–559.
88. Aucoin PJ, Kotilainen HR, Gantz NM, et al: Intracranial pressure monitors: Epidemiologic study of risk factors and infections. *Am J Med* 1986; 80:369–376.
89. Aucoin PJ, Kotilainen HR, Gantz NM, et al: Intracranial pressure monitors: Epidemiologic study of risk factors and infections. *Am J Med* 1986; 80:369–376.
90. Mayhill CG, Archer NH, Lamb VA, et al: Ventriculostomy-related infections. A prospective epidemiologic study. *N Engl J Med* 1984; 310:553–559.
91. Barnett GH, Chapman PH: Insertion and care of intracranial pressure monitoring devices, in Ropper AH, Kennedy SF (eds): *Neurological and Neurosurgical Intensive Care*, ed 2. Rockville, Md, Aspen Publishers, Inc, 1988, pp 43–55.
92. Lundberg N: Continuous recording and control of ventricular fluid pressure in neurosurgical practice. *Acta Psychiatr Neurol Scand* 1960; 149(suppl):1–193.
93. Risberg J, Lundberg N, Ingvar DH: Regional cerebral blood volume during acute transient rises of the intracranial pressure (plateau waves). *J Neurosurg* 1969; 31:303–310.
94. Matsuda M, Yondea S, Handa H, et al: Cerebral hemodynamic changes during plateau waves in brain tumor patients. *J Neurosurg* 1979; 50:483–488.
95. Brue DA, Alvi A, Bilanuik L, et al: Diffuse cerebral swelling following head injuries in children: The syndrome of malignant brain edema. *J Neurosurg* 1981; 54:170–178.
96. Zimmerman RA, Bilanuik LT, Bruce DA, et al: Computed tomography of pediatric head trauma: Acute general cerebral swelling. *Radiology* 1978; 126:403–408.
97. Povlishock JT, Becker DP, Sullivan HA, et al: Vascular permeability alterations to horseradish peroxidases in experimental brain injury. *Brain Res* 1978; 1533:223–239.
98. Povlishock JT, Becker DP, Miller JD, et al: The morphopathologic substrates of concussion. *Acta Neuropathol* 1979; 47:1–11.
99. Klatzo I: Presidental address: Neuropathological aspects of brain edema. *J Neuropathol Exp Neurol* 1967; 26:1–14.
100. Klatzo I: Pathophysiological aspects of brain edema, Reulen HJ, Schurman K (eds): in *Steroids and Brain Edema*. Berlin, Springer-Verlag, 1972, pp 1–8.
101. Long DM: Traumatic brain edema. *Clin Neurosurg* 1982; 29:174–202.
102. Costa JL, Ito U, Spatz M, et al: 5-Hydroxytryptamine accumulation in cerebrovascular injury. *Nature* 1974; 248:135–136.
103. Demopoulos HB, Flamm ES, Seligman ML, et al: Membrane perturbations in central nervous system injury: Theoretical basis for free radical damage and a review of the experimental data, in Popp AJ, et al (eds): *Neural Trauma*. New York, Raven Press, 1979.

104. Fenske A, Sinterhauf K, Reulen HJ: The role of monoamines in the development of cold-induced edema, in Pappius HM, Feindel W (eds): *Dynamics of Brain Edema*. Berlin, Springer-Verlag, 1976, pp 150–154.
105. Flamm ES, Demopoulos HB, Seligman ML, et al: Barbiturates and free radicals, in Popp AJ, et al (eds): *Neural Trauma*. New York, Raven Press, 1979.
106. Sloan TB: Neurologic monitoring. *Crit Care Clin* 1988; 4:543–557.
107. Swedlow DB, Schreiner MS: Management of Reye's syndrome. *Crit Care Clin* 1985; 1:285–311.
108. Borel C, Hanley D: Neurologic intensive care unit monitoring. *Crit Care Clin* 1985; 1:223–239.
109. Mihm FG: Barbiturates for intracranial hypertension and focal and global ischemia, in Newfield P, Cottrell JE (eds): *Handbook of Neuroanesthesia: Clinical and Physiologic Essentials*. Boston, Little, Brown & Co, 1983, pp 61–98.
110. Brain Resuscitation Clinical Trial I Study Group: Randomized clinical study of thiopental loading in comatose survivors of cardiac arrest. *N Engl J Med* 1986; 314:397–403.
111. Ward JD, Becker DP, Miller JD, et al: Failure of prophylactic barbiturate coma in the treatment of severe head injury. *J Neurosurg* 1985; 62:383–388.
112. Nemoto EM: Barbiturate therapy for the ischemic brain. *N Engl J Med* 1986; 315:397–398.
113. Slogoff S: Barbiturate therapy for the ischemic brain. *N Engl J Med* 1986; 315:398.
114. Yatsu FM: Barbiturate therapy for the ischemic brain. *N Engl J Med* 1986; 315:397.
115. Dampney RAL, Kumada M, Reis DJ: Central neural mechanisms of the cerebral ischemic response. *Circ Res* 1979; 44:48–62.
116. Maire FW, Patton HD: Neural structures involved in the genesis of preoptic pulmonary edema, gastric erosions, and behavior changes. *Am J Physiol* 1956; 184:345–350.
117. Samuels MA: Cardiopulmonary aspects of neurological catastrophes, in Ropper AH, Kennedy SF (eds): *Neurological and Neurosurgical Intensive Care*, ed 2. Rockville, Md, Aspen Publishers, Inc, 1988, pp 99–108.
118. Blessing WW, Sved AF, Reis DJ: Destruction of noradrenergic neurons in rabbit brainstem elevates plasma vasopressin, causing hypertension. *Science* 1982; 217:661–662.
119. Rosell S: Neuronal control of microvessels. *Annu Rev Physiol* 1980; 42:359–371.
120. Apuzzo MLJ, Weiss MH, Petersons V, et al: Effect of positive end expiratory pressure ventilation on intracranial pressure in man. *J Neurosurg* 1977; 46:227–232.
121. Burchiel KJ, Steege TD, Wyler AR: Intracranial pressure changes in brain-injured patients requiring positive end-expiratory pressure ventilation. *Neurosurgery* 1981; 8:443–449.
122. Cooper KR, Boswell PA, Choi SC: Safe use of PEEP in patients with severe head injury. *J Neurosurg* 1985; 63:552–555.
123. Burchiel KJ, Steege TD, Wyler AR: Intracranial pressure changes in brain-injured patients requiring positive end-expiratory pressure ventilation. *Neurosurgery* 1981; 8:443–449.
124. Cooper KR, Boswell PA: Reduced functional residual capacity and abnormal oxygenation in patients with severe head injury. *Chest* 1983; 84:29–35.
125. Frost EAM: Effects of positive end-expiratory pressure on intracranial pressure and compliance in brain-injured patients. *J Neurosurg* 1977; 47:195–200.
126. Born JD, Hans P, Smitz S, et al: Syndrome of inappropriate secretion of antidiuretic hormone after severe head injury. *Surg Neurol* 1985; 23:383–387.
127. Greger NG, Kirkland RT, Clayton GW, et al: Central diabetes insipidus. *Am J Dis Child* 1986; 140:551–554.
128. Bowerman JE, Heslop IH: Diabetes insipidus associated with maxillofacial injuries. *Br J Oral Surg* 1971; 8:197–202.
129. Kern KB, Meislin HW: Diabetes insipidus: Occurrence after minor head trauma. *J Trauma* 1984; 24:69–72.
130. Porter RJ, Miller RA: Diabetes insipidus following closed head injury. *J Neurol Neurosurg Psychiatry* 1948; 11:258–262.
131. McLaurin RL, King LR: Metabolic effects of head injury, in Vinkien PJ, Bruyn GW, Braakman R (eds): *Handbook of Clinical Neurology*, vol 23. *Injuries of the Brain and Skull*, part I. Amsterdam, Elsevier Science Publishers, 1975, pp 109–131.
132. Oppenheimer DR: Microscopic lesions in the brain following head injury. *J Neurol Neurosurg Psychiatry* 1968; 31:299–306.
133. Glauser FL: Diabetes insipidus in hypoxic encephalopathy. *JAMA* 1976; 235:932–933.
134. Keren G, Schreiber M, Aladjem M: Diabetes insipidus indicating a dying brain. *Crit Care Med* 1982; 10:798–799.
135. Outwater KM, Rockoff MA: Diabetes insipidus accompanying brain death in children. *Neurology* 1984; 34:1243–1246.
136. Plum F, Posner JB: Supratentorial lesions causing coma, in *The Diagnosis of Stupor and Coma*, ed 3. Philadelphia, FA Davis Co Publishers, 1980, pp 87–116, 153–157.

137. Roberson GL: Posterior pituitary, in Felig P, Baxter JO, Broadus AE (eds): *Endocrinology and Metabolism*, ed 2. New York, McGraw-Hill International Book Co, 1987, pp 338–385.
138. Decaux G, Waterlot Y, Genette F, et al: Treatment of the syndrome of inappropriate secretion of antidiuretic hormone with furosemide. *N Engl J Med* 1981; 304:329–330.
139. Miller PD, Linas SL, Schrier RW: Plasma demeclocycline levels and nephrotoxicity: Correlation in hyponatremic cirrhotic patients. *JAMA* 1980; 243:2513.
140. Oster JR, Epstein M, Ulano HB: Deterioration of renal function with demeclocycline administration. *Curr Ther Res* 1976; 20:794–801.
141. Longstreth WT Jr, Koepsell TD, Yerby MS, et al: Risk factors for subarachnoid hemorrhage. *Stroke.* 1985; 16:377–385.
142. Kassell NF, Drake CG: Timing of aneurysm surgery. *Neurosurgery* 1982; 10:514–519.
143. Alexander MSM, Dias PS, Uttley D: Spontaneous subarachnoid hemorrhage and negative cerebral panangiography: Review of 140 cases. *J Neurosurg* 1986; 64:536–542.
144. Sacco RL, Wolf PA, Bharucha NE, et al: Subarachnoid and intracerebral hemorrhage: Natural history, prognosis, and precursive factors in the Framingham Study. *Neurology* 1984; 34:847–854.
145. Schisano G, Franco A: Primary non traumatic intracranial hemorrhage: 139 consecutive cases treated at an emergency regional hospital. *J Neurosurg Sci* 1982; 26:199–204.
146. Ducker TB: Spontaneous intracerebral hemorrhage, in Wilkins RH, Rengachary SS (eds): *Neurosurgery*, vol 2. New York, McGraw-Hill International Book Co, 1985, pp 1510–1517.
147. Sano K: Cerebral vasospasm and aneurysm surgery. *Clin Neurosurg* 1983; 30:13–58.
148. Ropper AH, Zervas NT: Outcome 1 year after SAH from cerebral aneurysm: Management morbidity, mortality, and functional status in 112 consecutive good-risk patients. *J Neurosurg* 1984; 60:909–915.
149. Shepard RH: Prognosis of spontaneous (non-traumatic) subarachnoid hemorrhage of unknown cause: A personal series 1958–1980. *Lancet* 1984; 1:777–778.
150. Peerless SJ: Intracranial aneurysms: Neurosurgery, in Newfield P, Cottrell JE (eds): *Handbook of Neuroanesthesia: Clinical and Physiologic Essentials*. Boston, Little, Brown & Co, 1983, pp 173–183.
151. Freckman N, Noll M, Winkler D, et al: Does the timing of aneurysm surgery neglect the real problems of subarachnoid haemorrhage? *Acta Neurochir* 1987; 89: 91–99.
152. Byer E, Ashman R, Toth LA: Electrocardiogram with large upright T wave and long Q-T intervals. *Am Heart J* 1947; 33:796–801.
153. Hugenholtz PG: Electrocardiographic abnormalities in cerebral disorders: Report of six cases and review of the literature. *Am Heart J* 1961; 63:451–461.
154. Levine HD: Non-specificity of the electrocardiogram associated with coronary artery disease. *Am J Med* 1953; 15:344–350.
155. Plum F, Posner JB: The pathologic physiology of signs and symptoms of coma, in *The Diagnosis of Stupor and Coma*, ed 3. Philadelphia, FA Davis Co Publishers 1980, pp 1–86.
156. Bahandari AK, Scheinman M: The long QT syndrome. *Mod Concepts Cardiovasc Dis* 1985; 54:45–50.
157. Kistler JP, Crowell RM, Davis KR, et al: The relation of cerebral vasospasm to the extent and location of subarachnoid blood visualized by CT scan: A prospective study. *Neurology* 1983; 33:424–436.
158. Fisher CM, Kistler JP, Davis JM: Relation of cerebral vasospasm to subarachnoid hemorrhage visualized by computerized tomographic scanning. *Neurosurgery*, 1980; 6:1–9.
159. Harder DR, Dernbach P, Waters A: Possible cellular mechanism for cerebral vasospasm after experimental subarachnoid hemorrhage in the dog. *J Clin Invest* 1987; 80:875–880.
160. Chyatte D, Sundt TM: Cerebral vasospasm after subarachnoid hemorrhage (review). *Mayo Clin Proc* 1984; 59:498–505.
161. Kagstrom E, Greitz T, Hanson J, et al: Changes in cerebral blood flow after subarachnoid haemorrhage. *Excerpta Medica International Congress Series* 1966; 110:629–633.
162. James IM: Changes in cerebral blood flow and in systemic arterial pressure following spontaneous subarachnoid haemorrhage. *Clin Sci* 1968; 35:11–22.
163. Heilbrun MP, Olesen J, Lassen NA: Regional cerebral blood flow studies in subarachnoid haemorrhage. *J Neurosurg* 1972; 37:36–44.
164. Nilsson BW: Cerebral blood flow measurements in subarachnoid hemorrhage with intravenous ^{99}Tc technique, in Wilkins S (ed): *Cerebral Arterial Spasm: Proceedings of the Second International Workshop*. Baltimore, Williams & Wilkins, 1980, pp 320–324.
165. Pitts LH, Macpherson P, Wyper DJ, et al: Effects of vasospasm on cerebral blood flow after subarachnoid hemorrhage, in Wilkins RH (ed): *Cerebral Arterial Spasm: Proceedings of the Second International Workshop*. Baltimore, Williams & Wilkins, 1980, pp 333–337.
166. Grubb RL Jr, Raichle ME, Eichling JO, et al: Effects of subarachnoid hemorrhage on cerebral blood volume, blood flow, and oxygen utilization in humans. *J Neurosurg* 1977; 46:446–453.

167. Symon L, Ackerman R, Bull JWD, et al: The use of xenon clearance method in subarachnoid hemorrhage: Post-operative studies with clinical and angiographic correlation. *Eur Neurol* 1972; 8:8–14.
168. Heilbrun MP, Olesen J, Lassen NA: Regional cerebral blood flow studies in subarachnoid hemorrhage, in Wilkins RH (ed): *Cerebral Arterial Spasm: Proceedings of the Second International Workshop.* Baltimore, Williams & Wilkins, 1980, pp 314–319.
169. Zingesser LH, Schechter MM, Dexter J, et al: On the significance of spasm associated with rupture of a cerebral aneurysm: The relationship between spasm as noted angiographically and regional blood flow determinations. *Arch Neurol* 1968; 18:520–528.
170. Aaslid R, Huber P, Nornes H: Evaluation of cerebrovascular spasm with transcranial Doppler ultrasound. *J Neurosurg* 1984; 60:37–41.
171. Sekhar LN, Wechsler LR, Yonas H, et al: Value of transcranial Doppler examination in the diagnosis of cerebral vasospasm after subarachnoid hemorrhage. *Neurosurgery* 1988; 22:813–821.
172. Seiler RW, Grolimund P, Aaslid R, et al: Cerebral vasospasm evaluated by transcranial ultrasound correlated with clinical grade and CT-visualized subarachnoid hemorrhage. *J Neurosurg* 1986; 64:594–600.
173. Chan RC, Durity FA, Thompson GB, et al: The role of the prostacyclin-thromboxane system in cerebral vasospasm following induced subarachnoid hemorrhage in the rabbit. *J Neurosurg* 1984; 61:1120–1128.
174. Chyatte D, Sundt TM: Response of chronic experimental cerebral vasospasm to methylprednisolone and dexamethasone. *J Neurosurg* 1984; 60:923–926.
175. Chyatte D, Rusch N, Sundt TM: Prevention of chronic experimental cerebral vasospasm with ibuprofen and high-dose methylprednisolone. *J Neurosurg* 1983; 59:925–932.
176. Espinosa F, Weir B, Shnitka T, et al: A randomized placebo-controlled double-blind trial of nimodipine after SAH in monkeys, Part 1: Clinical and radiological findings. *J Neurosurg* 1984; 60:1167–1175.
177. Espinosa F, Weir B, Shnitka T, et al: A randomized placebo-controlled double-blind trial of nimodipine after SAH in monkeys, Part 2: Pathological findings. *J Neurosurg* 1984; 60:1176–1185.
178. Welty T: Use of nimodipine for prevention and treatment of cerebral arterial spasm in patients with subarachnoid hemorrhage. *Clin Pharm* 1987; 6:940–946.
179. Allen GS, Hyo SA, Preziosi TJ, et al: Cerebral arterial spasm—A controlled trial of nimodipine in patients with subarachnoid hemorrhage. *N Engl J Med* 1984; 308:619–624.
180. Pritz MB, Giannotta SL, Kindt GW, et al: Treatment of patients with neurological deficits associated with cerebral vasospasm by intravascular volume expansion. *Neurosurgery* 1978; 3:364–368.
181. McGillicuddy J, Kindt G, Giannotta S, et al: Focal cerebral blood flow in cerebral vasospasm: The effect of intravascular volume expansion. *Acta Neurol Scand* 60(suppl 72):490–491, 1979.
182. Keller TS, McGillicuddy JE, LaBond VA, et al: Volume expansion in focal cerebral ischemia: The effect of cardiac output on local cerebral blood flow. *Clin Neurosurg* 1982; 29:40–50.
183. Finn SS, Stephensen SA, Miller CA, et al: Observations on the perioperative management of aneurysmal subarachnoid hemorrhage. *J Neurosurg* 1986; 65:48–62.

12/Nontraumatic Coma

JEFFREY I. FRANK, M.D.
SCOTT L. HELLER, M.D.

The intensive care unit (ICU) harbors numerous patients with disorders of consciousness spanning the continuum from lethargy to coma. Consequently, a basic understanding of altered states of consciousness is crucial to any physician assessing and managing patients in a critical care setting. Figure 12–1 provides a schematic approach to management of patients presenting with altered consciousness.

The coma examination requires a systematic approach to assessing various levels of function in the central neuraxis. In general, when the various components of the examination localize a lesion to *one* level of the central nervous system (CNS), this is suggestive of a focal process such as infarction, hemorrhage, neoplasm, or infection. When the examination reveals abnormalities at *multiple* levels of the central neuraxis, a toxic-metabolic disorder (e.g., overdose/withdrawal, electrolyte abnormalities, hypercalcemia, diffuse ischemia/anoxia, hypothyroidism, and hepatic encephalopathy) is likely. Table 12–1 provides a basic outline of neurologic assessment of the comatose patient.

LEVEL OF CONSCIOUSNESS

In general, conscious behavior can be impaired by alterations in arousability and/or thought content. Arousability is predominantly controlled by a network of neurons traversing the brain stem and thalamus that is called the ascending reticular activating system (ARAS).[1, 2] Wakefulness is maintained by ARAS stimulation of deep cortical and thalamic structures. Disruption of this system affects conscious behavior by depression of arousability. The ARAS may be disrupted by torque forces as seen with head trauma, supratentorial or infratentorial pressure, and intrinsic brain stem lesions. Also, severe toxic or metabolic disturbances may depress function of the ARAS because they concomitantly affect the cerebrum diffusely.

Although conscious functioning depends heavily on the state of arousability provided by the ARAS, arousability by no means guarantees normal consciousness. After all, in the extreme, a wakeful patient without cognitive functioning is unable to exhibit conscious behavior. This aspect of conscious behavior that correlates with cognitive functioning is often referred to as the content of consciousness. It is most useful to consider that there must be bilateral cortical dysfunction in order to significantly impair cognition and, in turn, content of consciousness. Bilateral cortical

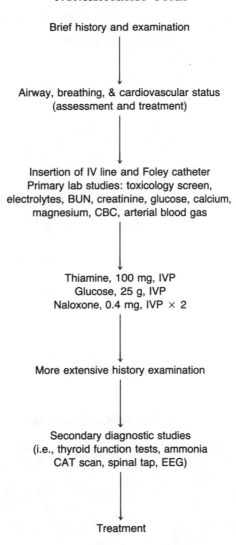

FIG 12–1.
Schematic outline of an approach to management of patients with nontraumatic coma. *BUN* = blood urea nitrogen; *CBC* = complete blood cell count; *IVP* = intravenous push; *CAT* = computed axial tomography; *EEG* = electroencephalography.

TABLE 12–1.

Neurologic Assessment of the
Comatose Patient

Level of consciousness
  Arousability
  Content
Brain stem function
  Respiratory rate and pattern
  Blood pressure and heart rate
  Pupil size and reactivity
  Eye position and movements
    Doll's eyes maneuver
    Cold caloric testing
  Corneal reflexes
  Facial symmetry
Motor function
  Posturing
  Tone
  Spontaneous movements
  Withdrawal to noxious stimulus
  Deep tendon reflexes

dysfunction is most often due to toxic-metabolic disturbances that diffusely affects brain function. In short, normal conscious behavior is dependent on arousability and content, and this can be altered by ARAS and/or bilateral cortical dysfunction.

Assessment of Consciousness

It should now be obvious that a determination of the level of consciousness depends on analyzing arousability and content. Initially, observe whether the patient appears asleep (eyes closed or wakeful spontaneous eye opening). If in a sleeping state, quantify how much stimulation is required to arouse the patient, if at all possible. Once aroused, determine the patient's ability to remain wakeful as well as respond in a coherent manner. Table 12–2 presents the meaning of several terms that describe various levels of consciousness.

TABLE 12–2.

Clinical Levels of Altered Consciousness

Terms	Eyes	Arousability	Content
Lethargy	Closed	Arousable	Mildly impaired
Stupor	Closed	Arousable with effort	Markedly impaired
Coma	Closed	Unarousable	Not applicable
Akinetic mutism* (abulic state, coma vigil)	Open	Wakeful	Impaired
Locked-in syndrome†	Open	Wakeful	Normal

*Secondary to bilateral frontal/basal forebrain dysfunction.
†Secondary to basis pontis dysfunction.

Lethargy, stupor, and coma represent different points on a continuum of decreasing levels of consciousness. Patients in each of these states appear to be sleeping with eyes closed. In contrast, patients with akinetic mutism and locked-in syndrome appear to be awake with eyes opened.

In addition to these terms used to describe patients with altered consciousness, the Glasgow Coma Scale (GCS) is used to assign a numerical description of consciousness, most often in the setting of trauma (Table 12–3). The GCS is a 0- to 15-point scale that assesses reactivity of eye opening (i.e., level of consciousness) and best verbal and motor responses.[3]

CASE STUDY 1

A 49-year-old black man was brought to the emergency room (ER) by paramedics. The patient's coworkers thought he was "acting strangely." The paramedics found him supine on the floor without signs of trauma. Vital signs showed a blood pressure (BP) of 230/140 mm Hg, a pulse of 50/min, and a respiratory rate (RR) of 40/min. His airway was patent, and his cardiovascular status was stable. The paramedics noted the pupils to be very small with an undetectable response to light. The patient was given 25 g glucose and 0.4 mg Naloxone intravenously (IV) in the field and 100 mg thiamine IV upon arrival to the ER. The vital signs were unchanged, and cardiovascular stability was confirmed. An accompanying friend indicated no history of alcohol or drug abuse, diabetes, hypertension, seizures, or

TABLE 12–3.

The Glascow Coma Scale*

Response	Points
Eye opening	
Spontaneously	4
To speech	3
To pain	2
Never	1
Best verbal response	
Oriented	5
Confused	4
Inappropriate	3
Garbled	2
None	1
Best motor response	
Obeys commands	6
Localizes pain	5
Withdrawal	4
Abnormal flexion	3
Extension	2
None	1
	15

*The lower the GCS score, the more severe the head injury.

TABLE 12–4.

Useful Physical Examination Findings in Comatose Patients

Exam Focus	Specific Features	Suggested Condition
Skin	Petechiae, splinter hemorrhage	Coagulopathy; SBE*
	Icteric	Hepatic encephalopathy
	Needle tracks	Drug overdose or withdrawal
	Cyanotic	CO_2 narcosis
Lymph nodes	Adenopathy	Infectious etiologies; immunocompromised hosts
Head	Contusion; postauricular ecchymosis (Battle's sign)	Trauma
	VP* shunt	Hydrocephalus; shunt malfunction
Eyes	Periorbital ecchymosis (raccoon eyes)	Trauma
	Papilledema	Increased intracranial pressure
Ears	Hemotympanum	Trauma
Nose	Excessive discharge	Trauma
Neck	Stiff	Subarachnoid hemorrhage, infection
	Enlarged thyroid	Dysthyroidism
Cardiovascular	Arrhythmia, etc.	Hypoxic/ischemic encephalopathy
Abdomen	Small hard liver	Hepatic encephalopathy
Misc.	Acetone, alcohol breath	Ketoacidosis; alcohol intoxication
	Fever	Infection
	Tongue laceration; incontinence	Postictal state

*SBE = subacute bacterial endocarditis; VP = ventriculoperitoneal.

trauma. The patient apparently complained of a severe posterior headache hours before the incident in association with vomiting and mild confusion. A general physical examination was unremarkable. The neck was supple.

Discussion

Brief History and Examination

Although these patients often present with limited information, there is usually historical information and examination findings that may be useful in prioritizing initial management steps. Some historical and general examination details useful in the diagnosis of these patients are outlined in Table 12–4.

Initial Management

Coma may reflect a profound threat to CNS viability and consequently requires emergent initial management steps. A more thorough effort can be made to pursue further history or perform a more extensive examination once initial management steps have been performed. As in any emergency medical situation, the priorities are airway procurement, ventilatory assessment and support if needed, and cardiovascular stabilization. Of course, maintenance IV fluid therapy and insertion of a Foley catheter to monitor urine output should be provided. Blood and urine should be obtained for early detection of some of the common reversible toxic-metabolic causes of coma (see Fig 12–1). There are three reversible causes of altered consciousness that are readily treatable. These include Wernicke's encephalopathy,* hypoglycemia, and narcotic overdose, which are treated with thiamine, glucose, and naloxone, respectively (Fig 12–1). Glucose administration may precipitate Wernicke's encephalopathy in a thiamine-deficient patient. Thus, the protocol is to administer thiamine followed by glucose and naloxone. Once these management steps have been completed, it is time to proceed with more extensive history and examination.

History

History is always helpful in developing a differential diagnosis for the individual patient presenting with altered consciousness. Unfortunately, such patients are often unaccompanied and unable to provide useful history themselves. Nonetheless, an aggressive attempt should be made to obtain relevant historical information, at times even requiring a search through the patient's personal effects. For example, it is relevant to determine any history of alcoholism, drug abuse, seizures, diabetes, as well as other medical conditions that increase the risk of CNS insult.

The patient's friend provided important historical information, The patient did not abuse alcohol or drugs and was not diabetic, which makes drug intoxication/withdrawal, Wernicke's encephalopathy, and hypoglycemia unlikely. The history of headache and nausea raises the possibility of increased intracranial pressure in this patient. Intracranial hemorrhage becomes a common etiology in this setting.

CASE STUDY 1 CONTINUED

The patient was hyperventilating with an RR of 40/min with regular rate and depth. Occasional hiccups were noted. The pupils were small (1.5 mm) but reactive to light. Funduscopic examination was unrevealing. Conjugate deviation of the eyes to the left was noted without spontaneous eye movements. The doll's eye maneuver and cold caloric testing failed to produce any change in eye position. The left corneal reflex was intact, but there was a diminished response on the right. In addition, the right facial musculature showed decreased movement, and asymmetrical grimacing was noted after noxious stimulation. The muscle tone was diminished in all extremities, with bilateral extensor posturing to painful stimuli. The patient was hyperreflexic bilaterally, and bilateral Babinski signs were noted.

---

*Wernicke's encephalopathy occurs secondary to thiamine deficiency in malnourished patients such as chronic alcoholics and is manifested by a variety of symptoms including confusion, memory loss, nystagmus, ocular motility problems, ataxia, and depression of consciousness.

Discussion

Neurologic Assessment in Coma

Respiratory control.—The cerebral cortex and forebrain are important in control of regular respiration. Damage to the cortex and forebrain bilaterally (usually toxic-metabolic in origin) often causes a breathing pattern characterized by a crescendo and then a decrescendo in the depth of breathing followed by brief apneic periods (i.e., Cheyne-Stokes respiration). Midbrain and upper pontine lesions may cause a central hyperventilation syndrome with persistent hyperventilation.[4] Lesions of the mid and/or lower pons are characterized by deep prolonged inspiration followed by a long pause referred to as apneustic breathing.[5] Ataxic breathing is an irregular respiratory pattern that occurs with lesions in the dorsomedial medulla and may be accompanied by hypersensitivity to respiratory depressants. Figure 12–2 summarizes these respiratory patterns and their neuroanatomic localizing significance. When assesssing a comatose patient, the rate and pattern of respiration should be observed. In addition vomiting and hiccups should be noted because they may result from intrinsic brain stem pathology or transmitted pressure on the brain stem.

This patient's respiratory pattern suggests midbrain dysfunction. The hiccups may be a manifestation of concurrent brain stem involvement.

Pupillary size and reactivity.—Pupillary size is controlled by the autonomic nervous system and is dictated by the balance between sympathetic and parasympathetic input to the pupillary dilators and constrictors, respectively. The parasympathetic efferents to the pupil originate from the Edinger-Westphal nucleus in the

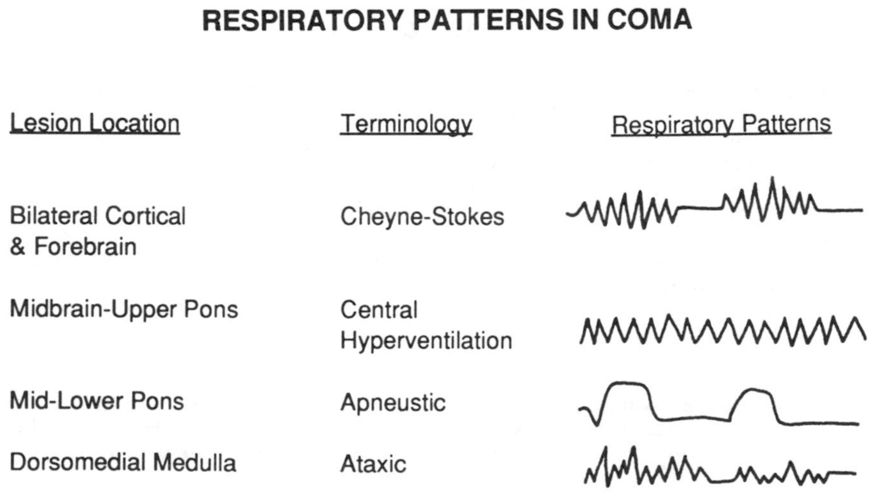

RESPIRATORY PATTERNS IN COMA

Lesion Location	Terminology	Respiratory Patterns
Bilateral Cortical & Forebrain	Cheyne-Stokes	
Midbrain-Upper Pons	Central Hyperventilation	
Mid-Lower Pons	Apneustic	
Dorsomedial Medulla	Ataxic	

FIG 12–2.
Respiratory patterns in coma.

upper midbrain and travel with the ipsilateral third cranial nerve (oculomotor). Dysfunction within this pathway will produce unopposed sympathetic input to the pupil and relative pupillary dilatation ipsilateral to the lesion. The sympathetic efferents to the pupil originate in the hypothalamus, descend through the brain stem and cervical spinal cord, and exit the upper thoracic spinal cord (T1–T3 levels). From there they ascend the carotid sheath and follow the vasculature to the pupil. Any disruption of the sympathetic fibers along this loop can lead to unopposed parasympathetic pupillary activity and subsequently an ipsilateral small (miotic) pupil. Since the midbrain is the one location in the brain stem where parasympathetic and sympathetic pupillary fibers are adjacent, a midbrain lesion classically results in intermediate pupil size. Lesions rostral or caudal to the midbrain may disrupt descending sympathetics and produce small pupils due to unopposed parasympathetic activity.

Obviously, many drugs affect the autonomic nervous system and therefore affect pupillary size. For example, parasympatholytics (anticholinergic agents) and sympathomimetics (adrenergic agents) lead to pupillary dilation. Parasympathomimetics (cholinergic agents) and sympatholytics (antiadrenergic agents) lead to pupillary constriction.

Pupillary light reflexes.—Normal pupillary reflexes depend on the integrity of afferent and efferent connections. A light stimulus to one eye, through a network of connections, sends input to both Edinger-Westphal nuclei, which produces constriction of the pupil ipsilateral (direct response) and contralateral (consensual response) to the stimulus. Table 12–5 summarizes the pupillary changes commonly seen in coma and their significance.

The unilaterally dilated, unreactive pupil in an unresponsive patient is worthy of mention. This may be caused by herniation of the ipsilateral temporal uncus through the tentorium, which compresses the ipsilateral oculomotor nerve and its parasympathetic fibers. In this setting, the large pupil is eventually accompanied by other evidence of cranial nerve (CN) III disruption (ipsilateral eye deviation, inferolater-

TABLE 12–5.

Pupillary Changes in Coma

Size	Reactivity	Comments
Bilateral		
Normal or small	Normal	Toxic-metabolic disturbance
Midposition (3–5 mm)	Poor	Midbrain dysfunction; drugs (glutethimide [Doriden])
Small (pinpoint)	Poor	Pontine dysfunction; drugs (narcotics)
Large	Poor	Toxic-metabolic disturbance (anoxia); drugs (anticholinergics)
Unilateral		
Large	Unreactive	Ipsilateral midbrain pathology or compression of ipsilateral CN III: uncal herniation, posterior communicating artery aneurysm
Small	Minimal	Ipsilateral sympathetic dysfunction

ally). This temporal herniation syndrome is due to an increase in intracranial pressure in, or transmitted to, the affected temporal lobe due to edema from a variety of pathologic processes. Prompt identification of this phenomenon is imperative because it represents a neurologic emergency.

In this case, the patient's small pupils may be consistent with disruption of the descending sympathetic fibers, rostral or caudal, to the midbrain.

Eye position and movements.—The eye muscles are controlled by three sets of cranial nerves, CN III (oculomotor), CN IV (trochlear), and CN VI (abducens), their nuclei being located in the upper midbrain, lower midbrain, and pontomedullary junction, respectively. Proper eye movement control requires a network of interconnections between these nuclei so that the eyes move conjugately. This interconnection is referred to as the medial longitudinal fasciculus (MLF), which is also integrated with the vestibular nuclei and allows for reflex conjugate eye movement in response to head positional changes.

Figure 12–3 displays the relevant anatomy accounting for horizontal conjugate eye movements. Each frontal eye field controls gaze to the contralateral side by stimulating the contralateral pontine paramedian reticular formation (PPRF) at the pontomedullary junction. The PPRF provides input to its ipsilateral abducens nucleus (abducting the ipsilateral eye) and sends input via the MLF to the contralateral oculomotor nucleus–medial rectus portion (adducting the contralateral eye).

Lesions of the frontal eye fields or the PPRFs lead to *conjugate* eye deviation, provided that the MLF is intact. Therefore, a lesion of the right frontal eye field or left PPRF impairs leftward gaze, and in turn, the eyes conjugately deviate to the right (Fig 12–3, lesions 1 and 2). Similarly, lesions of the left frontal eye field or right PPRF leads to conjugate eye deviation to the left (Fig 12–3, lesions 3 and 4). In short, the eyes turn toward the lesion with frontal eye field dysfunction and away from the lesion with PPRF dysfunction. In contrast, MLF lesions are manifested as poor adduction of the eye ipsilateral to the MLF lesion. Spontaneous "roving" eye movements in all directions in the comatose patient demonstrates integrity of a significant portion of the brain stem. If no spontaneous eye movements are observed, the intactness of the interconnections responsible for eye control are in question. Since comatose patients are unable to follow commands, maneuvers that take advantage of vestibular input to ocular control must be utilized.

Oculocephalic reflexes–doll's eye maneuvers.—The doll's eye maneuver is performed by rapidly rotating the head from side to side and observing the patient's eye positional changes (Fig 12–4). The normal response in the comatose patient with an intact brain stem is for the eyes to remain fixed on the same point in space. Thus, when the head is turned rightward, the eyes remain conjugate to the left. When the head is turned leftward, the eyes remain conjugate to the right. This normal response is referred to as "doll's eyes." If a comatose patient does not have normal doll's eyes, a disruption of brain stem ocular and vestibular connections may be present.

Of course, in the setting of trauma, the head should not be rotated due to the possibility of cervical spine injury. In this situation or when doll's eye maneuvers are inconclusive, cold water calorics are helpful.

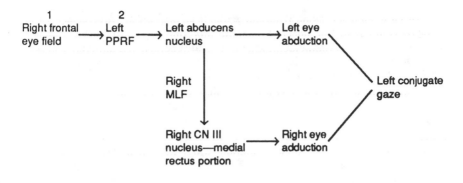

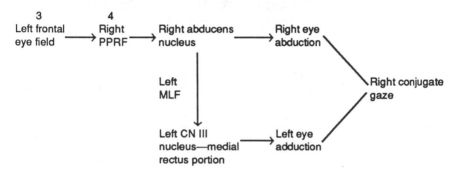

FIG 12–3.
Schematic representation of the neurologic pathways controlling horizontal conjugate gaze.
PPRF = pontine paramedian reticular formation; *MLF* = median longitudinal fasciculus; *CN III* = third cranial nerve; *1, 2, 3, 4* = sites of possible pathologic lesions (see the text).

Oculovestibular reflexes—cold water caloric testing.—Cold water calorics depend on vestibular system stimulation by altering endolymphatic flow in the semicircular canals. The change in endolymphatic flow is achieved by instilling ice-cold water in the external auditory canal, thereby cooling the mastoid process and, in turn, the semicircular canal. Prior to performing this test, examination of the external auditory canal should be performed in order to confirm intactness of the tympanic membrane and remove any impacted cerumen. The head should then be flexed 30 degrees above the horizontal. This position orients the lateral semicircular canal vertically and maximizes the response obtained from cold water. A functional apparatus for instilling the water is a butterfly catheter (with the needle removed) connected to a syringe containing approximately 100 cc of cold water (30°C). The cold water should be instilled slowly into the external auditory canal.

The responses to cold water calorics in patients with various lesions are summarized in Figure 12–4. In normal *wakeful* patients the response is horizontal nystagmus, with the slow component toward and the fast component away from the stimulated side and with minimal eye movement from the midline. With diminishing consciousness in patients without structural brain stem damage, the fast component of the nystagmus disappears, and the eyes tend to conjugately deviate toward the stimulated side. In order to ensure proper interpretation of cold water caloric testing, the opposite side should not be stimulated until 5 minutes after the initial side. Although simultaneous stimulation of both sides can occasionally be diagnostically helpful, a discussion of such maneuvers goes beyond the scope of this text.[6]

This patient's conjugate eye deviation to the left could be due to a contralateral brain stem lesion or an ipsilateral lesion of the frontal eyefield. The doll's eye maneuver and cold caloric testing differentiated between these two possibilities. The persistent conjugate eye deviation without any response to these maneuvers identified the lesion to be in the contralateral (right) brain stem, at the level of the pontomedullary junction.

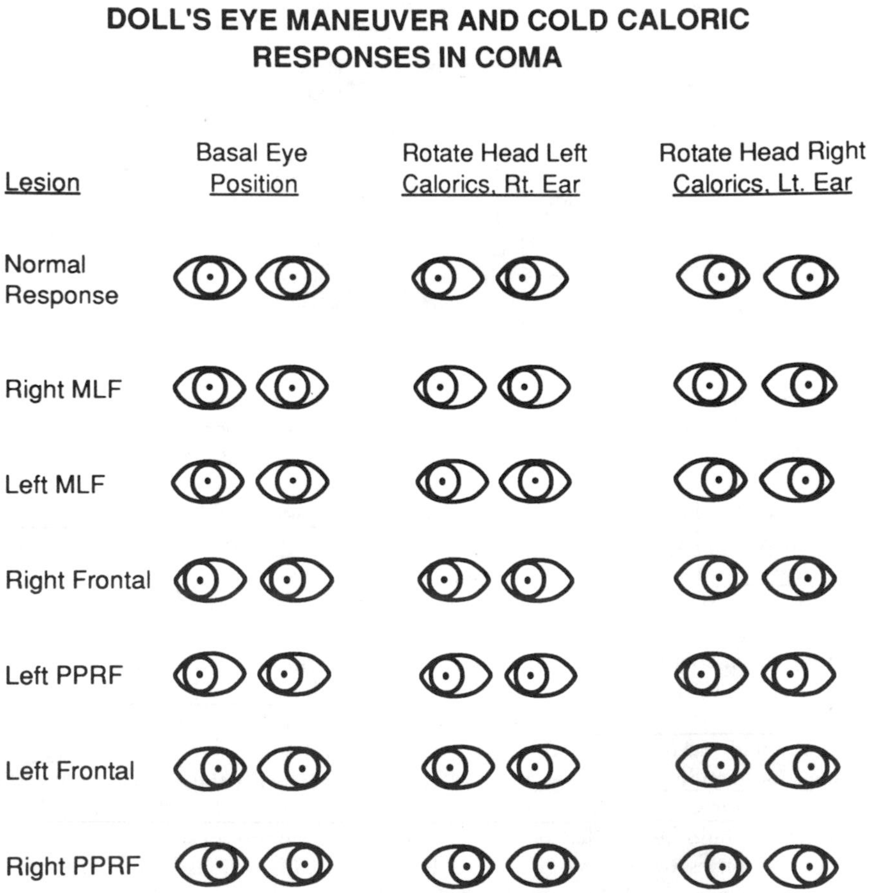

DOLL'S EYE MANEUVER AND COLD CALORIC RESPONSES IN COMA

Lesion	Basal Eye Position	Rotate Head Left Calorics, Rt. Ear	Rotate Head Right Calorics, Lt. Ear
Normal Response			
Right MLF			
Left MLF			
Right Frontal			
Left PPRF			
Left Frontal			
Right PPRF			

FIG 12–4.
Eye positions in the doll's eye maneuver and with cold caloric testing in coma. *MLF* = median longitudinal fasciculus; *PPRF* = pontine paramedian reticular formation.

Corneal reflex.—The corneal reflex is an important protective mechanism for the cornea. Essentially, it is a blinking reflex triggered when the cornea is presented with a noxious stimulus. Similar to other reflexes, it has an afferent and efferent limb. The afferent limb is via the trigeminal nerve (CN V), and the efferent limb is via the facial nerve (CN VII). Although corneal reflexes assess brain stem function, they have limited localizing value.

Each cornea, in sequence, should be lightly tapped with a wisp of cotton and the response observed. If the patient's eyelids are closed, they should be gently held open, the response being interpreted by "feeling" the reflex contraction of the orbicularis oculi. Focal lesions that disturb the trigeminal afferent or facial nucleus/ nerve efferent limbs of the corneal reflex arc may produce unilateral abnormalities of the normal response. Diffuse brain stem injury or depression secondary to hypothermia or structural or toxic-metabolic causes may lead to an absence of corneal reflexes bilaterally.

Facial musculature function.—Initially, the patient's face should be observed for symmetry. This may require removal of tape covering the mouth and lower portion of the face of the patient with an endotracheal tube in place. Lower facial weakness may be manifested as a depressed nasolabial fold or a depressed corner of the mouth. Upper facial weakness may be manifested as assymetry of forehead furrowing or incomplete eye closure. Since facial assymetry may be old (i.e., Bell's palsy) or constitutional, inquiring about past facial weakness and comparison with an old photograph may be helpful. Resting facial tone is observed, and then a grimace is elicited by providing a noxious stimulus to the supraorbital region. This maneuver may accentuate subtle weakness of facial musculature. Lower facial weakness alone implies a lesion involving the contralateral hemisphere or upper portion of the brain stem above the pontomedullary junction. Complete facial weakness suggests a lesion involving the ipsilateral facial nucleus or nerve at the level of the pontomedullary junction.

The diminished right corneal reflex response and right facial weakness remain consistent with a lesion localized to the right brain stem and involving the right facial nucleus.

Motor function.—The corticospinal tract predominantly originates from the frontal cortex and descends ipsilaterally through the corona radiata, the posterior limb of the internal capsule, and the cerebral peduncle of the midbrain and consolidates in the pyramids, the ventral swellings of the medulla. The pyramidal fibers decussate to the contralateral side at the junction of the medulla and spinal cord to form the lateral corticospinal tract.

Assessment of motor function.—Observation is the key to the motor examination in the comatose patient. The patient is observed for spontaneous movements or maintenance of particular postures.[7, 8] Lesions involving the corticospinal tract generally lead to diminished contralateral spontaneous activity. Upper midbrain or more rostral lesions may lead to *decorticate* posturing characterized by flexion of the contralateral arm at the elbow and hyperextension of the leg. Central midbrain and high pontine lesions, with a relatively intact brain stem inferiorly, may lead to *decerebrate* posturing characterized by contralateral arm and leg extension.[9] Such posturing may be caused by structural lesions or metabolic insults (e.g., postanoxia), and it is often mistaken for seizure activity. Also, the patient should be observed for the presence of tremor, myoclonus, or asterixis because these may be associated with toxic-metabolic encephalopathies.

After observing for spontaneous movements and posturing, motor tone should be assessed by passive flexion and extension of the extremities. Tone may be increased or decreased, depending on the location of the motor system involvement, and asymmetries in tone should be noted.

Noxious stimuli should then be applied to each limb and the supraorbital regions. Purposeful movement upon noxious stimulation suggests intactness of motor tracts to that limb, whereas decorticate or decerebrate posturing in response to noxious stimuli has the localizing significance mentioned above.

Acute corticospinal tract lesions may cause hyporeflexia because hyperreflexia may not occur for days to weeks after the injury. However, a Babinski sign, which is characterized by extension of the great toe (and fanning of the other toes) upon lateral plantar stimulation, may be present acutely with corticospinal tract lesions. Complete bilateral paralysis without any response to noxious stimuli usually indicates a grave prognosis. However, spinal cord injury and neuromuscular transmission blockade must be excluded because they may produce a similar state of complete paralysis.

CASE STUDY 1 CONTINUED

In summary, this patient's hyperventilation and pinpoint pupils suggested pontine dysfunction. Conjugate eye deviation to the left could have been secondary to a left frontal or right pontomedullary junction lesion. However, the lack of response to cold caloric testing localized the lesion to the right pontomedullary region. The bilateral Babinski signs were due to bilateral corticospinal tract involvement, and the decerebrate posturing localized the motor tract involvement to the brain stem below the lower part of the midbrain. Thus, the constellation of findings suggested a bilateral low-pontine lesion, with more involvement on the right. The right facial weakness and diminished corneal reflex were consistent with this localization.

The posterior headache, soon followed by coma, suggests a hemorrhagic process. The examination localized the hemorrhage to the posterior fossa predominantly affecting the right lower pons. The associated hypertension and bradycardia represents the "Cushing response," which is occasionally seen in the setting of increased intracranial pressure.

The patient was intubated and hyperventilated, and an emergent computed axial tomographic (CAT) scan of the head was performed with thin cuts through the posterior fossa. The CAT scan confirmed a large right cerebellar hemorrhage extending into the right pontine region with an associated mass effect. The neurosurgery team was notified, and the patient was emergently brought to the operating room for evacuation of the cerebellar hemorrhage. The etiology of the hemorrhage was not discovered, but the patient did well postoperatively, suffering minimal residual deficit due to prompt diagnosis and neurosurgical intervention.

TABLE 12–6.

Common Causes of Coma

Focal	Toxic Metabolic
Neoplasia	Hypoxic/anoxic
Hemorrhage	Ischemia
Subarachnoid	
Subdural/epidural	Hypoglycemia
Lobar	
Cerebellar	Electrolyte disturbance (Na, K, Ca, Mg)
Brain stem	
Cerebral infarction	Acid-base disturbance
Vasculitis	Hyperosmolar state
Infection	Nutritional deficiency (thiamine, B_2, B_6, B_{12})
Abscess	
Encephalitis (herpes)	
Empyema	Uremia
	Hepatic encephalopathy
	CO_2 narcosis
	Endocrine disorder (thyroid, parathyroid, etc.)
	Infections (encephalitis, meningitis)
	Drugs/toxins
	Hypothermia/hyperthermia

Discussion

The constellation of neurologic examination findings obtained should provide useful localizing information. When neuroanatomic localization indicates involvement at only *one* level of the central neuraxis, a focal pathologic process is likely. When the examination leads to the conclusion that the central neuraxis is affected at *multiple* levels or *diffusely*, the etiology is most likely of toxic-metabolic origin. Table 12–6 provides a list of common focal and toxic-metabolic processes that may produce coma.

Focal Etiologies of Coma

Intraparenchymal cerebral hemorrhage produces altered consciousness by the transmitted effects of increased intracranial pressure or by direct involvement of the brain stem as in the case of posterior fossa hemorrhages. There are numerous causes of cerebral hemorrhage, including hypertension, embolic stroke, vascular malformations, neoplasms, etc. The neuroanatomic localization may suggest the specific etiology. Patients with altered consciousness secondary to hemorrhage often progress gradually but rapidly. During the initial more wakeful stage, the patient may complain of severe headache located in the area referable to the location of the hemorrhage. The examination reveals findings suggesting a focal CNS disturbance. Hemorrhages are often associated with significantly elevated BP, and posterior fossa hemorrhages may be accompanied by vomiting. Subarachnoid hemorrhage, most commonly secondary to ruptured intracranial aneurysms, is often heralded by the acute onset of a severe headache followed by nuchal rigidity and altered consciousness.

Neoplasms can cause altered consciousness by two basic mechanisms. Supratentorial lesions can cause increased intracranial pressure due to their "space-occupying" effect within the closed cranial vault. Increased pressure can be transmitted to the brain stem causing disruption of the ARAS, and subsequently suppress arousability. Posterior fossa neoplasms may directly affect the ARAS due to the neoplasm's location contiguous with or intrinsic to the brain stem. Neoplastic processes are usually *insidious* in onset, as opposed to vascular phenomena, which may be *abrupt* in onset. Thus, the temporal profile of symptoms, prior to presentation, should be carefully sought. On occasion, intracranial neoplasms can be associated with hemorrhage, and this can account for an acute presentation.

Cerebral infarctions do not produce altered consciousness unless they involve the brain stem (affecting the ARAS directly) or are extremely large and associated with significant cerebral edema and increased intracranial pressure. Brain stem infarctions are often abrupt in onset and accompanied by cranial nerve dysfunction.

Altered consciousness with hemispheric infarctions usually occurs gradually since the cerebral edema and secondarily increased intracranial pressure responsible is gradual in onset. Thus, it should be clear that a sudden change in consciousness in a patient with a recent hemispheric infarction should raise the possibility of an incorrect localization (the infarct is actually in the brain stem), hemorrhage into the infarction, acute rise in intracranial pressure, or an additional process (i.e., new infarct, toxic effect of medications, electrolyte disturbance).

Secondary Diagnostic Testing

A variety of diagnostic tests are useful in evaluating comatose patients. CAT scanning of the head, a brain-imaging technique, is useful in detecting changes in brain density. It is utilized mainly to detect focal brain disease, being most sensitive for diagnosing acute hemorrhage, which appears as an area of increased density. Conversely, infarction shows up as an area of lucency. Neoplasms and abscesses are lucent on CAT but often accumulate IV contrast material due to alterations in the blood-brain barrier.

Magnetic resonance imaging (MRI) is the most sensitive way to image the brain in the vast majority of CNS diseases. The image resolution is much better than CAT, and it allows images of the CNS in multiple planes. MRI is particularly helpful for imaging posterior fossa structures, which often are poorly visualized on CAT due to bony artifact. MRI frequently displays pathologic processes earlier than CAT does, which may be critical for prompt initiation of appropriate therapy as in herpes encephalitis.

A spinal tap should be performed if CNS infection or subarachnoid hemorrhage is suspected. On occasion, CSF analysis is more sensitive than CAT is in documenting subarachnoid hemorrhage. Therefore, a lumbar puncture should be performed after a negative CAT scan when subarachnoid hemorrhage is clinically suspected. The major contraindication to performing a spinal tap is cerebral edema. Since processes associated with cerebral edema represent several of the etiologic considerations in the comatose patient, CAT should generally be performed prior to the spinal tap.

Electroencephalography (EEG) measures brain wave activity. It is useful in detecting focal cerebral dysfunction, seizures, encephalitis, and diffuse encephalopathy. In addition, it is often used as objective evidence in declaring "brain death."

CASE STUDY 2

A 37-year-old woman was found unarousable in the bathroom at work. The paramedics recorded her vital signs: BP, 100/50 mm Hg; pulse 60/min; and RR, 10/min. Oxygen was provided by mask. The pupils were small. She was given 25 g glucose and 0.4 mg naloxone IV before arrival at the ER. The patient was transported with a cervical collar on a spine board since trauma could not be completely excluded.

Upon arrival at the ER, the patient's vital signs were BP 90 mm Hg systolic pulse 60/min; RR 8/min; and temperature 35.5°C. There were no external signs of trauma. A screening general examination was only significant for very shallow spontaneous respirations. No needle "tracks" were noted. Due to the patient's shallow respirations, she was promptly intubated after "negative" cross-table cervical spine films. Blood was drawn for initial analysis, a Foley catheter was inserted, and IV fluids (normal saline, 150 cc/hr) were initiated. A fingerstick glucose level was 250 mg/dL. The patient was given 100 mg of thiamine by IV push, followed by naloxone, 0.4 mg × 2, and a neurologic consultation was ordered because the patient remained unresponsive.

Neurologic examination revealed an unresponsive, unarousable patient with eyes closed. The neck was supple, and there was no papilledema. Her pupils were 2 mm and reactive to light directly and consensually. The eyes were conjugately positioned in the midline, and no spontaneous eye movements were observed. A doll's eye maneuver and cold water calorics failed to reveal any response. Corneal reflexes were absent. The face appeared symmetrical and there was no grimacing to noxious stimulation. No spontaneous or extraneous movements of the extremities were noted. Tone was diminished throughout. The patient did not withdraw or posture to noxious stimulation, and she was diffusely hyporeflexic. No Babinski signs were elicited.

Discussion

Diffuse/Toxic-Metabolic Etiologies of Coma

In most critical care settings, toxic-metabolic disturbances are frequently responsible for coma. Because these disorders are often reversible but potentially lethal, recognition and prompt diagnosis is of utmost importance.

The onset of toxic-metabolic encephalopathies is usually characterized by a *gradual* deterioration in the patient's level of consciousness. Diffuse motor changes such as tremor, asterixis, and myclonus often accompany this group of disorders. Table 12–6 provides a list of the most common toxic-metabolic encephalopathies.

Drug intoxication and blood glucose alterations are common toxic-metabolic disturbances in acute care settings. A history of alcoholism, drug abuse, and their associated physical stigmata should be sought. A history of diabetes identifies the patients at most risk for both hypoglycemic and hyperosmolar states. The initial screening tests, including alcohol level, toxicology screens, and blood glucose determination, allow for prompt identification and treatment of these disorders.

Chronic liver disease predisposes patients to altered consciousness mainly due to altered amino acid metabolism. Hepatic encephalopathy usually occurs in patients with cirrhosis and can be precipitated by a large protein meal or gastrointestinal bleeding. These patients often have diffuse motor changes, incuding asterixis. Reye's syndrome is an encephalopathy associated with acute hepatic dysfunction often following a viral illness, and it should be suspected in children less than 12 years old presenting with altered consciousness.

Coma due to hypothyroidism is usually associated with hypothermia, bradycardia, thyromegaly, and hyporeflexia, whereas hyperthyroidism tends to cause an *agitated delirium* with tremulousness, tachycardia, and diffuse hyperreflexia.

Alterations in blood urea, sodium, calcium, magnesium, and more rarely, phosphate can lead to altered consciousness. Hyponatremia, hypocalcemia, and hypomagnesemia additionally predispose patients to seizures. The initial blood work should allow ready identification of these disorders even though the specific etiology may initially appear obscure.

Infectious etiologies can cause altered consciousness with either focal or diffuse examination findings. Cerebral abscesses are similar to neoplasms in their "space-occupying" characteristics and consequently cause coma by similar mechanisms. Bacterial and viral infections typically produce a meningoencephalitis and are therefore associated with diffuse CNS abnormalities. Herpes simplex virus is commonly associated with altered consciousness, but is frequently found with focal findings and seizures. CNS infections are often associated with nuchal rigidity, fever, and an elevated leukocyte count.

Altered consciousness typically occurs after generalized seizures and may persist for up to 24 hours after a single seizure. Of course, prior history can be quite useful in this circumstance. Evidence of tongue biting or urinary incontinence provides indirect evidence of prior seizure activity. Generally, the neurologic examination is nonfocal. However, if the seizure has a focal onset, the patient may display a postictal focal paresis. "Todd's paralysis" occurs contralateral to a focal hemispheric seizure focus and may last up to 24 hours with subsequent complete resolution.

Persistent seizures (status epilepticus) may cause prolonged altered consciousness without any gross motor activity. At times only an EEG may allow the detection of seizure activity with certainty.

CASE STUDY 2 CONTINUED

The patient's neurologic examination could not be localized to a single level in the neuro-axis. Rather, it revealed *diffuse* involvement of the CNS. This was felt to be typical of a toxic-metabolic disturbance. The hypothermia, hypoventilation, and small reactive pupils were possibly consistent with drug intoxication. Consequently, a nasogastric tube was placed for the purpose of gastric lavage. No drug residue was noted. Initial laboratory findings were normal except for the arterial blood gases, which were consistent with an acute respiratory acidosis. A toxicology screen and thyroid function tests were pending.

The patient was transported to the ICU and supportive care provided. Once stable, a CAT scan of the head, without contrast, was performed and found to be unrevealing. An EEG revealed diffuse changes in brain wave activity that were suggestive of a toxic-metabolic disturbance. The specific finding of "fast activity" on the EEG was highly suggestive of barbiturate or sedative poisoning. The toxicology screen returned and confirmed a barbiturate intoxication.

Discussion

The normal CAT scan in this patient was not surprising, given the suspicion of a toxic-metabolic disorder. Nonetheless, the CAT scan is an important diagnostic tool even in the patient with diffuse abnormalities. Disorders presenting with multifocal areas of pathology (e.g., multiple cardiac emboli) can mimic toxic-metabolic encephalopathies. The CAT scan can help differentiate such conditions, which may subsequently alter the patient's management.

The EEG was helpful in this case in that it confirmed a *diffuse* disturbance of cerebral activity typical of a toxic-metabolic encephalopathy.

CASE STUDY 2 CONTINUED

The patient's family was eventually located and revealed that she had been very depressed because of a "breakup" with her boyfriend. There was no history of medical illness, drug abuse, or suicide attempts. The patient was comatose for approximately 10 days due to the very long half-life of phenobarbital. Her recovery was complete, and she was transferred to a psychiatry unit to address her suicide attempt.

CASE STUDY 3

A 72-year-old man was admitted to the coronary care unit with an acute anterior wall myocardial infarction. Telemetry recorded multifocal premature ventricular contractions (PVCs) that improved with lidocaine administration. Later that evening, he went into rapid ventricular tachycardia that deteriorated to ventricular fibrillation. A "code" was announced, and resuscitation efforts began within 1 to 2 minutes. The patient was intubated within 4 minutes and was bagged with 100% O_2 prior to intubation. Defibrillation quickly converted the rhythm to sinus tachycardia as the appropriate antiarrhythmic agents were administered. Atropine was not utilized.

The patient was unresponsive immediately after the cardiac arrest and resuscitation. Two hours later, the patient was still unarousable with his eyes closed and required mechanical ventilation. The pupils were 5 mm bilaterally and nonreactive to light. The eyes were conjugate, and there was no response to the doll's eye maneuver or cold caloric testing. Corneal reflexes were absent. The face was symmetrical. There was no grimace to supraorbital pressure. No spontaneous movement of the extremities was noted. However, decerebrate posturing was noted after noxious stimulation to the extremities and tracheal suctioning. Tone was diminished throughout. The reflexes were 2/4, bilaterally. There was no response to plantar stimulation. The decerebrate posturing was initially thought to represent seizure activity by the medical housestaff, but the neurology consultant alleviated this concern.

Discussion

This patient suffered from anoxic encephalopathy, probably secondary to the arrhythmia and cerebral hypoperfusion. Anoxic encephalopathy is a diffuse disorder of cerebral function, the result of metabolic changes produced by hypoxia/anoxia and compounded by ischemia. The patient's examination did not localize to one level in the neuroaxis but was consistent with *diffuse* cerebral dysfunction.

Anoxic/ischemic encephalopathy is most commonly due to cardiopulmonary arrest but may also occur with choking, suffocation, drowning, hanging/strangulation, pulmonary embolism, massive systemic hemorrhage, and carbon monoxide poisoning. The diagnosis is most often made by obtaining an accurate history and recognition that the coma is toxic-metabolic in origin.

Prognosis in Non-Traumatic Coma

The cause of this patient's comatose state is clear. In this setting, the main goal of neurologic consultation is to assist in the assessment and prediction of the patient's chance of reasonable recovery. This, in turn, helps guide both physician and family in regard to the appropriateness of continuing advanced life support measures. Of all patients with nontraumatic coma, 15% may achieve good recovery or moderate disability at 1 month. When scrutinized by etiology, moderate disability or good recovery is three times more likely to occur in patients with metabolic encephalopathies (an approximately 30% chance of favorable outcome) in contrast to coma secondary to subarachnoid hemorrhage, cerebral hemorrhage, cerebral infarction, and hypoxic-ischemic encephalopathy (an approximately 10% chance of favorable outcome).

In the past decade, several studies have helped delineate the prognostic implications of nontraumatic or drug-related coma by clinical signs on examination.[10–12] The study of most practical significance in the critical care setting was performed by Levy et al—a review of the experience of 500 patients with nontraumatic coma.[13]

In general, the neurologic examination findings do not have prognostic significance until at least 6 hours after a cardiac arrest.[14–17] This patient displayed no evidence of brain stem function and minimal motor function. However, the examination was performed at only 2 hours.

CASE STUDY 3 CONTINUED

Eight hours after the arrest, the neurologic examination was repeated. The pupils were 3.5 mm and unreactive to light. The eyes were conjugate, and no response was elicited by the doll's eye maneuver or cold caloric testing. Corneal reflexes were absent, and the face appeared symmetrical. No purposeful movements were noted. There was no response to noxious stimuli. The patient was areflexic, and no plantar response was elicited.

Discussion

The absence of pupillary, oculocephalic, vestibulo-ocular, and corneal reflexes (brain stem reflexes) clearly placed this patient in the gravest prognostic category. Patients who lose any two of these reflexes after 6 hours of coma have a startlingly poor prognosis. At 1 month, 97% of these patients will die, have no recovery, or will be in a persistent vegetative state. Of the remaining 3% of patients, 2% will be left with severe neurologic disability.

Three days after coma onset, the absence of any one of the brain stem reflexes is indicative of a grave prognosis and virtually no chance of good recovery. Ninety-six percent of these patients will have no recovery or remain in a persistent vegetative state, while the remaining 4% will sustain severe neurologic disability. However, 74% of patients with intact brain stem reflexes and some verbal response will achieve good recovery or only moderate disability. At 1 week, those patients who fail to have eye opening to pain have no chance of good recovery or moderate disability. If they do open their eyes to painful stimuli and have a localizing motor response, 75% will achieve good recovery or moderate disability, in contrast to 10% in those without localizing motor responses.

CASE STUDY 3 CONTINUED

The patient's grave prognosis was discussed at length with his family. Although the clinical situation and examination findings alone supported the diagnosis of brain death, an EEG was performed to provide objective documentation, "electrocerebral silence." The EEG failed to reveal any brain wave activity. However, there was excessive artifact because of the electrical monitoring equipment in the ICU.

The clinical examination and EEG findings were unchanged 24 hours later. On the family's request, a nuclear medicine cerebral blood flow study was performed to further substantiate the diagnosis of brain death. The study was consistent with an absence of cerebral blood flow, thus supporting the diagnosis of brain death.

An apnea test revealed a complete absence of spontaneous respiration despite a progressive rise in CO_2 level. Further supportive care was withheld at the family's request after discussion with the physicians.

Brain Death

Clinical and laboratory determination of brain death is a common issue addressed in critical care settings. In general, brain death *cannot* be declared if the patient shows any evidence of CNS function. Clinically, this implies that the patient is completely unresponsive to stimulation and demonstrates no evidence of brain stem activity on examination. Patients with brain death should have a total absence of respiratory drive, a brain stem reflex. This may be evaluated by performing an "apnea test." The apnea test is performed after providing the patient with 100% oxygen for several minutes. The patient is then removed from the ventilator. Apnea with a documented rise of pCO_2 greater than 70 mm Hg generally confirms a loss of respiratory drive and brain stem function. Because toxic-metabolic disorders including hypothermia and barbiturate intoxication may lead to reversible coma and a loss of brain stem function, these etiologies must be properly excluded.

Angiography and cerebral blood flow studies may support the clinical diagnosis by demonstrating an absence of cerebral blood flow. An EEG may support the diagnosis by demonstrating a complete absence of cerebral activity. However, confident EEG interpretation of electrocerebral silence is occasionally difficult in the critical care unit setting because ambient electrical artifacts are frequently encountered.

Numerous criteria exist that assist in the diagnosis of brain death. Most of them are based upon the clinical absence of CNS function and the use of some objective tests as described above.[18-22]

REFERENCES

1. Moruzzi G, Magoun HW: Brainstem reticular formation and activation of the EEG. *Electroencephalogr Clin Neurophysiol* 1949; 1:455–473.
2. Jasper HH, Proctor LD, Knighton RS, et al: *Reticular Formation of the Brain*. Boston, Little, Brown & Co, 1958, pp 729–738.
3. Teasdale G, Jennett B: Assessment of coma and impaired consciousness, a practical scale. *Lancet* 1974; 2:81–84.
4. Plum F, Posner JB, Hain RF: Central neurogenic hyperventilation in man. *Arch Neurol Psychiatry* 1959; 81:535–549.
5. Plum F, Alvord EC: Apneustic breathing in man, *Arch Neurol* 1964; 10:101–112.
6. Plum F, Posner JB: *The Diagnosis of Stupor and Coma*, ed 3. Philadelphia, FA Davis Co Publishers, 1980, pp 54–57.
7. Sherrington CS: Cateploid reflexes in the monkey. *Proc R Soc Lond* 1897; 60:411–414.
8. Plum F, Posner JB: *The Diagnosis of Stupor and Coma*, ed 3. Philadelphia, FA Davis Co Publishers, 1980, pp 65–70.
9. Schepelmann F: Human motor activity in decerebrate states and their sequelae. *Acta Neurochir* 1979; 46:185–217.
10. Varnell PR: Neurologic outcome of prolonged coma survivors of out-of-hospital cardiac arrest. *Stroke* 1976; 7:279–282.
11. Willoughby JO, Leach BG: Relation of neurological findings after cardiac arrest to outcome. *Br Med J* 1974; 3:437–439.
12. Plum F, Caronna JJ: "Can one predict outcome of medical coma?" in *Outcome of Severe Damage to the Central Nervous System*. CIBA Foundation Symposium no. 34. Amsterdam, Elsevier Science Publishers, 1975, pp 121–139.
13. Levy DE, Bates D, Caronna JJ, et al: Prognosis in nontraumatic coma. *Ann Intern Med* 1981; 94:293–301.
14. Snyder BD, Ramirez-Lassepas M, Lippert DM: Neurologic status and prognosis after cardiopulmonary arrest: I. A retrospective study. *Neurology* 1977; 27:807–811.
15. Snyder BD, Loewenson RB, Gumnit RJ, et al: Neurologic prognosis after cardiopulmonary arrest: II. Level of consciousness. *Neurology* 1980; 30:52–58.
16. Snyder BD, Hauser WA, Loewenson RB, et al: Neurologic prognosis after cardiopulmonary arrest: III. Seizure activity. *Neurology* 1980; 30:1292–1297.
17. Snyder BD, Gumnit RJ, Leppik, IE, et al: Neurologic prognosis after cardiopulmonary arrest: IV. Brainstem reflexes. *Neurology* 1981; 31:1092–1097.
18. Beecher HK: A definition of irreversible coma. Report of the Ad Hoc Committee of the Harvard Medical School to examine the definition of brain death. *JAMA* 1968; 205:85–88.
19. Conference of Royal Colleges and Faculties of the United Kingdom: Diagnosis of brain death. *Lancet* 1976; 2:1069–1070.
20. Ingvar DH, Widen L: Brain death: Summary of a symposium. *Lakartidningen* 1972; 69:3804–3814.
21. Walker AE: An appraisal of the criteria of cerebral death. A summary statement. A collaborative study. *JAMA* 1977; 237:982–986.
22. Black PM: Brain death (Part I & II). *N Engl J Med* 1978; 299:338–344, 393–400.

13/ Pulmonary Aspiration

JEFFREY VENDER, M.D.

The Greek poet Anacreon was believed to have died in 475 B.C. after aspirating a grape seed,[1] and death by aspiration has frequently appeared in the literature ever since. Aspiration has been a commonly described cause of morbidity and mortality from the earliest recorded medical literature to this day. Following Mendelson's classic description of postpartum aspiration pneumonitis,[2] clinical and laboratory research has established the existence of a broad spectrum of "pulmonary syndromes" resulting from aspiration of various materials under many conditions. Aspiration pneumonitis usually refers to the inflammation resulting from aspirated material and does not necessarily imply infection.

INCIDENCE AND DIAGNOSIS OF ASPIRATION

Aspiration is a major cause of anesthetic mortality,[3-5] a common cause of pulmonary disease in the hospitalized patient,[6, 7] and believed to be a major cause of morbidity and mortality in critically ill patients.[7, 8] The incidence of pulmonary aspiration is difficult to establish because it most commonly occurs when the airway protective reflexes (swallow, gag, laryngospasm, and cough) are obtunded so that the patient shows little or no distress. Furthermore, healthy, sleeping individuals often aspirate oral contents without any resulting pulmonary dysfunction.[9]

Pulmonary aspiration is most often a presumptive and/or retrospective diagnosis based on both the assumption of compromised airway defense mechanisms at the time of aspiration and pulmonary pathology attributable to the aspiration. Airway defense mechanisms are often deficient in altered states of consciousness, in gastrointestinal disorders, and following therapeutic interventions.

Altered Neurologic States

The neurologically intact and awake individual has airway protective reflexes, coughing and laryngospasm, that greatly reduce the likelihood of clinically significant aspiration. Clinical evaluation of pharyngeal (gag and swallow), laryngeal, tracheal (cough), and carinal reflexes are often helpful, although 10% to 15% of the normal population has diminished or absent gag responses, and these reflexes tend to be diminished in the geriatric patient.[10]

Obtundation is usually associated with depression of airway protective reflexes.

This altered neurologic state is commonly associated with cerebrovascular accidents, drug overdose, alcohol intoxication, postictal states, sedative administration, general anesthesia, cardiopulmonary resuscitation and severe debilitation as well as numerous specific central nervous system (CNS) disorders.[11–13] Comatose patients must be assumed to have depressed airway protective reflexes and often require intubation for airway protection.

Gastrointestinal Disorders

Increased gastric pressure secondary to intestinal obstruction, obesity, intra-abdominal masses, or a diminished gastric emptying time increases the potential for pulmonary aspiration.[14] Esophageal disorders such as achalasia, stricture or spasm, pharyngoesophageal diverticula, and hiatal hernia have been associated with an increased incidence of pulmonary aspiration.[15–17] Neurologic dysphagias have been shown to enhance the potential for pulmonary aspiration.[18]

Iatrogenic Factors

Mechanical disruption of airway defense mechanisms is common in critically ill patients. Nasogastric tubes may disrupt the cardiac sphincter and allow reflux in the presence of gastric dilation or obstruction.[19] Although properly inflated balloon cuffs on tracheal tubes offer significant protection from massive aspiration, small amounts of pharyngeal fluid may enter the trachea around the inflated cuff.[20–22] Although the clinical significance of this phenomenon is not clear, it indicates that precautions are necessary, despite the presence of a tracheal balloon cuff. Low-pressure, high-volume endotracheal and tracheostomy tube cuffs are recommended.

Tracheostomy tubes often prevent adequate glottic protection during swallowing by limiting the ability of the pharyngeal muscles to elevate the larynx.[23] This often requires an appropriately inflated cuff during oral feedings despite intact protective reflexes. Overinflation can impinge the cuff posteriorly obstructing the esophagus and impeding swallowing.

Nasogastric tube feedings frequently result in high residual volumes in the stomach that increase the risk of aspiration.[24] Although transpyloric feeding may decrease the incidence of feeding-associated aspiration, it may also increase gastric secretions and acidity. Many drugs may prolong gastric emptying time and result in larger gastric residual volumes and an increased possibility of aspiration.

PATHOPHYSIOLOGY FOLLOWING ASPIRATION

Pulmonary aspiration leads to a pathologic spectrum determined by numerous patient and non–patient related factors. The introduction of a foreign inoculum into the pulmonary tree is the common denominator in all aspiration syndromes. The clinical presentation, pathophysiology, and therapeutic approach will be greatly influenced by the nature, volume, frequency, and distribution of the aspirated inoculum.[25] Three distinct classifications of inocula exist: toxic, nontoxic, and bacterial.

Toxic Inocula

Toxic fluids of clinical significance include acids, alcohols, volatile hydrocarbons, oils, and animal fats. The severity of pulmonary damage is influenced by the acidity, volume, and composition of the aspirate.[26] The most common and best studied of this group is the chemical pneumonitis resulting from gastric acid aspiration (Mendelson's syndrome).[2] Pulmonary damage from toxic fluids may be immediate or may appear within a few hours.[26, 27] Gross changes include edema, necrosis, and atelectasis. Microscopic changes include degeneration of bronchial epithelium, peribronchial hemorrhage and exudate, necrosis of alveolar epithelium, and alveolar infiltration of polymorphonuclear cells.

The most important factor in toxic fluid aspiration appears to be acidity.[28] A small volume (0.3 mL/kg) of pH 1 fluid introduced into dog tracheas results in significant pulmonary reaction.[27] Available data suggest that toxic fluids with a pH less than 2.5 consistently result in pulmonary pathology whereas fluids with a pH greater than 2.5 seldom result in significant pathology.[8, 29–31] The acidity is neutralized within seconds after contact with the pulmonary mucosa, which leaves little validity to the concept of tracheal lavage following toxic fluid aspiration.[3, 8, 26, 32]

With 0.1N HCl (pH 1) solutions, the volume of aspirate appears to play a secondary role.[33] Volume may be significant when the pH of the aspirate is between 1.5 and 3.0[8, 27, 34] since it appears that aspirated volumes of such fluids must exceed 0.3 to 0.4 mL/kg to produce significant effects.[35, 36] Evidence in humans indicates that the greater the volume and pulmonary distribution of toxic fluid aspirate, the higher the morbidity and mortality.[6, 8, 27] This influence of the aspirate composition in humans is demonstrated by the near 100% mortality following fecal-gastric fluid aspiration.[28, 37]

Clinical Presentation

Following significant toxic fluid aspiration, the patient may manifest dyspnea, wheezing, rales, rhonchi, cough, fever, tachycardia, hypotension, and cyanosis. Initial findings may vary, and any or all may not be present for as long as 6 hours after the aspiration. The damage to bronchial epithelium can produce bronchospasm and a massive mucosal exudation that results in pink, frothy airway fluid, dyspnea, and wheezing, which are easily mistaken for cardiogenic pulmonary edema.[8, 27] The intravascular volume loss secondary to exudation can be quite significant.

X-ray studies commonly show patchy alveolar infiltrates limited to segments of lung that were gravity dependent at the time of aspiration.[3, 35, 38, 39] However, 25% to 40% of patients have diffuse bilateral infiltrates.[25, 40] Radiologic findings may be delayed 4 to 8 hours.[3]

A decreased arterial P_{O_2} is an early finding consistent with chemical pneumonitis and does not necessarily correlate with either the clinical or radiologic findings.[3] The etiology of the arterial hypoxemia is partly attributable to venous admixture secondary to bronchospasm and inflammation that is initially responsive to oxygen therapy. However, severe chemical pneumonitis involves significant true shunting[41] from factors such as reflex airway closure,[42, 43] altered surfactant activity,[25, 27, 44] and alveolar-capillary leak.[25, 45–47] High F_{IO_2} as well as positive end-expiratory pressure (PEEP) therapy may be required to maintain adequate arterial oxygenation.

Although the work of breathing is increased secondary to diminished pulmonary compliance,[44] alveolar ventilation is usually adequate (arterial P_{CO_2} <40 mm Hg). The potential for prolonged respiratory derangement has been reported,[8] and the need for ventilatory assistance must be continuously evaluated.

Secondary Bacterial Infection

The pulmonary pathology present in the first 24 hours following toxic fluid aspiration cannot be attributed to bacterial pneumonitis.[26, 28, 33] Acidic gastric contents are considered to be sterile. The volume and low pH of a gastric acid aspiration dilutes and sterilizes the initially introduced oropharyngeal organisms. Initial cardiorespiratory signs include tachypnea, tachycardia, wheezing and cyanosis. However, secondary bacterial pneumonitis (bacterial superinfection) has been reported to occur in 20% to 50% of patients within 24 to 72 hours following toxic fluid aspiration.[2, 48, 49] Chemical pneumonitis appears to leave the lung more vulnerable to infection.[50]

The pathogenic organisms of secondary bacterial pneumonia are almost always representative of the patient's oropharyngeal flora. Hospitalized patients have a progressive increase in *Staphylococcus aureus* and gram-negative bacilli colonizing the oropharynx[26, 51–54] due to the hospital environment, nutritional and immunologic factors, and therapeutic factors such as steroids and antibiotics. This explains the higher incidence of staphylococcal and gram-negative pneumonias following toxic fluid aspiration in the hospitalized patient. Although some evidence exists for the administration of prophylactic penicillin in patients who aspirate toxic fluid outside the hospital,[49, 55, ,56] there is no evidence that prophylactic antibiotics reduce the incidence of bacterial superinfection in the hospitalized patient.[6, 33, 48]

Adult Respiratory Distress Syndrome

This severe form of lung endothelial and epithelial damage is believed to be the result of severe systemic or pulmonary insult (see Chapter 18). Although definitive data are lacking, certain insults (sepsis, disseminated intravascular coagulation, multiple trauma, fat embolism) are associated with a high incidence of adult respiratory distress syndrome (ARDS). Some studies suggest that ARDS is a frequent sequela to toxic fluid aspiration.[25, 26, 57]

Nontoxic Inocula

Aspiration of nontoxic materials can be separated into two distinct categories: aspiration of nontoxic fluids (water, saline, milk, blood, barium, gastric fluid with pH >7.3) and aspiration of particulate matter. The degree of pulmonary dysfunction due to such aspiration is primarily determined by the volume and/or composition of the aspirate.[26] These events do not cause chemical pneumonitis but may result in secondary bacterial infection.

Nontoxic Fluid Aspiration

Aspiration of small amounts of nontoxic fluid usually provokes an acute nonspecific reaction such as coughing and breath holding. This is usually reversible and self-limited. There are no characteristic radiographic findings and seldom significant sequelae unless the hypoxemia and intrathoracic pressure variations of the acute reaction precipitate cardiovascular events. Near-drowning is a common example of massive aspiration of nontoxic fluid.

Near-Drowning

Near-drowning may be defined as water submersion after which the victim is in a potentially salvageable condition. Approximately 15% of near-drowning victims develop laryngospasm that prevents water aspiration.[58] Such "dry" drowning is a true asphyxiation without direct pulmonary damage.

Eighty-five percent of near-drowning victims have significant water aspiration. Most of these will survive with appropriate therapy if they are rescued before hypoxic brain damage occurs.[59] Cold water submersion produces hypothermia that results in metabolic and cardiovascular changes that make resuscitation possible even after 30 minutes of submersion.[60]

Largely determined by the volume and tonicity[61, 62] of the fluid aspirated, early pathophysiologic events in human near-drowning are hypoxemia, hypotension, and pulmonary edema. Saltwater drowning is associated with a high incidence of hypovolemic shock and hemoconcentration. Freshwater drowning is associated with hypervolemia, hemodilution, and occasionally hemolysis.[63] Pulmonary edema associated with saltwater near-drowning is largely the result of the hypertonicity of the aspirated fluid, whereas in freshwater near-drowning the edema is mainly attributable to hypervolemia.[30, 64] The hypoxemia associated with near-drowning is due to pulmonary edema, parenchymal cellular changes, and alterations in alveolar surfactant.

A postimmersion syndrome may occur within 24 to 48 hours and will be manifested by respiratory distress or apnea, hypoxemia, pulmonary edema, fever, and leukocytosis.[30] This usually occurs after the patient has been clinically stable and apparently unaffected by the near-drowning incident. Many near-drownings are associated with alcohol and drug ingestion, which may have obtunded airway protective reflexes; therefore, the possibility of concomitant toxic gastric fluid aspiration must be entertained.

Particulate Aspiration

Small particles (foodstuffs) and particulate antacids are often associated with gastric content aspiration. These cause partial obstruction and produce an immediate prolonged inflammation with granulomatous resolution.[29, 30, 65]

Large particulate (foreign body) aspiration produces symptoms dependent on the size of the aspirate and its location within the pulmonary tree.[66] Large particulate aspiration is most common in the pediatric age group.[67] Total obstruction of the proximal portion of the airway results in asphyxiation, while partial obstruction may present with dyspnea, hoarseness, stridor, cough, and cyanosis.[30, 68] A peripheral total obstruction causes atelectasis, while a partial obstruction may cause either atelectasis or a distal emphysema ("ball valve obstruction").[30] In general, the more peripheral the obstruction, the smaller the amount of functional lung occluded, and therefore the less life-threatening the event. After appropriate supportive therapy, definitive treatment requires removal of the foreign body by bronchoscopy. If the obstructing object is not removed, the probability of a distal pneumonitis developing is great.[33, 69]

Bacterial Inocula

Primary bacterial aspiration is the most common type of pulmonary aspiration. Normally the trachea and lower portions of the airways are sterile. This sterility is maintained by the previously discussed protective airway reflexes in addition to the mucociliary and macrophage activity of the pulmonary system. When these defense mechanisms are absent, dysfunctional, or overwhelmed, pulmonary infection due to the aspiration of pathogenic inoculum can occur. It is a difficult diagnosis that is often made in retrospect or by exclusion. Unlike the usually observed toxic and nontoxic aspiration associated with factors such as cough, choking, and laryngospasm, aspiration of bacteria usually involves a small volume and is relatively unnoticed. It is heralded by the onset of symptoms of bacterial pneumonia at least 24 hours after the aspiration. With repeated aspiration the presenting symptoms may be due to lung abscess, empyema, or necrotizing pneumonia 1 to 3 weeks after the initial insult. In patients with factors predisposing to aspiration, the appearance of new pulmonary infiltrates on chest x-ray films raises the possibility of primary bacterial aspiration.

The bacteria most frequently responsible are those present in the patient's oropharyngeal secretions.[51] Factors such as gingivodental disease and sinusitis significantly influence the virulence and number of oropharyngeal bacteria.[70, 71] Primary bacterial aspiration pneumonia typically involves polymicrobial isolates, including anaerobes.[51, 72] Host defense capabilities are important since normal people are known to occasionally aspirate pharyngeal secretions during sleep without sequelae.[9]

Reasonable criteria for making the diagnosis of primary bacterial aspiration include (1) a clinical status predisposing the patient to aspiration, (2) clinical evidence of bacterial pneumonitis including chest x-ray infiltrate, and (3) bacteriologic evaluation of pulmonary secretions.

MANAGEMENT OF ASPIRATION

The overall success of management depends on the early recognition of aspiration and institution of therapy to ensure adequate pulmonary gas exchange and limit pulmonary damage. Specific therapy includes (1) oxygen therapy; (2) airway protection and tracheobronchial hygiene; (3) airway pressure therapy (PEEP, continuous positive airway pressure [CPAP], positive-pressure ventilation); (4) drug therapy (bronchodilators, antibiotics); and (5) bronchoscopy.

PREVENTION OF ASPIRATION

Aspiration must be viewed as a preventable phenomenon that occurs frequently and can add considerably to the morbidity and mortality of critically ill patients. Every reasonable effort must be made to minimize the incidence of aspiration in the susceptible population. In addition to the various risk factors identified earlier, outpatient and emergency surgical procedures appear to have an increased risk of pulmonary aspiration.

Various physical and pharmacologic interventions are recommended for the prevention of pulmonary aspiration. Anticipation, vigilance, and prevention are more effective than is postaspiration therapy!

Patient position is important since gravity plays a crucial role in the regurgitation process. Although the supine or reverse Trendelenburg (head-up) position may diminish the incidence of passive regurgitation, it also encourages aspiration of pharyngeal contents. The ideal position to prevent both regurgitation and aspiration is the lateral Trendelenburg, which encourages oropharyngeal pooling and ready access for suctioning.[19, 73] However, factors such as intracranial disease and gastric motility disturbances commonly require a head-up position. When in doubt, the airway should be protected by intubation with a cuffed tube.

Care must be taken when using drugs such as muscle relaxants, anesthetics, narcotics, tranquilizers, and sedatives because these can diminish the protective airway reflexes as well as prolong gastric emptying time.[73] A nasogastric tube does not ensure an empty stomach, even when continuous suction is applied. Nasogastric feedings are best administered in small amounts with the patient in the head-up position.

A great deal of data exists concerning the alteration of gastric fluid pH to diminish the pulmonary injury if aspiration occurs.[74] *Oral antacids* are effective in maintaining acceptable gastric pH but are associated with increased gastric volume.[75] Some antacid formulas are associated with precipitate formation in gastric contents, e.g., aluminum and magnesium hydroxide, which, if aspirated, may cause pulmonary damage.[76-78] Sodium citrate is presently preferred since no precipitate is formed. In addition, Bicitra and Alka-Seltzer are two commercial antacid products reported to be effective in increasing gastric pH. Following antacid administration rotating the patient is recommended to facilitate mixing of gastric contents and enhance efficacy.[79]

Although an increased gastric pH reportedly reduces pulmonary injury, a recent study raises the issue of increased gastric bacterial colonization secondary to higher pH with a resultant increased potential for secondary bacterial pneumonias following aspiration.[80]

Histamine-2 (H_2) receptor antagonists have also been shown to increase gastric pH while reducing the volume of gastric secretions.[81] The primary mechanism of H_2-receptor antagonists is to competitively block acid production stimulated by histamine. These drugs were initially used in the treatment of peptic ulcer disease and are now used prophylactically for the prevention of gastric acid aspiration.

The prototype H_2-receptor antagonists are cimetidine and ranitidine. Numerous studies have demonstrated the efficacy of these drugs in the elective surgical patient when compared with a placebo for the preoperative alteration of gastric pH and volume. These agents are available in both oral and parenteral preparations. Speed of onset and efficacy is best achieved by intravenous (IV) administration. Because H_2-receptor antagonists do not immediately decrease the acidity of existent gastric fluid, oral antacids are preferable for acute therapy. It has been suggested that a combination of antacid and H_2-receptor antagonist therapy provides the greatest protection in reducing acid aspiration in susceptible patients. The dosage for H_2-receptor antagonists varies depending on the specific drug employed, the route of administration, and patient size.

Histamine-2-receptor antagonists are associated with a number of side effects. [82] Rapid IV injection has been reported to cause cardiovascular problems (e.g., arrest, hypotension, arrhythmia). Other side effects associated with short-term use include headache, fatigue, fever, muscle pain, and dizziness. Longer-term utilization reportedly can cause gynecomastia (men), galactorrhea (women), and bone marrow suppression. In addition, microsomal enzyme inhibition can cause an alteration in the clearance of several commonly used intensive care unit (ICU) drugs. [80] Clinically significant drug interactions have been described most frequently with theophyllin and warfarin. Drug levels should be closely monitored to avoid the adverse effects of these concurrently administered drugs.

Metoclopramide acts peripherally to increase lower esophageal sphincter tone, decrease pyloric tone, and increase gastrointestinal motility. [79] These actions tend to hasten gastric emptying. In addition, the drug has antiemetic properties. Extrapyramidal reactions have been noted, but this appears to be minimized by single-dose administration of this agent.

CASE STUDY

A 72-year-old man was brought to the emergency room after suffering a "seizure" at home. His wife reported that he vomited a significant quantity of yellowish liquid during the seizure. Past history revealed the presence of organic brain syndrome, hiatal hernia, and a mild "stroke" 1 year previously.

On admission the patient's sensorium appeared depressed. Vomitus was noted on his clothing. His blood pressure (BP)was 122/90 mm Hg; pulse rate, 124 beats per minute and regular; respiratory rate, 42/min and unlabored; and temperature, 36.2°C. Residual vomitus was noted in the oropharynx, and severe periodontal disease was present. On chest examination bilateral rales were heard with mild expiratory wheezing. No cardiac or abdominal abnormalities were noted. The patient was arousable but somnolent when undisturbed.

Initial laboratory tests revealed a hemoglobin concentration of 14 g/dL and a white blood cell (WBC) count of 9,800 mm^{-3} with a mild leftward shift. An electrocardiogram revealed sinus tachycardia with occasional premature atrial contractions and nonspecific ST segment and T-wave abnormalities. Chest x-ray studies revealed mild bilateral patchy alveolar infiltrates greatest at the right base, and arterial blood gas analysis showed a pH of 7.49, a P_{CO_2} of 31 mm Hg, and a P_{O_2} of 46 mm Hg on room air.

Discussion

Toxic fluid aspiration must be assumed. A history of vomiting during seizure (unprotected airway), the x-ray findings, and the arterial blood gas values are all compatible and suggest the diagnosis. Decisions must be made pertaining to airway management, oxygen therapy, and steroid and antibiotic therapy.

Airway Management

The oropharynx should be suctioned immediately to help clear the airway, stimulate coughing, and confirm the diagnosis. Airway protective reflexes must be evaluated and the advisability of intubation considered. A nasotracheal intubation with only topical anesthesia would be ideal since central drug depression could be avoided and the nasal tube would be best tolerated as the patient's level of consciousness improved. Bronchoscopy does not appear immediately necessary unless particulate matter is suspected in the aspirate.

Pulmonary lavage with a neutral or alkaline solution has been recommended by some following intubation. There appear to be few or no data to support this procedure since the acid media is neutralized within seconds of contact with pulmonary mucosa. Furthermore, studies have demonstrated an increase in the area of lung injury and altered pulmonary compliance following pulmonary lavage with alkaline solutions.[32, 83, 84] Present recommendations support only the instillation of small aliquots of sterile saline (5 to 10 mL) in an effort to stimulate coughing and enhance pulmonary toilet.[35]

Oxygen Therapy

Hypoxemia is a common result of aspiration and can contribute to tachypnea and tachycardia. The early pulmonary insults lead to hypoxemia that is relatively responsive to oxygen therapy (venous admixture). Thirty percent to 50% inspired oxygen concentrations should result in an acceptable arterial Po_2 and often a decrease in respiratory rate. Oxygen therapy is indicated, with or without the placement of an endotracheal tube. Mechanical ventilation is not required unless the patient is in acute or impending ventilatory failure. Early institution of PEEP/CPAP may be considered because it can restore pulmonary function to nearly normal within 24 to 48 hours by increasing the functional residual capacity and improving the ventilation-perfusion relationships.[81]

Corticosteroids

Since toxic fluid aspiration results in a pulmonary inflammatory response, steroids have been recommended to reduce the degree of inflammation.[28, 35, 84, 85] Studies demonstrating stabilization of lysosomal membranes and prevention of leukocyte and platelet agglutination in the lungs have been cited as further rationale for early administration of steroids following aspiration.[83, 86, 87]

Despite a plethora of studies, the information on corticosteroids remains conflicting, anecdotal, uncontrolled, and controversial.[25, 88, 89] If steroids are indicated at all, they must be administered within "minutes" of the insult to have a significant effect.[25, 40] Although large doses administered for fewer than 36 hours do not appear to alter defense mechanisms or enhance colonization, some animal studies suggest that steroid therapy interferes with lung healing and promotes granuloma and abscess formation.[65]

Justification for steroid therapy following aspiration is entirely theoretical and must be weighed against the potential harm to each patient.[26, 90, 91] Indiscriminate use of steroids is probably best avoided until well-controlled experimental data are available to support their use.[48]

Antibiotics

Although the evidence supporting the use of prophylactic antibiotics following toxic and nontoxic fluid aspiration is scanty, many physicians continue the practice. In the critically ill patient population this practice appears to be ineffective[48] and potentially harmful because it may increase the incidence of antibiotic-resistant, gram-negative organisms responsible for the secondary bacterial pneumonia and expose the patient to the risk of drug reactions.[3, 40, 53, 92] Antibiotics can potentially eliminate from the oropharyngeal flora *Streptococcus viridans*, which normally inhibits the colonization of more virulent gram-negative bacilli and staphylococci.[2] One exception to this general rule is aspiration of intestinal fluid with a high bacterial count, which demands immediate administration of the appropriate antibiotics.

A logical approach is to anticipate a secondary bacterial infection and serially monitor the tracheobronchial secretions, chest x-ray findings, and clinical condition. Evidence of pulmonary infection 24 hours after aspiration should be specifically treated on the basis of microbiologic evidence of colonization of tracheal secretions. The avoidance of antibiotic therapy in the first 24 to 48 hours limits the potential risks of inappropriate antibiotics and provides the framework for rational antibiotic therapy.[3] If prophylactic antibiotics are to be employed, both aerobic and anaerobic coverage should be included.

Bronchodilators

Wheezing is a common sign associated with aspiration. Aerosolized and IV bronchodilators may be administered, assuming a therapeutic response is demonstrated.

CASE STUDY CONTINUED

The patient was given 40% oxygen by air entrainment mask. Assessment of the patient's airway revealed obtundation of airway protective reflexes. Following administration of topical anesthesia to the right nostril and nasopharynx with 10% cocaine and breathing an aerosol mist of 2% lidocaine for 5 minutes, an 8-mm endotracheal tube was placed via the nasal route without difficulty. Following manual ventilation and preoxygenation, the trachea was repeatedly suctioned until the return was clear. The patient's condition stabilized with a BP of 118/85 mm Hg, a heart rate of 118 beats per minute, and a respiratory rate of 32/min. Arterial blood gas analysis with the patient breathing 40% oxygen revealed a pH of 7.46, a Pco_2 of 32 mm Hg, and a Po_2 of 88 mm Hg.

Approximately 3 hours after admission the patient had frothy pink sputum and complained of increasing shortness of breath. His BP was 108/58 mm Hg, pulse was 128 beats per minute, and respiratory rate was 44/min. Diffuse rhonchi were heard bilaterally, and the chest x-ray film revealed a diffuse pulmonary edema pattern. Heart tones were normal without an S_3 or S_4. Arterial blood gas analysis with an Fio_2 of 0.4 revealed a pH of 7.44, a Pco_2 of 32 mm Hg, and a Po_2 of 52 mm Hg.

Discussion

Although cardiogenic edema must be considered and ruled out, a more likely diagnosis is noncardiogenic edema secondary to toxic fluid aspiration. The significant deterioration in arterial oxygenation on 40% supplemental oxygen (88 to 52 mm Hg) suggests increasing right-to-left shunting (true shunting). This is most likely secondary to factors such as surfactant destruction, dilution, or alteration by the aspirated acid with consequent alveolar collapse and alveolar edema.[81] Since this process can be expected to worsen over the next several hours, there is little chance that increasing the FIO_2 will ensure adequate arterial oxygenation.

Airway Pressure Therapy

There is no reason to institute mechanical assistance of ventilation at this point. However, this may become a reasonable alternative if other measures do not improve the patient's complaint of dyspnea. CPAP/PEEP has therapeutic value in the management of noncardiogenic edema, and some investigators contend that early application can lessen the severity of the disease process.[93, 94]

Fluid Therapy

The development of noncardiogenic edema secondary to increased endothelial permeability makes the lung sensitive to small increases in vascular pressure. There is controversy concerning the ideal fluid to use in patients with endothelial cell damage. The use of various osmotic agents has been recommended but may be deleterious.[35, 95] A balance between a vascular volume sufficient for organ perfusion and a vascular pressure that will not promote further fluid extravasation into the interstitium must be achieved. In patients with preexisting cardiac disease or an unstable fluid balance, a pulmonary artery catheter should be employed to evaluate vascular pressure and measure cardiac output. Ideally, the pulmonary artery occluded pressure should be maintained at the lowest value compatible with an acceptable cardiac and urine output.

CASE STUDY CONTINUED

The patient received 10 cm H_2O PEEP, and 450 mL of crystalloid solution was administered IV. His BP was 115/78 mm Hg, pulse 115 beats per minute, and respiratory rate 28/min without a complaint of shortness of breath. Arterial blood gas values on an FIO_2 of 0.35 were as follows: pH, 7.44; PCO_2, 35 mm Hg; and PO_2, 70 mm Hg.

Over the next 2 days the pulmonary edema pattern on x-ray studies improved, and the CPAP was decreased to 5 cm H_2O with an FIO_2 of 0.28. Arterial blood gas analysis showed a pH of 7.41, a PCO_2 of 38 mm Hg, and a PO_2 of 72 mm Hg. His BP was 122/80 mm Hg, pulse was 105 beats per minute, and respiratory rate was 20/min. The patient's sensorium was markedly improved. He was extubated without event and maintained the same vital signs and blood gas values on an oxygen flow of 2 L/min via nasal cannula.

Eighteen hours after extubation ($3^{1}/_{2}$ days after aspiration) the patient had a spiking temperature of 39.3°C rectally. The WBC count rose from 11,000 to 17,000 mm^{-3}, and the chest x-ray film showed a new infiltrate in the right lower lobe. His heart rate and respiratory rate had trended upward. Arterial Po₂ had declined to 55 mm Hg with oxygen delivered via the nasal cannula.

Discussion

All evidence suggests the appearance of a secondary bacterial pneumonia. Predicted on sputum specimens previously obtained for culture and sensitivity, specific antibiotic therapy was instituted. A 35% air entrainment mask was used, and the patient's ability to cough and breathe deeply was assessed frequently. Antipyretic agents were administered.

CASE STUDY CONTINUED

Within 12 hours the patient's temperature was below 38°C without antipyretics. His pneumonia resolved without incident, and he was able to cough up secretions with some assistance and encouragement.

REFERENCES

1. Broe PJ, Toung TJK, Cameron JL: Aspiration pneumonia. *Surg Clin North Am* 1980; 60:1551–1564.
2. Mendelson CL: The aspiration of stomach contents into the lungs during obstetric anesthesia. *Am J Obstet Gynecol* 1946; 52:191–205.
3. Little JW: Pulmonary aspiration. *West J Med* 1979; 131:122–129.
4. Bannister WK, Sahilaro AJ: Vomiting and aspiration during anesthesia. *Anesthesiology* 1962; 23:251–264.
5. Edwards G, Morton HJV, Pask EA, et al: Deaths associated with anesthesia: Report of 1,000 cases. *Anesthesia* 1956; 11:194–220.
6. Cameron JL, Mitchell WH, Zvidema GD: Aspiration pneumonia: Clinical outcome following documented aspiration. *Arch Surg* 1973; 106:49.
7. Cameron JL, Zvidema GD: Aspiration pneumonia: Magnitude and frequency of the problem. *JAMA* 1972; 219:1194.
8. Awe WL, Fletcher WS, Jacob SW: The pathophysiology of aspiration pneumonitis. *Surgery* 1966; 60:232–239.
9. Huxley EJ, Vinoslav J, Gray WR, et al: Pharyngeal aspiration in normal adults and patients with depressed consciousness. *Am J Med* 1978; 64:564–568.
10. Pontoppidan H, Beeche HK: Progressive loss of protective reflexes in the airway with the advance of age. *JAMA* 1960; 174:2209–2213.
11. Greenberg HG: Aspiration pneumonia after cardiac arrest and resuscitation. *J Am Geriatri Soc* 1967; 15:48–52.
12. Brown M, Glassenberg M: Mortality factors in patients with acute stroke. *JAMA* 1973; 224:1493–1495.
13. Mrazek SA: Bronchopneumonia in terminally ill patients. *J Am Geriatr Soc* 1969; 17:969–973.
14. Chase HF: Role of delayed gastric emptying time in the etiology of aspiration pneumonia. *Am J Obstet Gynecol* 1948; 56:673–679.
15. Belsey RH: Pulmonary complications of esophageal disease and their treatment. *Br J Dis Chest* 1960; 54:342–348.
16. Cohen S: Motor disorders of the esophagus. *N Engl J Med* 1979; 301:184–192.
17. Chernow B, Johnson LF, Janowitz WR, et al: Pulmonary aspiration as a consequence of gastroesophageal reflux. *Dig Dis Sci* 1979; 24:839–844.
18. Smith RA, Norris FH: Symptomatic care of patients with amyotrophic lateral sclerosis. *JAMA* 1975; 234:715–717.
19. Cameron JL, Zvidema GD: Aspiration pneumonia: Magnitude and frquency of the problem. *JAMA* 1972; 219:1194–1196.
20. Culver GA, Makel HP, Beecher HK: Frequency of aspiration of gastric contents of the lungs during anesthesia and surgery. *Ann Surg* 1951; 133:289–292.

21. Spray SB, Zvidema GD, Cameron JL: Aspiration pneumonia: Incidence of aspiration with endotracheal tubes. Am J Surg 1976; 131:701–703.
22. Pavlin EG, Van Nimwegan D, Hornbein TF: Failure of high compliance low pressure cuff to prevent aspiration. Anesthesiology 1975; 42:216–219.
23. Cameron JL, Reynolds J, Zvidema GD: Aspiration in patients with tracheostomies. Surg Gynecol Obstet 1973; 136:68–70.
24. Matheny NA, Eisenberg L, Speiss M: Aspiration pneumonia in patients fed through naso-enteral tubes. Heart Lung 1986; 15:256.
25. Stewardson RH, Nyhus LM: Pulmonary aspiration. Arch Surg 1977; 12:1192–1197.
26. Wynne JW, Modell JH: Respiratory aspiration of stomach contents. Ann Intern Med 1977; 87:466–474.
27. Greenfield LJ, Singleton RP, McCaffree DR, et al: Pulmonary effects of experimental graded aspiration of hydrochloric acid. Ann Surg 1969; 170:74–86.
28. Hamelberg W, Bosomworth PP: Aspiration pneumonitis: Experimental and clinical observations. Anesth Analg 1964; 43:669–677.
29. Teabeaut JH: Aspiration of gastric contents: An experimental study. Am J Pathol 1952; 28:51–67.
30. Ribaudo CA, Grace WJ: Pulmonary aspiration. Am J Med 1971; 50:510–520.
31. Schwartz DJ, Wynne JW, Gibbs CP, et al: The pulmonary consequences of aspiration of gastric contents at pH values greater than 2.5. Am Rev Respir Dis 1980; 121:119–126.
32. Wamberg K, Zeskov B: Experimental studies on the course and treatment of aspiration pneumonia. Anesth Analg 1966; 45:230–236.
33. Bartlett JG, Gonbach SL: The triple threat of aspiration pneumonia. Chest 1975; 68:560–566.
34. Cameron JL, Caldini P, Toung JK, et al: Aspiration pneumonia: Physiologic data following experimental aspiration. Surgery 1972; 72:238–245.
35. Broe PJ, Toung TJK, Cameron JL: Aspiration pneumonia. Surg Clin North Am 1980; 60:1551–1564.
36. Hupp JR, Peterson LJ: Aspiration pneumonitis: Etiology, therapy, and prevention. J Oral Surg 1981; 39:430–435.
37. Vilinskas J, Schweizer RT, Foster, JH: Experimental studies on aspiration of contents of obstructed intestines. Surg Gynecol. Obstet 1972; 135:568–570.
38. Kross DE, Effman EL, Putman CE: Adult aspiration pneumonia. Am Fam Physician 1980; 22:73–78.
39. Wilkins RA, DeLacey GJ, Flor R, et al: Radiology in Mendelson's syndrome. Clin Radiol 1976; 27:81–85.
40. LeFrock JL, Clark TS, Davies B, et al: Aspiration pneumonia: A ten year review. Am Surg 1979; 45:305–313.
41. Moseley RV, Doty RB: Physiologic changes due to aspiration pneumonitis. Ann Surg 1970; 171:73–76.
42. Halmagyi DFJ, Colebatch JHJ, Starzecki B: Inhalation of blood, saliva, and alcohol: Consequences, mechanism, and treatment. Thorax 1962; 17:244–250.
43. Colebatch HJH, Halmagyi DFJ: Reflex airway reaction to fluid aspiration. J Appl Physiol 1962; 17:787–794.
44. Cameron JL, Caldini P, Toung JK, et al: Aspiration pneumonia: Physiologic data following experimental aspiration. Surgery 1972; 72:238–245.
45. Glausen FL, Millen JE, Falls R: Effects of acid aspiration on pulmonary alveolar epithelial membrane permeability. Chest 1979; 76:201–205.
46. Brigham KL: Factors affecting lung vascular permeability. Am Rev Respir Dis 1977; 115:165–169.
47. Jones JG, Grossman RF, Slavin MB, et al: Alveolar–capillary membrane permeabiity: Correlation with functional, radiographic, and postmortem changes after fluid aspiration. Am Rev Respir Dis 1979; 120:399–410.
48. Bynum LJ, Pierce AK: Pulmonary aspiration of gastric contents. Am Rev Respir Dis 1976; 114:1129–1136.
49. Arms RA, Dines DE, Tinstman TC: Aspiration pneumonia. Chest 1974; 65:136–139.
50. Johanson WG, Jay SJ, Pierce AK: Bacterial growth in vivo: An important determinant of the pulmonary clearance of Diplococcus pneumoniae in rats. J Clin Invest 1974; 53:1320–1325.
51. Bartlett JG, Gorbach SL, Finegold SM: The bacteriology of aspiration pneumonia. Am J Med 1974; 56:202–207.
52. Wolfe JE, Bone RC, Ruth WE: Effects of corticosteroids in the treatment of patients with gastric aspiration. Am J Med 1977; 63:719–722.
53. Johanson WG, Pierce AK, Sanford JP: Changing pharyngeal bacterial flora of hospitalized patients: Emergence of gram-negative bacilli. N Engl J Med 1969; 281:1137–1140.
54. Johanson WG, Pierce AK, Sanford JP: Nosocomial respiratory infections with gram-negative bacilli: The significance of colonization of the respiratory tract. Ann Intern Med 1972; 77:701–706.
55. Bartlett JG: Aspiration pneumonia: Clinical notes. Respir Dis 1980; 18:3–8.

56. Murray HW: Antimicrobial therapy in pulmonary aspiration. *Am J Med* 1979; 66:188–190.
57. Horovitz JH, Carrico CJ, Shires GT: Pulmonary response to major injury. *Arch Surg* 1974; 108:349–355.
58. Spitz WO, Blanke RV: Mechanism of death in fresh water drowning. *Arch Pathol* 1961; 71:661–668.
59. Redding JS, Cozine RA, Voight C, et al: Resuscitation from drowning. *JAMA* 1961; 178:1136–1139.
60. Siebke H, Breiver H, Rod T, et al: Survival after a 40 minute submersion without cerebral sequelae. *Lancet* 1975; 1:1275–1277.
61. Kylstra JA: Survival of submerged mammals. *N Engl J Med* 1965; 272:198–200.
62. Donald KW: Drowning. *Br Med J* 1955; 2:155–160.
63. Model J: Near drowning. *Int Anesthesiol Clin* 1977; 15:107–115.
64. Modell JH, Graves SA, Ketover A: Clinical course of 91 consecutive near-drowning victims. *Chest* 1976; 70:231–238.
65. Wynne JW, Reynolds JL, Hood IC, et al: Steroid therapy for pneumonitis induced in rabbits by aspiration of foodstuff. *Anesthesiology* 1979; 51:11–19.
66. Brooks JW: Foreign bodies in the air and food passages. *Ann Surg* 1972; 175:720–732.
67. Kim LG, Brummett WM, Humphrey A, et al: Foreign body in the airway: A review of 202 cases. *Laryngoscope* 1973; 83:347–354.
68. Haugen RK: The cafe coronary: Sudden deaths in restaurants. *JAMA* 1963; 186:142–143.
69. Lansing AM, Jamieson WG: Mechanisms of fever in pulmonary atelectasis. *Arch Surg* 1963; 87:184–192.
70. Lorber B, Swenson RM: Bacteriology of aspiration pneumonia. *Ann Intern Med* 1974; 81:329–331.
71. Bartlett JG, Finegold SM: Anaerobic infections of the lung and pleural space. *Am Rev Respir Dis* 1974; 110:56–77.
72. Johanson WG, Harris GD: Aspiration pneumonia, anaerobic infection, and lung abscess. *Med Clin North Am* 1980; 64:385–394.
73. Turndorf H, Rodis ID, Clark TS: Silent regurgitation during general anesthesia. *Anesth Analg* 1974; 53:700–703.
74. Taylor G, Pryse-Davies J: The prophylactic use of antacids in the prevention of the acid aspiration syndrome. *Lancet* 1965; 1:288–297.
75. Stoelting RK: Response to atropine glycopyrrolate, and Riepan of gastric pH and volume of adult patients. *Anesthesiology* 1978; 48:367–369.
76. Kuchling A, Joyce TH, Cooke S: The pulmonary lesion of antacid aspiration, (abstracted) in *Proceedings of the Annual Meeting of the American Society of Anesthesiologists*. Philadelphia, JB Lippincott, 1975, p 281.
77. Gibb CP, Schwartz DJ, Wynne JW, et al: Antacid pulmonary aspiration in the dog. *Anesthesiology* 1979; 51:380–385.
78. Bond VK, Stoelting RK, Gupta CD: Pulmonary aspiration syndrome after inhalation of gastric fluid containing antacids. *Anesthesiology* 1979; 51:452–453.
79. Joyce TH: Prophylaxis for pulmonary aspiration. *Am J Med* 1987; 83:46–52.
80. Driks MR, Craven DE, Celli BB, et al: Nosocomial pneumonia in intubated patients given sucralfate as compared with antacids or histamine type 2 blockers: The role of gastric colonization. *N Engl J Med* 1987; 317:1376–1382.
81. Støelting RK: Gastric fluid pH in patients receiving cimetidine. *Anesth Analg* 1978; 57:675–677.
82. Freston JW: Safety perspectives on parenteral H_2-receptor antagonists. *Am J Med* 1987; 83:58–67.
83. Lewinski A: Evaluation of methods employed in the treatment of the chemical pneumonitis of aspiration. *Anesthesiology* 1965; 26:37–44.
84. Bosomworth PP, Hamelberg W: Etiologic and therapeutic aspects of aspiration pneumonitis. *Surg Forum* 1962; 13:158–159.
85. Dines DE, Titus JL, Sessler AD: Aspiration pneumonitis. *Mayo Clin Proc* 1970; 45:347–360.
86. Starling JR, Rudolf LE, Ferguson W, et al: Benefits of methylprednisolone in the isolated perfused organ. *Ann Surg* 1973; 177:566–571.
87. Wilson JW: Treatment and prevention of pulmonary cellular damage with pharmacologic doses of corticosteroid. *Surg Gynecol Obstet* 1972; 134:675–681.
88. Chapman RL, Downs JB, Modell JH, et al: The ineffectiveness of steroid therapy in treating aspiration of hydrochloric acid. *Arch Surg* 1974; 108:858–861.
89. Downs JB, Chapman RL, Modell JH, et al: An evaluation of steroid therapy in aspiration pneumonitis. *Anesthesiology* 1974; 40:129–135.
90. Lowrey LD, Anderson M, Calhoun T, et al: Failure of corticosteroid therapy for experimental acid aspiration. *J Surg Res* 1982; 32:168–172.
91. Lee M, Sukumavan M, Berger HW, et al: Influence of corticosteroid treatment on pulmonary function after recovery from aspiration of gastric contents. *Mt Sinai J Med* 1980; 47:341–346.
92. Sprunt K, Leidy GA, Redman W: Prevention of bacterial overgrowth. *J Infect Dis* 1971; 123:1–10.

93. Schmidt GB: Prophylaxis of pulmonary complications following abdominal surgery, including atelectasis, ARDS, and pulmonary embolism. *Ann Surg* 1977; 9:29–73.
94. Chapman RL, Modell JH, Ruiz BC, et al: Effect of continuous positive pressure, ventilation, and steroids on aspiration of hydrochloric acid in dogs. *Anesth Analg* 1974; 53:556–562.
95. Toung TJ, Cameron JL, Kimura T, et al: Aspiration pneumonia: Treatment with osmotically active agents. *Surgery* 1981; 89:588–593.

14/Acute Renal Failure

FRANK A. KRUMLOVSKY, M.D.
NANCY A. NORA, M.D.

Acute renal failure (ARF) can be defined as an acute deterioration in renal function. This may occur over hours, days, or even weeks. Prompt recognition and management of ARF are of critical importance since the severity and duration of failure and the ultimate degree of recovery depend largely on prompt institution of appropriate therapy, which in turn depends on a determination of etiology and an understanding of pathophysiologic mechanisms.

CLASSIFICATION

Acute renal failure is most appropriately divided into prenatal, postrenal, and intrarenal types. As indicated above, it is of critical importance to classify a given case of ARF by etiology and pathogenesis as promptly as possible since success in modifying the severity or reversing the cause depends on appropriate therapy based on pathophysiologic mechanisms.[1-3]

Prerenal azotemia, probably the most common type of ARF, is caused by renal hypoperfusion as a result of decreased effective renal blood flow; this in turn is almost invariably secondary to hypotension, intravascular hypovolemia, or poor cardiac output. Hypotension is relative and is related to preexisting blood pressure (BP), age, and preexisting status of the renal macrovasculature and microvasculature. Thus, an apparently normal BP may in fact represent hypotension in an elderly or previously hypertensive patient. Intravascular hypovolemia is most commonly the result of acute blood loss, third-space losses, sepsis, overdiuresis, gastrointestinal losses (vomiting, diarrhea, nasogastric suction), or hypoalbuminemia. A continuous spectrum exists between prerenal azotemia secondary to renal hypoperfusion and ischemic acute tubular necrosis (ATN); thus, prompt recognition and appropriate management of prerenal status can abort progression to ischemic ATN or minimize its severity and duration should it occur.

Postrenal azotemia refers to complete or incomplete obstruction of the urinary tract at any point along its course. It must be emphasized that a normal urine output does not rule out obstructive uropathy. Acute renal failure secondary to incomplete obstruction may be manifested by severe azotemia and normal urine volume or even polyuria.[4] Thus obstruction must be ruled out in all patients with ARF who do not respond promptly and completely to correction of prerenal factors.[5, 6]

Acute tubular necrosis is the most common type of intrarenal ARF and can be subclassified into ischemic and nephrotoxic types. Ischemic ATN represents a progression of prerenal azotemia in which prolonged or severe renal hypoperfusion has resulted in structural renal damage. Recent data suggest that prolonged mild hypotension may be even more injurious to the kidney than more severe hypotensive episodes of limited duration. Nephrotoxic ARF is less common but of great importance as withdrawal of the offending agent may permit prompt recovery. Just as in the case of incomplete obstruction, ATN may present a nonoliguric form in which worsening azotemia and eventually the full-blown uremic syndrome may be seen in the presence of a normal urine output. A partial listing of commonly encountered nephrotoxic drugs is given in Table 14–1.[7–9] Many drugs, especially the aminoglycoside antibiotics, are direct tubular toxins, and toxicity is dose related. Heme pigments are also direct tubular toxins; thus intravascular hemolysis or rhabdomyolysis with myoglobinuria may produce ATN.

Acute renal failure secondary to iodinated contrast media is commonly seen[10–12] and is multifactorial, resulting from a direct tubular toxic effect as well as initial vasodilatation followed by prolonged vasoconstriction. Patients with preexisting renal insufficiency, renal hypoperfusion from any cause (dehydration, congestive heart failure [CHF], diabetes mellitus, multiple myeloma, or recent iodinated contrast studies) have an increased risk of contrast-induced ARF. Recent evidence suggests that the newer nonionic or low-osmolar agents, while much more expensive, are no less nephrotoxic,[13] although they may be associated with a lower incidence of systemic allergic reactions.

Other agents may cause an allergic interstitial hypersensitivity nephritis that is not dose related (see Table 14–1). Drug-induced hypersensitivity nephritis may be recognized by the findings of eosinophilia, eosinophiluria, fever, and/or skin rash, although at times none of these is present.

Acute renal failure related to the administration of nonsteroidal anti-inflammatory drugs is being seen with increasing frequency.[14–19] These agents are prostaglandin inhibitors and decrease renal blood flow. In a setting of preexisting renal hypoperfusion, they are likely to further decrease renal blood flow since in this situation maintenance of renal perfusion is increasingly dependent on the vasodilator prostaglandins. These agents are also capable of causing acute interstitial nephritis, which may be associated with the nephrotic syndrome and ATN.

Space permits only brief mention of other less commonly encountered causes of intrarenal ARF.[20] Acute renal failure secondary to acute glomerulonephritis or systemic vasculitis can usually be recognized by active urine sediment (red blood cells [RBCs], RBC casts, and/or proteinuria), which is not typical of ATN. The hepatorenal syndrome appears to be related to intrarenal arteriolar vasoconstriction and resembles severe prerenal azotemia in many respects, although it does not respond well to appropriate therapeutic measures for prerenal azotemia; a LeVeen shunt may be helpful in some cases. Intratubular precipitation of sulfonamides, myeloma protein, or urates represents variants of intrarenal obstruction. Acute cortical necrosis may result from disseminated intravascular coagulation (DIC) secondary to gram-negative sepsis or obstetric accidents. Presumably, the clotting mechanism is activated as part of a generalized Shwartzman-like reaction as a result of sepsis and bacterial endo-

TABLE 14–1.
Nephrotoxic Drugs (Partial Listing)

Direct Tubular Toxin	Acute Allergic Interstitial Nephritis	Intratubular Obstruction	Vasoactive Mechanisms	Glomerulonephritis, Nephrotic Syndrome, or Tubular Basement Membrane Disease
Amphotericin	Allopurinol	Acyclovir	Captopril	Gold
Cephalosporins	Azathioprine	Allopurinol	Cisplatin	Heroin
Cisplatin	Carmustine	Lithium	Enalapril	Lomustine
Colistin	Cephalosporins	Methotrexate	Iodinated contrast media	Mercury
Cyclophosphamide	Cimetidine	Methoxyflurane	Nonsteroidal anti-inflammatory	Mesantoin
Cyclosporine	Clofibrate	Penthrane	drugs	Nonsteroidal anti-inflammatory drugs
Enflurane	Enflurane			Penicillamine
Iodinated contrast	Furosemide			Probenecid
media	Gold			Streptozocin
Lithium	Lomustine			
Mercury	Nonsteroidal anti-inflammatory			
Methoxyflurane	drugs			
Polymyxin	Penicillins			
Streptozocin	Phenytoin			
Tetracyclines	Rifampin			
Vancomycin	Sulfonamides			
	Tetracyclines			
	Thiazides			
	Vancomycin			

toxemia or by the release of thromboplastin, as may occur in abruptio placentae. The patient is usually severely oliguric or anuric. Also, ARF may occur secondary to thrombotic microangiopathy (hemolytic-uremic syndrome, thrombotic thrombocytopenic purpura, idiopathic postpartum ARF).

DIFFERENTIAL DIAGNOSIS

The first steps in establishing the differential diagnosis (Fig 14–1) are a history and physical examination. In the case of prerenal azotemia, the latter will usually reveal signs of intravascular hypovolemia (orthostatic hypotension and/or tachycardia, flat neck veins and/or low central venous pressure [CVP] or pulmonary capillary wedge pressure [PCWP]), hypotension (relative to the patient's usual BP), or evidence of CHF. The history will provide clues as to possible recent hypotensive insults (trauma, surgery, sepsis, myocardial infarction), recent or current exposure to nephrotoxic drugs, or the presence of symptoms or conditions indicative or causative or urinary tract obstruction.

The urine should next be examined.[21] In prerenal or postrenal azotemia, the urinalysis findings are characteristically within normal limits. In ATN, dirty brown epithelial cell casts may be seen, although the urinalysis may at times be normal. The presence of an active sediment (macroscopic or microscopic hematuria, RBC casts, and/or proteinuria) argues against prerenal or postrenal azotemia or ATN and suggests glomerulonephritis, systemic vasculitis, or DIC. The presence of eosinophiluria raises the question of acute allergic interstitial nephritis, although the urinalysis is often normal in this condition.

Renal ultrasound should be performed routinely to rule out obstruction and eval-

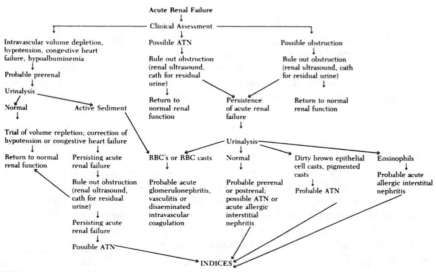

FIG 14–1.
Differential diagnosis of acute renal failure.

TABLE 14–2.

Urinary Indices in Acute Renal Failure

Index	Value	
Urine Na (mEq/L)	<20–30	>30–40
Urine specific gravity	>1.108	<1.018
Urine osmolality	>400	<400
Urine/plasma osmolality ratio	1.2–3.0	0.9–1.2
Urine/plasma creatinine ratio	>30–40	<20–30
Renal failure index*	<1	>1
Fractional excretion of sodium†	<1	>1
Serum BUN:creatinine ratio	>10:1	~10:1
	↓	↓
	Probably prerenal—treat with optimization of intravascular volume; if no immediate response, mannitol, dopamine, and/or furosemide (see the text on treatment of early ATN)	Probably established ATN, possibly chronic obstruction, acute interstitial nephritis—treat as for prerenal or early ATN initially; if no response, treat as established renal failure (see the text)

*Renal failure index $= \dfrac{\text{urine Na}}{\text{urine/plasma creatinine}}$.

†Fractional excretion of sodium $= \dfrac{\text{urine Na/plasma Na}}{\text{urine Cr/plasma Cr}} \times 100$.

uate gross renal anatomy in all patients who have not responded promptly to correction of prerenal factors.[5, 6] If there is any question of vascular trauma or occlusion, renal isotope scans should be obtained as well.

At the same time, it is appropriate to review the urinary indices. (Table 14–2).[21–27] These must be determined, if possible, prior to any therapeutic intervention since results may be made uninterpretable following many therapeutic measures such as the administration of mannitol or furosemide. A random sample of urine will provide data of comparable validity to a longer-timed collection, and results can be made available almost immediately. In prerenal azotemia, results will be consistent with renal hypoperfusion with well-preserved tubular function (high urine specific gravity and osmolality, high urine/plasma osmolality and creatinine ratios, low renal failure index, low fractional excretion of sodium [FeNa] and high blood urea nitrogen [BUN]/creatinine ratio). Conversely, in ATN, the ability to conserve sodium and water is decreased because of tubular damage, and this results in lower urine specific gravity and osmolality, low urine/plasma osmolality and creatinine ratios, a high renal failure index, a high FeNa, and normal BUN/creatinine ratio. The urine sodium, renal failure index and fractional excretion of sodium appear to be the most reliable and discriminatory of these tests. Urinary indices in other types of ARF are less characteristic. Values in obstructive uropathy, especially if chronic, resemble those seen in ATN, but acute obstruction may be manifested by a prerenal picture. Cortical necrosis and hepatorenal syndrome typically are associated with prerenal indices. Some types of ATN, especially those due to iodinated contrast media or myoglobinuria, as well as some cases of nonoliguric ATN may be manifested by prerenal indices.[23, 24, 27] The reason for this is not totally clear but may relate to a patchy process in which most of the glomerular filtrate is formed in nephrons with intact tubules or possibly to intrarenal (intratubular) obstruction or to contrast-induced vasoconstriction, which may precede the development of ATN. Indices may not be totally diagnostic or even internally consistent in every case[25]; in the majority of cases, however, urinary indices provide a valuable guide to etiology, pathophysiology, and appropriate management in patients with ARF.

PATHOPHYSIOLOGY OF ACUTE TUBULAR NECROSIS

Space does not permit an adequate discussion of this complex topic. Suffice it to say that considerable evidence exists that supports the role of both tubular obstruction and renal arteriolar vasoconstriction in the pathophysiology of the oliguria of ATN.[28, 29] Therapeutic efforts are directed toward both of these mechanisms.

THERAPY

In the case of obstructive uropathy, management is simple and obvious; the obstruction must be relieved. For this reason, obstruction must be ruled out in all cases of ARF that do not respond promptly and completely to a correction of prerenal factors. Obstruction is usually ruled out most easily by renal ultrasound. Occasionally, if the renal ultrasound is nondiagnostic or the index of suspicion is high, more invasive measures with a higher degree of risk, such as retrograde pyelography, will be necessary.

In the case of prerenal azotemia, initial management consists of optimizing the intravascular volume and BP so as to maintain renal perfusion. Adequacy of intravascular volume status can usually be evaluated clinically (absence of orthostatic hypotension or tachycardia, neck veins filling from below to an estimated CVP of 5 to 6 cm H_2O), but occasionally, especially in the critically ill patient, insertion of a CVP line or Swan-Ganz catheter will be required to ensure optimal filling pressures. Cardiac output, if low, should be optimized as well. When evidence of volume depletion is present, normal saline or colloid should be administered to correct the problem.

The most critical point in the management of early ARF is the situation when prerenal azotemia is progressing along its continuous spectrum leading toward ATN or early ATN is developing but has not yet become established. Here, therapeutic interventions are of greatest potential value. Optimizing the intravascular volume and cardiac output has already been mentioned. If intravascular volume status permits, mannitol, 12.5 g intravenously (IV) initially, followed by 12.5 g IV every 2 to 4 hours until a total of 50 g has been given or until CVP or PCWP have optimized or until signs of adequate intravascular volume, as outlined above, are present, may be of benefit via several mechanisms. It may cause a solute diuresis and increase the intratubular pressure and flow rate, which may relieve or prevent tubular obstruction[30, 31]; it may also decrease glomerular afferent arteriolar and endothelial cell swelling, thus potentially improving renal blood flow. Finally, it may help correct intravascular volume depletion. Unfortunately, the use of mannitol is often limited by increased intravascular volume or elevated left atrial filling pressures.

Dopamine has been shown to produce renal cortical vasodilation and increased renal cortical blood flow in experimental hemorrhagic shock and, in dopaminergic doses (1 to 3 μg/kg/min), may be of great benefit in the management of early ischemic ATN.[32]

Loop diuretics, furosemide in particular, may be of benefit in several ways. The solute diuresis resulting from their use may result in increased intratubular pressure and flow, thus relieving or minimizing the tubular obstructive component of early ATN.[30, 31] Loop diuretics may also convert some cases of oliguric ATN to nonoliguric ATN[33]; this facilitates clinical management but probably does not alter the eventual course of ATN. Obviously, diuretics should not be administered in the setting of intravascular volume depletion until the latter has been corrected.

Dopamine (3 μg/kg/min) and furosemide used together have been shown to have a synergistic protective effect in experimental ARF in normotensive, normovolemic animals.[34] Possible mechanisms include blockade of glomerulotubular feedback with decreased renal renin release, renal vasodilatation secondary to furosemide-induced prostaglandin release, and induction of a solute diuresis. We have used this combination with considerable success in the early stage of clinical ATN.

Other modalities of intervention in early ATN are less generally accepted. There is evidence that calcium transport across the tubular cell may play a role in the genesis of ATN, and verapamil has been used to diminish the severity of ATN in experimental animals.[21, 35] To date this has not found general acceptance in the clinical situation.

Once ARF becomes established, management consists primarily of conservative fluid, electrolyte, and nutritional management, with dialysis if necessary, until renal function improves. Care must be taken to avoid volume overload. Urine electrolytes must be quantitated, as well as the electrolyte composition of other fluid losses (nasogastric suction, ostomy losses, etc.), and replaced appropriately to avoid hyponatremia or hypernatremia. Serum potassium must be monitored closely and high potassium levels treated appropriately with sodium polystyrene sulfonate (Kayexalate) or dialysis, with calcium gluconate, sodium bicarbonate, or glucose and insulin used if necessary.[36] Serum bicarbonate levels should be maintained at 15 mEq/L or higher by means of exogenous bicarbonate administration. At least 100 g of glucose and 30 to 40 g of high–biologic value protein should be administered daily to minimize endogenous catabolism and encourage a positive nitrogen balance. Hyperphosphatemia and hypocalcemia should be treated with aluminum hydroxide and calcium gluconate administration, respectively, as indicated. Indications for dialysis include volume overload, hyperkalemia, or metabolic acidosis that cannot be controlled by conservative management. Uremic pericarditis or uremic gastroenteritis with hemorrhage constitute almost absolute indications for dialysis. We prefer to dialyze patients with ARF aggressively and early (BUN, approximately 100 mg/dL) to attempt to avoid these serious complications.

Dosage adjustments of many drugs are required in renal failure. Excellent comprehensive guides for alteration of drug dosages in renal failure are available.[37-39]

CASE STUDY

A 42-year-old man was brought to the emergency room because of multiple traumas sustained after a 20-foot fall from a construction site. He had previously been in good health, except for some vague problems with high BP for which he had never been treated.

On admission he was obese, weighing 195 lb. The skin was cyanotic, pale, and cold. His BP was 78/40 mm Hg, his pulse was 132 beats per minute, respirations were 30/min and shallow, and his temperature was 34.5°C rectally. He was disoriented and confused. Bony deformities were obvious in the right shin and left thigh. He was diffusely tender to touch, more so over the left side of the chest. The insertion of a Foley catheter was difficult and revealed gross hematuria.

Laboratory tests revealed the following values: hemoglobin, 12.2 g/dL; hematocrit, 37%; and white blood cell (WBC) count, 11,200 mm^{-3}. Urinalysis revealed a pH of 6, a specific gravity of 1.018, 4+ occult blood, 1+ protein, and RBCs too numerous to count. Chest x-ray studies showed multiple rib fractures on the left with a 30% to 40% pneumothorax. His heart size was normal. An electrocardiogram (ECG) showed left ventricular hypertrophy. Serum electrolyte and amylase levels were normal. Arterial blood gas analysis showed a pH of 7.52, a Pco_2 of 26 mm Hg, and a Po_2 of 71 mm Hg on 3 L of oxygen by nasal cannula. Fractures were confirmed in the shafts of the left femur and right tibia and fibula by x-ray films. He also had fractures of the pubic rami with gross displacement.

He was treated with 2 units of packed RBCs and 4 L of saline. His BP came up to 112/68 mm Hg and rectal temperature to 35.8°C. His urine output was 55 mL over the next 90 minutes.

After a chest tube was inserted on the left an IV pyelogram was obtained that showed delayed visualization of the collecting system bilaterally but no parenchymal defect. A computed tomographic (CT) scan of the head with contrast infusion was normal. CT scanning of the abdomen showed some ascitic fluid and a probable hematoma of the spleen. Abdominal paracentesis revealed gross blood. An aortogram with a celiac angiogram revealed leakage of contrast material from the splenic artery but was otherwise normal. The abdomen was explored and a lacerated spleen removed. No other source for the liter of blood in the peritoneal cavity could be identified. During the operation the patient required 4 additional units of blood.

For the next 3 days his urine output averaged 40 to 50 mL/hr, and his mean arterial pressure (MAP) was 60 to 80 mm Hg. The patient was alert and communicative. The color of his urine became gradually lighter; however, the BUN rose to 65 mg/dL with a serum creatinine value of 4.5 mg/dL. Urinalysis showed a pH of 5.5, specific gravity of 1.011, 4+ occult blood with more than 100 RBCs per HPF, and numerous dirty brown granular casts, epithelial cells, and cellular debris. Other laboratory tests revealed the following values; serum calcium, 6.2 mg/dL; phosphorus, 8.2 mg/dL; uric acid, 12.3 mg/dL; lactic dehydrogenase (LDH), 473 IU; alkaline phosphatase, 360 IU; AST, 156 units/mL; and creatine phosphokinase (CPK), 12,000 IU. Urine Na$^+$ was 42 mEq/L; K$^+$, 31 mEq/L; Cl$^-$, 30 mEq/L; urine creatinine, 52 mg/dL; and urine osmolality, 370 mOsm/kg. During this period the patient underwent internal fixation of the lower extremity fractures and wiring of the pelvis.

The renal service was consulted because of increasing BUN and creatinine levels.

Discussion

The patient had evidence of ARF with a BUN of 65 mg/dL and a serum creatinine level of 4.5 mg/dL. The renal failure had developed in the setting of good urine volumes and a normal serum potassium level.

There are several potential causes for ARF in this setting, as described below.

1. Urinary obstruction is a possibility in a patient with multiple traumas; disruption of the urethra, compression of the ureters by pelvic or retroperitoneal hematoma, or ureteral obstruction from blood clots are all possibilities to be considered. A good urine volume does not exclude obstruction since obstruction could be partial or intermittent. Another related possibility is leakage of urine into neighboring structures (pelvis, peritoneum, or groin). Obstruction can be easily and reliably excluded by renal ultrasound,[2] an excellent screening test for obstruction since it does not rely on renal function for visualization[3] and avoids the risks of a dye load. False negative renal ultrasound in the presence of obstruction may occasionally be seen, especially early in the course. If obstruction remains a consideration, the ultrasound should be repeated in 2 to 3 days; if the findings remain negative and obstruction is still a consideration, retrograde pyelography may be necessary to definitively rule out obstruction, although this will rarely be required. Urinary tract obstruction as a cause of ARF must always be excluded because it can so readily be diagnosed and treated and because it may, if missed, result in irreversible loss of renal function. Ordering an ultrasound in ARF should be almost as automatic as doing a urinalysis.[4]

2. Physical damage to the renal tissue or its vasculature secondary to trauma was excluded by the angiogram. In every patient with ARF following major abdominal trauma, renal blood flow should be evaluated promptly, at least by isotope renal scan and if necessary by angiography. Any delay in the diagnosis of renal artery thrombosis may result in irreversible total loss of renal function.[40, 41]

3. Acute tubular necrosis is the most common cause of an acute deterioration in renal function. In this particular patient, contributory factors, alone or in any combination, include (1) hypotension with ischemia of the kidneys (prerenal azotemia that has progressed to ATN, especially likely in the setting of preexisting hypertension by history and (ECG); (2) pigment nephropathy due to myoglobinuria or hemoglobinuria; (3) radiocontrast dye toxicity; and (4) other toxins, such as methoxyflurane during general anesthesia.

The absence of oliguria is totally compatible with a diagnosis of ATN. In a recent series of 92 prospectively studied patients with ATN, 59 had a nonoliguric picture.[33] This subgroup is characterized by lower morbidity and mortality and a less frequent need for dialysis. Others have also published similar results.[42, 43]

The urine sodium level of 43 mEq/L and FeNa of 2.8% are typical of ATN.[21-35] However, these findings are also compatible with obstruction of the urinary tract.

Pigment nephropathy is a very likely possibility. The evidence for rhabdomyolysis and myoglobinuria in this patient includes extensive muscle trauma in a male with large muscle mass, hypothermia, possible tenderness, impressive elevation of CPK as well as other enzyme levels, hyperphosphatemia, and hypocalcemia.[44, 45] The classical finding on urinalysis is 3–4+ occult blood with no or few RBCs seen on microscopy. This was not seen here, probably because of coincident trauma to and bleeding from the urinary tract. Some further diagnostic studies to reinforce the diagnosis of myoglobinuria include (1) centrifugation of the urine and then detecting occult blood in the supernatant and (2) testing urine for myoglobin and serum for aldolase and creatine. The problem with myoglobin measurements, however, is that present techniques are not specific for the presence of hemoglobin. In our experience myoglobinuria severe enough to result in ATN is usually associated with CPK values in excess of 10,000 IU. Hemoglobinuria due to a transfusion reaction is also a possibility.[46] The citrated blood would also explain the lower serum calcium value. However, hemoglobin, because of its molecular weight of 68,000 daltons and its binding in the serum to hepatoglobin, is not freely filtered at the renal glomerulus, in contrast to myoglobin, which has a molecular weight of only 17,000. In general, if a patient has enough hemoglobin in the serum to cause ATN, one should see pink discoloration of serum due to hemoglobinemia, which was not observed.

Iodinated contrast toxicity is a major cause of ATN.[10, 13, 47, 48] Predisposing risk factors in this patient include volume depletion, hyperuricemia, and the large dose of contrast material required for multiple procedures (angiography, IV pyelography, CT scan).

Anesthesia records must be reviewed to see whether methoxyflurane was used. Acute tubular necrosis with large urine volumes is the classical presentation.[49] However, with the increasing awareness of its nephrotoxic potential, this agent has now been almost abandoned. Also, the urinalysis report did not mention oxalate crystals.

4. Acute uric acid nephropathy is possible but unlikely because of the low serum level.[50] To exclude this possibility, a spot sample of urine should be sent for uric acid and creatinine analysis. Whenever the uric acid:creatinine ratio exceeds 1.0, uric acid nephropathy is likely.[51]

CASE STUDY CONTINUED

Based on the assumption that the patient had ATN caused by a combination of hypotensive ischemia, myoglobinuria, and contrast nephropathy, a forced alkaline diuresis with acetazolamide, IV sodium bicarbonate, and mannitol was started. Over the next 5 days the patient continued to improve, and his BUN and creatinine levels declined. The urine pH was consistently above 7.

Ten days after admission his BP again dropped to 90/48 mm Hg, and his urine output decreased. His temperature was 38°C, with a pulse of 122 beats per minute; his weight was 198 lb. He was confused and somewhat agitated. The axillae and tongue were dry. The neck veins were flat at 30 degrees, and at 60 degrees the BP dropped to 60/palpable. Generalized abdominal distension and tenderness were noted and were marked on the left. The abdominal wound looked clean, and no drainage was visible. Bowel sounds were generally hypoactive. The Foley catheter was draining small amounts of light-colored urine, with almost no increase after the administration of furosemide, 40 mg IV.

Laboratory studies revealed the following values: WBCs, 12,200 mm^{-3}, with 64% segmented neutrophils and 12% band forms. Serum sodium was 130 mEq/L; chloride, 95 mEq/L; bicarbonate, 18 mEq/L; potassium, 6.5 mEq/L; BUN, 38 mg/dL; glucose, 195 mg/dL; serum creatinine, 1.4 mg/dL; CPK, 7,000 IU; and calcium, 7.8 mg/dL. Arterial blood gas analysis on room air showed a pH of 7.28, a Pco$_2$ of 29 mm Hg, and a Po$_2$ of 66 mm Hg.

Urinalysis revealed a pH of 7.8, a specific gravity of 1.023, 2+ occult blood, 2 to 5 RBCs and 15 to 20 WBCs per HPF, a few dirty brown granular casts, and 3+ bacteria. A chest x-ray showed blunting of the left costophrenic angle and atelectasis in the left lower lung field. An ECG showed an increase in amplitude of the T waves in leads V2 to V4.

The patient was given 50 mEq of IV sodium bicarbonate, 50 mL of 50% dextrose in water, plus 10 units of regular insulin and 300 mL of normal saline. An hour later his BP remained at 84/45 mm Hg, and his pulse was 135 beats per minute with occasional premature atrial contractions. His temperature rose to 38.4°C. Urine output continued to be poor (<20 mL/ hr). The urine sodium concentration was 43 mEq/L; chloride, 16 mEq/L; potassium, 32 mEq/ L; and creatinine, 25 mg/dL. FeNa was 1.9%.

Discussion

Oliguria and hyperkalemia complicated an otherwise uneventful recovery from ATN. Whenever this occurs, one must reevaluate the patient as one would a new case of ARF, with particular consideration of obstruction, renal hypoperfusion, or superimposed drug nephrotoxicity.

In this case the lower supine BP with a further orthostatic drop, poor skin turgor, recent forced diuresis, and elevated BUN-creatinine ratio all suggest renal hypoperfusion. However, the fact that the patient had gained 3 L since admission as well as a urine Na+ of 44 mEq/L and an FeNa of 1.9% contradict this; the latter are usually strong arguments against renal hypoperfusion. We must, however, remember that the patient had recently received furosemide, and this makes urinary indices uninterpretable.

A saline challenge was given with negligible response, also arguing against intravascular volume depletion. Since the patient was now oliguric, further fluids could have precipitated pulmonary edema. On the other hand he was in shock, and therefore his intravascular volume may have become severely depleted and required replacement. Thus, faced with conflicting data, a critical decision must be made regarding volume status and volume repletion. Additional data, namely, central filling pressures, become imperative.

The explanation for the hyperkalemia at this point is probably multifactorial: (1) an increased load from tissue breakdown after trauma and rhabdomyolysis, (2) efflux of potassium from cells in response to acidosis, and (3) the inability of the kidneys to excrete the excess load of potassium due to a decrease in urine volume. If all other variables remain constant, urinary potassium excretion varies in direct proportion to urine volume. This is because distal tubular potassium secretion is dependent on the potassium concentration gradient between the intracellular fluid in the distal tubular cell and the lumen. Large urine volumes and flow rates past the distal tubular cell maintain a steep potassium gradient and promote kaliuresis.[52] The appropriate immediate therapy for hyperkalemia was employed.[36] Since ECG changes were not significant and the patient's cardiographic status was not being monitored, calcium was not given. Potassium ion exchange resins do not have an immediate effect. However, they are superior to the other modalities employed here in that the potassium load is removed, not merely transferred into the cell to present a problem later.

A point worth mentioning in the management of this and other cases of ARF is the advisability of removing indwelling bladder catheters as soon as possible to minimize the risk of infection. In this patient this should have been done after the pelvis was wired.

CASE STUDY 1 CONTINUED

The patient was transferred to the intensive care unit and a flow-directed balloon-tipped catheter (Swan-Ganz) floated into the pulmonary artery. Recorded pressures were as follows: pulmonary artery, 26/6 mm Hg; PAOP, 5 mm Hg: cardiac output, 10.2 L/min; cardiac index, 4.9 L/min; total systemic resistance, 670 dynes-sec-cm^{-5}; and an arteriovenous oxygen content difference of 7.3 vols%. The serum lactate concentration was 35 mg/dL. Therapy with IV fluids, clindamycin, tobramycin, and ampicillin was begun. Eight hours later the MAP was 80 mm Hg, PAOP was 11 mm Hg, and cardiac output was 12.4 L/minute. The urine sodium concentration was now 5 mEq/L; chloride, 3 mEq/L; and potassium, 18 mEq/L. The creatinine level in urine was 65 mg/dL, and in serum it was 2.4 mg/dL. The serum sodium content was 142 mEq/L, and FeNa was 0.13%.

The next day the patient appeared better oriented. However, he complained of abdominal bloating. Examination revealed a distended abdomen with tenderness and guarding in the area of the splenectomy wound. No rebound tenderness or rigidity could be elicited. Bowel sounds were hypoactive. A flat plate of the abdomen did not show free air in the abdomen; however, there were dilated loops of bowel suggesting an ileus. Fever, tachypnea, and a low urine output persisted. Ultrasound of the abdomen revealed multiple cystic echoes in the left upper quadrant. The kidneys were normal in size and without hydronephrosis. The urine sodium concentration at this time was 18 mg/dL, with a serum creatinine level of 4.2 mg/dL. An exploratory laparotomy revealed 500 cc of pus in the splenic bed. Gram staining of the fluid revealed numerous gram-negative rods.

During the day following surgery the patient's course was complicated by hypoxemia, and a diffuse bilateral infiltrate was noted on chest x-ray films. Mechanical ventilation was instituted. He also developed a picture consistent with DIC.

Cultures of blood, pleural fluid, urine, and abdominal drainage all yielded gram-negative rods sensitive to ceftriaxone. Anaerobic cultures were negative, and so the patient continued to receive ceftriaxone alone. A random serum level of tobramycin before its use was stopped was reported as 6.5 µg/mL.

Subsequently, the patient became normotensive with a MAP of 80 mm Hg and a urine output of 20 to 25 mL/hr. His mental status remained poor. Rales up to the midlung fields and asterixis were noted.

Laboratory tests revealed the following values: serum sodium, 130 mEq/L; chloride, 98 mEq/L; bicarbonate, 13 mEq/L; potassium, 6.5 mEq/L; BUN, 165 mg/dL; glucose, 210 mg/dL; calcium 7.2mg/dL; albumin, 3.4 g/dL; creatinine, 7.2 mg/dL; urine sodium, 62 mEq/L; urine creatinine, 52 mg/dL; and calculated FeNa, 6.45%.

Discussion

The events that transpired between days 20 and 23 were primarily related to sepsis due to an intra-abdominal abscess accompanied by an adynamic ileus and sequestration of fluid in the bowel. The hypotension and renal hypoperfusion that followed were reflected in the low urine sodium, chloride, and FeNa values. Earlier the furosemide masked this picture. The measurement of PAOP was very helpful in determining the correct fluid management. Appropriate therapy with antibiotics and drainage of the abscess resulted in general improvement. However, adult respiratory distress syndrome, DIC, and toxic tobramycin levels were noted. Because of the multiple insults of sepsis, hypotension, and probable aminoglycoside toxicity, full-blown ATN with overt uremia developed, as reflected in the most recent laboratory data.

Could this have been prevented? To some extent, yes. If the sequestration of fluid in the bowel with intravascular volume depletion and hypoperfusion had been recognized earlier and managed appropriately with volume repletion instead of furosemide, the progression of prerenal azotemia to ATN might have been prevented.

Tobramycin toxicity undoubtedly contributed to the development of ATN. In ARF, after the usual loading dose of aminoglycoside has been administered, the subsequent maintenance doses should be based not on the serum creatinine value, but instead initially on the assumption that the patient is anephric. For example, even when the serum creatinine level is only 2.0 mg/dL (and rising) in a patient with ATN, the glomerular filtration rate and hence the ability to excrete aminoglycosides may be essentially zero. With continuing renal failure, the serum creatinine level will eventually rise, but so will the serum drug levels unless due care with dosing is taken in the beginning. Frequent 2-hour measurements of creatinine clearance rates are helpful in estimating drug dosages in patients with ARF who are not functionally anephric.

At this point the therapeutic decision is simple. The patient has established ATN with clinical uremia, as manifested by fluid overload, a wide anion gap metabolic acidosis, hyperkalemia, and mental obtundation.[45]

CASE STUDY CONTINUED

Hemodialysis through a subclavian catheter was instituted. Administration of narcotic analgesics was discontinued. Three days later, after daily dialysis therapy, the patient was breathing comfortably at a rate of 18/min. The lungs were clear on examination, and his urine output had increased progressively. The patient began bedside physical therapy but complained bitterly of left hip pain, so ibuprofen therapy was started. Several days later the patient was noted to have decreasing urine output and edema; chemistries revealed mild hyperkalemia and an elevation in BUN and creatinine levels. Urinalysis showed 3 + protein but was negative for eosinophils. The ibuprofen therapy was discontinued. Three weeks later the patient was discharged from the hospital with normal BUN and creatinine values.

Discussion

Indications for dialysis in ARF have already been discussed. The acidosis and hyperkalemia could have been managed without dialysis; however, the administration of sodium bicarbonate and potassium ion exchange resins would have been required, both of which present a significant sodium load, which would have further jeopardized the patient's ventilatory status. Also, the deterioration in mental status was probably a result of uremia. Furthermore, risks of pericarditis and gastrointestinal bleeding secondary to uremia can be minimized by early dialysis. The diuretic phase sometimes seen during recovery from ATN is conspicuously absent here. This is probably due to the fact that the osmoles (urea, creatinine, etc.) that accumulate during the oliguric phase of ATN had in this case been largely removed through dialysis. In the absence of osmoles, the osmolar diuresis that contributes to the polyuric phase is absent. Narcotics were withheld as they can contribute to mental deterioration. Also, narcotics may cause a drop in BP, which can create problems during hemodialysis. It 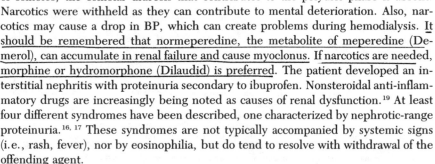 should be remembered that normeperedine, the metabolite of meperedine (Demerol), can accumulate in renal failure and cause myoclonus. If narcotics are needed, morphine or hydromorphone (Dilaudid) is preferred. The patient developed an interstitial nephritis with proteinuria secondary to ibuprofen. Nonsteroidal anti-inflammatory drugs are increasingly being noted as causes of renal dysfunction.[19] At least four different syndromes have been described, one characterized by nephrotic-range proteinuria.[16, 17] These syndromes are not typically accompanied by systemic signs (i.e., rash, fever), nor by eosinophilia, but do tend to resolve with withdrawal of the offending agent.

This patient's complicated hospital course emphasizes the transitions in renal pathophysiology that can occur from one day to the next. Only an appreciation of this fact and the meticulous medical attention that it demands will optimize management in this group of critically ill patients.

REFERENCES

1. Krumlovsky FA, Conn J: Acute renal failure, in Beal JM (ed): *Critical Care for Surgical Patients.* New York, Macmillan Publishing Co, Inc, 1981, pp 508–518.
2. Epstein FH, Brown RS: Acute renal failure. *Hosp Pract* 1988; 23:171–191.
3. Spiegel DM, Burnier M, Schrier RW: Acute renal failure. *Postgrad Med* 1987; 82:96–105.
4. Schlueter W, Batlle DC: Chronic obstructive nephropathy. *Semin Nephrol* 1988; 8:27–88.
5. Sanders RC, Berman S: B-scan ultrasound in the diagnosis of hydronephrosis. *Radiology* 1973; 108:375–382.
6. Qureshi N: Obstructive uropathy, in Earle DP (ed): *Manual of Clinical Nephrology.* Philadelphia, WB Saunders Co, 1982, pp 467–477.
7. Humes HD, Weinberg JM: Drug-induced nephrotoxicity. *DM* 1982; 28:1–81.
8. Fillastre JP, Mery JL, Godin M: Drug-induced glomerulonephrits. *Dial Transplant* 1981; 20:716–736.
9. van Ypersele de Strithou C: Acute oliguric interstitial nephritis. *Kidney Int* 1979; 16:751–765.
10. Krumlovsky FA, Simon NM, Santhanam S, et al: Acute renal failure associated with administration of radiographic contrast material. *JAMA* 1978; 239:125–127.
11. Byrd L, Sherman RL: Radiocontrast-induced acute renal failure. A clinical and pathophysiologic review. *Medicine (Baltimore)* 1979; 58:270–273.
12. Mason RA, Arbeit LA, Giron F: Renal dysfunction after arteriography, *JAMA* 1985; 253:1001–1004.
13. Nora NA, Berns AS: Renal failure following coronary angiography: A prospective study of diatrizoate and iopamidol abstracts. Presented at the 21st Annual Meeting, American Society of Nephrology, 1988.
14. Quigley MR, Ritchfield M, Krumlovsky FA, et al: Concurrent naproxen and penicillamine-induced renal disease in rheumatoid arthritis. *Arthritis Rheum* 1982; 25:1016–1019.
15. Garella S, Matarese RA: Renal effects of prostaglandins and clinical adverse effects of nonsteroidal anti-inflammatory drugs. *Medicine (Baltimore)* 1984; 63:165–181.
16. Pirson Y, van Ypersile de Strithon C: Renal side effects of nonsteroidal anti-inflammatory drugs. *Am J Kidney Dis* 1986; 8:338–344.
17. Clive DM, Stoff JS: Renal syndrome associated with nonsteroidal anti-inflammatory drugs. *N Engl J Med* 1984; 310:563–572.
18. Hart D, Lifschitz MD: Renal physiology of the prostaglandin and the effects of nonsteroidal anti-inflammatory agents on the kidney. *Am J Nephrol* 1987; 7:408–418.
19. Levin M: Patterns of tubulo-interstitial damage associated with nonsteroidal anti-inflammatory drugs. *Semin Nephrol* 1988; 8:55–61.
20. Brezis M, Rosens, Epstein FH: Acute renal failure, in Brenner B, Rector FC (eds): *The Kidney.* Philadelphia, WB Saunders Co, 1986.
21. Schrier RW: Acute renal failure. *JAMA* 1982; 247:2518–2525.

22. Miller TR, Anderson RJ, Linas SL, et al: Urinary diagnostic indices in acute renal failure. *Ann Intern Med* 1978; 89:47–50.
23. Steiner RW: Low fractional excretion of sodium in myoglobinuric renal failure. *Arch Intern Med* 1982; 142:1216–1217.
24. Fang LST, Sirota RA, Ebert TH, et al: Fractional excretion of sodium with contrast media induced acute renal failure. *Arch Intern Med* 1980; 140:531–533.
25. Oken DE: On the differential diagnosis of acute renal failure. *Am J Med* 1981; 71:916–920.
26. Espinel CH, Gregory AW: Differential diagnosis of acute renal failure. *Clin Nephrol* 1980; 13:73–77.
27. Diamond JR, Yourn DC: Nonoliguric acute renal failure associated with a low fractional excretion of sodium. *Ann Intern Med* 1982; 96:597–600.
28. Levinsky NG: Pathophysiology of acute renal failure. *N Engl J Med* 1977; 296:1453–1458.
29. Schrier RW, Conger JD: Acute renal failure: Pathogenesis, diagnosis, and management, in *Renal and Electrolyte Disorders*. Boston, Little Brown & Co, 1986, pp 423–494.
30. Cronin RE, del Torrente A, Miller PD, et al: Pathogenetic mechanisms in early norepinephrine-induced acute renal failure: Functional and histologic correlates of protection. *Kidney Int* 1978; 14:115–125.
31. Patak RR, Fadem SZ, Lifschultz MD, et al: Study of factors which modify the development of norepinephrine-induced acute renal failure in the dog. *Kidney Int* 1979; 15:227–237.
32. Nerberger RE, Passmore JC: Effects of dopamine on canine intrarenal blood flow distribution during hemorrhage. *Kidney Int* 1979; 15:219–225.
33. Anderson RJ, Linas SL, Berns AS, et al: Nonoliguric acute renal failure. *N Engl J Med* 1977; 296:1134–1138.
34. Lindner A, Cutler RE, Goodman WC: Synergism of dopamine plus furosemide in preventing acute renal failure in the dog. *Kidney Int* 1979; 16:158–166.
35. Schrier RW, Arnold PE, Van Putten VJ, et al: Cellular calcium in ischemic acute renal failure, *Kidney Int* 1987; 32:313–321.
36. Kunis KL, Lowenstein J: The emergency treatment of hyperkalemia. *Med Clin North Am* 1981; 65:165–176.
37. Bennett WM, Aronoff GR, Golper TA, et al: *Drug Prescribing in Renal Failure: Dosing Guideline for Adults.* Philadelphia, American College of Physicians, 1987.
38. Reed WE, Sabatini S: The use of drugs in renal failure. *Semin Nephrol* 1986; 6:259–295.
39. Van Scoy RE, Wilson WR: Antimicrobial agents in adult patients with renal insufficiency: Initial dosage and general recommendations. *Mayo Clin Proc* 1987; 62:1142–1145.
40. Stables DP, Fouche RF, Niekert DP, et al: Traumatic renal artery occlusion: 21 cases. *J Urol* 1976; 115:229–233.
41. Magilligan JD Jr, DeWeese JA, May AG, et al: The occluded renal artery. *Surgery* 1975; 78:730–738.
42. Myers C, Roxe DM, Hano JE: The clinical course of nonoliguric acute renal failure. *Cardiovasc Med* 1977; 2:669–672.
43. Vertel RM, Knochel J: Nonoliguric acute renal failure. *JAMA* 1967; 200:598–602.
44. Gabow PA, Kaehny WD, Kellebev SD: The spectrum of rhabdomyolysis. *Medicine (Baltimore)* 1982; 61:141–152.
45. Honda N: Acute renal failure and rhadomyolysis. *Kidney Int* 1983; 23:888–898.
46. Schmidt PJ, Holland PV: Pathogenesis of acute renal failure associated with incompatible transfusion. *Lancet* 1967; 2:1169–1172.
47. Hou SH, Bushinsky DA, Wish JB, et al: Hospital acquired renal insufficiency: A prospective study. *Am J Med* 1983; 74:243–248.
48. D'Elia JA, Gleason RE, Arday M, et al: Nephrotoxicity from angiographic contrast material: A prospective study. *Am J Med* 1982; 72:719–725.
49. Mazze RI, Shne GL, Jackson SH: Renal dysfunction association with methoxyflurane anesthesia. *JAMA* 1971; 216:278–288.
50. Kjellstrand CM, Campbell DC, VonHartitzsch B, et al: Hyperuricemic acute renal failure. *Arch Intern Med* 1974; 133:349–359.
51. Kelton J, Kelly WN, Holmes EW: A rapid method for the diagnosis of acute uric acid nephropathy. *Arch Intern Med* 1978; 138:612–615.
52. Good DW, Wright FS: Luminal influences on potassium secretion: Sodium concentration and fluid flow rate. *Am J Physiol* 1979; 236:192–205.

15/ Acute Myocardial Ischemia

DAN FINTEL, M.D.
KERRY KAPLAN, M.D.

Myocardial infarction is caused in most cases by thrombotic occlusion of a coronary artery. Following the demonstration by DeWood and colleagues[1] that the prevalence of total thrombotic occlusion of the infarct-related artery is 85% in the first 4 to 6 hours of a myocardial infarction, intense interest focused on using pharmacologic and mechanical means to recanalize occluded infarct arteries. From the era of the intracoronary administration of thrombolytic agents such as streptokinase,[2, 3] we have now moved to the administration of these agents via the intravenous (IV) route. As summarized in Table 15–1, efficacy approaches 55% for streptokinase administered IV and increases to 80% for IV tissue plasminogen activator (tPA), which is an endogenous human plasminogen activator now synthesized by bioengineering techniques. Table 15–1 summarizes the available thrombolytic agents, common clinical doses, side effects, and reduction in mortality associated with their early administration. Several large randomized placebo-controlled trials have demonstrated that thrombolytic therapy administered IV in the first 4 hours of evolving myocardial infarction can result in a 25% to 50% reduction in mortality at end points ranging from 2 to 6 weeks following the myocardial infarction.[4–14] These significant reductions in mortality and recurrent nonfatal myocardial infarction are present in most studies at 1 year of follow-up. Current research efforts are underway to determine the optimum time window for the administration of thrombolytic drugs as well as the value of "cocktails" or mixtures of thrombolytic agents such as tPA and urokinase.[8, 15]

The major adverse effect of thrombolytic therapy is bleeding. Serious, major organ bleeds are quite rare—0.5% to 1% rate of intracranial hemorrhage, 6% to 10% upper gastrointestinal (GI) bleeding—but bleeding at arterial and venous access sites is relatively common. Streptokinase has the additional adverse effect of hypotension if administered too rapidly and, rarely, anaphylaxis. Because of the 10% to 20% prevalence of reocclusion following recent thrombolytic therapy, most infarct management protocols include aspirin and anticoagulation with heparin. Contraindications to thrombolytic therapy include recent surgery, bleeding diathesis or active therapy with warfarin, a history of recent GI bleeding or active peptic ulcer, cerebrovascular event, severe uncontrolled hypertension with blood pressure (BP) greater than 180/120, recent trauma, prolonged cardiopulmonary resuscitation lasting greater than 1 minute, or a recent attempted placement of a central venous catheter.

TABLE 15–1.

Comparison of Thrombolytic Agents*

Feature	tPA	SK	APSAC	UK
Dose (IV)	100 mg	1.5 mU	30 units	2 mU
Recanalization rates (%)	70–80	35–55	50–60	50–60
Bleeding risk	Yes	Yes	Yes	Yes
Allergic reaction; hypotension	No	Yes	Yes	No
Duration of effect	Short	Long	Long	Long
	(1 hr)	(18–24 hr)	(18–24 hr)	(18–24 hr)
Cost	High	Low	High	High
Mortality reduction (%)	25–50	10–30	35–50	—

*APSAC = anisoylated plasminogen streptokinase activator complex; SK = streptokinase; tPA = tissue plasminogen activator; UK = urokinase.

Aspirin therapy initiated soon after infarction provides another significant contribution to mortality reduction. The large, multinational ISIS-II Trial[7] demonstrated that aspirin alone was associated with a 23% reduction in vascular events within 6 weeks of a suspected myocardial infarction. The Thrombolysis in Myocardial Infarction Phase IIB Trial (TIMI IIB)[16] demonstrated that mortality 6 weeks following infarction could be reduced to 5% by using a combination of IV tPA, aspirin, heparin, β-blockade and angioplasty in patients who manifest recurrent ischemia.

CASE STUDY 1

A 66-year-old white woman with no cardiac history was admitted with 3 hours of severe chest pain and precordial ST segment elevation compatible with an acute anterior wall myocardial infarction (day 1). Her past medical history was remarkable for insulin-dependent diabetes mellitus, a quiescent peptic ulcer, and inflammatory bowel disease.

Physical examination revealed a dyspneic, anxious female with a BP of 115/70 mm Hg and a regular pulse of 85/min. There were crackles present a third of the way up both posterior lung fields, and cardiac examination revealed soft heart tones, an S_3, and a grade I/VI systolic ejection murmur at the lower left sternal border. The rectal examination was negative for occult blood. The patient was treated with 100 mg of IV tPA administered over a 3-hour period: 60 mg in the first hour and 20 mg each in hours 2 and 3. A second IV line was inserted through which the patient received a 100-mg bolus of lidocaine followed by infusion at 2 mg/min as prophylaxis for ventricular tachyarrhythmias. A third IV line was established for the administration of IV nitroglycerin titrated to a dose of 100 μg/min and heparin in a 5,000-unit bolus followed by a 1,000-unit/hr infusion. Oxygen was administered by nasal cannula at 3 L/min with resultant arterial blood gas values of pH 7.44, a Pco_2 of 36 mm Hg, and a Po_2 of 62 mm Hg, and oral aspirin at 80 mg/day was initiated.

One hour after tPA infusion, electrocardiographic (ECG) monitoring revealed a 2-minute run of accelerated idioventricular rhythm, rate 75. The chest pain resolved over the following 2 hours, and an ECG obtained the following morning revealed resolution of previous ST segment elevation in the anterior precordial leads and preserved R waves in leads V1–3 compatible with an evolving anterior nontransmural myocardial infarction. Serum creatine phosphokinase (CPK) values peaked at 1,200 units/L with a 9% MB fraction 12 hours following admission.

Discussion

This patient is a nearly ideal candidate for thrombolytic therapy. The presence of anterior precordial ST segment elevation involving several leads and the signs of early congestive heart failure suggest a significant amount of myocardium at risk. Such patients derive the greatest benefit from early aggressive pharmacologic intervention. The prior history of peptic ulcer disease and inflammatory bowel disease are relative but not absolute contraindications to lytic therapy and illustrate how the physician must balance the potential risk of bleeding with the known benefits of thrombolytic therapy.

Although earlier trials with IV nitroglycerin provided little evidence of benefit in terms of reduction of infarct size or reduced mortality in acute myocardial infarction, more recent data[17] suggest early and lasting improvement in left ventricular function following the use of nitroglycerin therapy. Moreover, the early signs of vascular congestion suggest that benefit could result from preload reduction with nitrates. Nitrates act primarily by increasing venous capacitance, decreasing venous return to the heart, and thus reducing left ventricular wall tension. These drugs also increase coronary artery blood flow and, by relaxing vascular smooth muscle, may prevent the occurrence of coronary artery spasm.[18] IV nitroglycerin offers several advantages over topical or oral forms of nitroglycerin in the setting of the coronary care unit, including ease of administration, high bioavailability, and ability for rapid dose titration, features that have made IV nitroglycerin particularly beneficial in patients with unstable angina.[19] IV nitroglycerin infusions are started at a dose of 25 μg/min and increased by 25 μg/min every 5 minutes if no side effects occur, with an initial goal of 100 to 200 μg/min. The infusion is titrated for a clinical response, generally defined as a 10% to 15% decrease in systolic arterial pressure, or for prevention of further ischemic symptoms. The major potential adverse reaction is hypotension and/or reflex tachycardia, which can, however, be treated with cautious fluid therapy.

Early IV β-blockade was not appropriate in this case because of the presence of congestive heart failure as evidenced by the signs of moderate pulmonary congestion. The administration of β-blockers following myocardial infarction has been shown to reduce subsequent mortality by approximately 30% in several well-performed large randomized clinical trials.[20] The immediate IV administration of relatively $β_1$ selective β-blockers such as metoprolol or atenolol has been associated with an even further reduction in early mortality ranging from 18% at 2 weeks with atenolol[21] to 36% at 3 months with metoprolol.[22] The TIMI IIB trial[16] has demonstrated that following tPA, immediate IV metoprolol, when compared with oral metoprolol at discharge, was associated with a reduction in reinfarction rate and recurrent ischemia at hospital discharge but no overall reduction in mortality or relative improvement of left ventricular function. However, study patients who were eligible for β-blockade had substantially less mortality when compared with patients who were thought not to be candidates for immediate β-blockade. Table 15–2 lists clinical criteria that suggest eligibility for early IV β-blocker therapy.

Lidocaine is standard therapy for ventricular tachyarrhythmias in most coronary care units, although the prophylactic administration of lidocaine has not been shown to reduce mortality in several large patient series.[23] Systemic anticoagulation with a

TABLE 15–2.

Criteria for Eligibility for Intravenous β-Blocker Therapy

1. Heart rate > 55 bpm
2. Blood pressure > 100 mm Hg systolic
3. PR interval ≤ 0.26 seconds and absence of second- or third-degree heart block
4. Absence of significant pulmonary congestion (rales > 1/3 way up lung fields)
5. Absence of wheezing on examination or a history of asthma or chronic obstructive pulmonary disease

bolus of heparin followed by infusion is a standard component of thrombolytic therapy and is thought to reduce the risk of reocclusion. In this patient, a further and perhaps more important indication was the prevention of mural thrombus formation, which occurs frequently in the early hours of an acute anterior wall myocardial infarction.[24] Echocardiography has been very important in detecting the presence of mural thrombi. Echocardiographic features that are associated with increased embolic risk include mobility and protrusion of the thrombus into the ventricular cavity. Even if a thrombus is absent, in the presence of anterior wall akinesis or dyskinesis, heparin administration is continued until oral anticoagulation with warfarin has been accomplished.[25–27]

Mild arterial hypoxemia is common in the early phases of myocardial infarction due to "V/Q" mismatching. Because an adequate arterial oxygen content is critical in minimizing the amount of damaged myocardium, a reasonable practice is to maintain arterial oxygen saturation at 90% or greater.[28] Oxygen demands are reduced by placing the patient at bed rest and supplying an easily digested meal, usually clear liquids, during the first day of the infarction. Hemodynamically stable patients are encouraged to use a bedside commode because it is less strenuous, less likely to cause vagal stimulation, and associated with a milder Valsalva effect than is the use of a bedpan.[29]

Early peaking of the CPK concentration, defined as less than 18 hours after the onset of myocardial infarction, is suggestive but not diagnostic of successful recanalization of the infarct artery with the thrombolytic agent. The most uniformly reliable criterion of early recanalization is total resolution of ST segment elevation, which occurs in fewer than 15% of patients receiving thrombolytic therapy for acute infarction.[30] This patient's ECG revealed preservation of R waves, which suggests interruption of the transmural necrotic process due to successful opening of the infarct-related coronary artery.

CASE STUDY 1 CONTINUED

On the second hospital day, the patient developed recurrent chest pain with new ECG changes of ST segment depression in leads V2 to V4. The discomfort was relieved by sublingual nitroglycerin and further treated by an increase in the rate of infusion of IV nitroglycerin to 150 μg/min. A second episode occurred later that day, again relieved with nitroglycerin and sublingual nifedipine.

Repeat cardiac enzymes failed to show any evidence of infarct extension. Diltiazem therapy was begun at a dose of 30 mg orally every 6 hours. Cardiac catheterization performed later that day revealed a severe 95% occlusion in the proximal left anterior descending (LAD) and a 50% occlusion in the midright coronary artery followed by a 50% to 70% occlusion at the takeoff of one of the posterior descending branches. Although there were no other discrete lesions, the coronary arteries appeared to be diffusely diseased. Successful angioplasty of the LAD stenosis was performed, after which substantial resolution of the anterior ischemic changes followed.

Discussion

Recurrent myocardial ischemia after infarction is a marker for unfavorable outcomes. New ECG changes in a myocardial region "distant" from the infarction are associated with a particularly unfavorable prognosis.[31] Persistent pain at rest and ECG changes are often a marker for infarct extension. Pathophysiologic mechanisms for postinfarction angina include reocclusion of the infarct-related coronary artery, which occurs in 10% to 15% of patients receiving early thrombolytic therapy, vasospasm, and the development of new lesions or thrombosis elsewhere in the coronary arterial tree.

The initial response to postinfarction angina should include augmentation of medical therapy or even repeated thrombolytic therapy if the patient presents with recurrent ST-segment elevation and chest pain that persists for more than 30 minutes. Oral diltiazem started within 48 hours of non-Q infarction has been shown to significantly reduce the incidence of postinfarction angina and recurrent nonfatal infarction.[32]

Postinfarction angina unresponsive to medical management almost always requires relatively urgent myocardial revascularization. In the early period following a myocardial infarction, angioplasty of the infarct-related coronary artery only is performed, even if other significant stenoses are present. Although disease was present in this patient in the distribution of the right coronary artery, an angioplasty-related complication compromising flow in the distribution of the right coronary artery might convert a modest anterior infarct into a much more global and probably life-threatening event. Early-phase angioplasty following thrombolytic therapy of acute myocardial infarction can be expected to have an 80% to 90% success rate[33-35] and a complication rate of 5% to 10%. The preferred treatment strategy in the recently completed large multicenter trial (the TIMI IIB trial[16]) reserved early angiography and angioplasty for patients who manifested spontaneous or exercise-provoked ischemia, as exemplified by this patient.

CASE STUDY 1 CONTINUED

The next morning (day 3), heparin administration was stopped for several hours, which permitted removal of the femoral sheath. Shortly thereafter, the patient experienced severe chest pain accompanied by anterior ST-segment elevation that did not respond to sublingual nitroglycerin. She was taken to the cardiac catheterization laboratory within 1 hour where angiography was performed via access from the left femoral artery because of the presence of a hematoma at the previous site of sheath placement. Cardiac catheterization revealed reocclusion of the LAD at the site of the previously successful angioplasty 1 day earlier. The anterior descending was rapidly recanalized with a guide wire and subsequent angioplasty, with swift resolution of the chest pain and improvement of anterior precordial ST-segment elevation. Subsequent CPK determination revealed a peak of 196 units/L with a 6% MB fraction 10 hours after the onset of chest pain. The ECGs obtained the next morning revealed a loss of R waves in V1 through V3 that was compatible with anteroseptal extension of her previous non-Q myocardial infarction.

Discussion

Reocclusion of the infarct-related coronary artery is an important but infrequent complication of angioplasty. The use of aspirin begun shortly after suspected infarction is associated with a reduction in mortality nearly identical to that of thrombolytic therapy in one large multinational trial (ISIS-II[7]). Aspirin probably acts by preventing reocclusion due to platelet aggregation. Despite successful recanalization with thrombolytic therapy and angioplasty, this patient did reocclude the infarct artery when heparin use was briefly discontinued 1 day following angioplasty. Early recognition of reocclusion is important because mechanical reopening or repeat thrombolytic therapy can usually restore blood flow. Each episode of infarct artery reocclusion is generally associated with extension of the infarction and progressive myocardial injury.

Hematoma at angiographic access sites occurs frequently after thrombolytic therapy and the aggressive anticoagulation therapy that continues for the next few days. This complication has been documented in up to 50% of patients submitted to this form of therapy in the early days of the myocardial infarction.

CASE STUDY 1 CONTINUED

The next morning, a two-dimensional echocardiogram revealed hypokinesis of the anterolateral left ventricle, with an akinetic left ventricular apex. A protruding mass was noted at the apex that was compatible with a left ventricular thrombus. The patient was weaned off IV nitroglycerin and diltiazem, and begun on oral isosorbide dinitrate, captopril, and sodium warfarin (Coumadin).

When the prothrombin time reached 16 seconds, heparin use was discontinued. A stress test performed on the 10th hospital day was stopped at 4 minutes because of severe shortness of breath and fatigue. The ECG revealed no significant changes but was limited because of the level of inadequate stress attained. She was discharged on the 14th hospital day on a regimen of isosorbide dinitrate, 40 mg three times daily (TID); captopril, 25 mg TID; digoxin, 0.25 mg daily; furosemide (Lasix), 40 mg daily; Coumadin, 5 mg daily; and aspirin, 80 mg daily. Follow-up stress testing 6 weeks later revealed improved exercise performance and no ECG signs of ischemia.

Discussion

When echocardiography demonstrates a definite intracavitary mass in the left ventricle following myocardial infarction, it is appropriate to maintain anticoagulation for a 3- to 6-month period with warfarin compounds. Because of the effect of aspirin upon platelet adhesion and aggregation upon the intraventricular thrombus, many clinicians add low-dose aspirin (60–120 mg daily). Because the greatest embolic risk is present in the first weeks following the myocardial infarction, it is prudent to repeat the echocardiogram at approximately 3 months and stop warfarin anticoagulation if the thrombus has resolved.

Left ventricular remodeling occurs during the healing phase of a myocardial infarction. Infarct expansion refers to progressive dilatation of the left ventricle in the region of the infarction. Animal experimental data and now a recent angiographic study in patients with anterior infarction[36] demonstrate improved hemodynamics and reduction of infarct expansion when afterload reduction therapy with an angiotensin-converting enzyme inhibitor, captopril, is used. This form of vasodilator therapy is now being tested in several multicenter trials of postinfarction patients. Thus, captopril was added to this patient's regimen following the echocardiographic demonstration of an extensive area of left ventricular akinesis. Results from the multicenter postinfarction trial of diltiazem[37] suggested that patients with evidence of vascular congestion did not benefit from chronic oral therapy with this calcium blocker following the myocardial infarction, and thus diltiazem use was discontinued in the hospital.

Predischarge exercise stress testing has proved very useful for risk stratification; patients who have evidence of easily provocable ischemia are at increased risk of recurrent ischemic events. Patients with a low-level predischarge test positive for ischemia should be considered for early angiography to define the coronary anatomy. Bypass surgery was avoided in this patient because she became stable with intensive medical therapy and angioplasty of the infarct-related coronary artery.

Cardiogenic Shock

Cardiogenic shock may occur as the end stage of any form of heart disease but most often follows an acute myocardial infarction. In fact, since the advent of coronary care units and the vigorous treatment of arrhythmias, cardiogenic shock has become the most frequent cause of mortality following myocardial infarction. Cardiogenic shock occurs when enough myocardial contracting function is acutely lost that the cardiac output is inadequate to meet the body's needs, and it is associated with a reduction of blood flow to vital organs. In contrast, patients with chronically impaired left ventricular function have made circulatory adjustments that preserve critical organ perfusion, even with ejection fractions as low as 15%.

Approximately 50% of patients who develop cardiogenic shock following myocardial infarction do so within 24 hours.[38] In other patients, up to a week's delay in the onset of cardiogenic shock may reflect ongoing myocardial ischemia and infarct extension.[38, 39] Cardiogenic shock occurs more frequently with anterior than with inferior infarcts, probably because anterior infarcts tend to involve more left ventricular muscle.[40] Autopsy studies confirm that the severity of heart failure increases with the size of the infarct and that if 40% of the left ventricular muscle is lost, cardiogenic shock will result.[41] If circulatory support and urgent myocardial revascularization are not instituted, cardiogenic shock is usually fatal within a short time (55% to 85% mortality within 24 hours).[38,42–44]

Cardiogenic shock is diagnosed when the clinical manifestations of shock are present (hypotension, oliguria, altered sensorium, cool clammy skin) in the absence of significant persistent chest pain, arrhythmias, or diminished left ventricular filling pressure. Hemodynamic monitoring is necessary to make the diagnosis, institute appropriate therapy, and monitor the results of therapy. Intra-arterial pressure monitoring is advocated because BP determined with the cuff method underestimates the true pressure in patients with shock and high systemic vascular resistance.[45] It also allows easy access for frequent blood tests and arterial blood gas determinations. Insertion of a flow-directed pulmonary catheter is necessary to exclude inadequate left ventricular filling and to monitor the results of therapy. In cardiogenic shock the cardiac index (CI) is decreased while the left ventricular filling pressure is increased. Patients with a CI of less than 2.0 L/min/m^2 and a left ventricular filling pressure (left ventricular end-diastolic pressure or pulmonary arterial end-diastolic pressure) greater than 15 mm Hg have a very high mortality.[46] Pulmonary artery end-diastolic pressure has been shown to correlate closely with left ventricular end-diastolic pressure in patients in shock.[47]

Although cardiogenic shock in the setting of myocardial infarction most commonly develops secondary to a progressive loss of myocardial function, there are other causes. It may be related to mechanical factors such as rupture of the ventricular septum or a papillary muscle. Infarction of the right ventricle may result in inadequate filling of the left ventricle and is treated by expanding the intravascular volume and β_1-agonist pressor support.[48, 49] Pharmacologic agents such as β-receptor blockers or calcium channel blockers may cause shock that reverses over time when administration of the drug is stopped or an antagonist to the drug's effect is administered.

The initial goal of therapy in patients with cardiogenic shock is to maximize cardiac output at a minimum left ventricular filling pressure while maintaining a positive balance between diminished myocardial oxygen supply and demand. The major determinants of cardiac output and myocardial oxygen demand are the same: they both increase with increases in heart rate, contractility, and left ventricular filling pressure. Oxygen consumption increases, and cardiac output falls as peripheral vascular resistance increases. Therefore, the balance between limited oxygen supply and augmented demand must be considered during any therapeutic intervention in patients with myocardial infarctions. Unless the hemodynamic derangements rapidly normalize, recent data suggest that reperfusion of the ischemic myocardium via thrombolytic therapy, angioplasty, urgent surgical revascularization, or a combination of the above offers the best chance for survival.[44, 48, 49]

CASE STUDY 2

A 58-year-old black man was admitted to the coronary care unit (day 1) after three episodes of substernal chest pain radiating to the left shoulder, each lasting 20 minutes and associated with shortness of breath and light-headedness. These episodes began 36 hours prior to admission. On physical examination the BP was 90/60 mm Hg, the pulse was 54 beats per minute (bpm) and regular, and respirations were 24/min and mildly labored. Jugular venous pulsations were noted 2 cm above the clavicle at 30 degrees. End-inspiratory rales were audible over both bases. S$_1$ and S$_2$ were normal in intensity and splitting, and a soft S$_3$ was present at the apex and left lower sternal border. No murmurs were audible. The patient's abdomen was soft, nontender, and without organomegaly. All pulses were present and symmetrical. No pitting edema was present.

An ECG revealed sinus bradycardia at a rate of 50/min; 3 mm of ST-segment elevation in leads II, III and aVF, and 2 mm of ST-segment depression in leads V2–4. A chest x-ray film showed a normal-sized heart without signs of pulmonary venous congestion. Arterial blood gas determination on room air disclosed a pH of 7.47, a P_{CO_2} of 34 mm Hg, a P_{O_2} of 72 mm Hg, and an O_2 saturation of 95%.

Nitropaste 0.5 in. was administered every 6 hours; aspirin, 325 mg daily; subcutaneous heparin, 5,000 units TID; and oxygen, 30% by face mask. The pulse remained in the 50s while the patient was awake and fell to the low 40s when he was asleep. He had no further chest pain, shortness of breath, or lightheadedness.

Discussion

Although the patient had no prolonged episodes of chest pain, his presentation was consistent with an evolving inferior wall myocardial infarction, now probably 36 hours old. The initial ECG picture was consistent with this diagnosis and localized the infarct to the inferior wall. Anterior precordial ST-segment depression is frequently seen during inferior infarction and may reflect coexisting anterior ischemia or may be a reciprocal ECG manifestation of the inferior injury pattern.[50–52] Because the patient presented for evaluation 36 hours after the onset of symptoms, thrombolytic therapy is not indicated. In the presence of hypotension and bradycardia, acute IV or oral β-blockade would also not be appropriate. Similarly, oral calcium channel blockade is usually not initiated in the early hours of a transmural myocardial infarction.

Bradyarrhythmias are common after inferior wall myocardial infarction. They most commonly reflect increased vagal tone and sinoatrial or atrioventricular (AV) nodal ischemia and usually respond to IV atropine. Attempts to increase the heart rate should be made only if the patient becomes symptomatic. Signs of diminished cardiac output (cold clammy skin, decreased cerebral perfusion, decreased urine output), pulmonary edema, or refractory ventricular ectopy are indications for intervention. Atropine can be given IV in 0.4- to 0.5-mg boluses every 3 to 5 minutes to a total dose of 2 mg, depending on the response. Because of the difficulty in closely controlling the heart rate with atropine and because of its frequent and occasionally troubling side effect (central nervous system [CNS] stimulation, urinary retention, tachycardia, hyperpyrexia), a temporary pacemaker may be preferable to control the heart rate. In experienced hands, insertion of a temporary transvenous pacemaker can be accomplished safely, although ventricular fibrillation requiring cardioversion may occur in patients with right ventricular infarction.[53] Transcutaneous pacing electrodes can be applied within seconds during an emergency situation and can provide safe and reliable pacing until a transvenous pacemaker can be inserted. Alternatively, in patients with threatened but still-functioning cardiac conduction, prophylactic placement of transcutaneous pacing electrodes provides the ability to pace the ventricle if sudden symptomatic AV dissociation or profound bradycardia develops. The availability of this technique has made the insertion of prophylactic temporary transvenous pacemakers much more infrequent.

CASE STUDY 2 CONTINUED

The patient was awakened the next morning (day 2) by a return of chest discomfort accompanied by persistent inferior ST-segment elevation. The ECG revealed Q waves in leads 2, 3 and AVF and persistent ST-segment elevations in those leads. An IV nitroglycerin drip was initiated and titrated upward to a dose of 150 μg/min. The BP fell from 110/70 to 100/65 mm Hg with a pulse of 66 bpm and regular; respirations were 22/min and unlabored. Jugular venous distension was evident 5 cm above the clavicle at 30 degrees. Rales were heard over a third of the posterior portion of the thorax. A grade II/VI late systolic decrescendo murmur was heard along the lower left sternal border and radiated to the apex, where an S_3 was audible. There was no peripheral edema. Arterial blood gas determination on 30% oxygen by face mask revealed a pH of 7.42, a Pco_2 of 38 mm Hg, a Po_2 of 68 mm Hg, and an O_2 saturation of 94%.

Evaluation of the cardiac enzymes revealed a CPK value on admission of 850 units/L with 12% CPK-MB; this fell to 350 the following morning. A repeat chest x-ray film showed no cardiomegaly but slight pulmonary vascular redistribution. Ten milligrams of IV furosemide led to a brisk diuresis of 600 cc. Repeat lung examination 2 hours later revealed only basilar rales, and the respiratory rate had decreased to 16/min. The patient was allowed to sit at his bedside to take a soft solid diet, and the oxygen therapy was switched to 2 L/min via nasal cannula.

Discussion

The development of Q waves and falling CPK values are consistent with a recent inferior myocardial infarction. The presence of new ischemic pain prompted an augmentation of therapy, the addition of IV nitroglycerin. As discussed in case study 1, postinfarction angina should be vigorously treated and often suggests the presence of persistent ischemic jeopardized myocardium that survived necrosis following the initial vessel occlusion.

More than half of myocardial infarction patients will develop a soft, high-pitched, apical systolic descrescendo or holosystolic murmur due to papillary muscle dysfunction in the first several days. These murmurs occur more often with inferior than with anterior infarcts and are caused by the failure of a papillary muscle or its supporting ventricular muscle to shorten appropriately as the left ventricle contracts during systole.[54]

The pulmonary rales and S_3 were suggestive of congestive heart failure (CHF) and raise the issue of treatment with diuretics or digitalis. An acute myocardial infarction causes a localized area of left ventricular dysfunction that, if large enough, necessitates high left ventricular diastolic filling pressures to maintain an adequate cardiac output. Rales, which reflect the increased pulmonary vascular pressures, are not an uncommon finding in the first several days following a myocardial infarction. Diuretic agents are indicated in this patient because of signs of increased pulmonary water as noted on the physical examination and chest x-ray film as well as signs of increased work of breathing secondary to decreased pulmonary compliance. Orally or IV administered potassium will prevent the hypokalemia that frequently follows aggressive IV diuresis. As an infarct heals, left ventricular compliance increases, which allows lower filling pressures, and rales frequently disappear over the next several days.

Two-dimensional echocardiography with Doppler flow imaging may be very useful in this clinical setting. Global and regional left ventricular function can be studied, and acute mitral regurgitation or even the turbulent flow associated with rupture of the intraventricular septum can be detected. This information can be extremely helpful in distinguishing between pump failure due to diffuse myocardial disease or an acute mechanical problem.

In the past, physicians were concerned with the hemodynamic, metabolic, and arrhythmogenic effects of digitalis in the setting of an acute myocardial infarction. It is currently accepted that digitalis can be safely used during acute myocardial infarction when indicated for the control of supraventricular arrhythmias or CHF.[55] In the face of mild CHF one must consider the effects of any drug on the myocardial oxygen supply-demand ratio. If digitalis is used in a patient who has a normal-sized heart, it will cause increased oxygen consumption by increasing contractility and possibly systemic vascular resistance without direct effects on left ventricular wall tension or heart rate. However, if cardiomegaly is present, digoxin may cause some reduction in left ventricular size, which reduces oxygen consumption.[56]

CASE STUDY 2 CONTINUED

Later that afternoon (day 2) the patient experienced the acute onset of shortness of breath. He became confused and disoriented but denied chest pain. His BP was barely audible at 80/40 mm Hg, his pulse was 105 bpm, and respirations were 34/min and severely labored. On physical examination, the skin was cold and clammy. Neck veins were visible 9 cm above the clavicle. Pulmonary examination revealed rales over half of the posterior portion of the thorax bilaterally and a grade III/VI harsh holosystolic murmur loudest at the apex and radiating to the axilla and the left sternal border. There was a loud S_3 but no palpable thrill. Arterial blood gas analysis revealed a pH of 7.27, a Pco_2 of 44 mm Hg, a Po_2 of 44 mm Hg and an oxyhemoglobin saturation of 73%. The patient was treated with furosemide, 40 mg IV, oxygen by face mask with an Fio_2 of 0.5, and a dopamine drip titrated to a systolic BP of 90 to 100 mm Hg.

An emergency two-dimensional and Doppler color flow echocardiogram was obtained. Overall left ventricular function was fair, with severe hypokinesis of the inferoposterior wall. The left ventricle was slightly increased in size, but all other cardiac chambers appeared normal. The color flow study revealed a large jet of blood directed from the left ventricle into the left atrium during systole that was confirmed by the continuous-wave Dopper flow study.

Discussion

When an acute change in mental status occurs in the days after an infarct, drug toxicity, cerebral hypoxia, and inadequate cerebral perfusion must be considered. Hypoxia may be very difficult to judge clinically and, if suspected, should be confirmed by a determination of arterial blood gas values. Patients with decreased cerebral blood flow will usually have associated signs of poor systemic perfusion.

The patient had clinical and hemodynamic evidence of shock, more specifically of cardiogenic shock complicating acute myocardial infarction. Table 15–3 lists reversible causes of hypotension following myocardial infarction. Sudden, painless cardiovascular collapse associated with a new systolic murmur is an uncommon but

TABLE 15–3.

Reversible Causes of Hypotension
Following Myocardial Infarction

Myocardial ischemia
Bradyarrhythmia or tachyarrhythmia
Increased vagal tone
Hypoxemia
Acidosis
Drug toxicity
Surgically correctable lesions (PMR, VSR)*
Pericardial tamponade
Hypovolemia

*PMR = papillary muscle rupture; VSR = ventricular septal rupture.

ominous event following myocardial infarction. The differential diagnosis is between papillary muscle rupture and interventricular septal rupture. The patient should be stabilized and the diagnosis sought as quickly as possible. The finding of a new systolic murmur, the clinical setting of a recent inferoposterior myocardial infarction, and the Doppler demonstration of significant mitral regurgitation are all compatible with the development of acute mitral regurgitation.

Papillary muscle rupture is found in approximately 1% of patients dying of an acute myocardial infarction. It occurs more frequently with inferior than anterior myocardial infarction because of the relatively poor collateral blood supply to the posterior papillary muscles.[57] The prognosis following papillary muscle rupture without surgical intervention is poor, with less than half of patients alive after 24 hours. Rupture through the body of a papillary muscle almost always results in death, whereas rupture at the tip of a papillary muscle involves fewer chordae tendineae, causes less mitral regurgitation, and results in a greater chance of survival.[58]

Papillary muscle rupture occurs most commonly in the first week following an myocardial infarction. Examination reveals signs of pulmonary edema and low cardiac output. A loud, harsh holosystolic murmur is usually heard at the apex and radiates toward the left sternal border and base.[59] In this patient, the absence of a flail mitral leaflet on the two-dimensional echocardiogram is compatible with ischemic mitral valve dysfunction rather than rupture of the tip of the papillary muscle.

Interventricular septal rupture is responsible for 1% to 2% of deaths following an myocardial infarction. It occurs most commonly in the first week, has an equal incidence in anterior and inferior wall myocardial infarctions, and is often associated with right ventricular infarction.[60] Survival without surgery is dismal, with 50% mortality in the first week. Like papillary muscle rupture, it is manifested by the painless onset of hypotension and pulmonary congestion. A loud, harsh holosystolic murmur is heard at the apex and lower left sternal border and not uncommonly radiates to the right precordium. A thrill is felt along the lower left sternal border in approximately 50% of patients.[59]

A differential diagnosis between papillary muscle rupture and interventricular septal rupture is best made by right-heart catheterization. With papillary muscle rupture large V waves will be seen in the pulmonary artery occluded tracing. A step-up in oxygen content of 1 vol% or greater between the right atrium and right ventricle or pulmonary artery suggests a left-to-right shunt of blood (such as an interventricular septal rupture) between these sites.[61] A two-dimensional echocardiogram may demonstrate discontinuity of the interventricular septum, and turbulent flow into the right ventricle may be seen when a Doppler examination is performed.

CASE STUDY 2 CONTINUED

An indwelling arterial catheter was inserted (day 2) to monitor arterial pressure and to facilitate serial blood gas sampling. A Foley catheter was placed in the bladder, and a flow-directed pulmonary artery catheter was inserted. Initial pressures were as follows: right atrial mean pressure, 12 mm Hg; right ventricular pressure, 45/14 mm Hg; pulmonary artery pressure, 45/22 mm Hg; and pulmonary artery occluded pressure (PAOP), 26 mm Hg with a V wave of 36 mm. Cardiac output by thermal dilution technique was 3.0 L/min with a CI of 1.7 L/min/m^2. The Ca-vo$_2$ difference was 5.9 vol/dL. Arterial blood gas analysis on 50% O$_2$ showed a pH of 7.30, a Pco$_2$ of 41 mm Hg, and a Po$_2$ of 62 mm Hg. Systemic vascular resistance was 1,280 dynes-sec-cm^{-5}. Blood samples drawn simultaneously from the right atrium, pulmonary artery, and radial artery failed to reveal any step-up in oxygen content from the right atrium to the pulmonary artery. During this time the mean arterial pressure (MAP) was 50 to 60 mm Hg, the urine output was less than 10 cc/hr, and the patient remained confused. Because the MAP remained in the 60s, dopamine infusion was initiated. The dose of IV nitroglycerin was increased with the goal of both reducing preload and mildly reducing afterload, thus favoring forward cardiac output. Repeat hemodynamic measurements revealed a mild increase in CI along with a narrowing of the Ca-vo$_2$ difference and an increase in arterial oxygenation. Preparations were made for insertion of an intra-aortic balloon followed by emergency cardiac catheterization.

Discussion

The optimal PAOP in patients with acute ischemic myocardial injury is 16 to 20 mm Hg. This value results in increased cardiac output in most patients, without the deleterious increase in myocardial oxygen demands that occurs with further left ventricular dilation and higher filling levels.[62] If an optimal left ventricular filling pressure is reached (defined as no further increase in cardiac output as PAOP is increased) and tissue perfusion is still inadequate, pharmacologic intervention is necessary to increase cardiac output and, it is hoped, tissue perfusion. If MAP is greater than 70 to 80 mm Hg and the systemic vascular resistance is increased, a vasodilator such as nitroprusside would be the first agent used. With a lower MAP, a sympathomimetic agent such as dopamine, dobutamine, or epinephrine should be used. In this patient, the high PAOP and V wave in the setting of a markedly reduced cardiac output reflected the large volume of regurgitant left ventricular flow.

Dopamine is the metabolic precursor of norepinephrine. Its pharmacologic effects are dose related. At infusion rates of 1 to 2 μg/kg/min it causes renal and splanchnic artery vasodilation (dopaminergic effects). As the infusion rate is increased to 2 to 10 μg/kg/min, β-adrenergic effects predominate, with increased heart rate and contractility. At levels above 10 to 12 μg/kg/min, α-adrenergic (vasoconstrictive) effects predominate. The infusion rates at which the various effects predominate vary from patient to patient and can be assessed by direct hemodynamic measurements. In general, the initial dosage should be low (1 to 2 μg/kg/min) and the rate increased as dictated by clinical response. Major complications from the use of dopamine are rare but include tachycardia, ventricular arrhythmias, and hypotension.[63]

Dobutamine is a synthetic catecholamine that acts predominantly to increase cardiac contractility without causing marked tachycardia or a major decrease in peripheral vascular resistance. Like dopamine, it must be given by continuous infusion because its serum half-life is approximately 2 minutes. The initial dosage is 2.5 μg/kg/min, and the infusion may be increased to 10 to 15 μg/kg/min, depending on the clinical response. At higher doses tachycardia and decreased systemic vascular resistance may become evident. Unlike dopamine, dobutamine does not directly dilate the renal arteries. The major complication is precipitation of ventricular arrhythmias.[64, 65]

Norepinephrine stimulates both α- and β-adrenergic receptors. At low doses it stimulates predominantly β-adrenergic receptors in the heart, while at higher doses α-adrenergic effects become evident. Infusion should be started at 1 μg/kg/min and titrated to the desired clinical response.[66] Norepinephrine may be the agent of choice in states of severe vascular collapse unresponsive to other pressors.[66]

CASE STUDY 2 CONTINUED

An intra-aortic balloon pump was inserted via the right femoral artery. With one-to-one augmentation, hemodynamic parameters were improved (see Table 15–4). The patient's respiratory rate had declined to 24/minute, and arterial blood gas analysis showed a pH of 7.34, a P_{CO_2} of 38 mm Hg, and a pO_2 of 68 mm Hg with FIO_2 of 0.5. The patient was taken to the cardiac catheterization laboratory where angiography revealed occlusion of the largest marginal branch of the circumflex coronary artery and a left dominant circulation. Overall left ventricular function was fair to good with a measured ejection fraction of 48%. There was severe hypokinesis of the posterolateral wall with 3+ mitral regurgitation. A guide wire crossed the occluded circumflex marginal easily and was followed by a dilating catheter. Angioplasty of the left circumflex marginal was successful, with residual 30% stenosis at the site of previous total occlusion. A follow-up ventriculogram revealed a reduction of the mitral regurgitation to 1+, and the patient was returned to the coronary care unit in satisfactory condition. He was weaned off intra-aortic balloon counterpulsation the following day and discharged from the hospital 1 week later in good condition.

Discussion

This patient remained hypotensive and in pulmonary edema despite aggressive pharmacologic therapy. Thus, intra-aortic balloon counterpulsation was initiated. Intra-aortic balloon counterpulsation reduces myocardial ischemia and improves left ventricular dysfunction by reducing afterload and increasing coronary artery blood flow. An intra-aortic balloon may be inserted in the femoral artery by a percutaneous approach using the Seldinger technique. A 30- to 40-cc balloon is advanced up the aorta and secured just distal to the origin of the left subclavian artery. Balloon inflation is timed to the ECG tracing such that inflation occurs at the onset of diastole (anacrotic

TABLE 15–4.

Hemodynamic Measurements and Arterial Blood Gas Values

Parameter	Baseline	Following Intra-Aortic Balloon Pump
Right atrium (mm Hg)	12	9
Pulmonary artery (mm Hg)	45/22	42/16
Pulmonary artery occluded (mm Hg)	26 (V wave, 36)	20 (V wave, 30)
Cardiac index (L/min/m^2)	1.7	2.2
Ca-vo$_2$ (vol%)	5.9	4.6
Mean arterial pressure (mm Hg)	60	65
Arterial blood gas:		
PH	7.27	7.34
Pco$_2$	44	38
Po$_2$	44	68

notch of the arterial pulse tracing). Balloon deflation occurs just prior to myocardial contraction, thereby reducing left ventricular afterload by the creation of a potential space and the initiation of blood flow in a centrifugal direction. Diastolic inflation of the balloon propels blood toward the heart and coronary arteries, although it is controversial whether blood flow to ischemic myocardium is actually increased. Although often extraordinarily beneficial in the acute management of patients with myocardial ischemia or shock, insertion of the intra-aortic balloon is associated with a high rate of complications, including thrombosis, ischemia, embolism, hemorrhage, and infection.[67] In this patient, the systolic unloading caused by intra-aortic balloon counterpulsation allowed a further increase in forward cardiac ejection and a reduction in regurgitant flow through the mitral valve.

Several recent studies have demonstrated that timely myocardial reperfusion using a combination of thrombolytic therapy, percutaneous transluminal angioplasty, or bypass surgery may strikingly reduce mortality in patients with cardiogenic shock following myocardial infarction.[44, 48, 49] Angiography in this patient revealed total occlusion of the largest branch of the circumflex coronary artery that supplied the myocardium in the posterior papillary muscle as well as the posterolateral region of the left ventricle. Despite preserved left ventricular function in other myocardial regions, this combination of ischemia and injury was sufficient to cause cardiogenic shock. Following stabilization with preload reduction, sympathomimetic agents, and intra-aortic balloon compensation, angioplasty of the responsible vessel restored sufficient blood flow to improve both regional left ventricular function and papillary muscle function. As a result, this patient improved dramatically and survived this life-threatening complication of his myocardial infarction. This case highlights the urgency of hemodynamic monitoring, aggressive pharmacologic and mechanical support of the failing circulation, and most important in patients who develop cardiogenic shock after acute myocardial infarction, definition of coronary anatomy and improvement of myocardial perfusion.

REFERENCES

1. DeWood MA, Spores J, Notske RN, et al: Prevalence of total coronary occlusion during the early hours of transluminal myocardial infarction. *N Engl J Med* 1980; 303:897–903.
2. Rentrop P, Blanke H, Karsch KR, et al: Acute myocardial infarction: Intracoronary application of nitroglycerin and streptokinase in combination with transluminal recanalization. *Clin Cardiol* 1979; 2:354–363.
3. Yusuf S, Collins R, Peto R, et al: Intravenous and intracoronary fibrinolytic therapy in acute myocardial infarction: Overview of results on mortality, reinfarction and side-effects from 33 randomized controlled trials. *Eur Heart J* 1985; 6:556–585.
4. Gruppo Italiano per lo studio della streptochinasi nell'infarcto miocardico (GISSI): Effectiveness of intravenous thrombolytic treatment in acute myocardial infarction. *Lancet* 1986; 1:397–401.
5. Chesebro JH, Knatterud G, Roberts R, et al: Thrombolysis in myocardial infarction (TIMI) trial, phase I: A comparison between intravenous tissue plasminogen activator and intravenous streptokinase. *Circulation* 1987; 76:142–154.
6. White HD, Norris RM, Brown MA, et al: Effect of intravenous streptokinase on left ventricular function and early survival after acute myocardial infarction. *N Engl J Med* 1987; 317:850–855.
7. ISIS-2 (Second International Study of Infarct Survival) Collaborative Group: Randomized trial of intravenous streptokinase, oral aspirin, both or neither among 17,187 cases of suspected acute myocardial infarction: ISIS-2. *Lancet* 1988; 2:349–360.
8. Topol EJ, Califf RM, George BS, et al: Coronary arterial thrombolysis with combined infusion of recombinant tissue-type plasminogen activator and urokinase in patients with acute myocardial infarction. *Circulation* 1988; 77:1100–1107.
9. Guerci AD, Gerstenblith G, Brinker JA, et al: A randomized trial of intravenous tissue plasminogen activator for acute myocardial infarction with subsequent randomization to elective coronary angioplasty. *N Engl J Med* 1987; 317:1613–1618.
10. Wilcox RG, Von Der Liffe G, Olsson CG, et al: Trial of tissue plasminogen activator for mortality reduction in acute myocardial infarction. Anglo-Scandinavian Study of Early Thrombolysis (ASSET). *Lancet* 1988; 2:525–530.
11. Van de Werf F, Arnold AER, and the European Cooperative Study Group for Recombinant Tissue-type Plasminogen Activator (rTPA): Effect of intravenous tissue plasminogen activator on infarct size, left ventricular function and survival in patients with acute myocardial infarction. *Br Med J* 1988; 297:1374–1379.
12. Mathey DG, Schofer J, Sheehan FH, et al: Intravenous urokinase in acute myocardial infarction. *Am J Cardiol* 1985; 55:878–882.
13. Anderson JL, Rothbard RL, Hackworthy RA, et al: Multicenter reperfusion trial of intravenous anisoylated plasminogen streptokinase activator complex (APSAC) in acute myocardial infarction: Controlled comparison with intracoronary streptokinase. *J Am Coll Cardiol* 1988; 11:1153–1163.
14. AIMS Trial Study Group: Effect of intravenous APSAC on mortality after acute myocardial infarction: Preliminary report of a placebo-controlled clinical trial. *Lancet* 1988; 1:545–549.
15. Collen D, Van de Werf F: Coronary thrombolysis with low dose synergistic combinations of recombinant tissue-type plasminogen activator (rt-PA) and recombinant single-chain urokinase-type plasminogen activator (rscu-PA) in man. *Am J Cardiol* 1987; 60:431–434.
16. TIMI Study Group: Comparison of invasive and conservative strategies after treatment with intravenous tissue plasminogen activator in acute myocardial infarction. Results of the thrombolysis in myocardial infarction (TIMI) phase II trial. *N Engl J Med* 1989; 320:618–627.
17. Jugdutt BI, Warnica JW: Intravenous nitroglycerin therapy to limit myocardial infarction size, expansion and complication: Effect of timing, dosage, and infarct location. *Circulation* 1988; 78:906–919.
18. Miller RR, Olson HG, Vismara LA, et al: Pump dysfunction after myocardial infarction: Importance of location, extent, and pattern of abnormal left ventricular segmental contraction. *Am J Cardiol* 1976; 37:340–344.
19. Kaplan K, Davison R, Parker M, et al: Intravenous nitroglycerin for the treatment of angina at rest unresponsive to standard nitrate therapy. *Am J Cardiol* 1983; 51:694.
20. The Beta Blocker Pooling Research Group: The beta-blocker pooling project (BBPP): Subgroup finding from randomized trials in post infarction patients. *Eur Heart J* 1988; 9:8.
21. ISIS-1 Collaborative Group: Mechanisms for the early mortality reduction produced by beta-blockade started early in acute myocardial infarction. *Lancet* 1988; 1:921.

22. Hjalmarson A, Elmfeldt D, Herlitz J, et al: Effect on mortality of metoprolol on acute myocardial infarction. *Lancet* 1981; 2:823–827.

23. Wise OG, Kellen J, Rudemaker AW: Prophylactic vs. selective lidocaine for early ventricular arrhythmias of myocardial infarction. *J Am Coll Cardiol* 1988; 12:507–513.

24. Meltzer RS, Visser CA, Fuster U: Intracardiac thrombi and systemic embolization. *Ann Intern Med* 1986; 104:689–698.

25. Chesebro JH, Fuster U: Antithrombotic therapy for acute myocardial infarction: Mechanism and prevention of deep venous, left ventricular, and coronary artery thromboembolism. *Circulation* 1986; 74:1.

26. Turpie AGG, Robinson JG, Doyle DJ, et al: Prevention of left ventricular mural thrombosis in acute transmural anterior myocardial infarction: A double blind trial comparing high dose with low dose subcutaneous calcium heparin. *N Engl J Med* 1989; 320:352–357.

27. Visser CA, Kan G, Meltzer RS, et al: Embolic potential of left ventricular thrombus after myocardial infarction: A two-dimensional echocardiographic study of 119 patients. *J Am Coll Cardiol* 1985; 5:1276–1280.

28. Danzig R: Current status of oxygen therapy in acute myocardial infarction. *Cardiovasc Med* 1979; 4:1245–1248.

29. Gregoratos G, Gleeson E: Initial therapy of acute myocardial infarction, in Karliner JS, Gregoratos G (eds): *Coronary Care*. New York, Churchill Livingstone, Inc, 1981, pp 127–166.

30. Califf RM, O'Neill WW, Stack RS, et al: Failure of simple clinical measurements to predict perfusion status after intravenous thrombolysis. *Ann Intern Med* 1988; 108:658–662.

31. Schuster EH, Bulkley BH: Early post-infarction angina: Ischemia at a distance and ischemia in the infarct zone. *N Engl J Med* 1981; 305:1101.

32. Gibson RS, Boden WE, Theroux P, et al: Diltiazem and reinfarction in patient with non-Q myocardial infarction: Results of a double blind, randomized multicenter trial. *N Engl J Med* 1986; 315:427–429.

33. Topol EJ, Califf RM, George BS, and the Thrombolysis and Angioplasty in Myocardial Infarction (TAMI) Study Group: A multicenter randomized trial of intravenous recombinant tissue plasminogen activator and immediate angioplasty in acute myocardial infarction. *N Engl J Med* 1987; 317:581–588.

34. The TIMI Research Group: Immediate vs delayed catheterization and angioplasty following thrombolytic therapy for acute myocardial infarction: TIMI II A results. *JAMA* 1988; 260:2849–2858.

35. Simoons ML, Arnold AE, Betriu A, and the European Cooperative Study Group for Recombinant Tissue-Type Plasminogen Activator (rt-TPA): Thrombolysis with tissue plasminogen activator in acute myocardial infarction: No additional benefit from immediate percutaneous coronary angioplasty. *Lancet* 1988; 1:197–202.

36. Pfeffer MA, Lamas GA, Vaughn DE, et al: Effect of captopril on progressive ventricular dilatation after anterior myocardial infarction. *N Engl J Med* 1988; 319:80–88.

37. The Multicenter Diltiazem Postinfarction Trial Research Group: The effect of diltiazem on mortality and reinfarction after myocardial infarction. *N Engl J Med* 1988; 319:385–392.

38. Scheidt S, Ascheim R, Killip T: Shock after acute myocardial infarction: A clinical and hemodynamic profile. *Am J Cardiol* 1970; 26:556–564.

39. Gutovitz AL, Sobel BE, Roberts R: Progressive nature of myocardial injury in selected patients with cardiogenic shock. *Am J Cardiol* 1978; 41:469–475.

40. Miller RR, Olson HG, Vismara LA, et al: Pump dysfunction after myocardial infarction: Importance of location, extent and pattern of abnormal left ventricular segmental contraction. *Am J Cardiol* 1986; 37:340–344.

41. Page DL, Caulfield JB, Kastor JA, et al: Myocardial changes associated with cardiogenic shock. *N Engl J Med* 1971; 285:134–137.

42. Wackers FJ, Lie KI, Becker AE, et al: Coronary artery disease in patients dying from cardiogenic shock or congestive heart failure in the setting of acute myocardial infarction. *Br Heart J* 1976; 38:906–910.

43. Mason DT, Amsterdam EA, Miller RR, et al: Pathophysiology of myocardial infarction shock, in Eliot RS, Wolf FL, Forker AD (eds): *Cardiac Emergencies*. Mt Kisko, NY, Futura Publishing Co, Inc, 1977, pp 11–39.

44. Lee L, Bates ER, Pitt B, et al: Percutaneous transluminal coronary angioplasty improves survival in acute myocardial infarction complicated by cardiogenic shock. *Circulation* 1988; 78:1345–1351.

45. Cohn JN: Blood pressure measurement in shock. *JAMA* 1976; 199:118–122.

46. Weber KT, Batshin RA, Janicki JS, et al: Left ventricular dysfunction following acute myocardial infarction: A clinicopathologic and hemodynamic profile of shock and failure. *Am J Med* 1973; 54:697–705.

47. Scheinman M, Evans GT, Weiss A, et al: Relationship between pulmonary artery end-diastolic pressure and left ventricle filling pressure in patients in shock. *Circulation* 1973; 57:317–324.

48. Gunnar RM: Cardiogenic shock complicating acute myocardial infarction. *Circulation* 1988; 78:1508–1510.
49. Schreiber TL, Miller TH, Zola B: Management of myocardial infarction shock: Current status. *Am Heart J* 1989; 117:435–443.
50. Little WC, Rogers EW, Sodums MT: Mechanisms of anterior ST-segment depression during acute inferior myocardial infarction. *Ann Intern Med* 1984; 100:26.
51. Lew AS, Weiss AT, Shah PK, et al: Precordial ST-segment depression during acute inferior myocardial infarction: Early thallium-201 scintigraphy evidence of adjacent posterolateral or inferoseptal involvement. *J Am Coll Cardiol* 1985; 5:203.
52. Tzivoni D, Chenzbraun A, Keren A, et al: Reciprocal electrocardiographic changes in acute myocardial infarction. *Am J Cardiol* 1985; 56:23–26.
53. Sclarovsky S, Zafrir N, Strasberg B: Ventricular fibrillation complicating temporary ventricular pacing in acute myocardial infarction: Significance of right ventricular infarction. *Am J Cardiol* 1981; 48:1160–1166.
54. Heikkila J: Mitral incompetence complicating acute myocardial infarction: *Br Heart J* 1967; 29:162–169.
55. Rahimtoola SH, Gunnar RM: Digitalis in acute myocardial infarction: Help or hazard? *Ann Intern Med* 1975; 82:234–240.
56. Mason DT: Digitalis pharmacology and therapeutics: Recent advances. *Ann Intern Med* 1974; 80:520–530.
57. Sanders RJ, Neubeurger KT, Rabin A: Rupture of papillary muscles: Occurrence of rupture of the posterior muscle in posterior myocardial infarction. *Dis Chest* 1957; 31:316–323.
58. Vlodaver A, Edwards JE: Rupture of ventricular septum or papillary muscle complicating myocardial infarction. *Circulation* 1977; 55:815–822.
59. Kaplan K, Talano JV: Systolic murmurs following myocardial infarction. *Pract Cardiol* 1979; 5:25–39.
60. Cummings RG, Reimer KA, Califf R, et al: Quantitative analysis of right and left ventricular infarction in the presence of postinfarction ventricular septal defect. *Circulation* 1988; 77:33–42.
61. Meister SG, Helfant RH: Rapid bedside differentiation of ruptured interventricular septum from acute mitral insufficiency. *N Engl J Med* 1972; 287:1024–1025.
62. Baim DS, Baron MG, Barry WH, et al: Hemodynamics in acute myocardial infarction, in Braunwald E (ed): *Heart Disease*. Philadelphia, WB Saunders Co, 1988, pp 1273–1280.
63. Goldberg LI: Dopamine: Clinical uses of an endogenous catecholamine. *N Engl J Med* 1974; 291:707–710.
64. Sonnenblick EH, Frishman WH, LeJemtel TH: Dobutamine: A new synthetic cardioactive sympathetic amine. *N Engl J Med* 1979; 300:17–22.
65. Mason DT, Amsterdam EA, Miller RR: Treatment of myocardial infarction shock, in Eliot RS, Wolf GL, Forker AD (eds): *Cardiac Emergencies*. Mt Kisko, NY, Futura Publishing Co, Inc. 1977, pp 209–243.
66. Meadows D, Ffarcs J, Edwards D, et al: Reversal of intractable septic shock with norepinephrine therapy. *Crit Care Med* 1988; 16:663–666.
67. McEnany MT, Kay HR, Buckley MJ: Clinical experience with intra-aortic balloon pump support in 728 patients. *Circulation* 1978; 58(suppl 1):1124–1132.

16/ Gram-Negative Bacteremia and Shock

RICHARD DAVISON, M.D.

Bacteremia caused by gram-negative bacilli knows no medical specialty boundary in its steadily increasing frequency. It is presently the most commonly encountered serious infection in American hospitals. Some of the factors responsible for this increment are the increasing age and severity of illness in hospitalized patients, the widespread use of antibiotics, and the ever-growing population of immunocompromised individuals.

One fourth to one third of all patients with documented gram-negative bacteremia (GNB) die. If this overall mortality is scrutinized more carefully, it becomes obvious that the majority of deaths occur in the 40% to 50% of patients with GNB who go into shock.[1, 2]

The hemodynamic and metabolic disturbances found in GNB complicated by shock have been extensively investigated.[3, 5] It is generally agreed that endotoxic lipopolysaccharides as well as other microbial products are responsible for the development of the three major components of this syndrome: vasodilatation, diffuse intravascular coagulation, and generalized capillary damage. To a different degree and, in a varying sequence of events, end-organ damage eventually becomes irreversible and makes recovery of the patient impossible. Equally apparent is that the above phenomena are not the result of a direct action of endotoxin on tissues but rather a consequence of the induction by these bacterial products of the syntheses and release of a variety of chemical mediators and cytokines.[6] Some of the mechanisms that have been invoked include histamine,[7] β-endorphins,[8] kinins,[9] anaphylatoxins,[10] and most recently, cachectin.[11] *TNF (Tumor necrosis factors)*

CASE STUDY

A 76-year-old man with a history of untreated chronic lymphocytic leukemia was admitted via the emergency room complaining of a 48-hour history of weakness, malaise, and cough productive of blood-tinged sputum. Initial vital signs showed a regular pulse of 110/min, a rectal temperature of 35.8°C, a blood pressure by cuff measurement of 105/60 mm Hg, and respirations of 30/min. The patient was alert, and his skin was warm and dry. On examination of the lung fields, fine inspiratory rales were noted over the right lower lung field, and there were decreased breath sounds and dullness to percussion over that area. Cardiac and abdominal examinations were unremarkable. The rectal examination was noncontributory; stools were negative to guaiac. A complete blood count showed normal hemoglobin and hematocrit values, a white blood cell count of 18,600 mm^{-3} with 60% mature-looking lymphocytes and 5% band forms; and a platelet count of 210,000 mm^{-3} Chest x-ray films showed a normal cardiac silhouette and a patchy infiltrate involving the right lower lung field. The electrocardiogram was noncontributory, as were the serum electrolytes. Arterial blood gas analysis on room air showed a Po_2 of 65 mm Hg, a Pco_2 of 20 mm Hg, and a pH of 7.42. A Gram stain of purulent sputum that the patient spontaneously produced showed many white cells with a monotonous flora composed of small, gram-negative coccobacilli. In the emergency room appropriate cultures were obtained and, with the presumptive diagnosis of *haemophilus influenzae* pneumonia, therapy initiated with ceftriaxone. Two liters of normal saline were rapidly infused intravenously (IV).   *(Rocephin)*

Discussion

The history, physical findings, and initial laboratory determinations were compatible with a diagnosis of the sepsis syndrome.[12] This clinical entity is composed of a constellation of findings that express the systemic response to a serious infection. Fifty percent of patients so defined will be found to be bacteremic; within 24 hours 70% will have developed shock, and eventually 25% will develop the adult respiratory distress syndrome (ARDS). Therefore, criteria that describe the sepsis syndrome (Table 16–1) identify a patient population with a high propensity to develop septic shock and ARDS and with an overall mortality of 25%. It is thus an extremely valuable concept that promotes the early treatment of a high-risk group of patients.

As soon as baseline cultures are obtained, antibiotic treatment should be started promptly and fluid administration initiated on the assumption that the patient's blood volume is deficient secondary to increased capillary permeability and vasodilatation. The choice of fluids for this purpose—colloids vs. crystalloids—is not easy.[13] It is generally accepted that smaller total amounts of colloid solutions are required to restore an effective blood volume. Critics point out that the risk of volume overload is greater, that colloids are expensive, and that, in conditions associated with an enhanced capillary permeability, the egress of colloids into the interstitial tissues (such as those of the lung) can be deleterious. Conversely, lowering of the plasma colloid osmotic pressure following the infusion of large amounts of crystalloid solutions has been incriminated in the development of "noncardiogenic" pulmonary edema.[14] More recently, the use of a hypertonic saline albumin-containing fluid has been

TABLE 16–1.

Criteria for Diagnosis of the Sepsis Syndrome

Hypothermia (<96°F) or hyperthermia (>100°F)
Tachycardia (>90 beats per min)
Tachypnea (>20 breaths per min)
End-organ dysfunction (at least one of the
  following):
  Altered cerebral function
  Hypoxemia (Pao_2, <75 mm Hg)
  Elevated plasma lactate
  Oliguria (urine, <30 ml/hr)

proposed as an alternative that minimizes interstitial edema during fluid resuscitation.[15] In fact, there are no currently available data to indicate that the agent used for fluid resuscitation has any influence on the eventual outcome.

If colloid volume expansion is chosen, it would appear that the frequently expressed concern that the use of hydroxyethyl starch in a septic patient could result in added disturbance to the coagulation profile and increased bleeding is not supported by the existing literature.[16]

The concurrent results of two independently performed, large clinical trials have now firmly established the lack of indication for the use of high-dose corticosteroids in the management of the septic syndrome and bacteremic shock. In fact, one of these studies demonstrated that in the subgroup of individuals with failing renal function, steroids actually had a deleterious effect.[17, 18]

CASE STUDY CONTINUED

The patient was taken to the intensive care unit. Pulmonary and radial artery catheters were inserted, and the following hemodynamic values were obtained: cardiac output, 5.2 L/min; mean right atrial pressure, 5 mm Hg; mean pulmonary artery pressure, 25 mm Hg; mean pulmonary artery occluded pressure (PAOP), 10 mm Hg; Ca-vo$_2$, 4.0 vol%; and mean arterial pressure (MAP), 55 mm Hg. The systemic vascular resistance (SVR) was 692 dynes-sec-cm^{-5}. The arterial lactate level was reported as 43 mg/dL. Urine output for the previous hour was 15 cc. In the next 3 hours the patient received another 3 L of a crystalloid solution, and the urine output averaged 25 cc/hr. At this point repeat measurement of hemodynamic parameters demonstrated a cardiac output of 4.8 L/min, a mean right atrial pressure of 10 mm Hg, a mean pulmonary artery pressure of 32 mm Hg, a mean PAOP of 16 mm Hg, a Ca-vo$_2$ of 4.4 vol%, and a MAP of 50 mm Hg. SVR now was 567 dynes-sec-cm^{-5}. The serum lactate concentration had risen to 58 mg/dL. Further volume expansion resulted in an increase in PAOP but failed to correct any of the abnormal parameters.

Discussion

Taken in isolation, the initial hemodynamic measurements, other than for a modestly depressed MAP, are not alarming. But when integrated with the rest of the clinical data, indications of early tissue hypoperfusion become evident. Seriously ill, febrile patients increase their oxygen delivery to a greater extent than the tissue O$_2$ uptake via a hyperdynamic circulation that results in a narrow arteriovenous oxygen content difference.[19] In this setting a "normal" Ca-vo$_2$ suggests that a deficient blood flow is being compensated for by an increased tissue oxygen extraction. Consistent with this interpretation is the finding of an elevated serum lactate level and a poor urinary output since curtailment of renal blood flow occurs very early in the course of low perfusion states.

Diastolic volume, or preload, is one of the main determinants of myocardial function, the other two being afterload and the contractile state of the myocardium (see Chapter 1). In the clinical circumstance there is no practical method to obtain serial determinations of diastolic volume; therefore, this value is inferred from a measurement of the filling pressures, that is, PAOP. Human studies have shown that the normal resting left ventricle in the supine position has a filling pressure in the upper limits of normal (about 10 mm Hg). This pressure provides a diastolic volume that places the left ventricle close to its peak performance. Further elevation of the left ventricular end-diastolic pressure results in relatively minor increases in diastolic volume.[20] Unlike the normal heart, volume loading that raises PAOP well above normal values has been shown to improve the output of the ischemic left ventricle.[21] This is an expression of the disturbed diastolic pressure volume relationship, or compliance of the diseased myocardium. Because of this fact, in any instance other than the normal state, an isolated PAOP measurement gives little information on the degree of diastolic left ventricular filling unless the value obtained is below normal. A poor correlation between PAOP and left ventricular diastolic volumes has been well demonstrated in seriously ill septic and cardiac patients.[22] It is only by assessing the cardiac output response to an induced modification in the filling pressures that a valid estimation can be made of the ventricular preload at that particular point in time. If, with the increased PAOP, the cardiac output improves, the range of filling pressures at which the change takes place will provide a rough approximation of the ventricular compliance and identify valid end points for future manipulations of the intravascular volume.

In the present case, the cardiac output was initially recorded as being within the upper limits of normal. In the context of an acutely ill individual who is septic and has an elevated oxygen consumption and decreased peripheral vascular resistance, a "normal" cardiac output must be considered an inadequate cardiac response to the illness.

CASE STUDY CONTINUED

An IV infusion of 5 µg/kg/min of dopamine was initiated, and hemodynamic parameters were measured as follows: cardiac output, 6.6 L/min; mean right atrial pressure, 9 mm Hg; mean PAOP, 15 mm Hg; MAP, 65 mm Hg; and Ca-vO_2, 3.6 vol%. The urine output increased to 60 to 80 cc/hr. The calculated SVR was 606 dynes·sec·cm^{-5}. The arterial serum lactate level was measured at 50 mg/dL. These data suggest that the dopamine was exerting a positive inotropic effect as well as probably inducing renal vasodilatation by direct dopaminergic stimulation.

Discussion

A severe and persistent decrease in SVR is one of the hallmarks of bacteremic shock. In fact, there is well-documented evidence in the human condition that the degree of peripheral vasodilatation is directly related to the severity of the condition, to the extent that the greater the drop in SVR, the lesser the chance of survival.[23] This has led to the concept of septic shock as an example of shock due to "maldistribution" of what would otherwise be a perfectly adequate blood flow. In our patient, this fact is suggested by the elevated lactate level indicating both an inadequate provision of oxygen to tissues and an inability of a poorly perfused liver to dispose of this anion—truly "starvation in the midst of plenty."

Another cardinal feature of GNB shock that is well illustrated by the case study is the development of myocardial depression. This is demonstrated by the subnormal response of the ventricular performance to an increase in the preload, a finding that has been well documented in the setting of human gram-negative shock.[24] It is probably one of the earliest manifestations of the myocardial depression found in this condition and has recently also been demonstrated to occur when endotoxin is experimentally administered to normal humans.[25] Myocardial depression during sepsis has long been recognized and is most probably not the result of a direct effect of the bacteria or its toxins on the myocardium but rather is mediated by plasma factors.[26] Although the origin, character, and even existence of the "myocardial depressant factor(s)" have been quite controversial,[27] there is good evidence that irreversible myocardial dysfunction develops 4 to 6 hours after the induction of endotoxin shock in dogs.[28] Earlier studies that were unable to demonstrate myocardial failure in the isolated, perfused heart had not exposed the preparation to blood from an animal in septic shock for a long enough time.[29, 30] Certainly, these findings coincide with the clinical observation of a time dependent deterioration in cardiac function in the course of human GNB with shock. Serial radionuclide and hemodynamic determinations in the course of human GNB have demonstrated progressive left ventricular dilatation with an associated profound reduction in ejection fraction. Myocardial depression usually first develops within 24 hours of the onset of shock and can be totally reversible over a 7 to 10-day period.[23] Once myocardial dysfunction develops, the addition of β-adrenergic agents such as dopamine is considered standard therapy, although evidence is lacking that their administration modifies the prognosis. In the case study, the introduction of a catecholamine improved cardiac function and resulted in a better urine output but did not significantly affect the serum lactate level, which remained elevated, an indicator of poor prognosis.[31]

CASE STUDY CONTINUED

The patient became progressively more tachypneic, and diffuse, fine rales were heard over both lung fields. A chest roentgenogram now showed bilateral infiltrates with an "alveolar" pattern. On an FIO_2 of 0.6, arterial blood gas values were as follows: PO_2, 46 mm Hg; PCO_2, 38 mm Hg; pH, 7.22; Qsp/Qt, 30%; and Ca-vo_2, 4.2 vol%. Other pertinent findings on physical examination were a dulled sensorium, easily palpable peripheral pulses, cyanotic nail beds, and a cool clammy skin. Endotracheal intubation was performed and abundant serous secretions suctioned. With the addition of 15 cm H_2O of continuous positive airway pressure (CPAP), the arterial blood PO_2 rose to 88 mm Hg, and Qsp/Qt was measured at 20%. The significant reduction in intrapulmonary shunting and improvement in oxygenation with CPAP supports the diagnosis of ARDS (see Chapter 18). A possible contribution of the dopamine to the mounting pulmonary hypertension was suggested, and a switch to dobutamine was attempted. On 5 μg/kg/min of dobutamine the following parameters were recorded: cardiac output, 6.0 L/min; mean right atrial pressure, 8 mm Hg; MAP, 48 mm Hg; and mean pulmonary artery pressure, 27 mm Hg. The SVR dropped to 427 dynes·sec·cm^{-5}. The serum lactate concentration was 62 mg/dL, Ca-vo_2 was 4.2 vol%, and the urine output had decreased to 10 cc/hr (Table 16–2). The patient was placed back on dopamine.

TABLE 16–2.
Hemodynamic Data*

Parameter	Baseline	After Volume Loading	On Dopamine, 5 µg/kg/min	On Dobutamine, 5 µg/kg/min
Mean right atrial pressure	5	10	12	8
Mean pulmonary artery pressure	25	32	35	27
Mean pulmonary artery occluded pressure	10	16	15	18 (on CPAP)
Mean arterial pressure	55	50	65	48
Ca-vo$_2$ (vol%)	4.0	4.4	3.6	4.2
Cardiac output (L/min)	5.2	4.8	6.6	6.0
Systemic vascular resistance (dynes-sec-cm^{-5})	692	567	606	427
Serum lactate level (mg/dL)	43	58	50	62
Urine output (cc/hr)	15	25	70	10

*All pressures are expressed in millimeters Hg; Ca-vo$_2$ = arteriovenous oxygen content difference.

Discussion

Patients with GNB and associated shock are at high risk for the development of ARDS and the closely related entity of noncardiogenic pulmonary edema.[32] Experimentally, the effects of GNB on the lung have been studied in the isolated perfused dog lung following the infusion of live gram-negative bacteria. There is a prompt rise in pulmonary vascular resistance, a marked decrease in surfactant activity, and a rapid onset of pulmonary venous hypoxemia. Examination of the lung parenchyma with the electron microscope demonstrates that large numbers of capillaries have become obstructed by platelet thrombi and leukocyte plugs and that extravasation of fluid has occurred around vessels and small airways.[33] Similar involvement of the human pulmonary microcirculation is probably responsible for the genesis of pulmonary hypertension in GNB. This is a common observation in septic patients; it is not secondary to elevated left ventricular filling pressures, hypoxemia, or acidosis and usually augurs a poor prognosis.[34] Dopamine has been shown to increase pulmonary artery pressures by raising pulmonary vascular resistance, a phenomenon not observed with dobutamine. Therefore, it was reasonable to attempt a switch to the latter. Not unexpectedly, systemic hypotension ensued, most likely related to the vasodilating effects of dobutamine.[35]

The finding of an Ca-vo₂ that remains narrow in the setting of a mounting metabolic acidosis is a most ominous sign. The most frequently invoked explanation is that the increasing vasoconstriction and diffuse damage to the microvasculature virtually limit blood flow to a "core perfusion." Thus, even though peripheral pulses may be easily palpable and the blood pressure maintained at satisfactory levels, manifestations of severe tissue hypoperfusion persist. An alternate hypothesis emphasizes a cellular defect in oxygen uptake rather than a diminished capillary blood flow to explain the impaired oxygen extraction seen in severe GNB.[36]

CASE STUDY CONTINUED

Controlled ventilation became mandatory with the development of ventilatory failure. The metabolic acidosis worsened and was only temporarily alleviated by the administration of sodium bicarbonate. The rate of the dopamine infusion had to be increased into the α-adrenergic range to maintain arterial pressure. Eventually ventricular fibrillation supervened and was refractory to resuscitative efforts.

Discussion

It is an unfortunate fact that a majority of seriously ill patients with shock-complicating GNB die, no matter how vigorously currently accepted therapy is administered. In the future, innovative approaches may prove that what has been traditionally accepted as irreversible shock may not truly be an irrevocable state. Along these lines, a significant reduction in the mortality of such high-risk patients has been reported after the early administration of endotoxin antiserum,[37] and experimental work in animal models suggests a potential role for nonsteroidal anti-inflammatory drugs.[38]

REFERENCES

1. Young LS, Martin WJ, Meyer RD, et al: Gram-negative rod bacteremia: Microbiologic, immunologic and therapeutic considerations. Ann Intern Med 1977; 86:456–471.
2. Kreger BE, Craven DE, Carling PC, et al: Gram-negative bacteremia: III. Reassessment of etiology, epidemiology and ecology in 612 patients. Am J Med 1980; 68:332–355.
3. Gunnar RM, Loeb HS, Winslow EJ, et al: Hemodynamic measurements in bacteremia and septic shock in man. J Infect Dis 1973; 128(suppl):295–298.
4. Siegel JH, Cerra FB, Coleman B, et al: Physiological and metabolic correlations in human sepsis. Surgery 1979; 86:163–193.
5. Nishijima H, Weil MH, Shubin H, et al: Hemodynamic and metabolic studies on shock associated with gram-negative bacteremia. Medicine (Baltimore) 1973; 52:287–294.
6. Morrison DC, Ryan JL: Endotoxins and disease mechanisms. Annu Rev Med 1987; 38:417–432.
7. Hinshaw LW, Vick MM, Jordan MM, et al: Vascular changes associated with development of irreversible endotoxin shock. Am J Physiol 1962; 202:103–110.
8. Faden AI, Holaday JW: Experimental endotoxin shock: The pathophysiologic function of endorphins and treatment with opiate antagonists. J Infect Dis 1980; 142:229–238.
9. Martinez-Brotons F, Oncins JR, Mestres J, et al: Plasma kallikrein-kinin system in patients with uncomplicated sepsis and septic shock—comparison with cardiogenic shock. Thromb Haemost 1987; 58:709–713.
10. Robinson JA, Klodnycky ML, Loeb HS, et al: Endotoxin, prekallikrein, complement and systemic vascular resistance. Am J Med 1975; 59:61–67.
11. Beutler B, Cerami A: Cachectin, cachexia, and shock. Annu Rev Med 1988; 39:75–83.
12. Bone RC, Fisher CJ Jr, Clemmer TP, et al: Sepsis syndrome: A valid clinical entity. Crit Care Med 1989; 17:389–393.
13. Shine KI, Kuhn M, Young LS, et al: Aspects of the management of shock. Ann Intern Med 1980; 93:723–734.
14. Stein L, Beraud JJ, Morissette M, et al: Pulmonary edema during volume infusion. Circulation 1975; 52:483–489.
15. Jelenko C III, Williams JB, Wheeler ML, et al: Studies in shock and resuscitation: I: Use of a hypertonic, albumin-containing, fluid demand regimen (HALFD) in resuscitation. Crit Care Med 1979; 7:157–167.
16. Falk JL, Rackow EC, Astiz ME, et al: Effects of hetastarch and albumin on coagulation in patients with septic shock. J Clin Pharmacol 1988; 28:412–415.
17. Bone RC, Fisher CJ, Clemmer TP, et al: A controlled clinical trial of high dose methylprednisolone in the treatment of severe sepsis and septic shock. N Engl J Med 1987; 317:653.
18. The Veterans Administration Systemic Sepsis Cooperative Study Group: Effect of high-dose glucocorticoid therapy on mortality in patients with clinical signs of systemic sepsis. N Engl J Med 1987; 317:659.
19. Harrison RA, Davison R, Shapiro BA, et al: Reassessment of the assumed A-V oxygen content difference in the shunt calculation. Anesth Analg 1975; 54:198–202.
20. Parker JO, Case RB: Normal left ventricular function. Circulation 1979; 60:4–12.
21. Crexels C, Chatterjee K, Dikshit K, et al: Optimal level of ventricular filling pressure in the left side of the heart in acute myocardial infarction. N Engl J Med 1973; 289:1263–1266.
22. Calvin JE, Driedger AA, Sibbald WJ: Does the pulmonary capillary wedge predict left ventricular preload in critically ill patients? Crit Care Med 1981; 9:437–443.
23. Parker MM, Shelhamer JH, Bacharach SL, et al: Profound but reversible myocardial depression in patients with septic shock. Ann Intern Med 1984; 100:483–490.
24. Ognibene FP, Parker MM, Natason C, et al: Depressed left ventricular performance: Response to volume infusion in patients with sepsis and septic shock. Chest 1988; 93:903–910.
25. Suffredini AF, Fromm RE, Parker MM, et al: The cardiovascular response of normal humans to the administration of endotoxin. N Engl J Med 1989; 321:280–287.
26. Raffa J, Trunkey DD: Myocardial depression in sepsis. J Trauma 1978; 18:617–621.
27. Lefer AM, Martin J: Origin of myocardial depressant factor in shock. Am J Physiol 1970; 218:1423–1427.
28. Hinshaw LB, Archer LT, Black MR, et al: Myocardial function in shock. Am J Physiol 1974; 226:357–366.
29. Hinshaw LB, Archer LT, Greenfield LJ, et al: Effect of endotoxin on myocardial performance. J Trauma 1973; 12:1056–1062.
30. Hinshaw LB, Greenfield LJ, Owen SE, et al: Cardiac response to circulating factors in endotoxin shock. Am J Physiol 1972; 222:1047–1053.
31. Weil MH, Afifi A: Experimental and clinical studies on lactate and pyruvate as indicators of the severity of acute circulatory shock. Circulation 1970; 41:989.

32. Kaplan RL, Sahn SA, Petty TL: Incidence and outcome of the respiratory distress syndrome in gram-negative sepsis. *Arch Intern Med* 1979; 139:867–869.
33. Harrison LH, Hinshaw LB, Coalson JJ, et al: Effects of *E. coli* septic shock on pulmonary hemodynamics and capillary permeabiity. *J Thorac Cardiovasc Surg* 1971; 61:795–803.
34. Sibbald WJ, Patterson NAM, Holliday RL, et al: Pulmonary hypertension in sepsis: Measurement by the pulmonary arterial diastolic-pulmonary wedge pressure gradient and the influence of passive and active factors. *Chest* 1978; 73:583–591.
35. Schreuder WO, Schneider AJ, Groeneveld ABJ, et al: The influence of catecholamines on right ventricular function in septic shock. *Intensive Care med* 1988; 14:492–495.
36. Wright CJ, Duff JH, McLean APH, et al: Regional capillary blood flow and oxygen uptake in severe sepsis. *Surg Gynecol Obstet* 1971; 132:637–644.
37. Ziegler EJ, McCutchan JA, Fierer J, et al: Treatment of gram-negative bacteremia and shock with human antiserum to a mutant *Escherichia coli*. *N Engl J Med* 1982; 307:1225–1230.
38. Jacobs ER, Bone RC, Balk R, et al: Increased survival in bacteremic sheep treated with ibuprofen. *J Crit Care* 1986; 3:142.

17 / Coagulopathies in the Critically Ill Patient

DAVID GREEN, M.D., PH.D.
BENJAMIN ESPARAZ, M.D.

A variety of serious clotting problems are encountered in the critical care setting. These include platelet disorders, hypoprothrombinemia, hypofibrinogenemia, and disseminated intravascular coagulation (DIC). Such disorders are rarely the primary reason for the patient's admission to the intensive care unit (ICU) but are usually secondary to other disease processes. However, these coagulopathies require accurate diagnosis and appropriate management lest they further compromise an already seriously ill individual. These disturbances of hemostasis will be the subjects of this chapter.

PLATELET DISORDERS

Thrombocytopenia

Many illnesses are accompanied by a decline in the platelet count. Perhaps the most common of these is sepsis. While the causes of thrombocytopenia in infection are multifactorial, accelerated platelet destruction is the most prominent. At least two mechanisms have been described. Goldblum et al[1] reported that a pneumococcal-derived substance was capable of inducing severe thrombocytopenia after infusion into rabbits, presumably by lysing platelets. This substance had a molecular weight of between 100,000 and 300,000 daltons, was heat and trypsin resistant, was complement independent, and did not induce DIC.

Immunologic platelet destruction is the second mechanism for the trombocytopenia of septicemia. Kelton et al.[2] demonstrated elevated platelet-associated IgG in 16 of 21 thrombocytopenic patients with either gram-positive or gram-negative septicemia. Serial testing showed an inverse correlation between platelet count and platelet-associated IgG. The investigators suggested that immune complexes consisting of bacterial products and their specific antibodies bind to platelets. Such platelets, heavily coated with these complexes, are readily removed from the circulation by phagocytes. The outcome of infection-associated thrombocytopenia is dependent on the success of antibacterial therapy for the underlying infection. Platelet transfusions are rarely indicated; they are of value mainly for bleeding patients with platelet counts of less than 20,000/µL. Full recovery (to platelet counts of over 150,000/µL) generally requires 7 to 10 days.

Human immunodeficiency virus (HIV) infection is emerging as a very common cause of thrombocytopenia. Karpatkin et al.[3] demonstrated the presence of complement-containing immune complexes on platelets in patients with this infection. Platelet counts are usually in the 20,000 to 50,000 range, and spontaneous bleeding is infrequent. However, these patients often need invasive procedures such as bronchoscopy, tracheostomy, and central line insertion that require adequate hemostasis. In this situation, the intravenous administration of γ-globulin, in daily doses of 1 g/kg, provides satisfactory platelet increments for surgical procedures.[4]

Thrombocytopenia in critically ill patients may be dilutional due to the administration of large volumes of colloid fluids such as fresh frozen plasma, albumin solution, or packed red blood cells that contain few platelets. In the actively bleeding adult subject, 10 units of platelets (each derived from a single blood donation) should be administered after every 5 units of packed red blood cells in order to ensure circulating platelet counts in the 50,000 to 100,000 range.

Drug-induced thrombocytopenias are also not infrequent in the heavily medicated ICU patient. The drugs usually implicated are antibiotics, anticonvulsants, and antiarrhythmics (examples would be penicillins, carbamazepine, and procainamide). While some agents such as carbamazepine depress platelet production by the bone marrow, most cause immunologic platelet destruction. An important example of this latter group is heparin. Severe thrombocytopenia occurs in approximately 1% to 2% of patients receiving heparin.[5] The exposure to the drug may be by intravenous doses, subcutaneous injections, or catheter flushes. Generally, the patient has either been exposed to heparin in the past or received the drug for more than 5 days. The onset of the thrombocytopenia is abrupt, with platelet counts falling from normal to severely thrombocytopenic levels within hours. However, contrary to expectation, there is thrombosis and tissue infarction rather than bleeding. There may be a new onset of stroke, myocardial infarction, pulmonary infarction, or occlusion of major peripheral arteries or veins. These thrombotic events are due to the heparin/antibody-mediated release of platelet thromboxane A_2, a potent aggregating agent and vasoconstrictor, and endothelial cell tissue factor, a major procoagulant.[6, 7] Successful management of these patients depends on prompt recognition of the role of heparin in inciting the thrombocytopenia and thrombosis, the discontinuance of heparin from all sources (intravenous flushes, etc.), and substitution of other antithrombotic agents such as aspirin and warfarin. Under investigation are new forms of heparin (fractionated heparin, heparin fragments) and prostacyclin derivatives that may provide a larger margin of safety than standard heparin does.

Thrombocytopenia also occurs in patients with adult respiratory distress syndrome (ARDS) and diseased or prosthetic heart valves, in those having aortic balloon counterpulsation, and in association with the use of mechanical bypass or shunt procedures. In ARDS, there is evidence that platelets are sequestered in the lungs[8]; in those with valvular disease they may be fragmented or become adherent to artificial surfaces. Often, there is an element of intravascular coagulation to account for some of the observed thrombocytopenia.

Finally, severe folic acid deficiency occasionally occurs in the ICU setting[9] and produces thrombocytopenia. Folic acid is available from dietary sources such as fresh vegetables, meats, and dairy products, and the liver contains a 3-week supply of the vitamin. Patients with no oral intake during this time period who are also receiving antibiotics (which eliminate the gut flora, a source of folic acid) are vulnerable to become folate deficient. Inflammatory, neoplastic, hepatic, and renal diseases may accelerate the development of this deficiency. The initial manifestations of this condition are hypersegmentation of the neutrophils and a declining leukocyte count. Subsequently, severe thrombocytopenia may develop. Supplementing ICU patients with 1 mg of folic acid daily will prevent this complication.

Platelet Function Disorders

Platelet function is altered by hepatic and renal disease, infections, and drugs. Bleeding usually takes the form of hematomas at venipuncture sites and bleeding around catheters placed in the nose, bladder, vessels, etc. The clinical test most informative about platelet dysfunction is the bleeding time, which is generally prolonged to greater than 20 minutes in patients with serious platelet dysfunction. A prolonged bleeding time occurs in almost every patient with a platelet count of less than $50,000/\mu L$, and therefore the test is of little value in such patients. Bleeding time results are poorly predictable in hepatorenal disease; for example, in individual patients little correlation is seen with serum creatinine levels or even clearance values. Similarly, those who have recently taken aspirin or other nonsteroidal anti-inflammatory agents may have normal or greatly prolonged bleeding times. Therefore, this test is best ordered in patients who have evidence of a hemorrhagic disorder and normal or only modestly decreased platelet counts. It is also useful as a preoperative screening test in those who have recently ingested platelet-inhibiting drugs or have evidence of renal failure.

Another class of drugs that interferes with platelet function and may be responsible for increased surgical bleeding are the β-lactam penicillins (see Fig 17–1).[10] These are usually administered in high doses to patients with endocarditis and infected valves. Prior to valve replacement, the bleeding time of such patients should be determined and antibiotic use discontinued if the test result is abnormal. The bleeding time usually returns to normal within 72 hours of stopping penicillin therapy.

ε-Aminocaproic acid, a drug that inhibits fibrinolytic activity, is occasionally given to patients with bleeding subarachnoid aneurysms to prevent rebleeding. We observed an increase in the bleeding time of such patients if the daily dose of the drug exceeded 24 g/day.[11] At high concentrations, ε-aminocaproic acid inhibited platelet aggregation in vitro.[12] We recommend that serial bleeding time tests be performed in patients exposed to high concentrations of this drug over prolonged time intervals.

HYPOPROTHROMBINEMIA

Earlier, a dietary deficiency of folic acid in the ICU setting was described. Similarly, vitamin K deficiency can develop rapidly in critically ill patients. As with

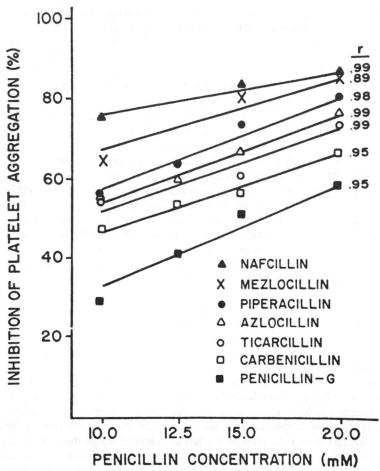

FIG 17–1.
Inhibition of epinephrine-induced platelet aggregation by various penicillins. (From Fletcher C, Pearson C, Choi SC, et al: *J Lab Clin Med* 1986; 108:217–223. Used by permission.)

folate, vitamin K is normally obtained from dietary staples, with a secondary source being the intestinal flora. A deficiency occurs in patients deprived of food who are also receiving antibiotics. The earliest manifestation of vitamin K deficiency is a prolongation of the prothrombin time (PT) in association with a normal partial thromboplastin time (PTT). This occurs because of a decline in factor VII levels. This clotting factor requires vitamin K for its synthesis, has a rapid turnover, and affects the PT but not the PTT. As vitamin K deficiency persists and intensifies, the other vitamin K–dependent clotting factors (prothrombin, factor IX, and factor X) decline, and the PTT also becomes prolonged. The coagulopathy associated with vitamin K deficiency is manifested by hematuria, gastrointestinal bleeding, hematomas of the skin and retroperitoneum, as well as bleeding from mucosal surfaces and other sites.

The diagnosis is suspected in patients who are nutritionally deprived, who are receiving antibiotics, and whose PT is prolonged. It is differentiated from other coagulopathies such as DIC by the fact that the platelet count is persistently normal. Treatment is tailored to the severity of the bleeding. For example, if the bleeding is mild and not life-threatening, 10-μg subcutaneous injections of soluble vitamin K (phytonadione [AquaMephyton] are all that is required. One or two doses will, within 24 hours, completely correct the coagulopathy and need be repeated at no more than weekly intervals. On the other hand, severe or life-threatening bleeding requires the use of fresh frozen plasma as well as phytonadione. The plasma is given intravenously in a dose of 15 mL/kg and supplies the prothrombin complex factors. It should be recognized that the corrective effects of plasma are incomplete because of the relatively low concentrations of the clotting factors in plasma, the diluting effects of the patient's plasma, and the rapid turnover of factor VII. Side effects are infrequently encountered with phytonadione; anaphylactic reactions are the most severe and require prompt recognition and appropriate management with epinephrine, steroids, etc. Such reactions are worse in patients receiving intravenous phytonadione, and therefore this route of administration should be avoided. Furthermore, the rapidity of correction of the PT is little affected by the route of administration of the drug since correction is dependent on the hepatic synthesis of the relevant clotting factors.

For patients in circulatory collapse due to massive hypoprothrombinemic bleeding, fresh frozen plasma and blood should be given along with subcutaneous vitamin K. The adverse effects associated with plasma include allergic and pyrogenic reactions, sensitization to plasma proteins, and transmission of infectious agents (non-A, non-B hepatitis viruses, HIV, etc.).

In recent years, it has been recognized that certain antibiotic agents are frequently associated with hypoprothrombinemia.[13] These antibiotics have an N-methyl-thiotetrazole ring and include cefoperazone, moxalactam, and cefamandole. In addition to inhibiting the gut flora, they interfere with the synthesis of the prothrombin complex factors. Patients most vulnerable to the hemorrhagic effects of these drugs are the elderly, the poorly nourished, and those with impaired renal function. Such patients should receive prophylactic doses of phytonadione, 10 mg weekly, to prevent hypoprothrombinemia.

DISSEMINATED INTRAVASCULAR COAGULATION

There are many causes of DIC in the critical care setting. The pathophysiology of DIC is complex and the management often dependent on the clinical situation. In this section, we present a patient with septic shock and DIC and discuss the pathogenesis and treatment.

CASE STUDY 1

A 60-year-old diabetic woman was brought to the emergency room with a 12-hour history of shaking chills, weakness, and diarrhea. Vital signs on admission were as follows: pulse,

120 beats per minute, temperature, 39.7°C; blood pressure (BP) by cuff, 90/60 mm Hg; and respirations, 36/min. The patient was alert but somnolent. The skin was warm and moist and the peripheral pulses weak but present. Lung fields were clear on auscultation and percussion. The cardiac examination was unremarkable. Pain was provoked on palpation of the left costovertebral angle, and there was abdominal distension with some diffuse tenderness and hypoactive bowel sounds. The complete blood cell count showed a normal hematocrit but a white blood cell count of 4,500 mm^{-3} with a marked shift to the left. She was given 2 L of intravenous normal saline, and appropriate antibiotic therapy for urinary tract infection was initiated. The patient was taken to the ICU. Pulmonary and radial artery catheters were inserted, but oozing from the puncture sites and emesis of coffee ground material were noted. Assessment of clotting parameters disclosed a platelet count of 52,000/μL; activated partial thromboplastin time (APTT), 60 seconds (control, 35 seconds); PT, 18 seconds (control, 11 seconds); and fibrin degradation products (FDP), greater than 40 μg/mL. The rapid onset of a hemorrhagic diathesis accompanied by thrombocytopenia, prolongation of the APTT and PT, and an increase in FDP is characteristic of DIC.

Discussion

In 1968, Corrigan et al[14] performed detailed coagulation analyses on 36 septic patients. They reported that various changes in the clotting mechanism were encountered irrespective of the infectious agent but apparently related to BP. The coagulation changes, regularly noted in patients with hypotension or shock, were interpreted as being secondary to DIC. Similar changes were not seen in patients with normal BP. Their conclusion that most patients with septicemia and low BP have DIC has been confirmed by many workers in the last 15 years.

The pathogenesis of the coagulopathy associated with septic shock requires the intravascular elaboration of thrombin. Thrombin is generated when either factor XII is activated or tissue factor is released. Endotoxin and bacterial coat lipopolysaccharides can activate factor XII.[15, 16] Activated factor XII converts prekallikrein to kallikrein, and kallikrein in turn further augments activation of factor XII. In patients with septic shock, the levels of factor XII, prekallikrein, and kallikrein inhibitors decrease.[17] Endotoxin stimulates monocytes to shed tissue factor[18] and granulocytes to release cytosolic procoagulant material.[19] In rabbits, depletion of granulocytes prevents the development of endotoxin-induced DIC.[20, 21]

When thrombin is generated, clotting factors V and VIII are consumed, and fibrinogen is converted to fibrin. The deposition of fibrin on endothelial cells leads to the release of plasminogen activator,[22] which converts plasminogen to plasmin.[23] Plasmin is a potent proteolytic enzyme that digests factors V and VIII and fibrinogen. Cleavage of fibrinogen results in the formation of FDP, which impair platelet aggregation, inhibit the action of thrombin on fibrinogen, and interfere with fibrin polymerization.

Thrombin induces platelet activation, and the activated platelets become adherent to areas of the vessel wall damaged by endotoxin. Platelets may also become coated with antigen-antibody complexes; as previously mentioned, these coated platelets are readily ingested by macrophages, thus contributing to the development of thrombocytopenia. Bleeding occurs in patients with septicemia because of endothelial cell injury due to endotoxin and/or antigen-antibody complexes, the depletion of platelets and clotting factors, an increase in systemic fibrinolytic activity, and the anticoagulant effects of FDP.

In some patients with septic shock, thrombosis rather than hemorrhage predominates. Hypotension results in impaired hepatic perfusion; the liver normally removes activated clotting factors from the circulation.[24] Retention of these activated clotting intermediates predisposes to continuing coagulation. Protein C and antithrombin III are two naturally occurring inhibitors of coagulation; they are rapidly depleted during the course of DIC.[25, 26] In addition, the levels of the potent vasoconstrictor and platelet-aggregating agent thromboxane A_2 (as reflected by measurements of thromboxane B_2) are markedly increased.[27] Intensive vasoconstriction and partial occlusion of the microcirculation by platelet-fibrin thrombi lead to tissue hypoxia, with release of tissue procoagulants and proteases, further endothelial cell damage, and fragmentation of erythrocytes. Adenosine diphosphate escaping from red cells may contribute to the formation of platelet thrombi.[28] The resulting microinfarcts contribute to multiple organ dysfunction. The effects of DIC on hemostasis are summarized in Table 17–1.

The diagnosis of DIC is based on the clinical picture and a characteristic constellation of laboratory abnormalities. Oozing from venipuncture sites, extensive ecchymoses, and bleeding from the gastrointestinal or genitourinary tract are typically observed. In the patient in whom thrombosis predominates, patchy areas of skin necrosis, gangrene of the tip of the nose, ears, or digits, and renal failure secondary to renal cortical necrosis will be observed. With either presentation, there will be thrombocytopenia[29] and elevated FDP levels; the latter will cause the thrombin time to be prolonged. In patients with severe sepsis, such as the subject of our case presentation, there will be hypofibrinogenemia and depletion of factors V and VIII, with marked prolongation of the APTT and PT. Antithrombin III titers will be

TABLE 17–1.

Effects of Disseminated Intravascular
Coagulation On Hemostasis

Hemorrhage
  Endothelial cell injury (hypoxia, endotoxin)
  Consumption of
    Platelets
    Factors V, VIII, XIII
    Fibrinogen
  Anticoagulant effects of FDP
  Depletion of antiplasmin
Thrombosis
  Elaboration of thrombin
    Platelet aggregation
    Fibrin formation
  Deposition of platelets and fibrin on injured
    vessel wall
  Consumption of
    Protein C
    Antithrombin III
    Plasminogen

reduced, and fragmented erythrocytes will be seen on peripheral smears. The differential diagnosis of DIC is shown in Table 17–2 and includes the disorders discussed earlier.

The management of DIC in the septic patient is directed toward the control of hemorrhage and the neutralization of thrombin. In the severely thrombocytopenic patient with persistent oozing of blood from the nose, gastrointestinal tract, or tracheostomy site, platelet transfusion should be given to maintain the platelet count above 20,000/μL. Platelets derived from a single blood donation ordinarily will increase platelet numbers by 5,000/μL; 10 units of platelets should provide a platelet count of 50,000/μL in the recipient. The platelet survival in these patients may be extremely abbreviated due to the presence of immune complexes, active bleeding, fever, etc., and daily transfusions may be required until the patient's condition has stabilized. Hypofibrinogenemia can be corrected by administering cryoprecipitate; each bag contains sufficient fibrinogen to increase fibrinogen levels by 5 mg/dL. A fibrinogen level greater than 50 mg/dL will generally provide adequate hemostasis. Clotting factors V and VIII may be supplemented by giving fresh frozen plasma; a dose of 15 to 20 mL/kg will raise factor levels by 25%, sufficient to prevent spontaneous bleeding.

A major concern is that thrombin generated by the underlying septic process will result in the continuing consumption of the transfused platelets and clotting factors, thereby resulting in additional platelet-fibrin thrombi in the microvasculature and further organ dysfunction. Therefore, efforts to neutralize thrombin have been attempted, usually by administering heparin. Originally, full-dose heparin therapy (5,000 to 15,000 units as in initial bolus, followed by 10,000 to 30,000 units/24 hours) was recommended,[30] but when reports of disastrous hemorrhage with such therapy were published,[31] the pendulum swung toward avoidance of heparin except for spe-

TABLE 17–2.

Hemostatic Abnormalities in Acutely Ill Patients That May be Misinterpreted as Signs of Disseminated Intravascular Coagulation

Abnormality	Probable Cause
Thrombocytopenia	Platelet-associated antigen-antibody complexes
	Secondary to major hemorrhage
	Bone marrow suppression
	Folate deficiency
	Drug induced (for example, heparin)
Prolongation of APTT and PT	Vitamin K deficiency
	Blood collection through heparin lock
Elevated FDP levels	Hematomas, pulmonary emboli
	Renal failure
All of the above plus hypofibrinogenemia	Liver disease

cific indications such as purpura fulminans or venous thromboembolism.[32] On the other hand, there is a rationale for the use of minidose heparin in DIC.[26] As previously mentioned, antithrombin III is depleted in DIC, and small amounts of heparin are known to potentiate antithrombin III activity.[33] Potentiation of antithrombin III would serve to neutralize thrombin and limit the extent of the intravascular coagulation. Furthermore, heparin in doses of 5,000 units subcutaneously every 12 hours does not appear to increase the bleeding tendency. In patients with very low levels of antithrombin III, the levels of this inhibitor may be supplemented with plasma infusions. Thus, the principles of management in the patient with septic shock and DIC are (1) vigorous treatment of the sepsis and hypotension, as previously described; (2) infusion of platelets and clotting factors to control hemorrhage; and (3) the use of minidose heparin to retard the ongoing intravascular coagulation.

CASE STUDY 1 CONTINUED

The patient received several units of fresh frozen plasma and two single-donor platelet transfusion, subcutaneous heparin at 5,000 units every 12 hours was started. With continued volume replacement as guided by central filling pressures, the BP normalized, and the urine output increased to 100 cc/hr. The following day, blood and urine cultures were positive for gram-negative organisms. The patient went on to an uneventful recovery.

BLEEDING IN LIVER DISEASE

Another serious hemorrhagic disorder observed in the critical care setting is gastrointestinal bleeding in the patient with liver disease. A typical example is described below, along with a discussion of the selection and interpretation of diagnostic tests and appropriate management strategies.

CASE STUDY 2

A 63-year-old unemployed salesman was admitted to the hospital with a history of vomiting bright red blood and collapsing. He had had several previous admissions to the alcohol rehabilitation program because of heavy drinking. On examination, his pulse was thready and BP barely discernible at 90 mm Hg systolic. The physical examination also disclosed mild scleral icterus, palmar erythema, spider angiomas over the chest wall, a liver span of 9 cm, and a palpable spleen tip.

Blood was obtained for type and crossmatch, a complete blood count and platelet count, PT, PTT, fibrinogen and fibrin(ogen) degradation products, euglobulin lysis time (ELT), and blood chemistry studies. An intravenous saline infusion was begun, and Swan-Ganz and arterial catheters were inserted. A fiber-optic esophagogastroduodenoscopic examination disclosed bleeding esophageal varices. Despite continuous peripheral intravenous infusions of vasopressin and iced saline lavage he continued to bleed, which prompted the institution of balloon tamponade with a Minnesota tube.

The admission laboratory tests revealed a hematocrit of 27%, a white cell count of 18,700/mm^{-3}, a platelet count of 35,000/mm^{-3}, a PT of 21 (10 to 13 seconds), and a PTT of 57 (25 to 35 seconds). The fibrinogen level was 92 (200 to 400 mg/dL); FDP, 20 to 40 (<10 μg/mL), and the ELT, 60 (>75 minutes). Blood studies revealed severely deranged hepatic function consistent with parenchymal liver disease (cirrhosis).

Discussion

Hemorrhagic disorders associated with alcoholism and cirrhosis are common, but the coagulopathy induced is complex.[34] The platelet count is usually decreased, there are reductions in clotting factor levels, and fibrinolysis is accelerated. The thrombocytopenia may be due to alcohol ingestion in some patients; the mechanism may be alcohol suppression of platelet production.[35, 36] Nutritional deficiencies (for example, folic acid) may also lead to thrombocytopenia. Liver disease is commonly associated with low platelet numbers, either on the basis of impaired synthesis of megakaryocyte growth factors[37] or platelet sequestration by a spleen enlarged from portal hypertension. During acute bleeds, platelet numbers are further decreased by dilution from the administration of fluids and non–platelet-containing blood products. Finally, platelets may be dysfunctional,[38] especially if aspirin has been taken along with alcohol.[39]

In the presence of cirrhosis, the coagulopathy is compounded by a clotting factor deficiency.[40] The liver is the organ of synthesis of virtually all of the coagulation factors; those most vulnerable are factors VII, IX, and X because of their relatively short half-lives. The PT is very sensitive to the factor VII level and thus can be used to gauge the severity of the hepatic damage.[41] The PTT is sensitive to the factor IX concentration and therefore also becomes prolonged as liver disease progresses. The liver has a great capacity to make fibrinogen; however, increases in the turnover of this factor as well as decreased synthesis can lead to deficiencies. Several workers[42–44] have shown accelerated fibrinolysis in cirrhosis. Two possible mechanisms are decreased clearance of circulating tissue plasminogen activator and decreased hepatic synthesis of the fibrinolytic inhibitors plasminogen activator inhibitior (PAI) and α_2-antiplasmin. The role of inhibitor deficiency is probably more critical than is a decreased clearance of activator.[45] Platelets also have PAI activity, and thus their deficiency may enhance fibrinolysis.[46] An increase in FDP and a shortened ELT are evidence of accelerated fibrinolysis. FDP have been shown to interfere with normal platelet aggregation[47] and may therefore contribute to the hemorrhagic diathesis.

CASE STUDY 2 CONTINUED

The patient was transfused with 8 units of packed red cells, 10 units of random donor platelets, and 10 units of cryoprecipitate. A continuous infusion of fresh frozen plasma was begun at a rate of 100 mL/hr. ε-aminocaproic acid (Amicar) was given intravenously in a dose of 5 g over a 20-minute period and then as a continuous infusion of 1 g/hr. He was also treated with vitamin K (Aquamephyton), 10 mg subcutaneously, and thiamine and folic acid parenterally.

On the second hospital day, bleeding subsided, and the hematocrit stabilized. The PT fell to 15 seconds and the PTT to 37 seconds while the fibrinogen level rose to 170 mg/dL and the ELT became >75 minutes. The platelet count gradually increased to 156,000/mm^{-3} by the eighth hospital day. The infusions of platelets, cryoprecipitate, and fresh frozen plasma were discontinued on the second hospital day, and the Amicar was switched to the oral route, 5 g every 6 hours, and continued until the patient was discharged.

Discussion

Platelet transfusions were administered to this patient because the low platelet count was associated with life-threatening hemorrhage. However, in general if the platelet count is in excess of $20,000/\mu L$ and there is no associated platelet dysfunction, platelet replacement is usually unnecessary. The platelets that appear in the circulation after alcohol consumption has ceased are mostly large platelets[36] that are functionally very potent. This is also probably true of the platelets generated from a marrow replenished with folic acid. Defects in platelet function may occur in patients with elevated FDP levels,[47] concomitant renal failure, or exposure to high doses of certain antibiotics (see the previous discussion), and in these instances, treatment with desmopressin in a dose of 0.3 $\mu g/kg$ given intravenously over a 20-minute period may decrease a prolonged skin bleeding time.[48]

Clotting factors were replaced in this patient by continuously infusing fresh frozen plasma. Such plasma contains approximately 1 unit/mL of most of the coagulation factors and specifically prothrombin and factors V, VII, IX, and X. However, these factors immediately become diluted in the patient's plasma, and simple calculations show that concentrations above 0.5 units/mL cannot be achieved. Furthermore, a loss of clotting activity because of consumption in stemming hemorrhage or due to circulating proteases additionally erodes plasma levels; in general, correction of PTs to about 1.3 to 1.5 times control is about the best that can be achieved.[49] Giving the plasma by continuous infusion provides a constant flow of coagulants and is less likely to cause pulmonary edema than if given by bolus infusion. Cryoprecipitate is an excellent source of fibrinogen and provides approximately 0.3 g per bag (each bag prepared from 200 to 250 mL of plasma). Ten bags will usually increase the fibrinogen level by at least 50 mg/dL and add no more than 100 to 150 mL of volume. Vitamin K is given initially with the intent of correcting any dietary vitamin deficiency that may be aggravating the hypoprothrombinemia due to the liver disease.

As previously indicated, patients with hepatic disorders often have increased fibrinolysis. Two fibrinolytic inhibitors are currently available, ϵ-aminocaproic acid (Amicar) and tranexamic acid (Cyklokapron). The latter is effective in a smaller dose than is the ϵ-aminocaproic acid (1.5 g every 8 hours as compared with 5 g every 6 hours), but the mode of action is similar: inhibition of plasminogen binding to fibrinogen, thereby impairing plasminogen activation. These agents are often very valuable in controlling bleeding[50, 51] and have few side effects when given to patients with cirrhosis; however, they are contraindicated in patients with DIC. Note that they do not correct the shortened ELT; this is because they are excluded from the euglobulin precipitate and therefore cannot affect the lysis of the euglobulin clot. Their effect is readily discernible if one does whole blood clot lysis times.

REFERENCES

1. Goldblum SE, Simon TL, Thilsted JP, et al: Pneumococcus-induced thrombocytopenia in rabbits. *J Lab Clin Med* 1985; 106:298–307.
2. Kelton JG, Neame PB, Gouldie J, et al: Elevated platelet-associated IgG in the thrombocytopenia of septicemia. *N Engl J Med* 1979; 300:760–764.
3. Karpatkin S, Nardi MA, Hymes KB: Immunologic thrombocytopenic purpura after heterosexual transmission of human immunodeficiency virus (HIV). *Ann Intern Med* 1988; 109:190–193.

4. Pollok AN, Janinas J, Green D: Successful intravenous immune globulin therapy for human immu-nodeficiency virus–associated thrombocytopenia. *Arch Intern Med* 1988; 148:695–697.
5. Green D, Martin GJ, Shoichet SH, et al: Thrombocytopenia in a prospective randomized double-blind trial of bovine and porcine heparin. *Am J Med Sci* 1984; 288:60–64.
6. Chong BH, Pitney WR, Castaldi PA: Heparin-induced thrombocytopenia: Association of thrombotic complications with heparin-dependent IgG antibody that induces thromboxane synthesis and plate-let aggregation. *Lancet* 1982; 2:1246–1249.
7. Cines DB, Tomaski A, Tannenbaum S: Immune endothelial cell injury in heparin-associated throm-bocytopenia. *N Engl J Med* 1987; 316:581–589.
8. Schneider RC, Zapol WM, Carvalho AC: Platelet consumption and sequestration in severe acute respiratory failure. *Am Rev Respir Dis* 1980; 122:445–451.
9. Amos RJ, Amess JAL, Hinds CJ, et al: Incidence and pathogenesis of acute megaloblastic bone marrow change in patients receiving intensive care. *Lancet* 1982; 2:855–859.
10. Fletcher C, Pearson C, Choi SC, et al: In vitro comparison of antiplatelet effects of β-lactum peni-cillin. *J Lab Clin Med* 1986; 108:217–223.
11. Glick R, Green D, Ts'ao C, et al: High dose ε-aminocaproic acid prolongs the bleeding time and increases rebleeding and intraoperative hemorrhage in patients with subarachnoid hemorrhage. *Neurosurgery* 1981; 9:398–401.
12. Green D, Ts'ao C, Cerullo L, et al: A clinical and laboratory investigation of the effects of ε-amino-caproic acid on hemostasis. *J Lab Clin Med* 1985; 105:321–327.
13. Mueller RJ, Green D, Phair JP: Hypoprothrombinemia associated with cefoperazone therapy. *South Med J* 1987; 80:1360–1362.
14. Corrigan JJ, Ray WL, May N: Changes in the blood coagulation system associated with septicemia. *N Engl J Med* 1968; 279:851–856.
15. Yoshikawa T, Tanaka R, Guze LB: Infection and disseminated intravascular coagulation. *Medicine (Baltimore)* 1971; 50:237–258.
16. Cronberg S, Skonsberg P, Nivenios-Larson K: Disseminated intravascular coagulation in septicemia caused by beta-hemolytic streptococci. *Thromb Res* 1973; 3:405–411.
17. Mason JW, Kleeberg U, Dolan P, et al: Plasma kallikrein and Hageman factor in gram-negative bacteremia. *Ann Intern Med* 1970; 73:545–551.
18. Edwards RL, Rickles FR, Bobrove AM: Mononuclear cell tissue factor; Cell of origin and require-ments for activation. *Blood* 1979; 54:359–370.
19. Niemetz J, Fani K: Role of leukocytes in blood coagulation and the generalized Schwartzman reac-tion. *Nature* 1971; 232:247–248.
20. Thomas L, Good RA: Studies on the generalized Schwartzman reaction: I. General observations concerning the phenomenon. *J Exp Med* 1952; 96:605–624.
21. Muller-Berghous G, Eckardt T: The role of granulocytes in the activation of intravascular coagula-tion and the precipitation of soluble fibrin by endotoxin. *Blood* 1975; 45:631–641.
22. Bernik MB, Kwaan HC: Plasminogen activator activity in cultures from human tissues: An immuno-logical and histochemical study. *J Clin Invest* 1969; 48:1740–1753.
23. Colman RW: Activation of plasminogen by human plasma kallikrein. *Biochem Biophys Res Commun* 1969; 35:272–279.
24. Wessler S: Studies in intravascular coagulation: III. The pathogenesis of serum-induced venous thrombosis. *J Clin Invest* 1955; 34:647–651.
25. Griffin JH, Mosher DF, Zimmerman TS, et al: Protein C, an antithrombotic protein, is reduced in hospitalized patients with intravascular coagulation. *Blood* 1982; 60:261–264.
26. Bick RL: Disseminated intravascular coagulation (DIC) and related syndromes, in Fareed J, Mess-more HL, Fenton JW, et al (eds): *Perspectives in Hemostasis*. New York, Pergamon Press, Inc, 1981, pp 122–138.
27. Reines HD, Cook JA, Halushka PV, et al: Plasma thromboxane concentrations are raised in patients dying with septic shock. *Lancet* 1982; 2:174–175.
28. Born GVR: Haemodynamic and biochemical interactions in intravascular platelet aggregation, in *Blood Cells and Vessel Walls: Functional Interactions*. Amsterdam, Excerpta Medica, 1980, pp 61–77.
29. Kreger BE, Craven DE, McCabe WR: Gram-negative bacteremia: IV. Reevaluation of clinical fea-tures and treatment in 612 patients. *Am J Med* 1980; 68:344–355.
30. Wolf PL: Disseminated intravascular coagulation: Principles of diagnosis and management, in Schmer G, Standjord PE (eds): *Coagulation*. New York, Academic Press, Inc, 1973, pp 17–44.
31. Green D, Seeler RA, Allen N, et al: The role of heparin in the management of consumption coagu-lopathy. *Med Clin North Am* 1972; 56:193–200.
32. Feinstein DI: Diagnosis and management of disseminated intravascular coagulation: The role of heparin therapy. *Blood* 1982; 60:284–287.
33. Rosenberg RD: Heparin, antithrombin and abnormal clotting. *Annu Rev Med* 1978; 29:367–378.

34. Stein SF, Harker LA: Kinetic and functional studies of platelets, fibrinogen, and plasminogen in patients with hepatic cirrhosis. *J Lab Clin Med* 1982; 99:217–230.
35. Cowan DH, Hines JD: Thrombocytopenia of severe alcoholism. *Ann Intern Med* 1971; 74:37–43.
36. Sahud MA: Platelet size and number in alcoholic thrombocytopenia. *N Engl J Med* 1972; 286:355–356.
37. Siemensma AB, Bathal PS, Penington DG: The effect of massive liver resection on platelet kinetics in the rat. *J Lab Clin Med* 1975; 86:817–833.
38. Thomas DP, Ream VJ, Stuart RK: Platelet aggregation in patients with Laennec's cirrhosis of the liver. *N Engl J Med* 1967; 276:1344–1348.
39. Deykin D, Janson P, McMahon L: Ethanol potentiation of aspirin-induced prolongation of the bleeding time. *N Engl J Med* 1982; 306:852–854.
40. Rapaport SI, Ames SB, Mikkelsen S, et al: Plasma clotting factors in chronic hepatocellular disease. *N Engl J Med* 1960; 263:278–282.
41. Suchman AL, Griner PF: Diagnostic uses of the activated partial thromboplastin time and prothrombin time. *Ann Intern Med* 1986; 104:810–816.
42. Goodpasture EF: Fibrinolysis in chronic hepatic deficiency. *Bull Johns Hopkins Hosp* 1914; 25:330.
43. Kwaan HC, McFadzean AJS, Cook J: Plasma fibrinolytic activity in cirrhosis of the liver. *Lancet* 1956; 1:132–136.
44. Fletcher AP, Biederman O, Moore D, et al: Abnormal plasminogen-plasmin system activity (fibrinolysis) in patients with hepatic cirrhosis: Its cause and consequences. *J Clin Invest* 1964; 43:681–695.
45. Hersch SL, Kunelis T, Francis RB Jr: The pathogenesis of accelerated fibrinolysis in liver cirrhosis: A critical role for tissue plasminogen activator inhibitor. *Blood* 1987; 69:1315–1319.
46. Kwaan HC, Suwanwela N: Inhibitors of fibrinolysis in platelets in polycythemia vera and thrombocytosis. *Br J Haematol* 1971; 21:313–322.
47. Kowalski E, Kopec M, Wegrzynowicz Z: Influence of fibrinogen degradation products (FDP) on platelet aggregation, adhesiveness and viscous metamorphosis. *Thromb Diath Hemorrh* 1964; 10:406–423.
48. Mannucci PM, Vicente V, Vianello L, et al: Controlled trial of desmopressin (DDAVP) in liver cirrhosis and other conditions associated with a prolonged bleeding time. *Blood* 1986; 67:1148–1153.
49. Spector I, Corn M, Ticktin HE: Effect of plasma transfusions on the prothrombin time and clotting factors in liver disease. *N Engl J Med* 1966; 275:1032–1037.
50. Stael V, Holstein C, Eriksson S, et al: Tranexamic acid as an aid to reduce blood transfusion requirements in gastric and duodenal bleeding. *Br Med J* 1987; 294:7–10.
51. Barer D, Ogilvie A, Coggon D, et al: Cimetidine and tranexamic acid in the treatment of acute upper gastrointestinal bleeding. *N Engl J Med* 1983; 308:1571–1575.

18/Acute Lung Injury and Positive End-Expiratory Pressure Therapy

BARRY A. SHAPIRO, M.D.
ROY D. CANE, M.B. B.CH

Severe physiologic stress potentially affects all organ systems, irrespective of the primary etiology or pathophysiology. The lungs are extremely vulnerable to such stress, which is why pulmonary dysfunction is so prevalent in critically ill patients. This chapter addresses two common lung sequelae of severe physiologic insult—noncardiogenic edema (NCE) and the adult respiratory distress syndrome (ARDS). The major supportive therapy for such pulmonary pathology is positive end-expiratory pressure (PEEP), which will be reviewed in that context.

PARENCHYMAL ANATOMY AND PHYSIOLOGY

Endothelial Permeability

The pulmonary endothelial cells are either joined together by adhesion at the luminal and medial surfaces or form gaps of about 4 nm between adjacent cells.[1]

Acute increases in capillary hydrostatic pressure (cardiogenic edema) result in increased movement of water into the interstitial space with no significant increase in protein flux. This increase in interstitial water results in decreased interstitial oncotic pressure while vascular oncotic pressure remains unchanged. Thus, the oncotic gradient is increased, which tends to offset the increased hydrostatic pressure gradient and serves to limit fluid translocation from the vascular to the interstitial space.[2] In this context pulmonary edema develops without abnormalities of endothelial permeability. If the selective permeability of the capillary endothelium is lost, both water and protein flux into the lung interstitium is increased (NCE). Interstitial oncotic pressures increase slightly and ablate the normal oncotic pressure gradient across the endothelium.

Lung Interstitium and Lymphatics

The interstitial space of the lung is composed primarily of hyaluronic acid molecules constrained within a network of collagen fibers.[3] Interstitial fluid is contained

321

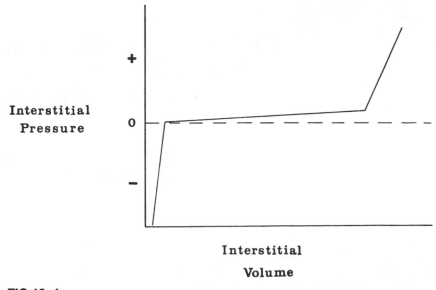

FIG 18–1.
Representation of the dynamic nature of the lung interstitial space compliance. Interstitial pressure is expressed relative to atmospheric pressure (760 mm Hg).

in and around the interstices of the collagen web to form a gel-like matrix that contains the alveoli. Gas exchange primarily occurs across the interstitial *tight space*—areas where capillary endothelium and alveolar epithelium come into close proximity. Most of the lung interstitium, however, exists as the *loose space* located in the alveolar septa adjacent to the tight space and surrounding the bronchioles, bronchial arteries, and veins. The loose space also contains lymphatic vessels, interstitial cells, smooth muscle, and nerve tissue[4] and has an extremely high compliance.

Normally, lung interstitial pressure is negative relative to atmospheric pressure, and the compliance of the interstitial space is low (Fig 18–1). However, as the interstitial pressure approaches atmospheric pressure, the compliance increases dramatically and enables large volumes of fluid to accumulate within the interstitial space without significant increases in interstitial pressures.[3] Interstitial water content can increase by at least 30% before significant increases in interstitial pressure occur.[5, 6]

The pulmonary lymphatic capillaries arise in the loose space as terminal sacs that become true lymphatic capillaries containing one-way valves. The lymphatic channels contain smooth muscle in their walls and eventually merge to become the larger collecting vessels that have an active peristaltic capability regulated by the autonomic nervous system.[7] Normal lung lymph flow is 5 to 6 mL/hr/100 g of lung tissue[6]; however, lymph flow has been demonstrated to increase by 20-fold.[2, 4, 6] This capability of increasing lymph flow in conjunction with the dynamic nature of the interstitial space compliance allows for increases of up to 300% in capillary hydrostatic pressures without physiologically significant increases in interstitial pressure.[2]

Lung Epithelium

Ninety percent of the alveolar surface is covered by type 1 alveolar cells, which play the major integumentary role in the maintenance of the air-blood barrier.[8] The cytoplasmic junctions between alveolar cells are extremely tight under normal conditions and are impermeable to water.[9] Alveolar type 2 cells (granular pneumocytes) constitute approximately 80% of alveolar epithelial cells[8] and produce the pulmonary surfactant and fluid that completely covers the alveolar epithelium.[10, 11] However, only 40% to 50% of the type 2 cell enzymatic activity can be accounted for by the production, storage, and secretion of the surfactant complex and the fluid lining.[12] It is highly probable that other functions exist that are not related to the formation of the surfactant system or the alveolar fluid lining.

Damage to alveolar epithelium has profound effects on lung function. Type 1 cells are extremely vulnerable to injury and limited in reparative capabilities.[13] At least three pathophysiologic phenomena accompany type 1 cell damage: (1) alveolar edema secondary to loss of the watertight barrier,[9, 14, 15] (2) atelectasis resulting from the loss of geometric alveolar stability secondary to alveolar fluid,[3, 4] and (3) decreased lung compliance due to atelectasis and loss of the type 1 cell stretchability.[8, 16]

Type 2 cells are far less susceptible to injury and have remarkable reparative capabilities.[13, 17–19] Severe injury to these cells may result in irreversible damage.[12, 19] Damage results in two predictable and clinically identifiable conditions: severely decreased lung compliance and alveolar atelectasis secondary to surfactant malfunction.

PULMONARY EDEMA

Pulmonary edema may be broadly defined as excessive vascular fluid egress with abnormal accumulation in the interstitial and air spaces of the lung. Such accumulation of extravascular water (EVW) affects pulmonary function and gas exchange to varying degrees, depending on both the site of accumulation (interstitial vs. alveolar) and the quantity of fluid involved.

Cardiogenic Edema

Pulmonary edema is most readily recognized when fluid cllects in the corners of the tetrahedron-shaped alveoli and causes geometric instability and rapid collapse.[4] Theoretically, *rapid* movement of fluid into the tight space results in sudden high pressures that may lead to destruction of the epithelium as an effective barrier to fluid passing into the alveolar space. Although this is speculative, it is a probable mechanism by which acute left ventricular failure (cardiogenic edema) results in alveolar fluid accumulation. The common clinical symptoms of dyspnea, rales, and severe hypoxemia are primarily attributable to the alveolar fluid accumulation.

Noncardiogenic Edema

In the absence of direct epithelial damage by toxic inhalants, the alveolar epithelium appears to remain an effective water barrier as long as *rapid* fluid movement is avoided. Most noncardiogenic causes of pulmonary edema (NCE) involve less rapid water movement than left ventricular failure does and therefore primarily involve interstitial accumulation of water without accumulation of alveolar fluid. Thus, the clinical symptoms are those of increased interstitial pressure impinging on bronchioles and blood vessels, which results in increased airway and vascular resistances leading to abnormal distribution of perfusion and ventilation.[6]

The most common genesis of pulmonary NCE in critically ill patients is believed to result from both increased permeability of the endothelium to proteins[20-23] and increased water conductance across the endothelial cells. Such abnormal endothelial cell function is identified in the animal model by increased pulmonary lymph flow with a concomitant increase in protein content.[4, 21, 23] Even though reliable laboratory models for the study of permeability in NCE are available,[4, 23] etiologies in humans are not clearly delineated. However, correlations between laboratory investigations and clinical observations allow the following generalizations to be made with a reasonable degree of confidence.

1. Certain blood-borne toxins such as bacterial endotoxins[24] and drugs[25-27] result in significant alteration of endothelial permeability. A high incidence of permeability edema is known to occur following sepsis in humans.

2. Microemboli produce endothelial humoral and cytoplasmic changes that affect permeability.[20-22, 28, 29] This is believed to be the primary mechanism of the development of NCE following disseminated intravascular coagulopathy (DIC) and fat emboli.[30-32]

3. Most investigators agree that the initial parenchymal damage from inhaled toxins is endothelial, which helps explain the NCE that often occurs in humans after exposure to inhaled toxins.[4, 20, 21, 23]

ADULT RESPIRATORY DISTRESS SYNDROME

Since the introduction of the term *adult respiratory distress syndrome* in 1967, *epithelial* cell involvement has been a consistent feature in the syndrome's morphologic description.[33-37] This epithelial cell involvement includes both type 1 cell sloughing and type 2 cell dysfunction.[38] The latter involves abnormal surfactant production resulting in reduced lung compliance and collapse of numerous gravity-dependent alveoli.[39, 40] Gravity-dependent alveolar collapse leads to an increase in unventilated but perfused areas of lung (zero V/Q), which will result in an arterial hypoxemia that is relatively refractory to increases in the inspired oxygen concentration.[41] The combination of refractory hypoxemia, severely decreased lung compliance, and diffuse involvement on chest x-ray studies has become the clinical hallmark of ARDS.[36,42-45]

TABLE 18–1.

Clinical Spectrum of Acute Lung Injury*

	Endothelial Cell Dysfunction ⌣ Increased Permeability		Epithelial Cell Dysfunction ⌣ Diminished Surfactant Function
Spectrum of ALI†	Mild ⟶	Moderate	⟶ Severe
Clinical diagnosis	NCE†		ARDS†
Degree of hypoxemia	Moderate		Severe
Response to Fio₂	Responsive		Refractory
Lung compliance	Moderate decrease		Severe decrease

*From Shapiro BA, Cane RD, Harrison RA: Chest 1983; 83:358. Used by permission.
†ALI = acute lung injury; NCE = noncardiogenic edema; ARDS = adult respiratory distress syndrome.

ACUTE LUNG INJURY

Acute lung injury (ALI) may be characterized as a spectrum of abnormal paren-chymal cell function that starts with predominately endothelial cell malfunction, which results in NCE; this progresses to both epithelial and endothelial cell mal-function, resulting in ARDS. Table 18–1 summarizes this concept.[46] Decreased com-pliance and hypoxemia are the two principal clinical concerns in ALI.

Lung Compliance

Figure 18–2 depicts normal pulmonary pressure-volume relationships, with the volume axis represented as a bar graph of total lung capacity (TLC). The first segment of the compliance curve occurs close to residual volume (RV) and is primarily influ-enced by intrinsic elastic properties. The second segment is the more linear portion and represents high compliance. Tidal ventilation normally occurs in this segment and allows for minimal work of breathing. Increases in interstitial water content would diminish the ease of alveolar expansion and tend to flatten this segment; abnormalities of the surfactant system would have profound "flattening" effects. The third segment represents the distensible limits of the alveolar structures and chest wall. Increases in interstitial water content would tend to lower the lung volume at which this segment occurs, while surfactant abnormalities would significantly lower the volume.

Refractory Hypoxemia

Severe arterial hypoxemia that is relatively unresponsive to increasing inspired oxygen concentrations must be attributed to a significant amount of true intrapul-monary shunting, i.e., blood that enters the left heart with the same oxygen content it possessed in the right heart. True shunting, resulting from pulmonary disease, represents significant areas of unventilated but perfused alveoli. This significant degree of alveolar collapse would result in a greatly reduced RV.

Noncardiogenic Edema

Increased EVW results in a less compressible interstitial matrix that limits alveolar expansion. This is illustrated in Figure 18–3 as the third segment of the compliance slope, occuring at a considerably lower lung volume, and there is some flattening of the second segment. Because dependent alveoli are initially prevented from collapsing due to normal surfactant function and airway closure mechanisms, the RV is not greatly affected, i.e., diminished TLC is related to diminished vital capacity (VC). Although the work of breathing is moderately increased, it is seldom a problem unless there is preexisting diminishment of ventilatory reserves. The fact that RV is near normal means that the dependent alveoli are not collapsed and therefore the hypoxemia should be relatively responsive to increases in FIO_2.

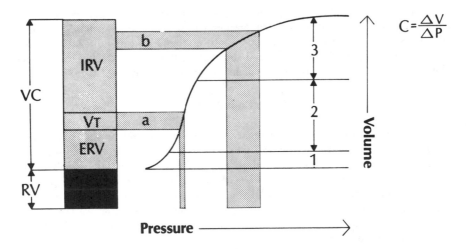

FIG 18–2.
Normal lung volume-compliance relationship. With normal functional residual capacity (FRC), tidal volume (VT) takes place on an advantageous portion of the compliance slope *a*, that is, the volume change necessitates a small pressure change; *b* represents the same volume change, but necessitating a larger change in pressure and representing a poor compliance. *1, 2,* and *3* delineate three segments of the pulmonary compliance curve. *IRV* = inspiratory reserve volume; *ERV* = expiratory reserve volume; *RV* = residual volume; *Vc* = vital capacity. FRC = ERV + RV. (From Shapiro BA, Harrison RA, Kacmarek RM, et al: *Clinical Application of Respiratory Care,* ed 3. Chicago, Year Book Medical Publishers, Inc, 1985. Used by permission.)

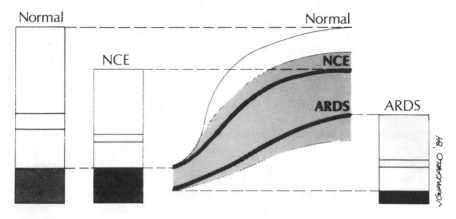

FIG 18–3.
The pulmonary compliance spectrum of noncardiogenic edema *(NCE)* to adult respiratory distress syndrome *(ARDS)*. (From Shapiro BA, Harrison RA, Kacmarek RM, et al: *Clinical Application of Respiratory Care,* ed 3. Chicago, Year Book Medical Publishers, Inc, 1985. Used by permission.)

Adult Respiratory Distress Syndrome

The greatly decreased lung elasticity secondary to epithelial damage and abnormal surfactant function results in a severe restriction of the TLC and a dramatic flattening of the second segment of the compliance curve (see Fig 18–3). The severe diminishment in RV is due to collapse of gravity-dependent alveoli secondary to surfactant malfunction. The significant increase in true shunting produces a refractory hypoxemia. This combination of refractory hypoxemia and severely decreased lung compliance is a clinical hallmark of ARDS.

Clinical Diagnosis of Acute Lung Injury

ALI is a term referring to the clinical spectrum of NCE to ARDS. The clinically relevant features are summarized in Table 18–1.

There appears to be general agreement that patients with multiple trauma, sepsis, and DIC are at high risk.[24, 30] Combinations of other physiologic insults (e.g., aspiration, drug injury, fat embolism, hypotension, interstitial pneumonia, multiple transfusions, operative procedures longer than 8 hours, poor nutritional status) have been suggested as predisposing factors.

The more severe form of ALI—ARDS—is readily identified by the following: (1) a compatible clinical history and physical findings, (2) refractory hypoxemia (arterial Po2 less than 60 mm Hg at an Fio2 of 0.5 or higher), (3) markedly diminished pulmonary compliance, and (4) a chest radiograph showing diffuse bilateral parenchymal infiltrates. The less severe or earlier form of this pathology—NCE—is more difficult to diagnose. The following features are reasonably reliable: (1) compatible clinical history, (2) FiO_2 of 0.35 or higher required to maintain an arterial Po_2 greater than 60 mm Hg, (3) absence of chronic lung disease and cardiogenic edema, and (4) chest radiograph compatible with NCE and without pneumonic infiltrate or atelectasis.

MANAGEMENT OF ACUTE LUNG INJURY

The initial factor leading to ALI is increased pulmonary endothelial permeability. There are presently no scientifically documented means of directly enhancing the ability of these cells to recover from the insult.[21] Therefore, therapy directed toward the underlying etiology (e.g., antibiotics in sepsis) must be emphasized, along with supportive pulmonary therapy to ensure an optimal milieu for patient survival as well as reversal of the pulmonary pathology. Essential goals of supportive therapy include (1) maintaining adequate vascular volume and perfusion, (2) ensuring tissue oxygenation by maintaining an adequate hemoglobin concentration and an arterial Po_2 of at least 55 to 60 mm Hg, and (3) limiting inspired oxygen concentrations to less than 50%.

Fluid Therapy and Acute Lung Injury

Relative hypervolemia results in elevation of capillary hydrostatic pressures and increased pulmonary EVW, a phenomenon that occurs to a greater extent and at lower hydrostatic pressures in the presence of NCE.[21, 47] Since there are no data suggesting that in the presence of NCE the increased EVW resulting from transient fluid overload is removed from the lung when euvolemia is reinstated, meticulous care must be taken to avoid relative hypervolemia.

Although it has been demonstrated that vigorous volume depletion with diuretics may limit the accumulation of EVW,[48] there is little evidence to suggest that severe volume depletion enhances mobilization of preexisting EVW. Since severe volume depletion may decrease cardiac output and perfusion, common sense dictates that maintaining a hypovolemic state in these patients is not desirable. It appears that careful titration of vascular volume and vascular space requirements to maintain euvolemia will provide adequate perfusion without excessive pulmonary microvascular pressures.

The administration of intravenous (IV) colloid solutions has been proposed as a therapy for NCE; this is based on the oversimplified rationale that increasing plasma oncotic pressures will prevent accumulation of interstitial lung water or possibly enhance removal of water from the pulmonary interstitium.[49] Since oncotic gradients are minimal in normal lung and nearly ablated in NCE, there can be no scientific validity to the assumption that colloid administration will remove EVW in this disease entity. Present knowledge of lung parenchymal function leads to the conclusion that colloid administration should lead to an increased net filtration of water and protein into the interstitium and therefore is inherently deleterious to the lung with NCE. The administration of albumin to burn patients has been shown to increase lung water.[50] The clinical decision to administer colloid to a patient with NCE must be based on specific indications that override the potential harm to the lungs.

Oxygen Therapy and Acute Lung Injury

Intracellular Oxygen Biochemistry

Cellular metabolism involves the stepwise reduction of oxygen to water, with the addition of an electron at each step: step 1 produces a superoxide molecule (O_2^-), step 2 produces hydrogen peroxide (H_2O_2), step 3 produces a hydroxyl ion (OH^-), and step 4 produces water. The free radicals O_2^- and OH^- are highly reactive molecules that tend to cause destructive and unregulated reactions of organic molecules. They are referred to as "toxic" oxygen radicals because they are capable of damaging cell membranes and mitochondria as well as inactivating many cytoplasmic and nuclear enzymes.[51] Mammalian cells contain enzyme systems that allow the stepwise reduction of oxygen to proceed quickly, thereby preventing an accumulation of toxic oxygen radicals. Intracellular hyperoxia is known to increase the rate of oxygen metabolism independent of energy demand.[52]

Alveolar Hyperoxia and Acute Lung Injury

Small mammals exposed to 100% oxygen atmospheres for several days manifest ALI. These animals are known to rapidly deplete enzymes involved in oxygen reduction and therefore accumulate toxic oxygen radicals when hyperoxic.[52] Lung endothelial cells are affected earlier and to a greater extent than epithelial cells.

Primates with normal lungs are known to have adequate enzyme reserves, which avoid toxic oxygen radical accumulation in hyperoxic conditions.[51] In certain circumstances, preexistent cellular damage appears to diminish this reserve so that hyperoxic conditions may result in toxic oxygen radical accumulation. The type 2 cell in primates is the last parenchymal cell to demonstrate abnormal function secondary to hyperoxia,[53] which partially explains the observation in humans that high inspired oxygen concentrations coincident with certain physiologic insults produce NCE while only later (coinciding with type 2 cell malfunction) does ARDS develop.

In persons with normal lungs, high alveolar oxygen tensions do not result in clinically significant abnormalities. However, previously damaged or stressed lung parenchyma may manifest significant abnormal function when confronted with alveolar oxygen tensions in excess of 250 mm Hg ($F_{IO_2} \approx 0.5$ ambient). There must be no doubt that F_{IO_2}s above 0.5 in critically ill patients are potentially damaging to the lung. The unanswered questions pertain to the extent and relative importance of this process when compared with other life-threatening processes affecting the patient and whether F_{IO_2}s below 0.5 may be damaging in some situations.

Chemically Mediated Toxic Oxygen Radicals

Neutrophils, mononuclear cells, and macrophages are consistent interstitial histologic findings in ARDS.[38] Polymorphonuclear leukocytes (PMNs) are closely associated with the inflammatory process, and their ability to adhere to endothelial cell membranes is believed important for migration from the vascular space.[54] Platelet destruction results in fibrin thrombi (microembolization) that has been clearly correlated with ARDS.

Activation of white blood cells (WBCs) (PMNs, neutrophils, mononuclear cells, and macrophages) and fibrin thrombi is associated with the release of at least three groups of substances: (1) a platelet-activating factor (acetyl glyceryl ethyl phosphoryl choline [AGEPC] that promotes the stasis of leukocytes and interstitial edema by activating blood complement factors[55]; (2) leukotrienes (arachidonic acid metabolites), which increase adhesion to endothelial cells and increase vascular permeability[56]; and (3) proteases, which tend to inactivate enzyme systems and produce toxic oxygen radicals.[57]

Figure 18–4 illustrates a simplified version of possible mechanisms by which bacterial sepsis or DIC may lead to lung parenchymal cellular damage by accumulation of toxic oxygen radicals.

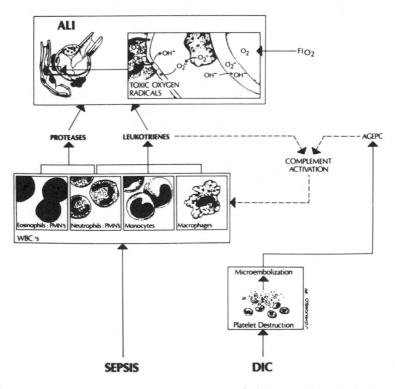

FIG 18–4.
A simplified schema showing probable pathways by which sepsis and DIC lead to the accumulation of toxic oxygen radicals in lung parenchyma. (From Shapiro BA, Harrison RA, Kacmarek RM, et al: *Clinical Application of Respiratory Care,* ed 3. Chicago, Year Book Medical Publishers, Inc, 1985. Used by permission.)

Positive End-Expiratory Pressure Therapy and Acute Lung Injury

Because specific therapy to prevent or reverse the cellular damge is not yet available, therapy in ALI must be aimed at treating the underlying pathology (sepsis, DIC, etc.) and maintaining oxygenation while creating as beneficial a milieu as possible for lung repair. The best available evidence suggests that this requires reexpansion of lung and FIO_2s below 0.4. These are attainable through appropriate application of PEEP therapy.[58]

POSITIVE END-EXPIRATORY PRESSURE THERAPY

For purposes of this discussion, PEEP shall refer to the existence of an airway pressure above ambient at the end of exhalation, independent of inspiratory dynamics.[58, 59] Continuous positive airway pressure (CPAP) shall refer to PEEP in conjunction with spontaneous ventilation through a device that provides inspiratory gas flow when minor airway pressures below the PEEP level are generated. Continuous positive-pressure ventilation (CPPV) shall refer to control or assist/control ventilation with PEEP.

Pulmonary Effects of Positive End-Expiratory Pressure

Three mechanisms have been postulated to explain the improvement in pulmonary function and gas exchange following PEEP therapy: (1) alteration of small airway ✓ closure in gravity-dependent lung areas; (2) decreased lung EVW, and (3) increased functional residual capacity (FRC).

Although it has been demonstrated that the lung volume at which small airway closure occurs often rises above FRC in anesthetized humans,[60, 61] the effect of PEEP on arterial oxygenation as related to the FRC–closing volume relationship is not well documented and is often conflicting.[62, 63] Although future studies may substantiate a beneficial relationship between PEEP and lung volumes at which airway closure occurs, the present data are inconclusive.

The direct effects of PEEP on extravascular lung water are difficult to evaluate because of the complex factors governing lung water distribution. However, there is sufficient evidence to support the statement that extravascular lung water is derived from both juxta-alveolar and extra-alveolar vessels and that the fluid flux varies with the degree of alveolar inflation, pulmonary artery pressure, and pleural pressures.[7-9] The overwhelming balance of evidence suggests that PEEP results in either ✓ a significant increase or no change in interstitial water.[64, 65]

Increased FRC

It is well documented that PEEP increases FRC, which appears to be the main mechanism by which pulmonary function and gas exchange are improved. However, to what extent the FRC improvement is accomplished by increases in alveolar volume or by alveolar recruitment is controversial.

Daly and associates[66] utilized incidence light photomicrography to study normal rat alveolar characteristics at various levels of PEEP. They demonstrated that (1) alveolar diameters increased linearly with 0 to 10 cm H_2O; (2) end-expiratory diameters increased to a greater degree than did end-inspiratory diameters; (3) beyond 10 cm H_2O PEEP, the increase in alveolar diameters progressively diminished and reached a plateau at approximately 15 cm H_2O PEEP; and (4) beyond 15 cm H_2O PEEP, alveolar pressure increased without a measurable increase in alveolar diameters. These data suggest that there is an upper limit to the distensibility of normal alveoli and that, within those limits, PEEP can increase FRC simply by increasing alveolar size.

Alveolar recruitment is a term commonly used to refer to an increase in FRC secondary to inflation of previously collapsed alveoli. Indirect evidence that PEEP may recruit alveoli was first presented in 1969 by McIntyre and associates,[67] who demonstrated that both arterial oxygenation and pulmonary compliance were rapidly improved when PEEP was applied to lung models with decreased surfactant activity. Recent studies[68] reaffirm this phenomenon occurring within minutes of the application of PEEP therapy.

Cardiac Effects of Positive End-Expiratory Pressure Therapy

Reduction of cardiac output coincident with PEEP therapy is due to a combination of mechanisms, of which reduction in right heart venous return is undoubtedly the primary and most frequently encountered.[69, 70] When PEEP therapy produces clinically significant reductions in cardiac output despite reasonable intravascular volume augmentation, an element of ventricular dysfunction most likely exists. Currently available information suggests that this is most often related to increased right heart afterload, with right ventricular dilation and leftward interventricular septal deviation resulting in decreased left ventricular output.[71, 72] Biventricular dysfunction has also been implicated.[73] Inotropic support is rarely necessary at PEEP levels less than 20 cm H_2O.[73] In each patient there appears to be a PEEP level at which reduction of cardiac output is of greater detriment to tissue oxygenation than the effects of improved arterial oxygen content are beneficial. Fortunately, these detrimental PEEP levels are usually above those that significantly improve the arterial oxygen content when the patient is not hypovolemic.

Therapeutic Positive End-Expiratory Pressure Levels

To determine the most desirable levels of PEEP, numerous clinical studies have been undertaken in patients with acute respiratory failure and clinical signs compatible with ALI.[74-78] These studies utilized an end point of achieving an arterial Po_2 above 60 mm Hg and an Fio_2 below 0.5 without detriment to the cardiac output. This end point is clinically valid in ALI because (1) the most readily monitored effect of PEEP in ALI is the improvement in arterial oxygen tension; (2) assuming adequate hemoglobin content and maintenance of adequate cardiac output, an arterial Po_2 of 60 mm Hg (90% oxyhemoglobin) is adequate for oxygen delivery to tissues; and (3) there are data to suggest that adequate arterial oxygenation at an FIO_2 below 0.5 may avoid cellular hyperoxic conditions that alter or depress pulmonary parenchymal metabolic function.

Table 18–2 summarizes data from six studies utilizing the above-described clinical end point for determining appropriate levels of PEEP therapy. The data demonstrate that only 5% of patients with ALI required PEEP levels above 30 cm H_2O and 80% required 20 cm H_2O or less. The required PEEP correlates with severity of lung injury, while correlations among these therapeutic PEEP levels and factors such as mortality, required fluid therapy, and incidence of pneumothorax are not well established.

Pulmonary Compliance and Positive End-Expiratory Pressure

Pulmonary compliance may be conveniently estimated in conjunction with control-mode positive-pressure ventilation by dividing the exhaled tidal volume (VT) by the pressure change from baseline to end-inspiratory plateau—a measurement referred to as effective static compliance (ESC). Some investigators noted that optimal PEEP levels and best pulmonary compliance often coincide and have suggested that ✓ ESC may be a useful clinical guide to determine optimal PEEP.

Although changes in *lung* compliance may correlate with the optimal PEEP level, utilization of the ESC measurement (a reflection of both lung and chest cage compliance) is not always reliable. Although chest wall compliance may remain relatively constant when comatose or paralyzed patients are being controlled by positive-pressure ventilation, it is subject to much variation when the patient breathes spontaneously on an intermittent mandatory ventilation (IMV) device, is on assist/control mode, or "fights" the ventilator for any reason.

Spontaneous Ventilation and Positive End-Expiratory Pressure

Zarins and associates[80] studied, in six normal primates, the effects on cardiac function of 20 cm H_2O PEEP in conjunction with both IMV and controlled mechanical ventilation (CMV). They found that all the animals manifested similar decreases in cardiac output irrespective of the presence of spontaneous ventilation. Considering that PEEP levels of 20 cm H_2O in normal lungs results in significant reduction of cardiac output without improvement in V/Q relationships,[81, 82] a logical explanation for the findings of Zarins et al. is that "excessive" PEEP decreases cardiac output without physiologic benefit, regardless of the mode of ventilation.

Downs et al.[83] compared CMV at a rate of 12/min without PEEP to IMV (2/min) with 0, 5, and 10 cm H_2O of PEEP and found that spontaneous ventilation associated with the IMV mode resulted in less positive intrapleural pressures. Venus and associates[84] reported similar findings in dogs following acid aspiration supported with 10 cm H_2O of PEEP in conjunction with both IMV and CMV. In addition, they found significantly less depression of cardiac output when spontaneous ventilation was present. Shah and associates[85] reported similar findings in nine patients convalescing from multiple trauma.

TABLE 18–2.

Therapeutic Positive End-Expiratory Pressure in Humans

Study	No. Patients	Probable Pathology*	Inspiratory Mode*	PEEP Range (Mean)
Downs et al.[74]	12	NCE-ARDS	IMV	6–20 (13.2)
Falke[75]	7	NCE-ARDS	CMV	5–15
Gallagher and Civetta[79]	315	Mixed	IMV	6–45 (15.3)
Kirby et al.[76]	28	ARDS	IMV	15–44 (25)
Suter et al.[77]	15	NCE-ARDS	CMV	0–15
Venus et al.[78]	15	NCE-ARDS	Spont	10–25

*NCE = noncardiogenic edema; ARDS = adult respiratory distress syndrome; IMV = intermittent mandatory ventilation; CMV = controlled mechanical ventilation; Spont = spontaneous ventilation.

The available data strongly support the thesis that spontaneous ventilation in conjunction with PEEP therapy enhances the pulmonary effects (increased transpulmonary pressures) while reducing detrimental alterations in cardiovascular function secondary to a rise in intrapleural pressures.

Early Application of Positive End-Expiratory Pressure Therapy

There is prospective evidence to suggest significant benefit from early application of low levels of PEEP when the inspired oxygen concentration is kept below 40% in surgical and trauma patients at risk of developing ARDS.[86, 87] In addition, McAslan and Cowley[88] reported on 1,676 major trauma patients who had routinely received 5 cm H_2O of PEEP on admission to the trauma center. The PEEP was increased as necessary to maintain an arterial Po_2 of 60 mm Hg at less than 0.4 Fio_2. PEEP of 10 cm H_2O was commonly required, while more than 15 cm H_2O was seldom necessary. This patient group was retrospectively compared with a similar group of major trauma victims in whom PEEP therapy had not been used until significant respiratory failure was clinically evident. The "early PEEP" group showed significantly diminished pulmonary morbidity.

It appears that serious consideration for applying early PEEP therapy should be given to patients at risk for ALI who require over 35% inspired oxygen to maintain an arterial Po_2 of 60 mm Hg or greater. Technical improvements in CPAP masks now make clinically practical the early application of low-level PEEP therapy to the unintubated patient at risk of developing ALI.

Clinical End Points of Positive End-Expiratory Pressure

Positive end-expiratory pressure therapy is believed generally beneficial for patients with acute lung injury because (1) arterial oxygenation is improved, (2) intrapulmonary physiologic shunting (Qsp/Qt) is reduced, (3) lung compliance is improved, and (4) inspired oxygen concentrations (Fio_2) can be reduced. However, the degree of PEEP therapy that provides the greatest benefit while producing the fewest nonbeneficial effects is difficult to define and complex to monitor clinically. To understand the various concepts of clinical "end points" for PEEP therapy as they relate to ALI, it is necessary to review the seven factors most commonly studied:

1. Arterial oxygen tension (Pao_2).—If we assume that the hemoglobin content is constant, a low Pao_2 represents a significant deficiency in oxygen content (oxyhemoglobin plus dissolved oxygen). Improvement in Pao_2 up to 80 mm Hg reflects significant physiologic increases in the oxygen content. A major goal of PEEP therapy is to improve the arterial oxygen content.

2. Cardiac output (Qt).—This measurement requires a pulmonary artery catheter. In nonprimate models the cardiac output is equal to or less than normal after injury, while in primates and humans with ARDS the cardiac output is usually greater than normal.[89, 90] There is no clear explanation for this discrepancy.

3. The arterial-venous oxygen content difference (Ca-vo$_2$).—This calculation re-

quires arterial and pulmonary arterial blood samples. It represents the volume of oxygen extracted from 100 mL of blood and is not necessarily reflective of total body oxygen extraction per minute ($\dot{V}O_2$). Acute stress has been demonstrated to commonly result in cardiac output increases in excess of increased oxygen demand, and this results in a Ca-$\bar{v}O_2$ less than normal (3 to 4 vol%). Untreated ARDS in humans usually produces Ca-$\bar{v}O_2$ less than 3.0 vol%.

4. Oxygen delivery (O_2 Del).—This calculation is cardiac output multiplied by the arterial oxygen content multiplied by 10. It is expressed as milliliters per minute and represents the total oxygen volume presented to the tissues per minute. O_2 Del is decreased in ARDS.

5. Intrapulmonary physiologic shunting (Qsp/Qt).—This calculation requires a measurement of FIO_2 plus arterial and pulmonary artery blood samples. The physiologic shunt is dramatically increased in ARDS, usually greater than 30%.

6. Dead-space ventilation (VD).—Dead-space ventilation can be quantified by calculation of the VD/VT ratio. This requires collection of exhaled gases over a period of time and an arterial blood sample. VD is increased in ARDS.

7. Lung compliance (CL).—A reflection of total pulmonary compliance is available by calculating ESC. Lung compliance and ESC are severely diminished in patients with ARDS.

Extrapolation of available data in both animals and humans allows for these seven factors to be placed in the general schema depicted in Figure 18–5. The graphs represent preinjury levels, postinjury stabilized levels, and levels after incremental applications of PEEP therapy. It is assumed that the FIO_2 remains 0.5, that the pH and PCO_2 remain acceptable, and that appropriate fluid therapy is administered. It has been our experience that in patients with ALI in whom intravascular volume and hemoglobin concentrations are appropriately maintained, the PEEP level at which a PaO_2 of 60 mm Hg is achieved with an FIO_2 of 0.4 or less corresponds to the classical PEEP end points of optimal PEEP, best PEEP, etc.

Summary of Positive End-Expiratory Pressure Therapy in Acute Lung Injury

Indications.—The principal clinical indication for PEEP therapy is the diagnosis of ALI. Initiation of PEEP therapy should be seriously considered as soon as the diagnosis is clinically evident.

Goals.—The primary goal of PEEP therapy in ALI is to accomplish adequate arterial oxygen content (adequate hemoglobin content plus an arterial PO_2 greater than 60 mm Hg) without a significant reduction in cardiac output at an FIO_2 below 0.5. This should provide adequate tissue oxygenation while avoiding potentially detrimental alveolar oxygen concentrations. Our experience is that an FIO_2 of 0.4 is an attainable and practical goal in most circumstances.

Therapeutic levels.—If the concept of ALI representing a spectrum of pulmonary damage from the less severe or earlier form (NCE) to the more severe form (ARDS)

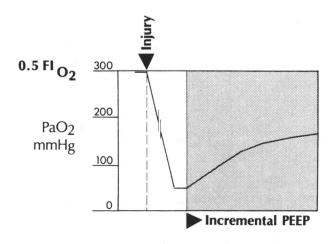

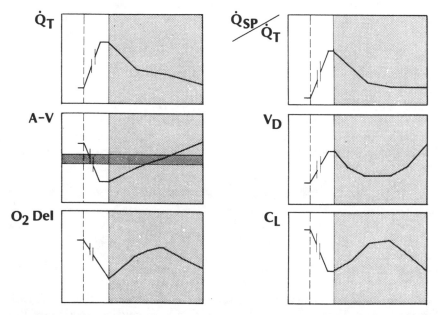

FIG 18–5.
Graphic depiction of seven factors recommended for use as clinical monitors to determine the required level of PEEP therapy in humans with ARDS. $\dot{Q}t$ = cardiac output. Although anesthetised animal models show a decreased cardiac output postinjury, available data and clinical experience demonstrate that humans respond with a significantly increased cardiac output. $A\text{-}V$ = the arterial–mixed venous oxygen content difference. The horizontal gray band represents 3 to 4 vol%. O_2 Del = oxygen delivery expressed as milliliters per minute (cardiac output × arterial oxygen context × 10). $\dot{Q}sp/\dot{Q}t$ = physiologic intrapulmonary shunt; V_D = dead-space ventilation; C_L = lung compliance. (From Shapiro BA, Harrison RA, Kacmarek RM, et al: *Clinical Application of Respiratory Care,* ed 3. Chicago, Year Book Medical Publishers, Inc, 1985. Used by permission.)

is used, NCE usually shows significant improvement in gas exhcange with 5 to 15 cm H_2O of PEEP, with most patients responding optimally by 10 cm H_2O PEEP; ARDS is usually improved with 10 to 30 cm H_2O of PEEP, and most of these patients manifest an optimal response between 10 and 20 cm H_2O of PEEP.

Methodology.—PEEP should be increased or decreased in increments of 3 to 5 cm H_2O, and effects should be evaluated within 20 minutes. We prefer increments of 5 cm H_2O since this is reliably attainable and rarely excessive. The patient should be allowed to breathe spontaneously to whatever degree is compatible with cardiovascular and clinical stability. Spontaneous breathing appears to be an advantage in PEEP therapy but by no means a necessity. Although PEEP is most consistently and reliably administered via endotracheal or tracheostomy tube, mask CPAP up to 15 cm H_2O PEEP is technically feasible and may prove beneficial in many unintubated patients.

Monitoring.—Essential monitoring includes vital signs, continuous electrocardiograms (ECGs), serial arterial blood gas measurement, and appropriate nurse/respiratory therapist availability. Appropriate monitoring of the respiratory equipment, inspired gas concentration, and system flow is essential since tehcnical malfunction is not uncommon.

A pulmonary artery flotation catheter is warranted when more than 20 cm H_2O of PEEP is required or there is uncertainty concerning the diagnosis of ALI, the cardiovascular status, or the intravascular fluid volume. The clinically useful information available by means of a pulmonary artery catheter in relation to PEEP therapy includes measurement of the arteriovenous oxygen content difference and cardiac output measurements to aid the assessment of tissue perfusion and oxygen extraction, intrapulmonary shunt calculations to aid assessment of the pulmonary effects of PEEP, and pulmonary artery occlusion pressures to aid in the assessment of intravascular fluid administration.

Cardiovascular support.—Correction of hypovolemia should ideally be achieved prior to initiation of PEEP therapy; however, intravascular volume augmentation is frequently required during or following the application of PEEP therapy. Reasonable IV fluid administration in conjunction with PEEP levels up to 20 cm H_2O usually compensates for reductions in cardiac output secondary to a reduction in venous return. PEEP therapy seldom requires inotropic support at levels below 20 cm H_2O.

Contraindications.—There are no absolute contraindications to the use of PEEP therapy in ALI. There do not appear to be data substantiating the concept that clinically appropriate levels of PEEP should be withheld for fear of producing barotrauma. While patients requiring PEEP therapy for severe ALI (ARDS) have an increased incidence of barotrauma, this appears to be related to the severity of the parenchymal disease rather than the level of applied airway pressure therapy.

CASE STUDY 1

A 59-year-old man was involved in a head-on motor vehicle accident at 10:00 P.M. The paramedics reported unfastening his seat belt and shoulder strap before removing him from the vehicle. They splinted his right leg, placed an 18-gauge IV catheter in the right forearm, and administered normal saline prior to bringing him to the emergency room.

He arrived in the emergency room at 10:30 P.M. awake but disoriented. His skin was cool and clammy to the touch; the blood pressure (BP) was 60 mm Hg systolic, the pulse was 130 beats per minute and regular, and his respiratory rate was 30/min and nonlabored. A 6 cm diameter echymosis without laceration was noted above the right eyebrow. His pupils were equal and reactive; the fundi were normal. His neck was supple. Clear breath sounds were present bilaterally. Heart tones were without murmurs or extra sounds. The abdomen was distended and tense but without bowel sounds. The right thigh was swollen, discolored, and painful; the skin was intact. He could move his foot and toes on command. Neurologic status was grossly intact.

Two 16-gauge peripheral IV catheters were inserted, and a central catheter placed via the right subclavian vein. A peritoneal tap returned blood that did not clot. Blood was obtained for typing, crossmatching, and other laboratory tests. The operating room staff was notified.

An ECG revealed sinus tachycardia. A right thigh x-ray film revealed a displaced femoral fracture. The hemoglobin content was 11 gm/dL and his WBC count was 8,500 cc^{-3}. The patient was placed on a 40% Venturi-type mask; arterial blood gas analysis revealed a pH of 7.41, a PCO_2 of 32 mm Hg, and a PO_2 of 95 mm Hg.

Over the next hour the patient received 4 units of whole blood, 1 L of hetastarch, and 2 L of crystalloid solution. On transfer to the operating room the patient was alert and oriented, with a BP of 100/50 mm Hg, a pulse of 110 beats per minute, a respiratory rate of 30/min, and a central venous pressure (CVP) of 8 cm H_2O.

In the operating room an inhalation anesthetic with muscle relaxant was administered without event. The induction was without any suspicion of aspiration. The BP remained over 100 mm Hg systolic, pulse 100 to 110 beats per minute; and CVP, 7 to 11 cm H_2O. A right radial arterial catheter was inserted. The spleen was removed and liver lacerations repaired. An open reduction of the right femur was accomplished. A nasogastric tube and a nasotracheal tube were inserted at the end of the operation.

The patient arrived in the surgical intensive care unit at 3:00 A.M. and was connected to a volume-limited ventilator. Fluids administered since admission were 6 units of whole blood, 10 units of packed RBCs, 3 L of hetastarch, and 7 L of crystalloid fluid, with an estimated blood loss in the operating room of 4,500 mL and a urine output of 700 mL. Assessment of cardiopulmonary function and arterial blood gases revealed the following: BP, 120/60 mm Hg; pulse, 100 beats per minute; respirations, 10/min; mechanical VT, 1,200 mL; pH, 7.42; PCO_2, 36 mm Hg; PO_2, 120 mm Hg; FIO_2, 0.50; CVP, 10 cm H_2O; temperature, 35°C; hemoglobin, 12 gm/dL; and normal serum electrolyte levels.

Discussion

The patient tolerated the surgery well and appeared to be no longer bleeding. There are a number of factors to consider in the immediate postoperative care that are important in decreasing the incidence of complications. The main factors are (1) maintaining adequate perfusion without fluid overload, (2) maintaining urine output above 50 ml/hr to reduce the chances of acute tubular necrosis (ATN), and (3) maintaining adequate arterial oxygenation without exposing the lungs to unnecessary hyperoxia. Additional factors are pain management and ventilator discontinuance.

The most reasonable clinical course is to assume that the patient is in adequate fluid balance since the hemodynamic and perfusion status are acceptable. Some overall plan for fluid administration is essential and must be based on the principle that urine and nasogastric fluid losses should be replaced with appropriate electrolyte solutions plus a minimal amount of free water. If the hemodynamic status should deteriorate, fluid challenges of 50 to 100 mL should be administered to reestablish an adequate vascular volume/vascular space relationship (see Chapter 1). Of course, frequent evaluation for further bleeding is essential.

A reasonable urine output should be maintained to diminish the incidence of ATN. Although controversial, a urine output above 50 ml/hr is a reasonable goal. Following assurance of adequate intravascular volume and, if needed, renal perfusion, dopaminergic stimulation or intermittent diuretic therapy can be employed singly or in combination.

Certainly an FIO_2 above 0.5 is undesirable, and one of 0.4 or less is preferred since some pulmonary parenchymal insult must be assumed because the patient's PaO_2 is only 120 mm Hg on 50% oxygen. Appropriate levels of PEEP (5 to 10 cm H_2O) should accomplish this goal with only small increments of additional vascular volume required to maintain cardiac output.

The patient should be warmed slowly by covering him with warm blankets. Shivering increases oxygen consumption and carbon dioxide production and should be avoided. The muscle relaxant (pancuronium) should be redistributed and excreted over the next several hours. Spontaneous ventilation should be evaluated as muscle strength returns. It is essential to remember that the patient will have pain as he emerges from the hypothermia and general anesthesia. Pain will raise catecholamine levels and create arteriolar and venous constriction. When narcotics are administered for pain relief, this catecholamine level will diminish, and hypotension may result. The best way to avoid this circumstance is to administer adequate analgesia from the beginning and avoid the pain and anxiety that lead to stress reactions. Morphine sulfate, 1 to 4 mg IV, may be administered each hour and as necessary to establish and maintain an adequte analgesic level without significantly depressing the respiratory drive. Conventional analgesic administration of larger doses of narcotics given intramuscularly results in widely fluctuating serum drug concentrations, poor pain control, and greater potential for adverse side effects.

CASE STUDY 1 CONTINUED

At 7:00 A.M. the patient was awake and oriented. He had received 2 mg of morphine sulfate IV on six occasions and complained only of mild right thigh pain. His urine output was 150 mL since returning from the operating room, and he had received 350 mL of 5% dextrose in 0.45% saline. His rectal temperature was 37.2°C. PEEP at 5 cm H_2O was added to the ventilator regimen and enabled a decrease in FIO_2 to 0.4.

Spontaneous ventilatory efforts began at 5:00 A.M., and the IMV rate was gradually decreased to 4/min. At this time the vital signs and blood gases were as follows: BP, 140/75 mm Hg; pulse, 90 beats per minute; respiratory rate: ventilator (V)—4/min, spontaneous (S)—20/min, TV(V)—1,200 mL, (S)—300 mL; minute volume (MV), 12.8 L; Vc, 1.4 L; pH, 7.44; PCO_2, 34 mm Hg; PO_2, 100 mm Hg; FIO_2, 0.40; and CVP, 9 cm H_2O.

The patient was switched from the ventilator to a CPAP system at 5 cm H_2O of PEEP with an FIO_2 of 0.4. His vital signs changed only in that the heart rate increased to 95 beats per minute. Arterial blood gas analysis after 20 minutes revealed a pH of 7.41, a PCO_2 of 38 mm Hg, and a PO_2 of 95 mm Hg.

Between 7:00 A.M. and 3 P.M. the patient received 1 L of 5% dextrose in water (D_5W)/ 0.45 saline plus 40 mEq of potassium chloride. His urine output was 650 mL with nasogastric drainage of 200 mL. Morphine sulfate, 4 mg IV, had been given each hour. A 2 µg/kg/min infusion of dopamine was running, and two 10 mg doses of furosemide had been given to maintain urine output. Six hours later assessment of the patient revealed a BP of 110/70 mm Hg, a pulse of 95 beats per minute, a respiratory rate of 22/minute, VT of 400 mL, MV of 8.8 L, pH of 7.43, P_{CO_2} of 38 mm Hg, P_{O_2} of 55 mm Hg, F_{IO_2} of 0.4, and CVP of 9 cm H_2O.

Heart tones were clear, and no murmurs were heard. Bilateral breath sounds were present with scattered rhonchi; no rales or wheezing were noted. A chest x-ray film revealed an appropriately placed endotracheal tube and no infiltrates or atelectasis.

Discussion

The patient was developing progressive hypoxemia that did not appear to be due to obvious hypervolemia, cardiogenic edema, pneumonia, atelectasis, or retained secretions. The most probable cause is NCE. If the P_{O_2} dropped further, it would be advisable to increase PEEP rather than increase F_{IO_2} because a low Pa_{O_2} on 40% oxygen implies a significant amount of lung with either very low V/Q ratios or zero V/Q ratios.

CASE STUDY 1 CONTINUED

At 3:30 P.M. the vital signs were unchanged, but the arterial P_{O_2} was 52 mm Hg. CPAP was increased to 10 cm H_2O without a change in vital signs or respiratory pattern. Arterial blood gas values were as follows: pH, 7.43; P_{CO_2}, 38 mm Hg; and P_{O_2}, 87 mm Hg on 40% inspired oxygen.

The remaining course was uneventful. The F_{IO_2} was decreased to 0.35 and the CPAP to 5 cm H_2O by the second postoperative day. The patient was extubated, placed on a 35% air entrainment mask, and had the following arterial blood gas values: pH, 7.41; P_{CO_2}, 39 mm Hg; and P_{O_2}, 82 mm Hg.

Careful titration of supportive therapy (fluids, diuretics, oxygen, PEEP, airway care) provided an optimal milieu for avoiding cardiac, pulmonary, and renal complications and ensuring a satisfactory outcome.

CASE STUDY 2

A 62-year-old woman with a 40-year history of malabsorption syndrome (nontropical sprue) experienced a 30-lb weight loss secondary to emotional stress and noncompliance with her glutin-free diet. After thorough investigation to rule out other causes for the weight loss, she was placed on a strict diet but did not gain weight over a 1-month period. It was decided to place her on parenteral nutrition, in response to which she gained over 10 lb in 14 days. On the 15th day she became febrile to 39.4°C, complained of chills and dizziness, and suffered mild hypotension. Empirical therapy for assumed gram-negative sepsis (subsequently confirmed by blood culture) consisted of an aminoglycoside and cephalosporin. Her fever defervesced the next day, but she was noted to bruise easily and had two episodes of hemoptysis. Coagulation studies confirmed a mild DIC. That evening she complained of dyspnea and an arterial blood gas analysis revealed a pH of 7.53, a P_{CO_2} of 32 mm Hg, and a P_{O_2} of 48 mm Hg (F_{IO_2} of 0.21). She was placed on 50% oxygen and transferred to the medical intensive care unit.

On admission to the intensive care unit she was awake, anxious, and alert, sitting up in bed and complaining of severe shortness of breath. She was markedly cachectic. Her BP was 90/50 mm Hg, her pulse was 120 beats per minute, and her respiratory rate was 28/min and labored, with a VT of 250 mL and a Vc of 1.4 L. She was using accesssory muscles to breath. Bilateral breath sounds were heard with no wheezes, rales, or rhonchi. Air entry was better as the apices than the bases. Attempts at coughing produced neither sputum nor relief. Heart tones were clear without murmers or extra sounds. On 50% inspired oxygen the pH was 7.51, the Pco₂ was 32 mm Hg, and the Po₂ was 42 mm Hg. Her hemoglobin concentration was 9.1 gm/dL; WBC count, 12,500 mm⁻³ (down from 21,000, 2 days earlier); and electrolytes, normal.

Discussion

This patient's cachexia, in addition to the recent sepsis and DIC, placed her at risk for ALI. Her refractory hypoxemia suggested significant areas of lung with zero V/Q ratios and intrapulmonary right-to-left shunting that, in the absence of pneumonia and/or atelectasis, made the most probable pulmonary diagnosis ARDS.

Since the sepsis was being adequately treated, the next most important factor is to ensure adequate perfusion and oxygenation while relieving the work of breathing and hopefully decreasing the FIO_2 to at least 0.4. Since it can be predicted that at least 15 cm H_2O of PEEP will be required to achieve these aims, an endotracheal tube is indicated. This will also allow safe tracheal suction and positive-pressure ventilation if the work of breathing is not sufficiently relieved by CPAP.

This patient's cardiovascular reserves are questionable because of her age and long-standing cachexia. A pulmonary artery catheter would be the safest and surest means of monitoring the cardiopulmonary response to her pathology and therapy. Additionally, an arterial line would facilitate blood gas monitoring and provide continuous BP monitoring.

Packed red blood cell (RBC) infusion will improve the oxygen-carrying capacity of the blood. However, it is advisable to transfuse after the pulmonary artery line is established so that careful hemodynamic monitoring can be accomplished during the transfusions.

CASE STUDY 2 CONTINUED

The entire situation was carefully explained to the patient and the need for her cooperation stressed. A right radial arterial catheter was inserted. Because of her inability to lie flat and because of the mild coagulopathy, a pulmonary artery catheter was placed via the right basilic vein by a cutdown procedure. After placement of the pulmonary artery catheter a no. 8 nasotracheal tube was inserted after adequate topical anesthesia had been established. The patient was placed on a CPAP system at 5 cm H_2O with an FIO_2 of 0.70. After allowing 15 minutes for the patient to stabilize, assessment revealed the following: BP, 90/60 mm Hg; pulse, 120 beats per minute; respirations, 30/min; VT, 250 mL; MV, 7.5 L/min; pH, 7.51; Pco₂, 32 mm Hg; Po₂, 41 mm Hg; FiO₂, 0.7; Pvo₂, 32 mm Hg; pulmonary artery occluded pressure (PAOP), 14 mm Hg; cardiac output, 7.0 L/min; Ca-vo₂, 2.2 vol%; Qsp/Qt, 43%; and hemoglobin, 9.2 gm/dL.

The CPAP was increased to 10 cm H_2O with essentially no changes occuring after 15 minutes. The CPAP was then increased to 15 cm H_2O, and 20 minutes later the patient indicated her breathing was easier. Approximately 500 mL of crystalloid solution had been administered since the intubation. At this time the patient's vital signs, hemodynamic parameters, and blood gas values were as follows: BP, 90/60 mm Hg; pulse, 110 beats per minute; respirations, 25/min; V_T, 250 mL; MV, 6.25 L/min; pH, 7.49; Pco_2, 35 mm Hg; Po_2, 65 mm Hg; Fio_2, 0.7; Pvo_2, 32 mm Hg; PAOP, 13 mm Hg; cardiac output 5.5 L/min; Ca-vo_2, 3.2 vol%; Qsp/Qt, 32% and hemoglobin, 9.2 gm/dL.

Discussion

The patient's pulmonary status had significantly improved. That she was not using accessory muscles to breathe indicated that it was much easier to breathe. The respiratory rate decreased, the arterial oxygenation markedly improved. The decrease in cardiac output was probably secondary to the improved arterial oxygenation, which was reflected in the markedly diminished intrapulmonary shunt. There can be no argument that PEEP was beneficial to this point; the critical question is whether or not it should then be increased further.

Two of the three clinical goals of PEEP therapy in ARDS have been met, namely, perfusion has been adequately maintained and the arterial Po_2 increased to above 60 mm Hg. However, the third goal, to decrease the Fio_2 to 0.4 or less, has not yet been met. One option is to wait and see whether the arterial Po_2 continues to improve, which will allow the Fio_2 to be decreased and at the same time allow transfusion with RBCs. However, this would ignore the overwhelming evidence that hyperoxic alveolar gas is detrimental to the lung parenchyma in this disease process. The other option is to increase the CPAP to 20 cm H_2O. Although many physicians are anxious about this level of PEEP therapy, there are few data to suggest that this level is deleterious in patients with severe disease.

CASE STUDY 2 CONTINUED

The CPAP was increased to 20 cm H_2O, and 20 minutes later reassessment revealed considerable improvement in oxygenation with no major hemodynamic changes. The arterial blood gas analysis and shunt study revealed an arterial pH of 7.43, a Pco_2 of 42 mm Hg, a Po_2 of 128 mm Hg (Fio_2 = 0.07) a Pvo_2 of 37 mm Hg; and a Qsp/Qt of 24%.

RBC transfusion was started and the Fio_2 decreased to 0.5, which resulted in an arterial Po_2 of 72 mm Hg. The patient remained comfortable. Four units of packed RBCs were administered over the next 2 hours. Reassessment revealed the following values: BP, 100/70 mm Hg; pulse, 100 beats per minute; respirations, 20/min; V_T, 220 mL; MV, 4.4 L/min; pH, 7.43; Pco_2, 42 mm Hg; Po_2, 84 mm Hg; Fio_2, 0.5; Pvo_2, 37 mm Hg; PAOP, 16 mm Hg; cardiac output, 5.1 L/min; Ca-vo_2, 3.8 vol%; Qsp/Qt, 22%; and hemoglobin, 11.3 gm/dL.

No rales were heard, and a repeated chest x-ray film showed increased lung volume with no new infiltrate or atelectasis. No S_3 or S_4 was noted. The Fio_2 was reduced to 0.4, and the Pao_2 was 64 mm Hg, with no significant change in any other clinical parameters.

The patient remained comfortable and stable for the next 18 hours, at which time her cardiovascular function remained unchanged, her Pao_2 was 80 mm Hg (Fio_2 = 0.4), and her Qsp/Qt was 18%.

The CPAP was reduced to 15 cm H_2O, which resulted in an acceptable Pao_2 of 68 mm Hg (Fio_2 = 0.4) and Qsp/Qt of 23%.

Four hours later the arterial Po_2 had risen to 79 mm Hg, and the Fio_2 was reduced to 0.35. The pulmonary artery catheter was removed. The next morning, on 15 cm H_2O CPAP, the patient had a BP of 100/60 mm Hg and a pulse of 90 beats per minute, was breathing comfortably with a VT of 275 mL, and had an arterial pH of 7.42, a PCO_2 of 38 mm Hg, and a PO_2 of 82 mm Hg (FIO_2 = 0.35).

The CPAP was reduced to 10 cm H_2O, and oxygenation remained satisfactory. The patient continued to improve, and the next day the CPAP was decreased to 5 cm H_2O and the patient extubated 3 hours later. She was discharged from the intensive care unit the following day and received 2 L of oxygen via a nasal cannula. Arterial blood gas values at that time were pH, 7.41; PCO_2 38 mm Hg; and PO_2 72 mm Hg.

REFERENCES

1. Scheeberger EE: Ultrastructural basis for alveolar-capillary permeability to protein. *Ciba Found Symp* 1976; 38:3.
2. Civetta JM: A new look at the Starling equation. *Crit Care Med* 1979; 7:84–91.
3. Zweifach BW, Silberberg A: The interstitial lymphatic flow system, in Guyton AC, Young DB (eds): *International Review of Physiology, Cardiovascular Physiology III.* Baltimore, University Park Press, 1979, pp 215–260.
4. Staub NC: Pulmonary edema. *Physiol Rev* 1974; 54:678.
5. Guyton AC, Granger HJ, Taylor AE: Interstitial fluid pressure. *Physiol Rev* 1971; 51:527.
6. Iliff LD, Green RE, Hughes JMB: Effect of interstitial edema on distribution of ventilation and perfusion in isolated lungs. *J Appl Physiol* 1972; 33:462.
7. Klika E: The ultrastructure of pulmonary lymphatic vessels and capillaries. *Acta Univ Carol [Med] (Praha)* 1975; 21:23.
8. Weibel ER, Gehr P, Haies D, et al: The cell population of the normal lung, in Bouhuys A (ed): *Lung Cells in Disease.* Amsterdam, Elsevier Science Publishers, 1976.
9. Staehlin LA: Structure and function of intracellular junctions. *Int Rev Cytol* 1974; 39:191.
10. Kikkawa Y, Yoneda K, Smith F, et al: The type II epithelial cells of the lung: II. Chemical composition and phospholipid synthesis. *Lab Invest* 1975; 32:295.
11. Mason RJ: Phospholipid synthesis in primary culture of type II alveolar cells, (abstracted). *Am Rev Respir Dis* 1977; 115:352.
12. Fishman AP: Non-respiratory function of lung. *Chest* 1977; 72:84.
13. Bachoven M, Weibel ER: Basic pattern of tissue repair in human lungs following unspecific injury. *Chest* 1974; 65:145.
14. Kuhn C: The cells of the lung and their organelles, in Crystal RD (ed): *The Biochemical Basis of Pulmonary Function.* New York, Marcel Dekker, Inc, 1976, pp 3–48.
15. Naimark A: Clinical implications of research in lung disease, in Bouhuys A (ed): *Lung Cells in Disease.* Amsterdam, Elsevier Science Publishers, 1976, pp 315–328.
16. Rosenbaum RM, Picciano P: The type 1 alveolar lining cells of the mammalian lung. *Am J Pathol* 1978; 90:123.
17. Adamson IYR, Bowden DH: The type 2 cell as a progenitor of alveolar regeneration: A cytodynamic study in mice after exposure to oxygen. *Lab Invest* 1974; 30:35.
18. Evans MJ, Cabral LJ, Stephens RJ, et al: Transformation of alveolar type 2 cells to type 1 cells following exposure to NO_2. *Exp Mol Pathol* 1975; 22:142.
19. Lamy M, Fallat RJ, Koeniger E, et al: Pathologic features and mechanisms of hypoxemia in adult respiratory distress syndrome. *Am Rev Respir Dis* 1976; 114:267.
20. Fishman AP: Pulmonary edema: The water exchange function of the lung. *Circulation* 1972; 46:390.
21. Robin ED, et al: Medical progress: Pulmonary edema. Parts 1 & 2. *N Engl J Med* 1973; 288:239.
22. Hurley JV: Current views on the mechanics of pulmonary edema. *J Pathol* 1978; 125:59.
23. Staub NC: Pulmonary edema due to increased microvascular permeability to fluid and protein. *Circ Res* 1978; 43:143.
24. Bessa SD, Dalmasso AP, Goodale RL Jr: Studies on the mechanism of endotoxin-induced increase of alveolocapillary permeability. *Proc Soc. Exp Biol Med* 1974; 147:701.
25. Addington WW, Cugell DW, Bazeley ES, et al: The pulmonary edema of heroin toxicity: An example of stiff lung syndrome. *Chest* 1972; 62:199.
26. Karliner JS, Steinberg AD, Williams MH: Lung function after pulmonary edema associated with heroin overdosage. *Arch Intern Med* 1969; 124:350.
27. Burton W, Vender J, Shapiro BA: Adult respiratory distress syndrome following Placidyl abuse. *Crit Care Med* 1980; 8:48.
28. Malik AB, VanderZee H: Mechanisms of pulmonary edema induced by microembolization in dogs. *Circ Res* 1978; 42:72.
29. Malik AB, VanderZee H: Lung vascular permeability following progressive pulmonary embolization. *J Appl Physiol* 1978; 45:590.

30. Bone RC, Francis PB, Pierce AK: Intravascular coagulation associated with the adult respiratory distress syndrome. *Am J Med* 1976; 61:585.
31. Deykin D: Emerging concepts of platelet function. *N Engl J Med* 1974; 290:144.
32. Josephson S, Swedenborg J, Dahlgren SE: Delayed lung lesion in dogs after thombin-induced disseminated intravascular coagulation. *Acta Chir Scand* 1974; 140:431.
33. Bachoven M, Weibel ER: Alterations of gas exchange apparatus in adult respiratory insufficiency associated with septicemia. *Am Rev Respir Dis* 1977; 116:589.
34. Bergofsky EH: The acute respiratory insufficiency syndrome following nonthoracic trauma: The lung in shock. *Am J Cardiol* 1970; 26:619.
35. Blaisdell FW: Pathophysiology of the respiratory distress syndrome. *Arch Surg* 1974; 108:44.
36. Blaisdell FW, Schlobohm RM: The respiratory distress syndrome: A review. *Surgery* 1973; 74:251.
37. Nash G, Foley FD, Langlinais PC: Pulmonary interstitial edema and hyaline membranes in adult burn patients: Electron microscopic observations. *Hum Pathol* 1974; 5:149.
38. Katzenstein AA, Bloor CM, Leibow AA: Diffuse alveolar damage: The role of oxygen, shock, and related factors. A review. *Am J Pathol* 1976; 85:210.
39. Clements JA, Brown ES, Johnson RP, et al: Pulmonary surface tension and the mucous lining of the lungs: Some theoretical considerations. *J Appl Physiol* 1958; 12:262.
40. Collier C, Hackney JD, Rounds DE, et al: Alterations of surfactant in oxygen poisoning. *Dis Chest* 1965; 48:233.
41. James O: Respiratory failure after injury: A review and plea for accuracy. *Heart Lung* 1977; 6:303.
42. Dowd J, Jenkins IC: The lung in shock: A Review. *Can Anaesth Soc J* 1972; 19:309.
43. Petty TL, Ashbaugh DG: The adult respiratory distress syndrome: Clinical features, factors influencing prognosis and principles of management. *Chest* 1971; 60:233.
44. Rosen AJ: Shock lung: Fact or fancy? *Surg Clin North Am* 1975; 55:613.
45. Webb WR: Pulmonary complications of non-thoracic trauma: Summary of the national research council conference. *J Trauma* 1969; 9:700.
46. Shapiro BA, Cane RD, Harrison RA: Positive end-expiratory pressure in acute lung injury. *Chest* 1983; 83:358.
47. Rinaldo JE, Rogers RM: Adult respiratory disease syndrome: Changing concepts of lung injury and repair. *N Engl J Med* 1982; 306:900.
48. Robin ED, Carey IC, Grenvik A, et al: Capillary leak syndrome with pulmonary edema. *Arch Intern Med* 1972; 130:66.
49. DaLuz P, Shubin H, Weil MH: Pulmonary edema related to changes in colloid osmotic pressure and pulmonary artery wedge pressure in patients after acute myocardial infarction. *Circulation* 1975; 51:350.
50. Goodwin GW, Dorethy J, Lam V, et al: Randomized trial of efficacy of crystalloid and colloid resuscitation on hemodynamic response and lung water following thermal injury. *Ann Surg* 1983; 5:197.
51. Frank L, Massaro D: The lung and oxygen toxicity. *Arch Intern Med* 1979; 139:347.
52. Freeman B, Crapo J: Hyperoxia increases O_2 radical production in rat lungs and lung mitochrondria. *J Biol Chem* 1981; 256:10986–10988.
53. Cross C: The granular type H pneumocyte and lung antioxidant defense. *Ann Intern Med* 1974; 80:409–413.
54. Fox RB, Hoidal JR, Brown DM, et al: Pulmonary inflammation due to oxygen toxicity: Involvement of chemotactic factors and polymorphonuclear leukocytes. *Am Rev Respir Dis* 1981; 123:512–523.
55. Bone RC: The adult respiratory distress syndrome: Treatment in the next decade. *Respir Care* 1983; 29:249–262.
56. Tate RM, Repine JE: Neutrophils and the adult respiratory distress syndrome. *Am Rev Respir Dis* 1983; 128:552–559.
57. Shasby DM, Fox RB, Harada RN, et al: Granulocytes contribute to acute lung injury from hyperoxia. *J Appl Physiol* 1982; 52:1237–1244.
58. Shapiro BA, Cane RD, Harrison RA: Positive end-expiratory pressure therapy in adults with special reference to acute lung injury: A review of the literature and suggested clinical correlations. *Crit Care Med* 1984; 12:127–141.
59. Kacmarek RM, Dimas S, Reynold J et al: Technical aspects of positive and expiratory pressure: Parts I–III. *Respir Care* 1982; 27:1478.
60. Weenig CS, Pietak S, Hickey RF, et al: Relationship of preoperative closing volume to FRC and alveolar-arterial oxygen difference during anesthesia with controlled ventilation. *Anesthesiology* 1974; 41:3–7.
61. Hedenstierna G, Santesson J, Norlander O: Airway closure and distribution of inspired gas in the extremely obese, breathing spontaneously and during anesthesia with intermittent positive pressure ventilation. *Acta Anaesthesiol Scand* 1976; 20:334–342.
62. McCarthy GS, Hedenstierna G: Arterial oxygenation during artificial ventilation: the effect of airway closure and its prevention by positive end expiratory pressure. *Acta Anaesthesiol Scand* 1978; 22:563–569.

63. Wyche MD, Teichner RL, Kallos T, et al: Effects of continuous positive-pressure breathing on functional residual capacity and arterial oxygenation during intra-abdominal operations. *Anesthesiology* 1973; 38:68–74.

64. Demling RH, Staub NC, Edmonds LH: Effect of end expiratory airway pressure on accumulation of extra-vascular lung water. *J Appl Physiol* 1975; 38:907–912.

65. Caldini P, Leith JD, Brennan MJ: Effect of continuous positive pressure ventilation (CPPV) on edema formation in dog lung. *J Appl Physiol* 1975; 39:672–679.

66. Daly BDT, Edmonds CH, Norman JC: In vivo alveolar morphometrics with positive end expiratory pressure. *Surg Forum* 1973; 24:217–219.

67. McIntyre RW, Laws AK, Ramachandran PR: Positive expiratory pressure plateau: Improved gas exchange during mechanical ventilation. *Can. Anaesth Soc J* 1969; 16:477–486.

68. Rose DM, Downs JB, Heenan TJ: Temporal responses of functional residual capacity and oxygen tension to changes in positive end-expiratory pressure. *Crit Care Med* 1981; 9:79–82.

69. Qvist J, Pontoppidan H, Wilson RS: Hemodynamic responses to mechanical ventilation with PEEP. *Anesthesiology* 1975; 42:45–55.

70. Perschau RA, Pepine CJ, Nichols WN, et al: Instantaneous blood flow responses to positive end-expiratory pressure with spontaneous ventilation. *Circulation* 1979; 59:1312–1318.

71. Haynes JB, Carson SD, Whitney WP, et al: Positive end-expiratory pressure shifts left ventricular diastolic pressure area curves. *J Appl Physiol* 1980; 48:670–676.

72. Jardin F, Farcot J, Boisante L, et al: Influence of positive end-expiratory pressure left ventricular performance. *N Engl J Med* 1981; 304:387–392.

73. Liebman PR, Patten MT, Manny J, et al: The mechanism of depressed cardiac output on positive end expiratory pressure (PEEP). *Surgery* 1978; 83:594–598.

74. Downs JB, Klein EF, Modell JH, et al: The effect of incremental PEEP on Pao$_2$ in patients with respiratory failure. *Anesth Analg Curr Res* 1974; 52:210–215.

75. Falke KJ: Do changes in lung compliance allow the determination of "optimal PEEP"? *Anaesthesist* 1980; 29:165–168.

76. Kirby RR, Downs JB, Civetta JM, et al: High level positive end-expiratory pressure (PEEP) in acute respiratory insufficiency. *Chest* 1975; 67:156–163.

77. Suter PM, Fairley HM, Isenberg MD: Optimum end-expiratory airway pressure in patients with acute pulmonary failure. *N Engl J Med* 1975; 292:284–289.

78. Venus B, Jacobs HK, Lim L: Treatment of the adult respiratory distress syndrome with continuous positive airway pressure. *Chest* 1979; 76:257–261.

79. Gallagher TJ, Civetta JM: Goal-directed therapy of acute respiratory failure. *Anesth Analg* 1980; 59:831–834.

80. Zarins CK, Bayne CG, Rice CL, et al: Does spontaneous ventilation with IMV protect from PEEP induced cardiac output depression? *J Surg Res* 1977; 22:299–304.

81. Dueck R, Wagner PD, West JB: Effects of positive end-expiratory pressure on gas exchange in dogs with normal and edematous lungs. *Anesthesiology* 1977; 47:359–366.

82. Hammon JW, Wolfe WG, Moran JF, et al: The effect of positive end expiratory pressure on regional ventilation and perfusion in the normal and injured primate lung. *J Thorac Cardiovasc Surg* 1976; 72:680–689.

83. Downs JB, Douglas ME, Sanfelippo PM, et al: Ventilatory pattern, intrapleural pressure and cardiac output. *Anesth Analg Curr Res* 1977; 56:88–94.

84. Venus B, Jacobs KH, Mathru M: Hemodynamic responses to different modes of mechanical ventilation in dogs with normal and acid aspirated lungs. *Crit Care Med* 1980; 8:620–627.

85. Shah DM, Newell JC, Dutton RE, et al: Continuous positive airway pressure versus positive end-expiratory pressure in respiratory distress syndrome. *J Thorac Cardiovasc Surg* 1977; 74:557–562.

86. Schmidt GB, O'Neill WW, Kotb E, et al: Continuous positive airway pressure in the prophylaxis of the adult respiratory distress syndrome. *Surg Gynecol Obstet* 1976; 143:613–618.

87. Weigelt JA, Mitchell RA, Snyder WH III: Early positive end-expiratory pressure in the adult respiratory distress syndrome. *Arch Surg* 1979; 114:497–501.

88. McAslan TC, Cowley RA: The preventive use of PEEP in major trauma. *Am Surgeon* 1979; 45:159–167.

89. Dantzker DR, Brok CJ, Dehart P, et al: Ventilation-perfusion distributions in the adult respiratory distress syndrome. *Am Rev Respir Dis* 1979; 120:1039.

90. Dantzker DR, Lynch JP, Wed JA: Depression of cardiac output is a mechanism of shunt reduction in the therapy of acute respiratory failure. *Chest* 1980; 77:636.

19/Infection in the Immunocompromised Patient

JOHN P. PHAIR, M.D.

Infection represents a major cause of morbidity and mortality in patients with defects in the immune or inflammatory system.[1] Compromised ability to produce antibody, deficiencies in the lymphocyte-macrophage system of cell-mediated resistance, defects in the complement cascade, or an inadequate number or dysfunction of polymorphonuclear leukocytes (PMNLs) leads to invasion by a wide variety of microorganisms. Such defects in host defense against infection can be the result of congenital deficiencies, acquired disease, or therapy. Management of infection in the compromised host requires aggressive attempts to establish an etiology and prompt, effective, therapeutic intervention.

PATHOGENESIS OF INFECTION AND PRINCIPLES OF MANAGEMENT IN THE COMPROMISED HOST

There are several principles that are relevant to a rational approach to the management of infection in compromised patients. First, specific infectious agents are associated with specific defects in host defenses (Table 19–1). The absence of antibody is associated with infection due to the pyogenic encapsulated microorganisms such as *Streptococcus penumoniae, Neisseria meningitidis,* and *Haemophilus influenzae.*[2] The capsule of these organisms represents a virulence factor that enables the bacteria to resist phagocytosis in the absence of opsonins (antibody and/or complement). Examples include dysgammaglobulinemia, multiple myeloma, and chronic lymphocytic leukemia. A deficiency in cell-mediated immunity is associated with infection due to intracellular pathogens.[3] The classical association is tuberculosis or cryptococcal meningitis with Hodgkin's disease.

The complement system plays a central and complex role in the inflammatory response that has been recently reviewed.[4] This system is composed of 14 proteins, or complement components, that circulate as inactive precursors in serum and several biologically active and inactive factors that are released following activation of the sequence. A major facet of defense against infection provided by this humoral system is facilitation of phagocytosis of microorganisms. Opsonization, or coating of bacteria, aids the ingestion of the organisms by phagocytic cells and occurs after fixation of the first protein in the complement sequence, Clq, by antibody. The interaction of Clq with antibody follows the combination of antibody with antigen, in this case the

347

TABLE 19–1.

Some Host Defects, Disease States, and Microorganisms

Defect	Disease	Microorganisms
Absent or low antibody concentration	Multiple myeloma Chronic lymphocytic leukemia X-linked hypogammaglobulinemia Common variable hypogammaglobuli- nemia	*S. pneumoniae* *H. influenzae* *N. meningitidis*
Complement deficiency		
C3	Congenital absence	*S. aureus*
C5–9	Congenital absence	*N. gonorrhoeae*
Deficient or defective poly- morphonuclear leukocytes	Cirrhosis (chemotactic factor inactivator)	Aerobic gram-negative bacilli
	Chronic granulomatous disease (killing)	*S. aureus*
	Neutropenia (absence)	Fungi
	Diabetes (chemotaxis)	
	Corticosteroid therapy (adherence)	Aerobic gram-negative bacilli, gram-positive cocci
Deficient cell-mediated immunity	Hodgkin's disease	Fungi
	Corticosteroid therapy	*Mycobacterium*
	Acquired immunodeficiency syndrome	Herpes virus
	Sarcoidosis	Simplex
	Protein-calorie malnutrition	Zoster
	Postoperative state	Cytomegalovirus

surface of the invading microorganism. The fixation of Clq activates the classical complement pathway and results in deposition of the third component of the cascade, C3, on the cell wall of the microorganism. Phagocytic cells have receptors for C3 that facilitate attachment of the cell to the microorganism, thus initiating the process of engulfment. Some bacteria and fungi activate C3 directly and bypass the requirement for specific antibody. Activation of the terminal components of complement (C5 through C9) by this mechanism requires components of the so-called alternative or properdin pathway. In addition to facilitating phagocytosis, by-products of activated C3 and C5 attract PMNLs to areas of inflammation. Finally, the terminal components of this cascade, when activated and deposited on bacterial surfaces, are able to lyse susceptible organisms. Congenital absence of Clq results in multiple infections, as does a deficiency of C3. Kindreds that lack C2 have a high incidence of collagen-vascular disease, and individuals who lack terminal complement components are susceptible to recurrent meningococcemia and gonococcemia.

A defect in function or inadequate numbers of PMNLs result in an increased infection due to staphylococci, including both *Staphylococcus aureus* and *Staphylococcus epidermidis*, aerobic gram-negative bacilli, and fungi.[5] Such infections are common in the prototypic example of PMNL dysfunction, chronic granulomatous disease, a congenital defect in cellular oxidative metabolism resulting in a failure of intracellular killing of catalase-negative microorganisms.[6] However, the most common infectious problem associated with PMNL abnormalities is sepsis occurring in neutropenic patients.

The second principle requiring emphasis is the need for early, accurate diagnosis to facilitate the management of infection in compromised patients. There is solid evidence that in this group of patients, early appropriate therapy results in an improved prognosis. The survival of a bacteremic patient who receives two effective bactericidal antibiotics approaches 70%. If the organism is susceptible to only one agent or no effective antibiotic is given, survival decreases.[5] Similarly, survival of patients developing invasive pulmonary aspergillosis is totally dependent on early diagnosis and initiation of antifungal chemotherapy.[7]

A third point that must be borne in mind is that institution of therapy in specific situations must often be empirical. Waiting for results of culture and susceptibility testing before initiating antibiotics to a febrile neutropenic patient results in an unacceptable mortality.[5] In patients with defects in cell-mediated immunity, prompt therapy is also necessary, but there is not the same urgency as in the neutropenic individual.

Finally, following initiation of therapy, close observation of the patient must continue. The response to therapy, the search for superinfection, and need for alternate treatment must be reevaluated daily. Superinfection represents a major problem due to persistence of the underlying host defect and the alteration in the normal flora resulting from the use of antibiotics. In addition, "new" infections can arise during the initial treatment regimen. Examples include the development of *Pneumocystis carinii* pneumonia, disseminated herpes zoster, or tuberculosis. Presumably, these infections represent "reactivation" of previously dormant organisms, a common sequelae of corticosteroid or other immunosuppresive therapy, the stress of infection, or the basic disease state.

The following cases are presented to illustrate the decision analysis necessary for the care of the infected compromised patient.

CASE STUDY 1

A 45-year-old man presented with fatigue and a 5-lb weight loss over several weeks. The patient had noted minimal bleeding when brushing his teeth and some increase in bruising. Physical examination revealed pale mucus membranes and conjunctiva; there was no lymphadenopathy, splenomegaly, or hepatomegaly. A complete blood count was remarkable for a hemoglobin concentration of 8 g/dL and a total white count of 1,500 mm^{-3}. The differential white blood cell count revealed 30% segmented neutrophils and "blast" forms; a paucity of platelets was noted on the smear. The patient was admitted to the hospital where a bone marrow aspiration and biopsy confirmed the diagnosis of acute nonlymphocytic leukemia. Combination induction therapy consisting of doxorubicin (Adriamycin), cyclophosmamide, 6-thioguanine, and cytosine arabinoside was begun. There was a progressive fall in the total white cell count over the next 8 days. On the 10th day of hospitalization, the total white count was 100 mm^{-3}, and no segmented neutrophils were seen. The platelet count was 7,000 mm^{-3}, and bleeding at sites of intravenous lines was apparent. Platelet transfusions were administered. During the hospitalization, the patient had been gargling twice a day with nystatin (Mycostatin), which had been administered to prevent oropharyngeal fungal infection. On the 12th day, the patient's temperature rose to 39.8°C; no localizing symptoms were noted. A physical examination revealed no source of the fever. A chest radiograph was unchanged from admission; no infiltrates were noted. Blood and urine were obtained for culture. The patient was unable to produce sputum. Ticarcillin and amikacin were initiated as empirical antibiotic therapy.

Discussion

The appropriate decision was made to initiate empirical antibiotic therapy to this patient, specifically, a broad-spectrum β-lactam antibiotic and an aminoglycoside. Fever in the profoundly neutropenic patient, even in the absence of localizing signs or symptoms, must be treated as infection, even if blood products have been recently administered. In numerous studies approximately 20% of febrile neutropenic patients will be blood culture–positive, 20% will have bacteriologically documented but non-bacteremic infections, 20% will have clinically evident infections where an organism cannot be isolated, and in the remainder the fever will be unexplained.[8] The choice of antibiotics should be dictated by the flora isolated consistently from patients in the hospital unit. Oncology services should be monitored to determine the etiology of recent bacterial infections. Some units routinely obtain cultures of stool, skin, anterior nares, and oropharynx to determine the microorganisms most commonly colonizing patients. Organisms most frequently cited as causing bacteremia in neutropenic patients include *Pseudomonas aeruginosa, Klebsiella pneumoniae, Escherichia coli,* and more recently staphylococcal species.

Various combinations of antibiotics have been used as empirical therapy for the febrile neutropenic host. As reviewed by Young,[8] when evaluating published reports of results of therapeutic trials several issues should be kept in mind: first, the composition of the patients enrolled in the study must be ascertained. Are the arms of the trial equally weighted with patients with leukemia, of similar age, with bacteremia, or with indwelling venous catheters? Second, are the number of bacteremic and nonbacteremic infected patients large enough to make valid comparisons? It is well documented that patients whose fever is unexplained do well with any empirical antibiotic regimen. Third, is the control or comparison regimen one that is widely used and accepted by clinicians? It has become clear that an aminoglycoside used alone does not provide adequate therapy for established infection in the neutropenic host. However, a combination of an aminoglycoside with a β-lactam antibiotic does improve patient survival.[5]

The currently available aminoglycosides are, in order of introduction to clinical practice, gentamicin, tobramycin, and amikacin. Gentamicin, in clinical use since 1969, has the advantage of familiarity and a wide spectrum of activity against the majority of aerobic gram-negative bacilli including *P. aeruginosa* and staphylococci. The disadvantages of gentamicin include the development of significant resistance, especially among pseudomonads and in specific centers.[9] In addition, ototoxicity and nephrotoxicity occur with prolonged use of this agent or when the dose administered is too high for a given patient's renal status. Tobramycin, (the second broad-spectrum aminoglycoside introduced into practice), is approximately twice as effective as gentamicin against *P. aeruginosa* on a weight-for-weight basis but is less effective in the treatment of *Serratia marcescens* infection. Resistance to this agent in certain centers is also high. Well-controlled studies have demonstrated less nephrotoxicity in patients receiving tobramycin as compared with gentamicin. Amikacin, the most recently available aminoglycoside, has the widest spectrum of activity against aerobic gram-negative bacilli. In addition, the pharmacokinetics of this agent differ from gentamicin and tobramycin, and there is an increase in the therapeutic-to-toxic ratio. Thus, serum concentrations achieved with amikacin are usually well above the minimal concentrations required to inhibit growth of aerobic gram-negative bacilli and are below toxic levels. There are no well-designed studies comparing the nephrotoxicity of amikacin with that of tobramycin. It is generally felt that this agent is intermediate in toxicity between gentamicin and tobramycin.[10]

The majority of published studies of the treatment of febrile neutropenic patients have combined an aminoglycoside with a third-generation penicillin such as carbenicillin or ticarcillin. One multicenter study compared carbenicillin/gentamicin with cephalothin/gentamicin and cephalothin/carbenicillin. Overall, there was little difference between these three regimens; *Pseudomonas* infections responded better to the first combination and *Klebsiella* to the second. Interestingly, bacteremia due to *S. aureus* was treated effectively by the combination of carbenicillin and gentamicin.

Recently published reports have compared the use of the newly available, wider-spectrum cephalosporins (third-generation agents) imipenem-cilastatin and third- and fourth-generation penicillins plus aminoglycosides in the treatment of these patients. Trials of double β-lactam antibiotic combinations, monotherapy with a single broad-spectrum cephalosporin, and combinations including vancomycin have been published.[8, 12] Finally, trials comparing programmed modification of antibiotics have been performed.[13] In such trials a combination of a broad-spectrum cephalosporin and an aminoglycoside are begun, but the aminoglycoside therapy is discontinued. The overall outcome was similar to standard therapy unless the patient had bacteremia due to gram-negative bacilli. In this situation patients continuing to receive both the cephalosporin and aminoglycoside for the entire treatment course did much better. Reports of increasing numbers of infections due to staphylococcal species, especially in patients with indwelling venous catheters, have inhibited the widespread use of broad-spectrum β-lactam agents alone. These agents often have less activity against staphylococci. A recent publication comparing a regimen including vancomycin with one that lacked this antistaphylococcal agent noted breakthrough staphylococcal bacteremia in the latter arm of the trial.[12] See Table 19–2 for a list of available antibiotics.

It should be kept in mind that, in the absence of segmented neutrophils, the signs and symptoms that serve to identify the site of infection are often muted.[14] A perirectal abscess or urinary tract infection can be asymptomatic and present with none of the classical physical findings. The patient with pneumonia manifests cough and dyspnea, but sputum production is usually scanty and rarely contains inflammatory cells. The chest film, which demonstrates fluid exudation into alveoli, does reveal infiltrates even in the absence of segmented neutrophils.

After initiating empirical antibiotic therapy, the physician must continue to reevaluate the clinical situation. Usually if appropriate agents are chosen, the patient stabilizes. Ultimately, however, the prognosis depends upon the response of the bone marrow. Thus, patients who rapidly develop a leukocytosis do better than those whose granulocyte count remains below 500 mm^{-3}.[15]

CASE STUDY 1 CONTINUED

The patient, following initiation of antibiotic therapy, remained febrile; his temperature rose daily to 38.3°C or higher. Blood cultures obtained at the onset of fever and during antibiotic treatment were sterile. The number of segmented neutrophils remained under 100/mm^3. *Candida* stomatopharyngitis, which had been noted 3 days earlier, progressed in spite of continued Mycostatin gargles. The patient complained of difficulty swallowing and sticking of food at the level of the midsternum. A barium swallow confirmed the diagnosis of esophagitis.

A test dose of amphotericin B, 1 mg suspended in 125 mL of 5% dextrose and water, was infused over a 2-hour period. There was no reaction, and following premedication with acetylsalicyclic acid and prochlorperazine (Compazine), 15 mg of the antifungal agent in 250 mL of dextrose and water was administered intravenously over a 4-hour period. The following day 30 mg was given, again following premedication, and on day 8 of antibiotic therapy 50 mg of amphotericin B was given and continued on a daily basis. Serum creatinine and potassium were measured every third day to monitor renal toxicity and renal potassium wasting, known complications of amphotericin B therapy. A complete blood count was also frequently obtained because anemia due to ineffective erythropoiesis commonly occurs with amphotericin therapy.

After 10 days of antifungal treatment and a total of 17 days of antibiotic therapy, the patient noted less discomfort with swallowing, and the pharyngeal exudate had markedly decreased. The number of peripheral segmented neutrophils had increased to 500 mm^{-3}. On the 20th day of antibiotic therapy, the count had risen to 1,100 mm^{-3}. The patient's temperature had continued to rise daily to 38.3°C in association with the infusion of amphotericin. All antibiotic use was discontinued, and he became afebrile. A repeat bone marrow aspiration demonstrated a complete remission.

TABLE 19–2.

Antibiotics Useful in Neutropenic Patients

Agents	Spectrum	Adverse Effects
β-Lactam antibiotics		
Penicillins	*P. aeruginosa*	Allergy
Azlocillin	Enterobacteria	Hypokalemia
Mezlocillin	Streptococci	Inhibition of platelet
Ticarcillin		aggregation
(plus clavulanic acid)		
Piperacillin		
Cephalosporins	*S. aureus*	Allergy
1st generation	Enterobacteriaceae	Inhibition of platelet
Cephalothin	Streptococci	aggregation
Cefazolin		Prolonged prothrom-
2nd generation		bin time
Cefamandole		Superinfection
3rd generation		
Ceftizoxime		
Cefotaxime		
Ceftazidime	*P. aeruginosa**	
Cefoperazone		
Other		
Aztreonam	Enterobacteriaceae	
	P. aeruginosa	
Imipenem-Cilastatin	*S. aureus*	Seizures
	P. aeruginosa	Nausea/vomiting
	Anaerobic bacteria	
	Streptococci	
Antifolates		
Trimethoprim-sulfamethoxazole	Enterobacteriaceae	Allergy
	Streptococci	Superinfection
	S. aureus	Marrow suppression
Trimetrexate	*Pneumocystis carinii*	
Pyrimethamine/sulfadiazine	*Toxoplasma gondii*	
Aminoglycosides		
Amikacin	Enterobacteriaceae	Nephrotoxicity
Gentamicin	*S. aureus*	Ototoxicity
Tobramycin	*P. aeruginosa*	
Other		
Vancomycin	*S. aureus*	Phlebitis
	S. epidermidis	Nephrotoxicity
	Enterococcus	Allergy
	J-K Corynebacteria	
Antifungal		
Amphotericin	*Candida* sp.	Acute fever, chills,
	Aspergillus sp.	nausea, phlebitis
	Phycomycetes	Chronic: nephrotoxic-
	Cryptococcus neoformans	ity, anemia

Discussion

When a patient remains neutropenic and febrile after 5 to 7 days of antibiotic therapy, a second critical decision faces the physician. In the patient presented, there was good evidence of probable invasive fungal infection, which is extremely common in neutropenic patients. Involvement of the gastrointestinal tract and later dissemination is the usual course of this infection if unrecognized.[5] Diarrhea, renal insufficiency, and indurated erythematous skin lesions have been associated with disseminated *Candida tropicalis* infection.[16] This organism is more invasive than *Candida albicans* is, which more commonly colonizes mucus membranes of neutropenic patients. Daily funduscopic examinations should be carried out to look for evidence of *Candida endophthalmitis,* another sign of disseminated infection.

Amphotericin B represents the treatment of choice for fungal infection in the neutropenic patient. However, it does produce acute toxicity including nausea, vomiting, rigors, and fever. With rapid infusion, ventricular arrhythmias have been reported. Prolonged therapy results in renal insufficiency and ineffective erythropoiesis.[17]

When blood cultures are positive and the microbial isolate is susceptible to the antibiotics being administered, granulocyte transfusions have been reported to benefit patients with continued evidence of bacteremia.[18] To be useful, the granulocyte transfusions should be given daily. The ultimate prognosis again is dependent upon reversal of the marrow aplasia. With negative blood cultures, granulocyte transfusions are reported to be of less benefit.

Reevaluation of the patient must include repeated blood cultures and a renewed search for a focus of infection. Careful examination of the rectum, pharynx, sinus, and sites of intravenous lines, removal of those catheters in place for 3 or more days, culture of catheter tips, and blood cultures drawn through the long line, (i.e., Hickman catheters) should be carried out. Consideration of line removal is necessary if cultures are positive or if fever persists with no recognized cause. Organisms recently implicated as causes of sepsis in this situation include *S. epidermidis*[19] and the group CDC-JK Corynebacteria,[20] which have in the past been dismissed as contaminants. In some centers, the isolation of these organisms is frequent enough to justify the empirical addition of vancomycin to the antibiotic combination already in use. These bacteria are generally resistant to β-lactam antibiotics.

Currently, the safest approach to unexplained fever in the neutropenic patient is to continue the antibiotics rather than discontinue therapy and reevaluate the patient.[21] A more recent study provided evidence to support the addition of amphotericin B to the antibiotic regimen to treat probable fungal infections.[22] If the fever responds, therapy should be continued until the segmented neutrophil count returns to at least 1,000 mm^{-3}.

Alternately, the patient may have evidence of a focus of infection such as pneumonia. Some findings can suggest an etiology. For example, colonization of the nose with the *Aspergillus* species has preceded the development of pulmonary infection due to this organism.[23] Empirical initiation of amphotericin B with the development of signs of pulmonary infection in the presence of positive nasal cultures has been recommended. It is also well to keep in mind that *Aspergillus* infection of the lung may be associated with pleuritic pain and hemoptysis and may mimic pulmonary infarction.[7]

Commonly, however, pneumonia presents without providing clues as to the etiology. Cultures of the sputum and blood are often not helpful, and aggressive attempts to define the etiology are required. Bronchoscopy with brushing and transbronchial biopsy under coverage of platelet transfusions should be carried out before the patient is extremely hypoxemic. The range of potential etiologies is extremely broad. Total empirical therapy requires the use of many agents with a great potential for toxicity. Thus, an aggressive, diagnostic approach represents the most conservative management.

A discussion of the management of febrile neutropenic hosts is incomplete without mention of the current state of attempts to prevent infection in these patients. The only documented method of reducing risk to patients who are neutropenic while in the hospital is to ensure that the staff, including physicians, adhere rigorously to the practice of hand washing before examining the patient. Although there have been suggestions that flowers should be kept out of the patient's rooms and that the diet should include no raw vegetables or fruits, exposure to these items have not been documented as a source of infection. The majority of infections that develop in these patients are due to the patient's skin or bowel flora, and therefore attempts at protective isolation are usually unsuccessful.

In the past 15 years a literature has evolved that has evaluated the use of prophylactic antibiotics to reduce the frequency of infections in neutropenic patients. It is now clear that the number of bacterial infections can be reduced with the prolonged prophylactic use of trimethoprim-sulfamethoxazole (TMP-SMX) or the newer quinolones.[24, 25] The use of TMP-SMX, however, has been associated with an increase in the number of fungal infections and/or infections caused by TMP-SMX–resistant organisms. Evaluation of the quinolone antibiotics is too recent to have generated an extensive literature relevant to adverse effects of this form of prophylaxis.

CASE STUDY 2

A 25-year-old man with hemophilia A was admitted to the neurosurgical service following an episode of head trauma. He presented with obtundation and seizures. Computed axial tomography revealed a subdural hematoma. During hospitalization carbamazepine therapy was begun, and this controlled his convulsions. Ten days after discharge he returned to the emergency room with a severe sore throat and a fever of 39.1°C orally. Examination revealed a patient in moderate distress due to difficulty in swallowing. Severe stomatopharyngitis with whitish plaques in the pharynx and on the tongue and buccal mucosa was present. The remainder of the examination was noncontributory; specifically, the lung fields were clear. Laboratory studies revealed a total white count of 4,300 mm^{-3} with fewer than 10% segmented neutrophils. A chest radiograph was unchanged from the film obtained 2 weeks before; there were no infiltrates. The patient was admitted to the hospital. Intravenous ticarcillin and amikacin and Mycostatin mouth gargles were begun. Carbamazepine treatment was discontinued and phenobarbital substituted as anticonvulsant therapy. Within 96 hours, the patient's peripheral smear revealed metamyelocytes and band forms, thus indicating a return of the bone marrow to normal function. The highest daily temperature was 37.9°C orally, and the patient felt somewhat improved. It was decided to continue antibiotics until the patient's neutrophil count was 1,000 mm^{-3} or greater. On the seventh hospital day the white cell and differential count were normal; however, the patient's temperature rose to

38.8°C, and he developed cough and dyspnea. Arterial blood gas analysis revealed a pH of 7.45, a Pco_2 of 20 mm Hg, and a Po_2 of 50 mm Hg. A chest film revealed bilateral nodular densities. Bronchoscopic brushings were positive for *P. carinii*. Ticarcillin and amikacin therapy was discontinued and intravenous TMP-SMX initiated.

By the sixth day of therapy the patient's respiratory condition was improved; however, he had developed a rash, and his temperature had risen again. His total white cell count and absolute neutrophil count were within normal limits. It was elected to continue the TMP-SMX therapy. On the 8th day of therapy the macular rash had become confluent, and the temperature rose to 40.5°C. The patient complained of pruritus and generally felt miserable. His physicians discontinued the TMP-SMX therapy and substituted pentamidine, 4 mg/kg administered intravenously every 24 hours. Orders were given to administer this agent over a 60-minute period. A complete blood count and SMA-6 to monitor renal function and glucose levels were requested every third day. Hepatic enzymes were obtained every week. The patient completed a 21-day course of therapy, 8 days of TMP-SMX and 13 days of pentamidine, without incident. His rash cleared by the 12th day of therapy, and his temperature was normal during the final 10 days of therapy.

Following recovery, it was determined that the patient was anergic when skin tested with *Candida,* histoplasmin, mumps, *Trichophyton* antigens, and purified protein derivative. His absolute lymphocyte count was 1,488 mm^{-3}, and the ratio of T-helper to T-suppressor lymphocytes was 0.59 (normal range, 1.0 to 2.5). Assays for antibody for the human immunodeficiency virus (HIV) were positive.

Discussion

This patient illustrates the necessity for aggressive diagnostic efforts in infected patients who are immunocompromised even after initiating empirical broad-spectrum antibiotic therapy.

This individual, who received approximately 90,000 units/yr of factor VIII for hemophilia, had been infected with HIV, the cause of the acquired immunodeficiency syndrome (AIDS). This member of the retrovirus family infects cells of the immune system bearing the CD4 epitope on their surface including T-helper lymphocytes, a subset of monocytes/macrophages including glial cells, and B lymphocytes. When the T-helper lymphocyte is infected, the genomic material (RNA) of the virus transcribes DNA. This is mediated by the viral enzyme reverse transcriptase. The proviral DNA is then integrated into the DNA of the host cell. When the cell is stimulated, viral replication occurs and results in death of the T-helper cell. In addition, there are other mechanisms of virally mediated cell dysfunction and death.[26] In contrast to the depletion of T-helper cells induced by HIV infection, the infected macrophages and B cells are not killed but develop varying degrees of alteration in function. With the loss of T-helper cells over time, severe immunosuppression occurs; the median duration of AIDS-free time after infection is estimated to be approximately 8 years. HIV is spread by intimate sexual contact; exposure to blood through transfusions, factor therapy, and needle-stick accidents; exposure of broken skin or mucous membranes to blood; or sharing contaminated needles through illicit intravenous drug use. In addition, the virus is transmitted across the placenta and results in in utero infection of the fetus of an infected woman.[27] There is no evidence that HIV spreads through casual daily activities or through aerosolization. In the industrialized countries, homosexual/bisexual males, intravenous drug users, heterosexual contacts of these groups, and recipients of blood or blood products represent groups who have a high potential for exposure to HIV and account for more than 99% of the cases. In the Third World the great majority of infected individuals have been exposed through heterosexual activities.[28]

This patient's rehospitalization was initially due to stomatopharyngitis precipitated by neutropenia, which was an adverse response to the anticonvulsant therapy. With recovery of the bone marrow and appropriate broad-spectrum empirical antibiotics, this infection responded. However, during the hospitalization he developed pneumonia. The fact that this patient had hemophilia A in conjunction with the changes seen on a chest radiograph alerted his physician to the possibility of a second "opportunistic" infection. The appropriate test, bronchoscopy, was immediately performed, and TMP-SMX therapy was instituted.

As occurs in approximately 70% of patients with AIDS, the patient developed an allergic reaction to the TMP-SMX. The etiology of this enhanced hypersensitivity in HIV-infected patients has not been delineated. The other major adverse effect of TMP-SMX therapy is bone marrow suppression. The alternate therapy, pentamidine, which this patient received without difficulty, is also associated with neutropenia. Other adverse effects occurring with pentamidine include renal and hepatic toxicity and pancreatitis leading initially to hypoglycemia and ultimately diabetes. Finally, if the agent is infused rapidly, it can produce hypotension and/or arrhythmias.

The response in the first episode of *Pneumocystis carinii* pneumonia (PCP) approaches 90%. If a patient develops an adverse reaction to either TMP-SMX or pentamidine and the alternate agent is substituted, the response remains good. The substitution of either TMP-SMX or pentamidine for the other because of failure to improve results, however, in very poor survival rates. A new antifolate, trimetrexate, is currently being evaluated to determine whether the salvage rate in individuals who fail the usual therapy can be improved.

The results of positive airway pressure therapy to maintain oxygenation and/or ventilation also are discouraging. Fewer than 10% of individuals requiring intubation and mechanical ventilation survive. Currently the use of steroids is being evaluated to determine whether survival in these patients can be improved.

Acquired immunodeficiency syndrome is the consequence of the altered immune status caused by HIV. Infection due to specific facilitative intracellular pathogens and malignant diseases such as Kaposi's sarcoma or non-Hodgkin's lymphoma is diagnostic. In addition to *P. carinii*, common infections complicating AIDS include cytomegalovirus, herpes simplex, mycobacteria (especially of the *Mycobacterium avium-intracellulare* group), and fungi, particularly *Candida* sp. and *Cryptococcus neoformans*. In endemic areas disseminated histoplasmosis, blastomycosis, and coccidioidomycosis are also seen in HIV-infected patients.[29]

This pattern of infection is similar to that in patients with Hodgkin's disease or patients receiving corticosteroids and is due to an altered cell-mediated immune regulation. It should be noted that pneumonia due to *Legionella pneumophila* and related atypical bacteria also occurs with increased frequency in patients with Hodgkin's disease, those receiving corticosteroids, and transplant recipients, but less frequently in AIDS patients.

Protection of personnel who care for patients or handle clinical specimens obtained from persons with AIDS or HIV infection has been a major concern. Studies of families clearly indicate that nonsexual contact with infected individuals does not result in transmission of the virus. Contact with blood through spills, needle-stick accidents, or accidents in surgery or in the laboratory, however, does pose a hazard. Therefore, every effort must be made to reduce accidents and exposure to blood. The American Hospital Association and the Centers for Disease Control recommend that each institution review current phlebotomy practices, handling of sharp instruments, and disposal of needles and evaluate the need for universal precautions. Such precautions basically treat all blood, blood-contaminated specimens, semen, or cervical secretions as infected. Such specimens and secretions are treated as if they had been obtained from a patient with hepatitis B. Gloves are worn when drawing blood or handling specimens, and containers of specimens are bagged in impermeable plastic bags. Blood and fluids are centrifuged in screw-capped tubes. When procedures are performed that could result in exposure to blood or secretions, gowns, masks, and goggles should be worn. Full details of the current recommendations have been published.[30] The risk of transmission to health care personnel is extremely low but real. Therefore, every effort should be made to educate medical and hospital staffs as to risks and methods of minimizing these risks that are consistent with maintenance of good patient care.

It is not uncommon to be faced with a septic patient with multiple causes of increased susceptibility to infection who presents with pneumonia.[31] In such circumstances, although the chest radiograph can be suggestive, a definitive diagnosis can only be made by identification of a specific pathogen in induced sputum and bronchial washings, brushings, or tissue. It is especially useful to histologically demonstrate tissue invasion. The bronchoscopist in collaboration with the infectious disease consultant should decide which cultures are most appropriate for a specific patient. The number of specimens should be dictated by the differential diagnosis. If available, a shielded brush is essential to prevent contamination by the aerobic and anaerobic flora of the oropharynx. The shielded brush is disposable and can be clipped with sterile wire cutters and placed in appropriate media for culture. This technique usually provides a large specimen for staining and inoculation of appropriate media for culture. Quantitative cultures can help interpretation when there is a high suspicion that flora usually resident in the oropharynx is the cause of the pulmonary infection. Topical anesthesia should be administered via inhalation, not through the bronchoscope, to avoid contamination of the area to be sampled. The most useful smears and cultures can be secured by alerting the diagnostic microbiology laboratory that the procedure is imminent. Table 19–3 outlines the appropriate handling of specimens obtained by bronchoscopic washings and brushings. If definitive results are not immediately available, empirical therapy with intravenous TMP-SMX and erythromycin should be started. Alteration of therapy upon identification of the pathogen can be made within 24 hours.

Very hypoxemic patients who do not respond to oxygen therapy require an open lung biopsy because of the drop in Po_2 and the associated cardiac arrhythmias that can occur during bronchoscopy.[32, 33] Prolonged trials of empirical antimicrobial therapy result in a delay that is often associated with further worsening of the clinical situation, greater operative risk, and more confusion. Further, the use of empirical therapy alone without a diagnosis can be hazardous. As previously discussed TMP-

TABLE 19–3.

Microbiology Processing of Bronchoscopy Specimens Obtained From Immunocompromised Hosts

Microorganism	Specimen	Procedure	Handling
Anaerobic bacteria	1 brush in triple-lumen sheathed catheter	Anaerobic culture	Place brush in anaerobic prereduced broth with glass beads; vortex & culture on anaerobic media
Pneumocystis, yeasts	1 brush in triple-lumen sheathed catheter	Toluidine blue O, periodic acid–Schiff silver methenamine stain	Place brush in 0.5 mL of sterile saline, vortex; use cell suspension for smears
Legionella	1 brush in triple-lumen sheathed catheter	*Legionella* culture and fluorescent stain	Place brush in 1.0 mL of sterile H_2O, vortex; use cell suspension for smears, culture
Routine aerobic bacteria & fungi	1 brush in triple-lumen sheathed catheter	Routine aerobic and fungal culture & Gram stain	Place brush in 1.0 mL of sterile saline, vortex; use cell suspension for culture & smears
Virus	1 brush in triple-lumen sheathed catheter	Virus culture	Place brush in viral media, transport *promptly* to virology lab for tissue culture inoculation; if laboratory is closed, store in transport medium at 70°C
	1 brush, nondisposable	Fluorescent stains for virus identification	Make 6 smears of brushed bronchial cells at bedside for fluorescent stains; air-dry and bring to virology lab with culture specimen
Mycobacteria	1 brush or <5 mL of bronchial washings	Mycobacterial smear and culture	Place brush in 1.0 mL of Tween-albumin broth, vortex; use cell suspension for smear & culture; *or* process bronchial washings according to standard lab protocol

SMX has many adverse effects,[34] amphotericin B is nephrotoxic,[17] and erythromycin, isoniazid, and rifampin are hepatotoxic. Finally, in complicated cases, other entities can mimic pulmonary infection. Pulmonary pathology resembling infection can be due to earlier radiation, bleomycin therapy, hemorrhage, embolism, or progression of neoplastic disease.[35] Intelligent management of these ill patients requires knowledge of the cause of immunosuppression, careful evaluation of the therapy to date and the clinical situation, and appropriate use of invasive techniques.

REFERENCES

1. Allen JC: *Infection and Compromised Host.* Baltimore, William & Wilkens, 1976.
2. Hermans PE, Diaz-Buxo, JP, Stobo JD: Idiopathic late-onset immunoglobulin deficiency: Clinical observations in 50 patients. *Am J Med* 1976; 61:221.
3. Sharma S, Remington JS: The role of cell-mediated immunity in resistance to infection in the immunocompromised host, in Verhoef J, Peterson PK, Quie PK (eds): *Infection in the Immunocompromised Host. Pathogenesis, Prevention and Therapy.* Amsterdam, Elsevier Science Publishers, 1980, pp 59–76.
4. Frank MM: The complement system in host defense and inflammation. *Rev Infect Dis* 1979; 1:483.
5. Schimpff SC: Therapy of infection in patients with granulocytopenia. *Med Clin North Am* 1977; 61:1101.
6. Mills EL, Quie PC: Congenital disorders of the function of polymorphonuclear neutrophils. *Rev Infect Dis* 1980; 3:505.
7. Herbert PA, Bayer AS: Fungal pneumonia: Invasive pulmonary aspergillosis. *Chest* 1981; 80:220.
8. Young LS: Problems of studying infections in the compromised host. *Rev Infect Dis* 1986; 8(suppl 3):341–349.
9. Kauffman CA, Ramundo NC, Williams SG, et al: Surveillance of gentamicin-resistant gram-negative bacilli in a general hospital. *Antimicrob Agents Chemother* 1978; 13:918.
10. Smith CR, Lietman PS: Comparative clinical trials of aminoglycoside, in Whelton A, Neu HC (eds): *The Aminoglycosides: Microbiology Clinical Use and Toxicology.* New York, Marcel Dekker, Inc, 1982, pp 497–510.
11. The EORTC International Antimicrobial Therapy Project Group: Three antibiotic regimens in the treatment of infection in febrile granulocytopenic patients with cancer. *J Infect Dis* 1978; 137:14.
12. Shenep JL, Hughes WT, Roberson PK, et al: Vancomycin, ticarcillin, and amikacin compared with ticarcillin-clavulanate and amikacin in the empirical treatment of febrile, neutropenic children with cancer. *N Engl J Med* 1988; 319:1053–1057.
13. The EORTC International Antimicrobial Therapy Cooperative Group: Ceftazidime combined with a short or long course of amikacin for empirical therapy of gram negative bacteremia in cancer patients with granulocytopenia. *N Engl J Med* 1987; 317:1692–1698.
14. Sickles EA, Greene WH, Wiernik PH: Clinical presentation of infection in granulocytopenic patients. *Arch Intern Med* 1975; 135:715.
15. Bodey GP, Buckley M, Sathe YS, et al: Quantitative relationships between circulating leukocytes and infection in patients with acute leukemia. *Ann Intern Med* 1966; 64:328.
16. Winegard JR, Merz WG, Saral R: *Candida tropicalis:* A major pathogen in immunocompromised patients. *Ann Intern Med* 1979; 91:539.
17. Bennett JE: Chemotherapy of systemic mycoses. *N Engl J Med* 1974; 290:30.
18. Schiffer CA: Principles of granulocyte transfusion therapy. *Med Clin North Am* 1977; 61:1119.
19. Wade JC, Schimpff SC, Newman KA, et al: *Staphylococcus epidermidis:* An increasing cause of infection in patients with granulocytopenia. *Ann Intern Med* 1982; 97:503.
20. Lipsky BA, Goldberger AC, Tompkins LS, et al: Infections caused by nondiptheria corynebacterium. *Rev Infect Dis* 1982; 4:1220.
21. Pizzo PA, Robichaud KJ, Gill FA, et al: Duration of empiric antibiotic therapy in granulocytopenic patients with cancer. *Am J Med* 1979; 67:194.
22. Pizzo PA, Robichaud, KJ, Gill FA, et al: Empiric antibiotic and antifungal therapy for cancer patients with prolonged fever and granulocytopenia. *Am J Med* 1982; 72:101.
23. Aisner J, Murello J, Schimpff SC, et al: Invasive aspergillosis in acute leukemia: Correlation with nose cultures and antibiotic use. *Ann Intern Med* 1979; 90:4.
24. Gualtieri RJ, Donowitz CR, Kaiser DL, et al: Double blind randomized study of prophylactic trimethoprim/sulfamethoxazole in granulocytopenic patients with hematologic malignancies. *Am J Med* 1983; 74:934–940.

25. Karp JE, Merz WG, Hendricksen C, et al: Oral norfloxacin for prevention of gram-negative bacterial infections in patients with acute leukemia and granulocytopenia. *Ann Intern Med* 1987; 106:1–6.
26. Fauci AS: AIDS: Immunopathogenic mechanisms and research strategies. *Clin Res* 1987; 35:503–509.
27. Curran JW, Jaffe HW, Hardy AM, et al: Epidemiology of HIV infection and AIDS in the United States. *Science* 1988; 239:610–616.
28. Piot P, Cerael M: Epidemiological and sociological aspects of HIV infection in developing countries. *Br Med Bull* 1988; 44:1–21.
29. Fauci AS, Masur H, Gelmann PD, et al: The acquired immunodeficiency syndrome: An update. *Ann Intern Med* 1985; 102:800–813.
30. CDC Update: Universal precautions for prevention of transmission of human immunodeficiency virus, hepatitis B and other blood borne pathogens in the health-care setting. *MMWR* 1988; 37:377–388.
31. Phair JP, Reising KS, Metzger E: Bacteremic infection and malnutrition in patients with solid tumors. Investigation of host defense mechanisms. *Cancer* 1980; 45:2702.
32. Dubrausky C, Awe RJ, Jenkins DE: The effect of bronchofiberscopic examination on oxygenation status. *Chest* 1975; 2:137.
33. Katz AS, Michelson EL, Stawicki J, et al: Cardiac arrhythmias: Frequency during fiberoptic bronchoscopy and correlation with hypoxemia. *Arch Intern Med* 1981; 141:603.
34. Lawson DH, Pauce BJ: Adverse reactions to trimethoprim-sulfamethoxazole. *Rev Infect Dis* 1982; 4:429.
35. Pennington JE: Dilemma: Pneumonia in the immunocompromised patient. *J Respir Dis* 1982; 3:25.

20 / Gastrointestinal Tract Bleeding and Liver Failure

ARVYDAS VANAGUNAS, M.D.

GASTROINTESTINAL BLEEDING

Acute gastrointestinal hemorrhage is a common problem that results in at least 225,000 hospital admissions per year[1] and obviously directly impacts on the intensive care unit (ICU). Patients may have primary gastrointestinal bleeding and be admitted to the ICU for aggressive monitoring and treatment to ensure hemodynamic stability. Alternatively, gastrointestinal bleeding may be secondary or "stress" induced in patients acutely ill with ventilatory failure, sepsis, coma, or other critical conditions. Although major advances have been made in patient monitoring and intensive care, mortality from gastrointestinal bleeding has remained surprisingly stagnant at approximately 10% for the last 40 years.[2] This constant mortality rate, however, should be interpreted in light of an increasingly older and generally sicker population who would not have survived 10 or 20 years ago.[3]

UPPER GASTROINTESTINAL BLEEDING

CASE STUDY 1

A 30-year-old lawyer was brought to the hospital from his law office because of syncope. Although he was not totally coherent, he related that he had black stools last night and early this morning. He denied excessive alcohol intake, use of any medications, abdominal pain, or previous gastrointestinal bleeding. His blood pressure was 100/60 mm Hg, and his pulse was 100/min supine and 80/60 mm Hg and 130/min upright. His lung and heart examination was normal. He had dramatic spider agiomas on the anterior portion of his thorax and a firm, enlarged liver of 15 cm. There was no splenomegaly or ascites. A large-bore intravenous (IV) line was started, and he was given normal saline at 250 mL/hr. Blood was sent for crossmatch, electrolyte, chemistry, and coagulation studies. His hemoglobin was 8 g/dL. A nasogastric tube was inserted and revealed fresh red blood with clots that did not clear with 1 L of iced saline lavage.

Discussion

The approach to this patient should revolve around several questions. How risky is this patient's bleeding? What is the best way to diagnose the source of bleeding? What is the best initial therapy?

Not all acute gastrointestinal bleeding is life-threatening, and approximately 80% of all bleeding events are self-limited.[2] However, 20% of patients continue to bleed or rebleed under observation and have an unacceptable mortality rate in the range of 40%.[3] It is crucial to develop a profile that will simply and accurately identify this subgroup of patients at high risk of severe, persistent, or recurrent hemorrhage.

Some easily identifiable factors predict risk in acute gastrointestinal hemorrhage. Age above 60 years, severity of concomitant illness, initial hemoglobin below 8 g/dL, shock on presentation, and a transfusion requirement of more than 4 to 6 units of blood are parameters that directly correlate with a poorer outcome and should alert the clinician to a higher stage of vigilance.[3, 4] The simple maneuvers of inserting a nasogastric tube and directly examining the stool substantially aid in assessing severity and stratifying the risk of bleeding. A clear or "coffee ground" nasogastric aspirate implies less severe bleeding than a grossly bloody aspirate does. Melena is less worrisome if the nasogastric aspirate is clear. The combination of bloody nasogastric drainage and red rectal bleeding is particularly ominous and carries a mortality of 30%![3]

The etiology of the bleeding is also obviously a very important risk factor for continued bleeding. Gastric cancer, gastric ulcer, and duodenal ulcer have a higher rate of rebleeding (24% to 50%) and mortality (4% to 14%) when compared with the rebleeding (7% to 15%) and mortality (2% to 7%) of gastric erosions and Mallory-Weiss tears.[5] Although not the most common etiology of acute upper gastrointestinal bleeding, bleeding esophageal varices can be lethal and are the leading cause of severe, persistent, or intractable bleeding.[6] The clinical context of gastrointestinal bleeding is also very important. Whereas the majority of patients presenting to the hospital with gastrointestinal hemorrhage will spontaneously stop bleeding on admission, the onset of bleeding in a hospitalized patient is a very risky event, and only 67% of such bleeding is self-limited.[6]

The causes of acute upper gastrointestinal bleeding are multiple (Table 20–1) and can vary substantially from institution to institution depending on patient mix patterns. However, gastric and duodenal ulcers, acute gastric erosions, and gastroesophageal varices account for the vast majority (80%) of bleeding episodes and certainly are the key etiologies of severe or recurrent bleeding.[6]

Several features quickly establish that this patient has a serious gastrointestinal hemorrhage. The history of syncope, relative hypotension, bloody nasogastric aspirate, and a hemoglobin concentration of 8 g/dL prior to hydration are all factors that identify a high-risk patient. High-risk patients need to have the source of their bleeding accurately diagnosed. Although he is young and denies alcohol abuse, the presence of hepatomegaly and spider angiomas should immediately raise the possibility of cirrhosis and portal hypertension with bleeding gastroesophageal varices. Bleeding gastroesophageal varices are the leading cause of intractable gastrointestinal bleeding,[6] and because their treatment is complicated and potentially lethal, it should

TABLE 20–1.

Causes of Upper Gastrointestinal Bleeding

Diseases of the esophagus
    Esophagogastric varices
    Esophagitis
    Mallory-Weiss syndrome
    Malignant and benign tumors
Diseases of the stomach and duodenum
    Chronic peptic ulcer (gastric or duodenal)
    Stress ulcerations
    Gastric erosions
    Gastric neoplasms
    Hiatal hernia
    Dieulafoy's ulcer
    Stomal ulcer
    Osler-Weber-Rendu telangiectasia
    Duodenitis
Other
    Epistaxis or swallowed blood
    Hematobilia
    Rupture of aortic aneurysm or prosthetic graft
    Bleeding within the pancreatic duct

never be empirically undertaken. Urgent endoscopy is clearly indicated, and is the diagnostic procedure of choice.

Early gastrointestinal endoscopy has been routinely advocated for all patients with upper gastrointestinal bleeding. This approach certainly seems appropriate when data show that the average endoscopist is able to adequately complete the examination in 89% of actively bleeding patients, make a specific and accurate diagnosis more than 90% of the time, and perform the examination safely with a minimal complication rate of 0.9%.[3] Although there is little debate about the ability of making a safe and specific diagnosis with endoscopy, randomized, controlled trials in gastrointestinal bleeders of varying severity have not shown that emergency endoscopy influences the ultimate mortality, length of hospital stay, or frequency of gastrointestinal surgery.[1] It should be noted, however, that the role of endoscopy has not been fully evaluated in the 20% "high-risk" group of patients who do not stop bleeding spontaneously. Early identification of these patients would be a very important guide to management, especially with the increasing availability of simple endoscopic electrothermal treatment modalities. Indications are relative and conditioned by the urgency of the clinical situation, but endoscopy is certainly justified and strongly recommended early in the course of any patient deemed ill enough to be admitted to the ICU.

Gastrointestinal endoscopy has documented several visual predictors of rebleeding. These endoscopic stigmata in combination with the clinical parameters discussed earlier may be the most reliable predictors of risk. The presence of a protruding, red, 2- to 3-mm mound in the base of a peptic ulcer is of special importance. Initially thought to be a "visible vessel," this lesion is actually a small clot plugging a side hole in an aneurysmally dilated and inflamed artery.[7] It carries a rebleeding risk of 50% and should be a red flag to the clinician.[8] An adherent clot also carries an increased risk of continued or recurrent bleeding of 35%,[8] undoubtedly because of an underlying artery. A clean ulcer base, on the other hand, reliably predicts a negligible risk of further bleeding of 1%. Barium studies of the upper gastrointestinal tract can, on occasion, be used effectively to diagnose the cause of bleeding, but their use is more appropriate in the subacute or mild bleeder whose clinical profile does not suggest increased risk. This situation would be rare in the ICU setting.

Angiography can be useful in the infrequent patient with torrential upper gastrointestinal hemorrhage that cannot be adequately evaluated by upper endoscopy. Superselective angiography also has a therapeutic advantage in that bleeding vessels can be selectively embolized or infused with vasoconstrictors in an attempt to control bleeding.

Hemodynamic stability should be ensured prior to endoscopy. The general therapeutic approach to gastrointestinal bleeding demands synchronous clinical evaluation, fluid resuscitation, and attempts to minimize blood loss. The priorities should lie in appropriate fluid resuscitation. Placement of secure large-bore IV lines and immediate institution of IV saline or Ringer's lactate should be almost instinctive first steps. Sending blood for crossmatch, coagulation studies, a complete blood cell count (CBC), and chemistries are obviously appropriate. Placement of a vented nasogastric tube is essential. It provides immediate information on the severity of bleeding and helps localize the source. The information from nasogastric suctioning should be interpreted carefully, however. A clear or even bile-stained nasogastric aspirate is not an absolute guarantee that bleeding is below the ligament of Treitz.[3] Bleeding can be intermittent, and the nasogastric tube should remain in place for several hours to ensure that bleeding is not from the upper gastrointestinal tract. Iced water or saline lavage is frequently instituted, but there is no evidence that this maneuver is of any therapeutic advantage other than providing a clearer field for endoscopy. Early surgical referral is also appropriate in this patient as in any patient with gastrointestinal bleeding. This simple, pragmatic maneuver frequently pays worthwhile dividends in the overall management of the patient.

Central venous pressure measurement or pulmonary artery pressure monitoring may be needed in patients with underlying cardiopulmonary compromise.

Specifically directed therapy is available for treating bleeding gastroesophageal varices in the patient with portal hypertension, but most medical treatment aimed at controlling established gastrointestinal bleeding remains empirical and unproven. Although keeping the gastric pH at 4 or higher with the use of frequent antacids or histamine H_2 antagonists makes good physiologic sense and is routinely recommended in upper gastrointestinal bleeding, there is no evidence to conclusively prove the value of such therapy in controlling hemorrhage once gastrointestinal bleeding has started. The likelihood of getting definitive information in this area is limited. Unless studies were specifically targeted to only high-risk patients, it would require, for example, the randomization of at least 10,000 patients to detect even a modest improvement in survival in patients treated with histamine H_2 antagonists.[9] It should be noted, however, that prophylactic treatment with antacids, histamine H_2 antagonists, and sucralfate (Carafate) has been successful in preventing upper gastrointestinal bleeding in the high-risk ICU or postoperative patient.[10, 11]

Advancements in endoscopic technology may influence the natural history of gastrointestinal bleeding. Endoscopic therapy is now available to directly treat upper gastrointestinal bleeding. Emergent sclerotherapy can control acutely bleeding esophageal varices and is the treatment of choice when pharmacologic intervention fails.[12] Although endoscopic lasers can control bleeding, their substantial expense and small but definite risk of intestinal perforation or aggravation of bleeding have dampened initial enthusiasm about their usefulness. Portable and inexpensive thermal modalities such as heater probes and bipolar cautery units have been safely and successfully used in treating bleeding peptic ulcers and angiodysplasia and with time and more experience may be more widely applied.[13] Endoscopically directed injection of vasoconstrictors has stopped bleeding in patients with ulcers, Mallory-Weiss tears, and gastric carcinomas.[14] It should be stressed that these modalities, like any other therapy, should be constantly monitored for efficacy and not used indiscriminately.

CASE STUDY 1 CONTINUED

Emergency gastrointestinal endoscopy is performed on admission of the patient to the ICU. Large esophageal varices with active bleeding in the distal portion of the esophagus were noted. The stomach and duodenum were normal, and no gastric varices were seen. The patient had a prothrombin time that was 2 seconds prolonged over control, a normal partial thromboplastin time, and a platelet count of 110,000 mm^{-3}. His bilirubin was 8.1 mg/dL; alkaline phosphatase, 272 units/L; AST, 160 units/L; serum albumin, 2.5 mg/dL; and serum cholesterol, 95 mg/dL. Repeat hemoglobin measurement was 8.6 g/dL after 2 units of packed red blood cells and 1 L of saline.

Discussion

Upper gastrointestinal endoscopy certainly provided critical information for the proper management of this patient. Even though bleeding esophageal varices were noted, a complete evaluation of the stomach and duodenum was appropriately performed. Bleeding sources other than esophageal varices are found in 50% of patients with known portal hypertension,[15] thus underscoring the necessity of an accurate diagnosis. All of the risk factors for variceal hemorrhage are not completely known, but the size of varices seems to be the one finding that most directly predicts the risk of bleeding.[16] Although a portal pressure of at least 12 mm Hg is required for the development of varices, it is interesting that the level of portal pressure does not directly correlate with the risk of bleeding.[17] Local factors directly at the varix level such as the tension within the vessel wall itself seem to be important in the pathogenesis of bleeding. Physicians are frequently dissuaded from inserting a nasogastric tube in a patient with cirrhosis because of a fear of traumatizing esophageal varices. This position is overly conservative, and the need to know the severity and activity of gastrointestinal hemorrhages should certainly outweigh the minimal risk of a "diagnostic" nasogastric tube. Prolonged maintenance of a nasogastric tube, especially when the patient is stable, may give rise to problems, however, and should be avoided in the patient with varices.

The mortality of acute variceal bleeding is alarmingly high, with up to 67% of patients dying with each bleeding episode.[18] The popularity of various treatments has waxed and waned over the years, but the present consensus is that stabilization of the patient with pharmacologic treatment prior to institution of more definitive endoscopic sclerotherapy is the best approach. Although sclerotherapy can be done in the acutely bleeding patient, the technical aspects of properly guiding needle placement are obviously easier in a patient with a clear endoscopic field, and stabilization of the patient with vasopressin may improve the success of sclerotherapy.

Intravenous vasopressin lowers portal pressure and controls variceal bleeding 50% to 60% of the time.[19] Intra-arterial infusion of vasopressin has no advantage over constant IV infusion.[20] The infusion should be started at a dose of 0.2 units/min, with a maximum dose up to 0.6 units/min. Complications of vasopressin include hypertension, bradycardia, peripheral vasoconstriction, myocardial ischemia, mesenteric angina, cerebrovascular accidents, and hyponatremia with fluid retention. It should be administered with constant cardiac monitoring and is contraindicated in patients with coronary or systemic vascular compromise. The addition of IV nitroglycerin, 40 μg/min and titrated by 40-μg increments, to maintain a systolic blood pressure of 100 to 110 mm alleviates some of the systemic vasoconstrictive effects of vasopressin and protects against complications without a loss of effect on controlling variceal hemorrhage.[21]

If vasopressin succeeds in stabilizing the patient, endoscopic sclerotherapy can be done in a calmer environment. If bleeding continues, one should attempt sclerotherapy or proceed to balloon tamponade. Sclerotherapy involves an injection of small amounts of a sclerosing solution such as sodium morrhuate through an endoscopically placed 25-gauge needle directly into the varices. Although technical aspects may vary (type and amount of sclerosant used, paravariceal or intravariceal injection, etc.), sclerotherapy controls active bleeding in a substantial number of patients.[22, 23] The overall experience also suggests that sclerotherapy reduces the rebleeding rate and improves long-term survival in patients with bleeding esophageal varices when compared with the "standard" treatments. Sclerotherapy, however, is not beneficial in preventing bleeding in patients who have not bled and should not be performed prophylactically.[24, 25] Sclerotherapy is not an innocuous procedure, and complications such as esophageal perforation, pleural effusion, respiratory failure, bacteremia, and esophageal stricture have been infrequently described.[26]

Balloon tamponade of bleeding esophageal varices may be as effective as vasopressin in controlling bleeding[27] but, because of its risk and patient discomfort, should be reserved for patients not responding to sclerotherapy or vasopressin infusion. Triple (Sengstaken-Blakemore) or quadruple (Minnesota) lumen tubes contain a large-bore nasogastric tube with two inflatable balloons (Fig 20–1). The distal balloon is round, is situated in the stomach, and when pulled back and attached to traction, mechanically tamponades varices at the gastroesophageal junction. The proximal balloon is sausage shaped and lies in the esophagus. It is connected to a mercury blood pressure manometer by a Y connector and, when inflated to pressures above portal pressure (usually 25 to 45 mm Hg), impedes filling of esophageal varices. A

TRACTION AND
SUCTION

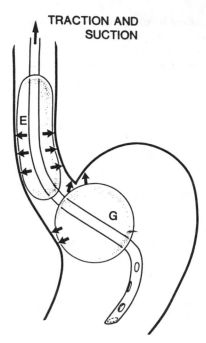

FIG 20–1.
Diagram showing placement of a Sengstaken-Blakemore tube. E = esophageal balloon; G = gastric balloon pulled into the gastroesophageal junction.

separate nasogastric tube is passed coaxially along the Sengstaken-Blakemore tube and positioned above the esophageal balloon to aspirate nasopharyngeal secretions. The Minnesota tube has a "built-in" proximal aspiration port as its fourth lumen. The gastric balloon should be filled with 50 mL of air and its position radiologically verified to be below the diaphragm prior to full inflation of 400 mL. The gastric balloon should be inflated and traction applied for at least 1 hour before going to esophageal balloon inflation. The gastric balloon may control bleeding and avoids the worrisome complications of pulmonary aspiration, esophageal necrosis, and rupture that can occur with inflation of the esophageal balloon. Pulmonary aspiration can be a major problem with these tubes, and every effort should be directed toward protecting the airway. Prophylactic airway intubation is an advisable precaution in almost every case. If hemostasis is achieved and persists for 24 hours, the esophageal balloon (if inflated) should be deflated, and traction should be released. If the patient remains stable over the next 6 to 12 hours, the gastric balloon should be deflated, but the tube should remain in place for a few additional hours in case bleeding recurs. Tamponade should not be maintained for more than 48 hours, and if bleeding recurs, other options, if not already attempted, should be tried.

Emergency surgery should be reserved for the minority of patients (15% to 25%) who continue to bleed despite treatment with vasopressin, endoscopic sclerotherapy, or balloon tamponade. Operative mortalities for emergency portosystemic decompression are substantial and directly correlate with the degree of hepatic compromise.

Patients with liver disease frequently have abnormal coagulation. Vitamin K administration is usually ineffective in parenchymal liver disease, but 3 to 4 units of fresh frozen plasma will usually correct the coagulopathy. Thrombocytopenia may need treatment with platelet transfusions.

Even though the patient is bleeding from esophageal varices, the potential for complications such as sepsis, pulmonary aspiration, or liver failure raise the possibility of developing diffuse erosive gastritis. Prevention of this lethal complication is crucial. Hourly antacids, histamine H_2 antagonists, or sucralfate have been successfully used in this setting.[10] Maintaining the gastric pH at levels above 4 probably provides the best insurance against developing significant gastric stress erosions. As a matter of fact, the early and nearly universal institution of such measures in the ICU has dramatically reduced the morbidity of this previously fatal complication.

CASE STUDY 1 CONTINUED

The patient was administered an infusion of vasopressin of 0.2 units/min and nitroglycerin at 40 μg/min. His bleeding decreased over the next 4 hours, and emergency sclerotherapy was performed. Multiple variceal columns at the gastroesophageal junction were injected with a total of 18 mL of 5% sodium morrhuate. Cimetidine, 300 mg IV every 6 hours, was also started, and the patient was given 3 units of fresh frozen plasma. A follow-up hemoglobin value was stable at 9 g/dL, and the nasogastric tube was removed. The patient was stable overnight and oriented but became progressively agitated and combative the next morning. His blood pressure and pulse were 110/80 mm Hg and 100/min without orthostatic changes. His respiratory rate was moderately increased at 22/min. His temperature was 37.3°C orally. Laboratory measurements revealed serum K, 4.6 mEq/L; serum Cl, 100 mEq/L; blood urea nitrogen (BUN), 23 mg/dL; glucose, 190 mg/dL; bilirubin, 2.8 mg/dL; hemoglobin, 9.2 g/dL; and prothrombin time 1 second above control. His white blood cell (WBC) count was 12,500 mm^{-3} with 12% band forms. Arterial blood gas analysis on room air revealed a pH of 7.48, a P_{CO_2} of 28 mm Hg, and a P_{O_2} of 86 mm Hg. Serum ammonia was 131 mg/dL (normal range: 11 to 35 mg/dL). Chest x-ray findings were normal except for some blunting of the left costophrenic angle.

Blood and urine were cultured, and cefoxitin, 2 g IV every 6 hours, was started. A tap water enema was administered, and lactulose, 30 mL orally every 6 hours, was administered.

Discussion

This patient demonstrates a very common problem seen in the cirrhotic patient with gastrointestinal hemorrhage. His agitation may be a manifestation of hepatic encephalopathy. Upper gastrointestinal bleeding loads the gut with a ready protein source for bacteria to catabolize and can precipitate hepatic encephalopathy. Although this patient's serum ammonia level is elevated and supports the diagnosis of hepatic encephalopathy, serum ammonia levels do not directly correlate with encephalopathy and may be normal.[28] Clinical judgment is critical. If you think that the patient may be encephalopathic, do not hesitate to treat for this while ruling out other causes of altered mentation.

Hepatic encephalopathy is a reversible condition that occurs in acute or chronic liver disease when the liver is unable to clear toxic products of intestinal origin. These toxic products dampen cerebral function and produce electroencephalographic (EEG) evidence of increased slow-wave activity. The clinical manifestations of hepatic encephalopathy are many and may be subtle. Early encephalopathy may be manifested by irritability, personality changes, or reversal of day-night sleep patterns.[29] As encephalopathy progresses, asterixis of the hands and tongue may develop, and the patient becomes increasingly lethargic. Ultimately, the patient lapses into deep coma, at times with decerebrate posturing.

The exact cause of hepatic encephalopathy is unknown. Multiple candidate toxins have been proposed and studied. Although ammonia has received the most scrutiny, it is probably not the only factor involved. False neurotransmitters,[30] mercaptans,[31] short-chain amino acids,[32] and γ-aminobutyric acid[33] have also been suggested as causes of hepatic encephalopathy. It is important to remember, however, that most of the candidate toxins are nitrogenous products of gut origin that bypass the cirrhotic liver and reach the brain. They undoubtedly act synergistically in depressing central nervous system (CNS) function. Furthermore, treatment directed at reducing intraluminal gut protein and bacterial action is successful in ameliorating hepatic encephalopathy.

The diagnosis of hepatic encephalopathy is usually made clinically. Although EEG evidence of slow-wave activity, especially over the frontal lobes, is suggestive, it is not specific and may be seen in a variety of metabolic encephalopathies. Measurement of ammonia levels may not always be reliable or clinically useful and is not a critical diagnostic feature of hepatic encephalopathy. There is frequently little correlation between the level of serum ammonia and the extent of encephalopathy, and hepatic encephalopathy may occur with normal ammonia levels.[34] Often the diagnosis of hepatic encephalopathy is best established by initiating therapy and observing the response.

A persistent search for percipitating factors is mandatory. Hepatic encephalopathy is not spontaneous except in the terminal stages of liver disease. Silent infections (especially spontaneous bacterial peritonitis), volume depletion, overuse of diuretics, sedatives, gastrointestinal bleeding, and excessive dietary protein can all cause hepatic encephalopathy, and each factor should be carefully excluded.

The treatment of hepatic encephalopathy involves several steps: (1) identify and correct any percipitating factors, as described above. (2) Limit the amount of dietary protein that can reach the intestine. If a patient is very ill, all feedings should be held. If alert enough to protect his airway, a protein-restricted diet (e.g.,. 40 g) can be given. Vegetable protein seems to be less comagenic than animal protein is.[35] (3) Cleanse the colon of nitrogenous waste and bacteria. The use of tap water enemas or laxatives such as citrate of magnesia can be very effective in initiating this process. The synthetic disaccharide lactulose, given orally at 15 to 30 mL three times daily (TID) or 300 mL diluted with 700 mL of tap water as an enema TID, should be administered. Lactulose passes unchanged into the colon, where it is fermented by bacteria into lactic acid and lowers stool pH. The osmotic effects of unabsorbed lactulose promote diarrhea, thereby emptying the colon of potential nitrogenous toxins. The acidic stool pH traps ammonia in its nonabsorbable state (NH_4^+), reduces its absorption, and also inhibits intestinal formation of short-chain fatty acids.[36] Neomycin, 1 g four times daily orally or by enema with a laxative, is as effective as lactulose in reducing the nitrogen load within the gut.[37] However, a minimal amount of neomycin may be absorbed, and there is some worry about nephrotoxicity and ototoxicity, especially in the patient with renal impairment. In the severely ill patient, lactulose and neomycin can be combined with some synergistic therapeutic benefit.[38]

Sepsis can be subtle in the cirrhotic. If you wait for such typical signs of sepsis as fever and impressive leukocytosis, the game could be lost, especially in the encephalopathic patient. Appropriate cultures, including paracentesis to rule out spontaneous bacterial peritonitis, should be done, and if the patient's condition is at all questionable, broad-spectrum antibiotics should be administered. Aminoglycosides carry an increased risk of nephrotoxicity in the cirrhotic and should be avoided, if possible.[39]

CASE STUDY 1 CONTINUED

The patient improved over the next 24 hours without evidence of continued gastrointestinal bleeding. He was fully oriented and appropriate. He had 6 to 7 watery bowel movements in 24 hours, the lactulose dosage was reduced to 15 mL orally every 8 hours, and he was given a regimen of clear liquids. His hemoglobin stayed at 9.2 g/dL, and his electrolyte levels were normal. The vasopressin and nitroglycerin infusions were stopped. The patient remained stable over the next 12 hours and was transferred to a general medical floor for continued treatment and investigation into the etiology of his chronic liver disease.

Discussion

The patient had an appropriate response to lactulose and was placed on a lower maintenance schedule. Once the mental status clears, the best way to titrate the lactulose dose is to adjust it according to the volume of diarrhea—aiming for 2 to 3 semisolid movements daily. Although frequently done, the vasopressin infusion does not have to be slowly tapered, and there is no evidence that continuing vasopressin therapy beyond 24 hours will prevent rebleeding from esophageal varices. The patient will need close follow-up, and a series of endoscopic sclerotherapy sessions to obliterate his varices should be planned.

LOWER GASTROINTESTINAL BLEEDING

Lower gastrointestinal hemorrhage is a disease of the elderly, with an average age of 65 years on presentation. The causes of lower gastrointestinal bleeding are also multiple (Table 20–2), but diverticular hemorrhage, bleeding colonic vascular ectasia, and clinically unsuspected upper gastrointestinal hemorrhage account for fully 90% of the cases.[40]

CASE STUDY 2

A 78-year-old woman was brought to the emergency room at 8 A.M. because of bright red rectal bleeding. The bleeding started suddenly and awakened the patient from sleep at

TABLE 20–2.
Causes of Lower Gastrointestinal Bleeding

Large-bowel lesions
  Diverticular disease
  Angiodysplasia
  Upper gastrointestinal bleeding
  Neoplasms
  Inflammatory bowel disease
  Ischemic colitis
  Anal fissure
  Hemorrhoids
  Radiation proctitis
Small-bowel lesions
  Aortoenteric fistula
  Crohn's disease
  Meckel's diverticulum
  Neoplasms (cancer and lymphoma)
  Potassium-induced ulcers
  Radiation enteritis
  Arteriovenous malformations and angiodysplasia
  Intussusception

6 A.M. She had three large bloody movements in the space of 2 hours and now felt dizzy and weak. She denied abdominal pain, vomiting, or previous gastrointestinal bleeding. She took no medications and did not use alcohol. Her blood pressure was 90/60 mm Hg, and her pulse was 120/min supine and 70/40 mm Hg and 140/min upright. Her heart and lung examination was normal, and the abdomen was benign. A large-bore IV line was inserted, and she was given normal saline at 250 mL/hr. Blood was sent for crossmatch, electrolyte, and coagulation studies. Her hemoglobin concentration was 7.2 g/dL. A nasogastric tube was inserted and revealed only bile-stained drainage.

Discussion

This patient presents the picture of acute lower gastrointestinal hemorrhage. The first priority lies in fluid resuscitation and correction of obvious hypovolemia. It should be remembered that gastrointestinal bleeding that is hemodynamically apparent indicates a loss of at least 15% of the blood volume and requires quick restitution of colloid. Warmed, packed red blood cell transfusions are the most appropriate, but on occasion in the massive bleeder, whole blood could be used. The coagulation status should be regularly checked, and each 6-unit administration of packed red blood cells suggests the need for a supplementary unit of fresh frozen plasma. Vitamin K, 10 mg IV or subcutaneously (SC), should be given if the prothrombin time is prolonged but is of little help in patients with severe parenchymal hepatic disease. Each 10-unit administration of packed red blood cells suggests the need for a 10-unit platelet transfusion. Calcium is an essential cofactor for coagulation, and citrate may chelate calcium in banked blood products. Transfusions over 50 mL/min may overwhelm calcium homeostasis and dictate a need for judicious calcium supplementation, especially in patients with depressed myocardial function. Potassium intoxication may occur if large quantities of banked blood are infused. The concentration of potassium in stored blood rises with time and may approach levels of 30 mEq/L. 2,3-Diphosphoglycerate concentrations are low in stored blood and may adversely effect the delivery of oxygen to the tissues.

The next priority is the expeditious diagnosis of the cause of bleeding. Lower gastrointestinal bleeding is notoriously intermittent and therefore difficult to accurately localize. By the time diagnostic forces are mobilized the patient may have stopped bleeding or slowed enough to be below the sensitivity of available diagnostic tests. It is usually far more important to know the general location of the lower gastrointestinal bleeding rather than the specific nature of the lesion, and the clinician can take comfort in the fact that 75% of even massively bleeding patients will stop bleeding spontaneously.[41] Nuclear imaging techniques may be helpful. Technetium–sulfur colloid is rapidly cleared from the intravascular space and can localize bleeding sites with bleeding rates as low as 0.05 mL/min.[42] Although the sensitivity of this test is excellent, the intermittency of bleeding and the rapid clearance of labeled sulfur colloid really limit its usefulness. Technetium-labeled red blood cells are cleared slowly. This type of labeling is theoretically more advantageous in that the patient can be scanned repeatedly for as long as 24 hours after a single injection and positive scans may correctly localize bleeding 91% of the time.[43] The realities of lower gastrointestinal bleeding, however, have not always supported the diagnostic accuracy of nuclear angiography. False negative and positive scans occur and may confuse the situation. Nuclear scanning, however may be a reasonable indicator of poor outcome and, because it seems to correlate with the severity of bleeding, may predict and guide successful angiography.[43]

Superselective angiography can localize bleeding with moderate bleeding rates of 2 mL/min and is probably the procedure of choice in active lower gastrointestinal bleeding.[44] Diverticular hemorrhage, arteriovenous malformations, and neoplasms can be recognized and potentially treated with vasoconstrictor therapy or embolization if the bleeding continues and surgery is not an acceptable option.

Emergency colonoscopy is an attractive option in acute lower gastrointestinal hemorrhage. When done in an unprepared patient, it is a laborious and inaccurate examination, but when done immediately after the administration of large-volume oral lavage solutions, it can establish the etiology and site of bleeding in nearly 90% of patients.[45] Unprepared flexible sigmoidoscopy or rigid proctoscopy can be a rewarding diagnostic first step when it reveals active perianal bleeding, but the difficulties in visualization and the ability of blood to reflux long distances in the colon mitigate against the clinical usefulness of this examination in severe lower gastrointestinal bleeding.

It is important to remember that 10% or more of lower gastrointestinal bleeding is from the upper tract even in the face of a clear nasogastric aspirate.[45] Upper gastrointestinal endoscopy may be an appropriate and time-saving diagnostic first step.

Barium studies of the colon should be avoided in the acute stage of lower gastrointestinal hemorrhage. Although diverticular disease and malignancy can be diagnosed, these lesions could be innocent bystanders and not the actual cause of bleeding. In addition, localization of specific bleeding sites would be impossible with angiography in the face of even minute amounts of retained barium.

CASE STUDY 2 CONTINUED

The patient was sent to the nuclear medicine department for an emergency technetium-labeled red blood cell scan, which suggested extravasation in the left lower quadrant. Angiography of the celiac axis and superior and inferior mesenteric arteries, however, failed to reveal any extravasation or potential bleeding sites. A catheter was left in the inferior mesenteric artery and secured in the groin, and the patient was transferred to the ICU. Observation over the next 24 hours did not support any recurrent gastrointestinal bleeding, and the arterial catheter was removed. The patient remained stable and underwent colonoscopy 3 days after admission. Colonoscopy revealed only extensive diverticulosis of the descending and sigmoid colons.

Discussion

Angiography can be a therapeutic option in some patients with uncontrolled hemorrhage who are deemed to have an unacceptable surgical risk. Obviously, the bleeding rate should be substantial, but a superselective intra-arterial infusion of vasopressin or embolization can be lifesaving in some patients. Although more frequently used in upper gastrointestinal bleeding, therapeutic angiography can also be beneficial in colonic diverticular bleeding. The risks for colonic ischemia always need to be remembered, however. Gastrointestinal bleeding is typically intermittent, and if the initial study does not reveal a bleeding source, the intra-arterial catheter may be left in place for 24 hours to permit easy reexamination if bleeding recurs. Colonoscopy documented extensive left-sided diverticulosis in this patient, but the diagnosis of diverticular hemorrhage remains presumptive because actual visualization of bleeding was not achieved.

LIVER FAILURE

Life-threatening complications of liver disease are not uncommon. Although these complications can be generically lumped under the category of "liver failure," they are distinct syndromes. Several complications are specifically encountered in the ICU: hepatic encephalopathy (see case 1), acute hepatic failure, and hepatorenal syndrome.

CASE STUDY 3

A 22-year-old man, a known heroin addict, came to the emergency room complaining of tremendous fatigue, low-grade fever, and yellow discoloration of his skin and eyes. Physical examination revealed a blood pressure of 110/90 mm Hg, a pulse of 90/min, a temperature of 37.8°C, and a respiratory rate of 12/min. His sclerae and skin were deeply icteric. His liver was soft but enlarged to 15 cm by percussion and somewhat tender. His spleen tip was palpable at the left costal margin. There was no ascites and no stigmata of chronic liver disease. He was oriented but lethargic and had mild asterixis of both hands. Multiple blood cultures were drawn, and the patient was admitted to the hospital with the diagnosis of acute hepatitis. Laboratory data revealed AST of 1,250 units/L, ALT of 1,125 units/L, alkaline phosphatase of 520 units/L, serum bilirubin of 13 mg/dL, prothrombin time 7 seconds prolonged over control, partial thromboplastin time 10 seconds prolonged over control, platelet count of 80,000 mm^{-3}, hemoglobin of 13 g/dL, and WBC count of 4,500 mm^{-3}. His BUN was 10 mg/dL, and serum creatinine was 0.9 mg/dL. Hepatitis serologies revealed a positive IgG antibody to hepatitis A, positive hepatitis B antigen, positive hepatitis E antigen, negative hepatitis E antibody, negative hepatitis B core antibody, and negative hepatitis B antibody. The administration of IV dextrose with 0.5 normal saline was needed because the patient vomited on attempted oral feeding. As the day progressed, he became more lethargic and wanted to be left alone so he could sleep. The next day he seemed more lethargic and was disoriented to place and time. The asterixis was more pronounced. His electrolyte levels were normal, but his blood glucose concentration was 50 mg/dL, and his prothrombin time was 10 seconds prolonged over control. He was given a bolus of 50 mL of 50% dextrose and transferred to the ICU for observation. A neurologic consultant recommended intracranial pressure monitoring.

Discussion

Acute fulminant hepatic failure is a lethal disease with an overall mortality of 50% to 90%.[46, 47] The most common cause is acute hepatitis resulting from infection with hepatitis B, non-A/non-B, and A viruses. Drug-induced necrosis from halothane or acetaminophen overdose constitutes the next largest group.[48] There has been some encouraging improvement in survival statistics over the last 15 years. This improvement is not the result of successful treatment of the primary liver disease but a consequence of modern techniques of critical care and management of complications. The initial enthusiasm about charcoal hemoperfusion has waned because controlled trials have failed to support its efficacy in fulminant hepatic failure.[49] Although the key to successful management of acute hepatic failure lies in the recognition and treatment of various systemic complications, it should be stressed that hepatic transplantation is certainly a viable option in some patients and contact with a liver transplant center early in a patient's course is recommended.

The effects of acute fulminant hepatic failure are multisystemic. Cerebral edema is a lethal complication in 50% to 80% of cases.[50] Increasing intracranial pressure will lead to respiratory arrest and death. The traditional signs of cerebral edema such as myoclonus, bradycardia, vomiting, and papilledema may be unreliable, and the use of intracranial pressure monitoring is strongly recommended.[51] Increasing intracranial pressure in the face of systemic hypotension and decreased cerebral perfusion may be especially lethal, and efforts should be directed toward maintaining intracranial pressure below 30 mm Hg and cerebral perfusion above 40 mm Hg. The etiology of cerebral edema in acute hepatic failure is uncertain, and its absence in hepatic encephalopathy is puzzling. The acute effects of hepatically uncleared toxins on the blood-brain barrier or vasogenic edema induced by increased brain vascular permeability are the leading theories.[52] Corticosteroids have not proved useful in reducing intracranial pressure, and the treatment of choice is IV mannitol.[53] Mannitol, 0.5 g/kg, is rapidly infused, and serum osmolarity is periodically monitored and kept at 310 to 320 mOsm.[53] Other measures that may be helpful in reducing intracranial pressure include elevation of the top half of the body at 30 degrees and aggressive treatment of hyperthermia.[52]

Acute hepatic failure depletes liver glycogen stores and blocks the liver's ability to respond to gluconeogenesis. The resultant hypoglycemia can be profound and may aggravate CNS depression. Large amounts of IV glucose may be needed to support glucose homeostasis.

Coagulopathy is a common problem in acute hepatic failure. The liver is the principal site of the synthesis of fibrinogen and factors II, V, VII, IX, and X. Whereas the half-life of the other factors is in the range of 1 to 3 days, factors V and VII can be depleted in a matter of hours, and changes in coagulation parameters may be sudden.[54] Frequent correction with infusions of fresh frozen plasma is recommended. Exchange plasmapheresis with fresh frozen plasma rapidly corrects coagulation defects and avoids the risk of fluid overload in these marginal patients.[28]

Respiratory problems are frequently encountered. Ventilatory failure with depression of the respiratory drive may occur and require mechanical ventilation. Noncardiogenic pulmonary edema is also a common problem that requires positive end-expiratory pressure (PEEP) therapy and appropriate invasive pulmonary artery pressure monitoring.

CASE STUDY 3 CONTINUED

The patient's blood pressure was 120/95 mm Hg, his pulse was 60/min, and his temperature was 101°F. Initial intracranial pressure was 45 mm Hg, and the patient was given 25 g of IV mannitol as a bolus. Three units of fresh frozen plasma were transfused, and a solution of 10% dextrose with 0.5 normal saline was infused at 100 mL/hr. A nasogastric tube was inserted, and the patient was given 30 mL of liquid antacid every hour in an attempt to keep the gastric pH above 4. The patient's lethargy and confusion continued over the next 24 hours. His intracranial pressure was maintained at 25 to 30 mm Hg with periodic infusions of mannitol. His urine output averaged 125 mL/hr for the first 24 hours but dropped to 40 mL/hr on the second ICU day. His BUN was 24 mg/dL, and serum creatinine was 1.8 mg/dL. The patient's fluids were increased to 200 mL/hr, and he was given 20 mg of IV furosemide as well as an additional 3 units of fresh frozen plasma. Despite the fluid challenge his urine output averaged 30 mL/hr over the next 4 hours. The patient's physical examination revealed a blood pressure of 100/60 mm Hg and a pulse of 88/min without orthostatic drop, and his neck veins were visible in the supine position.

Discussion

Progressive oliguria and a rising creatinine concentration have devastating consequences in a patient with liver disease. Hepatorenal syndrome is a unique form of oliguric renal failure seen in the presence of severe liver disease and in the absence of other causes of renal failure. It is most commonly encountered in fulminant hepatic failure or in decompensated cirrhosis with obvious portal hypertension and tense ascites. The clinical course is variable, but the mortality is uniformly high, approaching 100%.[55] Frequently accompanied by relative hypotension, it is diagnosed by excluding other causes of acute renal failure, a characteristic set of urinary electrolyte values, and the failure of fluid expansion to reverse the renal insufficiency. It mimics the picture of exaggerated prerenal azotemia and hypovolemia and is characterized by a very low urine sodium level (less than 5 Meq/L) and a urine-to-plasma creatinine ratio greater than 20.[56] Impairment of hepatic urea synthesis limits the reliability of BUN readings and BUN-to-creatinine ratios in chronic cirrhosis. Hepatorenal syndrome may occur spontaneously, but relative or absolute hypovolemia is a very frequent precursor. It is a rare event outside the hospital setting and is frequently iatrogenically induced. Precipitating factors such as excessive diuretic therapy, nephrotoxic antibiotics, nonsteroidal anti-inflammatory drugs, silent sepsis, gastrointestinal bleeding, and large-volume paracentesis are usually found. The precise pathogenesis of hepatorenal syndrome remains unknown, but intense intrarenal cortical vasoconstriction plays a critical role.[57] The etiology of the vasoconstriction is not clear, but reduced renal production of vasodilating prostaglandins[58] or circulation of hepatically uncleared vasoactive substances[59] are factors that have been incriminated. Although hemodialysis can buy time, direct treatment of established hepatorenal syndrome has uniformly failed except in a few unique instances. Hepatic transplantation has totally reversed the renal failure, may be an option in the properly selected patient, and may become the treatment of choice.[60] In spite of uniform renal vasoconstriction, the use of angiotensin-converting enzyme inhibitors and other vasodilators has not been successful and has caused hypotension.[61] Low-dose dopamine may improve the renal function of some cirrhotics,[62] but its efficacy in hepatorenal syndrome is doubtful. Since many patients teeter on the brink of hepatorenal syndrome, early and aggressive treatment of mild renal insufficiency in cirrhosis is imperative. Precipitating factors, as described earlier, need to be sought out and treated. All diuretic therapy should be stopped. Unrecognized sepsis is always a problem, and broad-spectrum, nonnephrotoxic antibiotics frequently need to be empirically started after appropriate cultures. It is critical to ensure adequate intravascular volume because intense prerenal azotemia can mimic all the clinical and laboratory features of hepatorenal syndrome. Infusion of saline and colloids (e.g., albumin, 25 g every 8 hours) should be done in each patient until clinical examination or, preferably, Swan-Ganz catheterization indicates an adequate intravascular fluid status. If significant ascites is present, peritoneovenous shunting with its immediate redistribution of ascitic fluid to the intravascular compartment has had some rare and anecdotal successes in reversing hepatorenal syndrome, but its use is controversial.[63]

CASE STUDY 3 CONTINUED

Urinalysis was unremarkable, and spot urine electrolytes revealed sodium at 1 Meq/L, chloride at 5 Meq/L, and potassium at 23 Meq/L. Fluids were increased to 250 mL/hr, and the patient was given 25 g of salt-poor albumin every 8 hours. In spite of these interventions his urine output remained at 20 to 30 mL/hr over the next day. Blood chemistries on the third ICU day revealed a BUN of 34 mg/dL and serum creatinine of 2.3 mg/dL. The lung fields on chest x-ray remained clear. Urine and multiple blood cultures were sent, and the patient was administered cefotetan, 2 g IV every 12 hours. In addition, IV dopamine at a dosage of 2 µg/kg/min was started in an attempt to improve renal perfusion. Despite these efforts, the patient's urine output continued to drop, and his mentation progressively decreased to the point of coma. Charcoal hemoperfusion through a femoral catheter was initiated. The patient's blood pressure dropped several times during the 10-hour hemoperfusion, and he required larger doses of dopamine. At the end of the hemoperfusion, the patient's level of coma was unchanged, and he was noted to have a melanotic stool and spontaneous skin and mucosal bleeding. At this time his hemoglobin content was 9 g/dL; platelet count, 33,000 mm^{-3}; prothrombin time, 13 seconds prolonged; activated partial thromboplastin time, 12 seconds prolonged; fibrin degradation products, greater than 40 μg/mL; BUN, 52 mg/dL; and creatinine, 3.1 mg/dL. The patient was transfused with 2 units of packed red blood cells, 10 units of random-donor platelets, and 4 units of fresh frozen plasma. Ranitidine, 50 mg IV every 8 hours, was administered. The patient developed progressive metabolic acidosis and sustained ventricular fibrillation that was refractory to resuscitation and died on the fifth ICU day.

Discussion

Unfortunately, the outcome of this patient with fulminant hepatic failure is not unusual. Patients with fulminant hepatic failure regardless of the etiology have a survival rate of only 20% or less with even the most intensive medical treatment. The development of hepatorenal syndrome was an especially ominous event. Although an initial experience with charcoal hemoperfusion in the treatment of fulminant hepatic failure was encouraging,[64] subsequent controlled trials have failed to document any benefit.[65] The mounting successful experience with hepatic transplantation makes this an increasingly important consideration in any patient with fulminant hepatic failure.[66] Although organ transplantation in the setting of a positive hepatitis B antigen guarantees ultimate infection of the transplanted liver, this treatment is lifesaving and offers an immediate survival rate of at least 55%.[67] With continuous improvement in technique and availability of donor livers, transplantation should be considered as a viable therapeutic alternative earlier than ever before.

REFERENCES

1. Peterson WL, Barnett CC, Smith HJ, et al: Routine early endoscopy in upper gastrointestinal tract bleeding. A randomized, controlled trial. N Engl J Med 1981; 304:925–929.
2. Allan R, Dykes P: A study of the factors influencing mortality rates from gastrointestinal hemorrhage. Q J Med 1976; 180:533.
3. Silverstein FE, Gilbert DA, Tedesco FJ, et al: The National ASGE Survey on Upper Gastrointestinal Bleeding. Parts I, II, III. Gastrointest Endosc 1981; 27:73–101.
4. Clason AE, Macleod DAD, Elton RA: Clinical factors in the prediction of further haemorrhage or mortality in acute upper gastrointestinal haemorrhage. Br J Surg 1986; 73:985–987.
5. Morgan AG, Clamp SE: OMGE International Upper Gastrointestinal Bleeding Survey 1978–82. Scand J. Gastroenterol 1984; 19(suppl):41–58.
6. Fleischer D: Etiology and prevalence of severe persistent upper gastrointestinal bleeding. Gastroenterology 1983; 84:538–43.
7. Swain CP, Storey DW, Brown SG, et al: Nature of the bleeding vessel in recurrently bleeding gastric ulcers. Gastroenterology 1986; 90:595–608.
8. Johnston JH: The sentinal clot/visible vessel revisited. Gastrointest Endosc 1986; 32:239–240.
9. Collins R, Langman M: Treatment with histamine H$_2$ antagonists in acute upper gastrointestinal hemorrhage. N Engl J Med 1985; 3134:660–666.
10. Borrero E, Bank S, Margolis I, et al: Comparison of antacid and sucralfate in the prevention of gastrointestinal bleeding in patients who are critically ill. Am J Med 1985; 79:62–64.
11. Shuman RB, Schuster DP, Zuckerman GR: Prophylactic therapy for stress ulcer bleeding: A reappraisal. Ann Intern Med 1987; 106:562–567.
12. Rikkers LF: Variceal hemorrhage. Gastroenterol Clin North Am 1988; 17:289–301.
13. Sanowski R: Thermal application for gastrointerstinal bleeding. J Clin Gastroenterol 1986; 8:239–244.

14. Hirao M, Kobayashi T, Masuda K, et al: Endoscopic local injection of hypertonic saline epinephrine solution to arrest hemorrhage from the upper gastrointestinal tract. *Gastrointest Endosc* 1985; 31:313–317.
15. Christensen E, Fauerholdt L, Schlichting P, et al: Aspects of the natural history of gastrointestinal bleeding in cirrhosis and the effect of prednisone. *Gastroenterology* 1981; 81:944–952.
16. Lebrec D, DeFleury P, Rueff B, et al: Portal hypertension, size of esophageal varices and risk of bleeding in alcoholic cirrhosis. *Gastroenterology* 1980; 79:1139–1144.
17. Garcia-Tsao G, Groszman RJ, Fisher RL, et al: Portal pressure, presence of gastroesophageal varices and variceal bleeding. *Hepatology* 1985; 5:419–424.
18. Conn HO: Cirrhosis, in Schiff L, Schiff ER (eds): *Disease of the Liver*, ed 5. Philadelphia, JB Lippincott, 1982, p 894.
19. Conn HO, Ramsby GR, Storer EH, et al: Intra-arterial vasopressin in the treatment of upper gastrointestinal hemorrhage: A prospective controlled trial. *Gastroenterology* 1975; 6:211–221.
20. Chojkier M, Groszmann RJ, Atterbury CE, et al: A controlled comparison of continuous intra-arterial and intravenous infusions of vasopressin in hemorrhage from esophageal varices. *Gastroenterology* 1979; 77:540–546.
21. Gimson AE, Westaby D, Hegarty J, et al: A randomized trial of vasopressin and vasopressin plus nitroglycerin in the control of acute variceal hemorrhage. *Hepatology* 1986; 6:406–409.
22. Barsoum MS, Bolous FI, El-Rooby AA, et al: Tamponade and injection sclerotherapy in the management of bleeding oesphageal varices. *Br J Surg* 1982; 69:760–778.
23. Korula J, Balart LA, Radvan G, et al: A prospective, randomized controlled trial of chronic esophageal variceal sclerotherapy. *Hepatology* 1985; 5:584–589.
24. Santangelo WC, Dueno MI, Estes BL, et al: Prophylactic sclerotherapy of large esophageal varices. *N Engl J Med* 1988; 318:814–818.
25. Sauerbruch T, Wotzka R, Kopke W, et al: Prophylactic sclerotherapy before the first episode of variceal hemorrhage in patients with cirrhosis. *N Engl J Med* 1988; 319:8–15.
26. Sanowski RA, Waring JP: Endoscopic techniques and complications in variceal sclerotherapy. *J Clin Gastroenterol* 1987; 9:504–513.
27. Correia JP, Alves-Martins M, Alexandrino P, et al: Controlled trial of vasopressin and balloon tamponade in bleeding esophageal varices. *Hepatology* 1984; 4:885–888.
28. Munoz SJ, Maddrey WC: Major complications of acute and chronic liver disease. *Gastroenterol Clin North Am* 1988; 17:265–287.
29. Gitlin N, Lewis DC, Hinkley L: The diagnosis and prevalence of subclinical hepatic encephalopathy in apparently healthy, nonshunted patients with cirrhosis. *J Hepatol* 1986; 3:75–82.
30. James J, Ziparo V, Jeppson B, et al: Hyperammonemia, plasma amino acid imbalance, and blood-brain amino acid transport: A unified theory of portal systemic encephalopathy. *Lancet* 1979; 2:504.
31. McClain CJ, Zieve L, Doizaki WM, et al: Blood methanethiol in alcoholic liver disease with and without encephalopathy. *Lancet* 1980; 21:318–323.
32. Mortensen PB, Rasmussen HS, Holtug K: Lactulose detoxifies in vitro short-chain fatty acid production in colonic contents induced by blood: Implication for hepatic coma. *Gastroenterology* 1988; 94:750–754.
33. Schafer DF: Hepatic coma: Studies on the target organ. *Gastroenterology* 1987; 93:1132–1134.
34. Munoz SJ, Maddrey WC: Major complications of acute and chronic liver disease. *Gastroenterol Clin North Am* 1988; 17:265–287.
35. Uribe M, Marquez A, Garcia-Ramos G, et al: Treatment of chronic portal-systemic encephalopathy with vegetable and animal protein diets: A controlled crossover study. *Dig Dis Sci* 1982; 27:1109–1116.
36. Elkington SG, Floch MH, Conn HO: Lactulose in the treatment of chronic portal systemic encephalopathy: A double blind clinical trial. *N Engl J Med* 1969; 281:408–412.
37. Atterbury CE, Maddrey WC, Conn HO: Neomycin-sorbitol and lactulose in the treatment of acute portal systemic encephalopathy. *Dig Dis Sci* 1978; 23:398–406.
38. Wever AJ, Fresard KM, Lally BR: Effects of neomycin and lactulose on urea metabolism in cirrhotic subjects. *Gastroenterology* 1982; 82:213–217.
39. Cabera J, Arroyo B, Ballesta AM, et al: Aminoglycoside nephrotoxicity in cirrhosis. Value of urinary beta-2-microglobulin to discriminate functional renal failure from acute tubular damage. *Gastroenterology* 1982; 82:97–105.
40. Potter GD, Sellin JH: Lower gastrointestinal bleeding. *Gastroenterol Clin North Am* 1988; 17:341–357.
41. Buchman TG, Bulkley GB: Current management of patients with lower gastrointestinal bleeding. *Surg Clin North Am* 1987; 67:651–664.
42. Alavi A, Ring EJ: Localization of gastrointestinal bleeding: Superiority of ^{99m}Tc sulfur colloid compared with angiography. *Am J Radiol* 1981; 137:741–748.
43. Markisz JA, Front D, Royal HD, et al: An evaluation of ^{99}Tc-labeled red blood cell scintigraphy for

the detection and localization of gastrointestinal bleeding sites. *Gastroenterology* 1982; 83:394–398.

44. Colacho TA, Forde KA, Patsos TJ, et al: Impact of modern diagnostic methods on the management of active rectal bleeding. *Am J Surg* 1982; 143:607–610.

45. Jensen DM, Machicado GA, Tapia JI: Emergent colonoscopy in patients with severe hematochezia. *Gastroenterology* 1983; 29:177.

46. Gimson AE, O'Grady J, Ede RJ, et al: Late onset hepatic failure: Clinical, serological and histological features. *Hepatology* 1986; 6:288–294.

47. Gimson AES, White YS, Eddleston A, et al: Clinical and prognostic differences in fulminant hepatitis A, B, and non-A, non-B. *Gut* 1983; 24:1194–1198.

48. Sherlock S: *Diseases of the Liver and Biliary System,* ed 7. London, Blackwell Scientific Publications, 1985, p 108.

49. Berk PD, Goldberg JD: Charcoal hemoperfusion: Plus ca change, plus c'est la même chose. *Gastroenterology* 1988; 94:1228–1230.

50. Ede RJ, Gimson AE, Bihari D, et al: Controlled hyperventilation in the prevention of cerebral edema in fulminant hepatic failure. *J Hepatol* 1986; 2:43–51.

51. Hanid MA, Davies M, Mellon PF, et al: Clinical monitoring of intracranial pressure in fulminant hepatic failure. *Gut* 1980; 21:866–869.

52. Ede RJ, Williams R: Occurrence and management of cerebral edema in liver failure, in *Liver Failure.* London, Butler & Tanner, Ltd, 1986.

53. Canalese J, Gimson AE, Davis C, et al: Controlled trial of dexamethasone and mannitol for the cerebral edema of fulminant hepatic failure. *Gut* 1982; 63:625–629.

54. Martinez J, Palascak JE: Homeostatic alterations in liver disease, in Zakin D, Boyer TD (eds): *Hepatology: A Textbook of Liver Disease.* Philadelphia, WB Saunders Co, 1982, p 546.

55. Ring-Larsen H, Palazzo U: Renal failure in fulminant hepatic failure and cirrhosis: A comparison between incidence, types, and prognosis. *Gut* 1981; 22:585–591.

56. Epstein M: Renal functional abnormalities in cirrhosis: Pathophysiology and management, in Zakin D, Boyer TD (eds): *Hepatology: A Textbook of Liver Disease.* Philadelphia, WB Saunders Co, 1982, p 456.

57. Guarner F, Hughes RD, Gimson AE, et al: Renal function in fulminant hepatic failure: Hemodynamics and renal prostaglandins. *Gut* 1987; 28:1643–1647.

58. Arroyo V, Rimola A, Gaya J, et al: Prostaglandins and renal function in cirrhosis. *Prog Liver Dis* 1986; 8:505.

59. Kew MC, Varma R, Williams H, et al: Renal and intrarenal blood flow in cirrhosis of the liver. *Lancet* 1979; 2:504.

60. Wood RP, Ellis P, Starzl TE: The reversal of the hepatorenal syndrome in four pediatric patients following successful orthotopic liver transplantation. *Ann Surg* 1984; 205:415–419.

61. Pariente E, Bataille C, Bercoff E, et al: Acute effects of captopril on systemic and renal hemodynamics and on renal function in cirrhotic patients with ascites. *Gastroenterology* 1985; 88:1255–1259.

62. Barnardo DE, Baldus WP, Haer FT: Effects of dopamine on renal function in patients with cirrhosis. *Gastroenterology* 1970; 58:524–531.

63. Epstein M: The Le Veen shunt for ascites and hepatorenal syndrome. *N Engl J Med* 1980; 302:628–630.

64. Gazzard BG, Portmann B, Weston MJ, et al: Charcoal haemoperfusion in the treatment of fulminant hepatic failure. *Lancet* 1974; 1:1301–1307.

65. O'Grady JG, Gimson AES, O'Brien CJ, et al: Controlled trials of charcoal hemoperfusion and prognostic factors in fulminant hepatic failure. *Gastroenterology* 1988; 94:1186–92.

66. Iwatsuki S, Esquivel CO, Gordon RD, et al: Liver transplantation for fulminant hepatic failure. *Semin Liver Dis* 1985; 5:325–340.

67. Stieber A, Ambrosino G, Van Thiel D, et al: Orthotopic liver transplantation for fulminant and subacute hepatic failure. *Gastroenterol Clin North Am* 1988; 17:157–165.

21 / Chronic Obstructive Pulmonary Disease

Jeffrey Glassroth, M.D.

Chronic obstructive pulmonary disease (COPD) is an imprecise term encompassing a wide variety of chronic respiratory conditions. In this chapter the acronym COPD is used to refer to *chronic bronchitis and emphysema,* although most of the information is applicable to other conditions such as asthma, cystic fibrosis, and bronchiolitis.

Regardless of type or degree of underlying pathology, all COPD patients demonstrate several common characteristics: (1) chronically increased airway resistance resulting in increased work of breathing[1]; (2) decreased efficiency of inspiratory muscles secondary to chronic thoracic hyperinflation[2]; and (3) impaired pulmonary gas exchange due to ventilation-perfusion (V/Q) mismatching and, particularly in emphysema, alveolar-capillary destruction.[3] There is reason to believe that some of these patients have central ventilatory drive dysfunction resulting in diminished responsiveness to increasing arterial Pco_2 or decreasing arterial Po_2.[4]

Patients with stable COPD often manifest arterial hypoxemia (arterial Po_2 <80 mm Hg on room air); however, CO_2 retention (compensated respiratory acidosis) is less common. Although CO_2 retention is most often seen in patients with severe COPD, some retain CO_2 with moderate disease, while others remain normocarbic despite severe airway obstruction. Some event or series of events, when superimposed on these gas exchange deficiencies, may destabilize this precarious homeostasis, exacerbate the patient's symptoms, and cause clinically significant deterioration. Acute respiratory failure superimposed on chronic respiratory failure is a common challenge in critical care medicine. This condition is compatible with arterial blood gas measurements revealing a Po_2 below 55 mm Hg, Pco_2 above 50 mm Hg, and a pH below 7.35, particularly when concomitant metabolic acidosis has been excluded.

Although acute respiratory failure superimposed on COPD is a catastrophic event, appropriate therapy is often lifesaving.[5, 6] Indeed, a 2-year survival rate as high as 72% may be expected when mechanical ventilation is not required.[7] Furthermore, there is evidence that these patients have a life expectancy comparable to that of stable outpatients with the same severity of COPD who have not experienced acute respiratory failure.[7]

PATHOPHYSIOLOGY OF ACUTE RESPIRATORY FAILURE IN CHRONIC OBSTRUCTIVE PULMONARY DISEASE

It is traditionally assumed that a specific event precipitates acute respiratory failure in the COPD patient. Most commonly these are bacterial or viral respiratory infections, myocardial failure, sedative drugs, dehydration, electrolyte imbalance, inappropriate oxygen therapy, air pollution, and less commonly, an increased metabolic demand due to a nonrespiratory febrile illness. Although the precise pathophysiologic mechanisms responsible for acute respiratory failure in COPD are poorly understood, a hallmark is the acute increase in arterial Pa_{CO_2}.

Respiratory Drive

It is commonly thought that stable COPD patients with hypercarbia simply make less effort to ventilate than do their counterparts who do not retain CO_2 because the "respiratory centers" of CO_2 retainers are somehow less responsive to increments in Pa_{CO_2}.[8, 9] There is controversy as to whether the respiratory drive is reduced or increased in COPD patients with CO_2 retention, and recent data suggest that this concept of central CO_2 hyporesponsiveness may be an oversimplification.[10] In any event, it is clear that suppression of the respiratory drive with sedative drugs is likely to have disastrous consequences. The potential role for respiratory stimulants is far less clear: if the respiratory drive is decreased, stimulants may be useful; if the respiratory drive is increased, stimulants at best may be ineffective and at worst may further increase the work of breathing. More information is required before any recommendations can be made.

Respiratory Pattern

A comparison of severe but stable COPD patients with and without CO_2 retention reveals no significant difference in minute ventilation, i.e., CO_2 retainers "breathe" just as much as their normocapneic counterparts. However, CO_2 retainers display a more shallow and rapid breathing pattern that results in significant increase in the physiologic dead space/tidal volume ratio (V_D/V_T).[11, 12] When these observations were extended to COPD patients with acute respiratory failure, it was found they also have relatively well maintained levels of minute ventilation but breathe in a rapid, shallow fashion. In addition, the respiratory drive of these acutely CO_2-retaining patients may far exceed that of normal subjects. As the acute respiratory failure and CO_2 retention subside, the ventilatory pattern normalizes (becoming slower and deeper), which reduces the proportion of dead-space ventilation.[13] Thus, regardless of responsiveness to CO_2 in the stable state, recent evidence suggests that many COPD patients in acute respiratory failure are expending great effort to breathe. The physiologically inefficient rapid, shallow breathing pattern may be the most significant factor responsible for the acute CO_2 retention and respiratory acidosis.

It is known that a rapid and shallow respiratory pattern can be produced experimentally by stimulating airway "irritant" receptors or the juxtacapillary (J) receptors of the interstitial space. Clinical counterparts of these experimental models would be acute bronchitis or air pollution triggering airway receptors and left heart failure producing interstitial edema to stimulate J receptors. Thus, we are starting to gain insights into the mechanisms by which precipitants of acute respiratory failure in COPD might act.

Ventilatory Muscle Fatigue

Rapid and shallow breathing patterns might also arise in an attempt to minimize ventilatory muscle work and thereby limit ventilatory muscle fatigue. Ventilatory muscles are subject to fatigue as are other skeletal muscles,[2, 14] and there is reason to believe that the COPD patient is even more susceptible to fatigue than are normal people. There is a maximum inspiratory pressure any individual can achieve. When normal subjects repetitively generate 50% to 60% of this maximum pressure with each breath, they consistently develop ventilatory muscle fatigue within several minutes. Hyperinflation of normal subjects reduces the critical ratio of inspiratory pressure to the maximum at which fatigue occurs.[14]

Chronic hyperinflation in COPD patients may well make them more prone to fatigue because the inspiratory muscles are at a disadvantageous position on their tension-length curve and this decreases the maximum inspiratory pressures attainable by these muscles.[2, 15] This may have an additive effect in reducing the absolute inspiratory pressure at which ventilatory muscle fatigue occurs. Although adequate inspiratory pressures might be achieved without fatigue in the stable COPD patient, the superimposition of factors such as increased airway resistance or increased ventilatory demand created by an acute febrile illness might produce ventilatory muscle fatigue. Clearly, much more information concerning these issues is required.

Nutritional Status

If ventilatory muscle fatigue is important to the development of respiratory failure, one ought to consider the availability of energy substrate to those muscles. Nutritional surveys demonstrate considerable malnutrition in advanced COPD.[16] Ventilatory muscles appear to be affected to the same extent as other muscle groups by nutritional depletion, with resultant impaired ventilatory muscle function and ventilatory mechanics.[17, 18] Moreover, it is now appreciated that nutritional preparations can affect CO_2 production as well as respiratory center sensitivity to CO_2.[19] It is not known whether nutritional factors alone are sufficient to produce respiratory failure in the COPD patient or whether it is possible to reverse nutritional deficiencies in the ventilatory muscles of the COPD patient.

THERAPY FOR ACUTE RESPIRATORY FAILURE IN CHRONIC OBSTRUCTIVE PULMONARY DISEASE

Specific management related to reversing the precipitants of acute respiratory failure is essential. However, hours to days are sometimes required for such therapy to produce substantial results. Therefore, immediate therapy to decrease airway resistance and improve pulmonary gas exchange is essential in all of these patients, regardless of precipitating events. Airway resistance is diminished by bronchodilator therapy and removal of secretions (bronchial hygiene therapy); gas exchange is improved by oxygen therapy and ventilatory assistance if required. The role of antibiotics remains somewhat controversial, but recent data suggest accelerated physiologic recovery when antibiotics are used to treat acute exacerbations of chronic bronchitis. [20]

Bronchodilator Therapy

Bronchodilators should be administered to all COPD patients in impending or acute respiratory failure. Although many COPD patients do not respond to bronchodilators during periods of relative stability, most of these patients develop some degree of bronchospasm when stressed. In addition, the various agents used to achieve bronchodilation have beneficial effects other than bronchodilation. For example, theophylline may improve diaphragmatic efficiency, [21] and inhaled β-agonists may improve the ciliary clearance of mucus. [22]

Aminophylline

Theophylline has been assumed to accomplish bronchodilation indirectly by inhibiting the enzyme (phosphodiesterase) that destroys bronchiolar smooth muscle cell cyclic adenosine monophosphate (AMP). Because the concentrations of theophylline required to achieve this effect in muscle preparations exceed the levels attained clinically, alternative mechanisms of theophylline action are being sought. The pharmacokinetics of theophylline are well known, and regimens for its safe administration have been developed. Intravenous (IV) administration of aminophylline is preferred with a loading dose of 3 to 6 mg/kg over a period of 20 to 30 minutes, followed by a constant infusion of 0.3 to 0.9 mg/kg/hr. A theophylline serum concentration between 10 and 20 μg/mL is recommended, with maximal physiologic response occurring at the higher range. The loading dose should be diminished or omitted and lower rates of infusion used in patients who have been taking theophylline up to the time of the acute exacerbation and in those with significant cardiac or liver dysfunction. Table 21–1 lists common drugs that interact with theophylline.

β₂-Agonists

β₂-agonists complement theophylline in bronchodilation by increasing the synthesis of bronchial smooth muscle cyclic AMP by stimulating the synthetic enzyme adenyl cyclase. Therefore, they are recommended for coincident administration with theophylline in the COPD patient in acute respiratory failure. Of particular benefit are the inhaled β₂-specific agents, which offer the best potential for benefit with the least chance of side effects. Currently available β₂ agents are listed in Table 21–2.

TABLE 21-1.

Interactions Between Theophylline and Commonly Used Drugs

Drug	Effect on Theophylline Concentration	Probable Theophylline Interaction
Barbiturates	Decreased	Microsomal enzyme induction
Cigarettes*	Decreased	Increased metabolism
Cimetidine	Increased	Microsomal enzyme inhibition
Erythromycin	Increased	Inhibition of metabolism
Phenytoin	Decreased	Enzyme induction (?)
Propranolol	Increased	Decreased clearance

*May be a factor despite recent cessation of smoking.

Inhalation bronchodilator treatments should be given every 2 to 4 hours during the acute phases of the patient's illness, depending on the anticipated half-life of the particular β_2-agonist used.

There are a number of delivery systems available for aerosolizing drugs. Intermittent positive-pressure breathing (IPPB) is seldom necessary since these patients are capable of initiating a reasonable inspiratory VT. In general, the simplest and cheapest means of delivering the drug aerosol is advised.

Corticosteroids

Adrenal corticosteroids have been claimed to be useful in reducing airflow resistance in COPD patients with acute exacerbations not caused by pneumonia. IV methylprednisolone sodium succinate (Solu-Medrol), 0.5 mg/kg every 6 hours for the initial 72 hours of hospitalization, has been shown to produce significant improvements in airflow.[23] The mechanisms by which corticosteroids produce this acute improvement is unknown. In appropriate patients corticosteroids should be given early since it is usually several hours before they begin to act. Early steroid use may obviate the need for mechanical ventilation in some patients. The use of steroids in this acute setting should not be confused with their use in stable COPD patients, in whom the potential benefit is not as well documented.

TABLE 21-2.

β_2-Agonists Currently Available for Aerosol Therapy

Generic Name	Brand Names	Duration of Effect (hr)
Albuterol	Ventolin, Proventil	2-6
Isoetharine	Bronkosol	1-4
Metaproterenol	Alupent, Metaprel	2-6

Anticholinergics

There is considerable evidence that ipratropium bromide, a congener of atropine, is an effective bronchodilator, particularly when used to treat patients with stable COPD. There is relatively little information available concerning the use of this agent in the management of acute exacerbations of COPD.[24]

Bronchial Hygiene Therapy

The COPD patient with acute pulmonary inflammation usually produces significant amounts of mucus that increase airflow resistance unless mobilized from the airways. An intact cough mechanism is undoubtedly the most efficient means of raising these secretions, and indeed, a vigorous directed cough is likely superior to most other physical therapy interventions in raising sputum.[25] Adequate systemic hydration is the second most important factor. Thick tenacious secretions can be rendered less viscous with hydration. Aerosol therapy may be used to facilitate this process, but only when appropriately administered in conjunction with bronchodilators, assistance in coughing and deep breathing, and adequate systemic hydration. Postural drainage and percussion is of no proven value in such patients and carries the risk of acutely reducing arterial oxygen tensions.[26]

When a COPD patient in acute respiratory failure is unable to mobilize secretions adequately despite optimal therapy, tracheal intubation may be required. This is seldom necessary and should be considered only after other therapies have been attempted.

Oxygen Therapy

All COPD patients with acute respiratory failure require oxygen therapy. The goal is to restore the patient's arterial oxygenation status to a level that ensures adequate hemoglobin saturation while approximating the patient's stable baseline. Usually this requires an arterial P_{O_2} of 50 to 60 mm Hg.

The classic explanation for CO_2 retention with oxygen administration has been suppression of the hypoxic drive. In its simplest form, this situation is thought to result from a central CO_2 response that is blunted by chronic CO_2 retention, which leaves only hypoxia-sensitive peripheral chemoreceptor mechanisms intact to drive ventilation.[4] When an increased FIO_2 results in augmentation of the arterial P_{O_2}, a decrease in hypoxic stimulation occurs and causes hypoventilation. Experience in acute respiratory care resulted in abandonment of that "traditional wisdom" in favor of a more complex concept in which additional factors such as changes in the work of breathing, hypoxic vasoconstriction, denitrogenation, and hemoglobin-oxygen affinity relationships are potentially involved.[10, 27]

Suffice it to say that oxygen administration, although clinically necessary, has the risk of augmenting CO_2 retention, and the risk increases with increasing concentrations of inspired oxygen. Since great care must be taken to avoid significant CO_2 retention, precise and consistent inspired oxygen concentrations (FIO_2) are essential.

It is recommended that premixed, high-flow gas delivery systems (e.g., air entrainment masks) be utilized until the patient's condition improves. It is generally prudent to initially administer an FIO_2 of about 0.24. If no significant increment in CO_2 retention results and the Pao_2 is still inadequate, the FIO_2 can be safely increased to 0.28. This procedure should be continued in increments of 0.03 to 0.05 FIO_2. The effects of each FIO_2 increment must be evaluated by clinical assessment as well as by arterial blood gas measurement.

CARDIOVASCULAR SUPPORT

Tissue oxygenation also depends on adequate cardiovascular function and blood flow. Thus, care must be taken to provide appropriate fluid therapy and inotropic support when necessary. These patients may be polycythemic despite adequate hydration. Hematocrits above 55% to 60% can result in hyperviscosity of the blood and can threaten blood flow and tissue oxygen delivery. Phlebotomy is recommended to reduce the red blood cell (RBC) volume to a hematocrit below 55%. No more than a single unit of blood should be removed in one 24-hour period. Phlebotomy should not be substituted for adequate hydration. If the patient has a significant anemia (i.e., hematocrit <30%), RBCs should be administered to optimize oxygen-carrying capacity and the cause of the blood loss evaluated.

VENTILATORY ASSISTANCE

The ability to treat acute respiratory failure in the COPD patient without initiating positive-pressure ventilation has contributed greatly to the long-term survival of this patient population. However, despite aggressive and appropriate therapy, a small but significant number of patients do require mechanical assistance of ventilation.

In the event that adequate levels of arterial oxygenation cannot be attained without an unacceptably high level of CO_2 retention and attendant respiratory acidosis, the institution of mechanical ventilation must be seriously entertained. Considerable attention has been given to identifying the characteristics of those COPD patients who will ultimately fail conservative management and require mechanical ventilation. It appears that patients with either marked hypoxemia (Pao_2 <45 mm Hg) or significant degrees of respiratory acidemia (pH <7.30), marked alterations of mental status, or obvious thoracoabdominal paradoxical breathing suggesting ventilatory muscle fatigue will frequently require mechanical ventilation.[28, 29] While it may still be reasonable to attempt management without mechanical ventilation, these patients will require very close observation, and if they do not begin to improve promptly, intubation and mechanical ventilation are probably indicated.

Once the physician is committed to positive-pressure ventilation, it is essential to maintain the patient's baseline arterial Pco_2. Such "eucapneic" support ensures appropriate acid-base and electrolyte maintenance and also facilitates the weaning process. It is recommended that a Pco_2 level providing a pH between 7.40 and 7.45 be maintained.

Arterial Po_2 levels above 55 mm Hg are of no consequence if the patient is receiving full ventilatory support. However, if only partial support is being provided (i.e., significant effective work of breathing is being provided by the patient), an arterial P_{O_2} approximating the patient's baseline must be maintained. With the above exceptions, principles of ventilator management are similar to those for the general intensive care patient. It is important to remember that the use of mechanical ventilation does not necessarily eliminate all of the patient's work of breathing. Each mechanical system will have its own characteristic elastic threshold loads and expiratory flow resistance. These are of considerable importance when patients are required to spontaneously contribute to the required alveolar minute ventilation, as with the use of intermittent mandatory ventilation (IMV) systems.[30] (See Chapter 3.)

CASE STUDY 1

A retired 63-year-old male truck driver with an 80-pack-year smoking history was brought to the emergency room by ambulance. He had a 6-year history of a chronic productive cough and had had numerous pulmonary function tests demonstrating severe airway obstruction that was not reversible following inhalation of bronchodilators. One year prior to admission his forced inspiratory volume in 1 second (FEV_1) was 0.78 L, and his forced vital capacity (FVC) was 2.2 L (FEV_1/FVC = 33%). On the basis of his chronic cough and pulmonary function test results he was diagnosed as having chronic bronchitis. Arterial blood gases measured 1 year prior to admission showed a P_{O_2} of 52 mm Hg, a P_{CO_2} of 54 mm Hg, and a pH of 7.42 on room air. He had been managed with inhaled bronchodilators and oral theophylline, which together provided some improvement in symptoms. He was relatively active and able to walk several blocks and bowl occasionally without distress. He had no other significant medical problems except for a peptic ulcer 20 years ago. He had no known allergies.

About 10 days prior to admission he noticed increased sputum production and dyspnea after walking less than one block, and his appetite decreased. His sputum became yellow and then somewhat gray, and he began to notice slight swelling in his legs. On the night of admission he began having difficulty raising sputum and complained of severe dyspnea. His wife noted that he was audibly wheezing and called a local ambulance company to transport him to the hospital.

On arrival in the emergency room he was somnolent but arousable. His rectal temperature was 38°C, his blood pressure (BP) was 170/100 mm Hg, his pulse was 110 beats per minute and regular, and respirations were 28/min and shallow. He was diaphoretic with decreased skin turgor. Head and upper respiratory tract examination showed conjunctival injection bilaterally. Diffuse expiratory wheezes were heard bilaterally. He was sitting up and using accessory muscles to breathe. Heart sounds were distant; no gallop was noted. Mild pretibial edema was present. The neurologic examination showed no evidence of abnormality.

Initial laboratory tests disclosed the following values: hemoglobin, 17 gm/dL; hematocrit, 52%; and white blood cell (WB) count, 12,200 mm^{-3} with 58% neutrophils, 5% band forms, 20% lymphocytes, 4% monocytes, and 3% eosinophils. An electrocardiogram (ECG) revealed a sinus tachycardia with right-axis deviation and low voltage in the limb leads. Electrolyte, blood urea nitrogen (BUN), and glucose levels were normal; the bicarbonate concentration was 34 mEq/L. Arterial blood gas values obtained shortly after admission on room air showed a pH of 7.32, a P_{CO_2} of 72 mm Hg, and a P_{O_2} of 44 mm Hg. No acute infiltrate was evident on an anterioposterior portable chest radiograph.

Discussion

The patient's presentation and history suggest chronic CO_2 retention secondary to severe COPD. Since the pH is 7.32 despite a high P_{CO_2}, preexisting metabolic alkalosis exists. Intubation and ventilatory assistance may be avoidable if (1) the work of breathing can be decreased, (2) myocardial work can be diminished, and (3) the ventilatory status can be improved.

A major step toward relieving both the work of breathing and myocardial work would be to improve the arterial oxygenation. The severe arterial hypoxemia and presumptive alveolar hypoxia may significantly increase pulmonary vascular resistance, thereby increasing the cardiac work load. Appropriate oxygen therapy may potentially decrease myocardial work and improve alveolar oxygen tensions without decreasing ventilation. To avoid variations in the F_{IO_2} as ventilatory patterns change, a Venturi-type device should be used to titrate the inspired oxygen concentration.

Decreasing the bronchospasm and facilitating the removal of airway secretions would greatly decrease airway resistance and the work of breathing. Evaluation and appropriate treatment of the presumed pulmonary infection are necessary. Despite dependent edema and cor pulmonale, there is evidence that the patient may be volume depleted. Adequate fluid management is essential.

A major point is that with proper therapy, cardiopulmonary collapse is not imminent. There is a good chance that intubation and ventilatory assistance may be avoided. However, the patient requires close cardiopulmonary monitoring and must be placed in an intensive care environment until his condition stabilizes.

CASE STUDY 1 CONTINUED

A 24% air entrainment mask was applied and an IV line established. A blood specimen was obtained for serum theophylline determination, and then a 3-mg/kg loading dose of aminophylline was administered over a period of 20 minutes, followed by a constant infusion of 0.5 mg/kg/hr. An acetaminophen suppository was administered, and the patient was transported to the intensive care unit. Although the patient was more alert, he was still audibly wheezing, preferred to sit up, and was using accessory muscles. A radial arterial line was inserted for BP monitoring and serial blood gas determinations. A coughed sputum specimen was obtained for wet preparation and Gram stain. Vital signs were as follows: BP, 150/90 mm Hg; pulse, 100 beats per minute and regular; and respirations, 24/min and less shallow. Arterial blood gas analysis with the patient breathing 24% oxygen disclosed a pH of 7.35, a P_{CO_2} of 66 mm Hg, and a P_{O_2} of 50 mm Hg.

Discussion

The patient remained alert and cooperative. Oxygen therapy improved arterial oxygenation without deterioration in the P_{CO_2}. Of course, some of this improvement may be attributed to the aggressive bronchodilator therapy. Many believe that steroid therapy is an important adjunct to bronchodilator therapy in this type of patient. Solu-Medrol, 0.5 mg/kg IV every 6 hours for 3 days, would be an acceptable regimen. Similarly, the administration of an aerosol bronchodilator every 2 to 4 hours may be helpful.

Two options are available at this point in terms of oxygen therapy: either 24% oxygen can be continued, or the FIO_2 can be increased to 0.28. This decision depends on the apparent rate of improvement and the clinical stability of the patient. As long as an arterial PO_2 above 55 to 60 mm Hg is not sought and careful evaluation of the ventilatory status is constantly accomplished, either option is appropriate.

CASE STUDY CONTINUED

The sputum wet preparation showed numerous polymorphonuclear cells, and the Gram stain showed mixed flora, including gram-negative diplococci consistent with *Haemophilus*. Trimethoprim-sulfamethaxazole (TMP-SMX) at a dose of 150 mg (of the trimethoprim component) IV every 6 hours, was initiated.

The FIO_2 was increased to 0.28, with arterial blood gas values determined after 30 minutes and then hourly (or immmediately if the clinical status were to deteriorate). Additionally, metaproterenol, 0.33 cc in 2.5 cc diluent, in conjunction with ultrasonic aerosol therapy was initiated every 4 hours when the patient was awake, and Solu-Medrol therapy was started.

Four hours after admission and 30 minutes following the ultrasonic treatment, the patient was perceptibly more comfortable. His use of accessory muscles had decreased, and he was able to cough up large amounts of yellow-green sputum. Diffuse expiratory wheezing was still present. Bedside spirometry showed an FVC of 1.3 L and an FEV_1 of 0.45 L. The serum theophylline level measured in the emergency room was reported as 7.8 µg/mL, and the aminophylline infusion rate was left at 0.5 mg/kg/hr. The BP was 130/90 mm Hg, the pulse rate was 95 beats per minute and regular, respirations were 20/min, and the temperature was 37.9°C. Arterial blood gas analysis on 28% oxygen disclosed a pH of 7.39, a PCO_2 of 55 mm Hg, and a PO_2 of 63 mm Hg.

Discussion

The patient's condition was obviously stabilizing. The primary concerns now are to optimize medical therapy and prepare for discharge from the intensive care unit to the general floor area. Specifically, the aminophylline infusion rate has to be adjusted, the aerosol therapy and inhaled bronchodilator therapy tapered, and the patient switched to oral fluid intake. Since the respiratory pattern was stable and the cardiopulmonary homeostasis improved, arterial blood gas monitoring should be decreased to an as-needed basis, with oxygen delivery attempted via a more comfortable mode (nasal cannula) as soon as appropriate. This should be accomplished prior to transfer from the intensive care unit.

CASE STUDY CONTINUED

Sixteen hours after admission the patient looked and felt much improved. He had slept several hours and was hungry. Although diffuse audible wheezes were present, the FVC had increased to 1.8 L and the FEV_1 to 0.6 L. A repeat serum theophylline level was 16.4 µg/mL, and the infusion rate was decreased to 0.3 mg/kg/hr. Arterial blood gas values on 1 L per nasal cannula were pH, 7.41; PCO_2, 58 mm Hg; and PO_2, 57 mm Hg.

Thirty hours after admission the patient remained stable and was transferred to the general medical service. He was switched to an oral theophylline preparation and oral antibiotics. Bronchodilator treatments were decreased to four times daily.

He continued to do well, and by the fourth hospital day arterial blood gas analysis on room air showed a pH of 7.41, a P_{CO_2} of 55 mm Hg, and a P_{O_2} of 52 mm Hg. However, on the sixth hospital day he complained of increased cough and shortness of breath and felt feverish. Physical examination revealed a rectal temperature of 38.6°C, a BP of 150/90 mm Hg, a pulse rate of 110 beats per minute and regular, and respirations of 26/min. Chest examination showed scattered expiratory wheezes and an area of increased breath sounds at the right base. A chest x-ray film confirmed the presence of a right lower lobe infiltrate. Arterial blood gas analysis on room air revealed a pH of 7.35, a P_{CO_2} of 60 mm Hg, and P_{O_2} of 46 mm Hg. One liter of oxygen was given via a nasal cannula, following which arterial blood gas values were pH, 7.36; P_{CO_2}, 58 mm Hg; and P_{O_2}, 53 mm Hg.

A sputum Gram stain revealed many neutrophils and clusters of gram-positive cocci. Blood and sputum cultures were obtained, and a tentative diagnosis of staphylococcal pneumonia was made. The TMP/SMX therapy was discontinued, and oxacillin, 1 g IV every 4 hours, was administered. Acetaminophen was given to reduce the fever, and ultrasonic nebulizer with bronchodilator treatments were increased from four times daily to every 4 hours while awake. A serum theophylline level obtained the previous day was 13.8 µg/mL.

Although the development of staphylococcal pneumonia represents a major setback for this patient, his ability to maintain near-baseline blood gas values and his general clinical condition led the physicians to decide to delay transfer to the intensive care unit. Over the next 16 hours the patient's rectal temperature remained below 38.5°C with antipyretic therapy. He began to raise less sputum with bronchial hygiene treatments. Arterial blood gas values remained stable while the tachypnea and tachycardia worsened. The patient began to appear fatigued and complained of increasing shortness of breath. The FVC had decreased to 1.1 L, while the FEV_1 was 0.55 L.

A decision was made to transfer the patient to the intensive care unit, where an arterial line was inserted and nasal oxygen changed to a high-flow Venturi system delivering 28% oxygen. Arterial blood gas values deteriorated over the next 8 hours to a pH of 7.32, a P_{CO_2} of 64 mm Hg, and a P_{O_2} of 44 mm Hg on 28% oxygen. Vital signs were BP, 155/100 mm Hg; pulse, 130 beats per minute; and respirations, 30/min. The patient had no appetite and was unable to sleep. A repeat chest x-ray film showed extension of the right lower lobe infiltrate.

Discussion

Although the patient's alveolar ventilation remained reasonable, it was being maintained at a significant cost in terms of the work of breathing. Several factors were quite different now compared with the previous acute episode in the emergency room. First, the oxygenation deficit was significantly worse; second, airway resistance and vascular volume deficits (which can be reasonably rapidly reversed) were already optimally treated; third, the hospital-acquired pneumonitis was most likely more virulent and more difficult to treat than the presenting acute bronchitis; and fourth, ventilatory muscle fatigue appeared to be a greater factor at this time than when the patient was first admitted to the hospital. Note that the FVC was less than on admission, although the FEV_1 was better. This most likely represented a significant diminution of ventilatory reserve.

The primary factors indicating the need for mechanical ventilation are that respiratory muscle fatigue is apparently developing and the acute pathology is not rapidly reversible. A decision to mechanically ventilate would offer the following advantages: (1) assume the work of breathing, thereby allowing the patient to rest the fatiguing ventilatory muscles; (2) decrease myocardial demands by assuming the work of breathing; (3) allow the patient to sleep; (4) allow aggressive bronchial hygiene therapy via the endotracheal tube; and (5) provide time for the antibiotic therapy to be effective.

Potential complications of such intervention are (1) difficulty with intubation; (2) embarrassment of venous return, requiring IV fluid loading; (3) contamination of the lower airways secondary to intubation; (4) barotrauma; and (5) difficulty weaning from the ventilator.

CASE STUDY CONTINUED

The procedure for a blind nasal intubation was explained to the patient, and adequate topical anesthesia of the nasopharynx, oropharynx, and larynx was accomplished. An 8.5-mm internal diameter tube was inserted without difficulty and positive-pressure ventilation initiated with a self-inflating hand ventilator. Within 2 minutes the patient was fully apneic and asleep, although easily arousable. His BP was 110/70 mm Hg, his pulse rate was 115 beats per minute, and 250 mL of crystalloid was infused over a 10-minute period, which resulted in a BP of 120/80 mm Hg and a pulse rate of 105 beats per minute.

The patient was placed on a volume-cycled ventilator with an IMV circuit at a V_T of 15 mL/kg, a rate of 9/min, and an F_{IO_2} of 0.35. Arterial blood gas analysis then showed a pH of 7.48, a P_{CO_2} of 46 mm Hg, and a P_{O_2} of 110 mm Hg. The ventilator rate was decreased to 8/min, and repeated arterial blood gas analysis showed a pH of 7.45, a P_{CO_2} of 50 mm Hg, and a P_{O_2} of 105 mm Hg. Vital signs were stable, and the patient was sleeping when not disturbed. A chest x-ray film confirmed placement of the endotracheal tube in the middle third of the trachea. The V_T was decreased to 13 mL/kg; repeated arterial blood gas analysis showed a pH of 7.41, a P_{CO_2} of 54 mm Hg, and a P_{O_2} of 101 mm Hg.

Discussion

Intubation was accomplished by the blind nasal technique with topical anesthesia and without sedation. The use of a fiber-optic bronchoscope to accomplish the intubation is appropriate, depending on the experience and preference of the intubating physician. The advantage of having the patient awake during the procedure is that the patient receives no sedation prior to intubation and continues to ventilate spontaneously. Thus, the chances of maintaining adequate gas exchange and cardiovascular function during the procedure are optimized, especially if difficulty is encountered in establishing the airway. A nasal tube is preferable because it is easier to stabilize and is better tolerated by the awake patient than an oral tube.

If an awake nasal technique is not desirable or possible, the next safest method is to preoxygenate and ventilate, administer IV sedation, and with or without muscle relaxation attempt oral intubation with direct laryngoscopy. When the patient's condition stabilizes, a nasal tube can be used to replace the oral tube.

Since a primary reason for instituting positive-pressure ventilation is to rest the respiratory muscles, full ventilatory support is preferable. This patient did what most patients with fatigue do—he became apneic shortly after the work of breathing was provided. With V_Ts of 12 to 15 mL/kg, ventilator rates of 8/min or more usually provide full ventilatory support. Since most patients will make some spontaneous breathing efforts from time to time, some flexibility in technology is desirable so that these efforts will not result in a need for heavy sedation and/or paralysis. This flexibility in administering full ventilatory support is accomplished by use of either assist/control, IMV, or synchronized intermittent mandatory ventilation (SIMV) modes.

The choices among these modes depend primarily on physican preference since most patients can be adequately supported with any of them. The role of the newer pressure support ventilation mode needs further definition. (See Chapter 5.)

It must be appreciated that maintaining the patient at *his* acid-base baseline is essential (eucapneic ventilation). This was accomplished by first decreasing the ventilator rate to 8/min and then decreasing the VT. As a rule, VTs of less than 12 mL/kg are not desirable.

As long as full ventilatory support is the goal, an arterial Po_2 above 60 mm Hg is not undesirable since it will tend to keep this patient's spontaneous efforts to a minimum. However, as soon as the patient is expected to do some of his work of breathing (partial ventilatory support), the FIo_2 should be decreased to bring the Po_2 to the 50–60–mm Hg range, which is normal for this individual.

CASE STUDY CONTINUED

During the next 48 hours the patient remained febrile, and the arterial Po_2 fell to the 60s on an FIo_2 of 0.35. Chest x-ray findings remained unchanged, and large amounts of sputum were suctioned from the endotracheal tube. Sputum cultures confirmed the presence of *Staphylococcus aureus* sensitive to oxacillin. A small-bore feeding tube was inserted to accomplish enteral alimentation with a goal of maintaining a slightly positive nitrogen balance.

By 72 hours following the initiation of ventilatory support there was significant evidence that the pneumonia was resolving in that (1) an afrebrile state for 24 hours ensued, (2) arterial Po_2 increased to 90 mm Hg with a consistent FIo_2 of 0.35, (3) the copious secretions from the endotracheal tube diminished and contained fewer WBCs, and (4) the WBC count had significantly diminished. The patient was able to produce an FVC of 0.9 L with a negative inspiratory force of − 15 cm H_2O, and when removed from the ventilator, his spontaneous respiratory rate was 32/min with a VT of 150 to 225 mL (2 to 3 mL/kg).

Discussion

All evidence suggested that the acute pneumonitis was resolving and that the patient was increasing his ventilatory reserves. However, there was still significant acute pulmonary pathology that would take several more days to reverse. Alimentation had begun to maintain a reasonable nutritional status.

Since it was not yet reasonable to expect the patient to assume all his work of breathing without significant cardiopulmonary stress, removal from the ventilator at this point would have been premature. However, some clinicians prefer to allow the patients to assume some of their work of breathing (partial ventilatory support), while others prefer to keep the patient on full support. Assist modes of ventilation do not allow for partial support; only IMV, SIMV, and pressure support ventilation allow partial support.

CASE STUDY CONTINUED

The patient was placed on an IMV of 4/min during the day and 6/min at night. The FIo_2 was decreased to 0.28, and the representative arterial bood gas values were pH, 7.42; Pco_2, 54 mm Hg; and Po_2, 55 mm Hg. His BP was 125/90 mm Hg, and the pulse was 100 beats per minute. Spontaneous ventilation ranged from 10 to 20/min with VTs of 150 to 400 mL.

On the sixth day of ventilatory support the decision was made that the patient should be able to maintain spontaneous ventilation because his FVC was 1.6 L with a negative inspiratory force of -30 cm H_2O. The chest x-ray film showed further resolution of the pneumonic infiltrate. The WBC count was normal, and the hemoglobin value was 14.6 gm/dL. The serum theophylline level was 13.0 μg/mL. He had been in a 50 degree head-up position during the day since partial ventilatory support had been instituted.

Following bronchial hygiene treatment with a bronchodilator and endotracheal suctioning, the patient was placed on a T piece circuit at an FIO_2 of 0.28. Both BP and pulse rate increased less than 10%, and the patient appeared comfortable without complaint. One hour after he was removed from the ventilator, arterial blood gas analysis showed a pH of 7.39, a PCO_2 of 57 mm Hg, and a PO_2 of 60 mm Hg. The patient was alert and did not desire to go back on the ventilator. The FIO_2 was decreased to 0.24, 1 hour later there was no change in vital signs, and arterial blood gas analysis showed a pH of 7.42, a PCO_2 of 52 mm Hg, and a PO_2 of 55 mm Hg. FVC was 1.6 L, and FEV_1 was 0.76 L after bronchodilator treatment.

The patient was extubated and a 24% air entrainment mask applied. Vital signs were unchanged, and he was very happy the tube was out and he could talk, even though it was in a hoarse whisper. He did well for the following 48 hours, including resuming eating, and was transferred from the intensive care unit 9 days after initiation of ventilatory support.

Discussion

There are several acceptable methods for "weaning" from the ventilator. However, none of these methods is successful until the patient's acute pathology has reversed and he possesses adequate ventilatory reserves. Once the decision to wean is made, the process should be accomplished as rapidly as is compatible with patient safety. The process seldom requires more than 4 hours unless (1) the baseline ventilatory reserve was borderline before the acute insult occurred, (2) the nutritonal status is poor, or (3) emotional factors produce a "fear" or "desire" resulting in wanting to stay on the ventilator.

Although patients with severe COPD often require prolonged weaning times, this is by no means the rule. With proper medical care and appropriate respiratory therapy, most of these patients readily come off the ventilator when the acute insult has been adequately reversed.

REFERENCES

1. Rochester DF, Braun NMT, Laine S: Diaphragmatic energy expenditure in chronic respiratory failure: The effect of assisted ventilation with body respirators. Am J Med 1977; 63:223–232.
2. Roussos C, Macklem PT: The respiratory muscles. N Engl J Med 1982; 307:786–797.
3. Wagner PD, Dantzker DR, Dueck R, et al: Ventilation-perfusion inequality in chronic obstructive pulmonary disease. J Clin Invest 1977; 59:203–216.
4. Tenney SM: Ventilatory response to carbon dioxide in pulmonary emphysema. J Appl Physiol 1954; 6:477–484.
5. Roger, RM, Weiler C, Ruppenthal B: Impact of the respiratory care unit on survival of patients with acute respiratory failure. Chest 1972; 62:94–97.
6. Petty TL, Lakshminarayan S, Sahn SA, et al: Intensive respiratory care unit: Review of ten years' experience. JAMA 1975; 233:34–37.
7. Martin RT, Lewis SW, Albert RK: The prognosis of patients with chronic obstructive pulmonary disease after hospitalization for acute respiratory failure. Chest 1982; 82:310–314.
8. Altose MD, McCauley WC, Kelsen SG, et al: Effects of hypercapnia and inspiratory flow-resistive loading on respiratory activity in chronic airway obstruction. J Clin Invest 1977; 59:500–506.

9. Mountain R, Zwillich C, Weil J: Hypoventilation in obstructive lung disease: The role of familial factors. N Engl J Med 1978; 298:521–525.
10. Milic-Emili J, Aubier M: Some recent advances in the study of the control of breathing in patients with chronic obstructive lung disease. Anesth Analg 1980; 59:865–873.
11. Sorli J, Grassino A, Lovange, G, et al: Control of breathing in patients with chronic lung disease. Clin Sci 1978; 54:295–304.
12. Javaheri S, Blum J, Kazemi H: Pattern of breathing and carbon dioxide retention in chronic obstructive lung disease. Am J Med 1981; 71:228–234.
13. Aubier M, Murciano D, Fournier M, et al: Central respiratory drive in acute respiratory failure of patients with chronic obstructive pulmonary disease. Am Rev Respir Dis 1980; 122:191–199.
14. Roussos CS, Fixley M, Gross D, et al: Fatigue of inspiratory muscles and their synergic behavior: J Appl Physiol 1979; 46:897–904.
15. Macklem PT, Roussos CS: Respiratory muscle fatigue: A cause of respiratory failure? Clin Sci Mol Med 1977; 53:419–422.
16. Hunter AM, Carey MA, Larsh HW: The nutritonal status of patients with chronic obstructive pulmonary disease. Am Rev Respir Dis 1981; 124:376–381.
17. Rochester DF, Braun NMT, Arora NS: Respiratory muscle strength in chronic obstructive pulmonary disease. Am Rev Respir Dis 1979; 119 (suppl, 2):151–154.
18. Askanazi J, Weissman C, Rosenbaum SH, et al: Nutrition and the respiratory system. Crit Care Med 1982; 10:163–172.
19. Rodriguez JL, Askanazi J, Weissman C, et al: Ventilatory and metabolic effects of glucose infusions. Chest 1985; 88:512–518.
20. Anthonisen NR, Manfreda J, Warren CPW, et al: Antibiotic therapy in exacerbations of chronic obstructive pulmonary disease. Ann Intern Med 1987; 106:196–204.
21. Aubier M, DeTroyer A, Sampson M, et al: Aminophylline improves diaphragmatic contractility. N Engl J Med 1981; 305:249–252.
22. Wanner A: Clinical aspects of mucociliary transport. Am Rev Respir Dis 1977; 116:73–125.
23. Albert RK, Martin TR, Lewis SW: Controlled clinical trial of methylprednisolone in patients with chronic bronchitis and acute respiratory insufficiency. Ann Intern Med 1980; 92:753–758.
24. Gross NJ: Ipratropium bromide. N Engl J Med 1988; 319:486–499.
25. Kirilloff LH, Owens GR, Rogers RM, et al: Does physical therapy work? Chest 1985; 88:436–444.
26. Aubier M, Murciano D, Milic-Emili V, et al: Effects of the administration of O_2 on ventilation and blood gases in patients with chronic obstructive pulmonary disease during acute respiratory failure. Am Rev Respir Dis 1980; 122:747–754.
27. Connors AF, Hammon WE, Martin RJ, et al: Chest physical therapy. The immediate effect of oxygenation in acutely ill patients. Chest 1980; 78:559–564.
28. Bone RC, Pierce AK, Johnson RL: Controlled oxygen administration in acute respiratory failure in chronic obstructive pulmonary disease. Am J Med 1978; 65:896–902.
29. Gilbert R, Ashutosh K, Auchincloss JH, et al: Prospective study of controlled oxygen therapy: Poor prognosis in patients with asynchronous breathing. Chest 1977; 71:456–462.
30. Christopher KL, Neff TA, Borman JL, et al: Intermittent mandatory ventilatory systems. Chest 1985; 87:625–629.

22/Acute Endocrine Emergencies

MARK STOLAR, M.D.

Although endocrine and metabolic disturbances are a frequent occurrence in the intensive care unit (ICU) setting, endocrine emergencies are somewhat less common. Acute adrenal insufficiency is uncommon and should be easily recognizable clinically, and treatment is very straightforward. Pituitary apoplexy, although dramatic, is quite rare and only occurs in the setting of an antecedent pituitary tumor. More common are acute diabetic emergencies and the frequent need to distinguish between myxedema coma and euthyroid sick syndrome. The subtleties between diabetic ketoacidosis (DKA) and hyperosmolar nonketotic coma (HNC) and between myxedema and euthyroid sick states have a profound impact on the management and outcome of these patients. This chapter will focus on these two classical endocrine emergencies.

DIABETIC KETOACIDOSIS AND HYPEROSMOLAR NONKETOTIC COMA

The development of DKA or the hyperosmolar state is the most critical and common of all endocrine emergencies. Since the advent of insulin therapy some 60 years ago, the importance of these disorders as a cause of death among diabetic patients has declined drastically. However, the mortality rate in DKA remains in the range of 5% to 15%,[1] and for HNC, the mortality rate is a surprising 20% to 50%,[2] usually because of the severity of the underlying illness. The most important point to remember in the treatment of patients with these problems is that death does not result from hyperglycemia but rather is due to the metabolic shifts that occur because of the deranged glucose metabolism. It therefore becomes important to be able to distinguish between DKA and HNC because there are subtle differences in the treatments of these two conditions and their attendant complications.

Pathogenesis

The development of DKA and the hyperosmolar state are somewhat different. Insulin exerts its metabolic effects primarily through improving glucose uptake by the periphery, decreasing hepatic gluconeogenesis, and suppressing lipolysis.[1, 3–5] Diabetic ketoacidosis is primarily a disorder of the type I, or insulin dependent, diabetic, although it can occur among type II, or non–insulin-dependent, "adult-onset" diabetic patients. Because of an absolute deficiency or absence of insulin, hepatic glucose output markedly increases, and lipolysis is no longer suppressed, which leads to the generation of high levels of free fatty acids. Because insulin-dependent tissues such as fat, muscle, and liver can no longer utilize glucose for their metabolic needs, fatty acids are metabolized to the organic acids, acetoacetate, and β-hydroxybutyrate.[6–8] Also, muscle tissue cannot use circulating ketone acids for metabolic needs. These acids as well as acetone accumulate in the blood and result in a clinical setting of metabolic acidosis due to the hyperketonemia. Hyperosmolarity occurs due to the hyperglycemia and attendant osmotic diuresis, and dehydration results both from free water loss as well as from the frequent vomiting that occurs with DKA.

Patients with HNC have a relative deficiency of insulin secretion often magnified by an underlying infection. Insulin levels remain adequate to suppress lipolysis but are not sufficient to suppress hepatic glucose output. Due to the underlying stress, there is increased secretion of hormones with insulin antagonistic action such as epinephrine, cortisol, glucagon, and growth hormone. These hormones increase gluconeogenesis and lipolysis, further exacerbating the metabolic derangement. Blood glucose levels gradually rise, and the resultant hyperglycemia leads to an osmotic diuresis that further elevates the blood sugar level. Acidosis that occurs in this situation is primarily due to lactic acidosis arising either from hypoperfusion due to the dehydrated state or secondary to some underlying infectious process, with up to 60% of all patients with this syndrome demonstrating lactic acidosis of some degree.

Although the degreee of abnormality of glucose and lipid metabolism in these two disorders is severe, the most frequent causes of morbidity and mortality in these patients are fluid and electrolyte imbalances. The osmotic diuresis seen in both illnesses generates not only a loss of free water but also of potassium and sodium. In DKA a lack of insulin also has a natriuretic effect.[9] Dehydration often proceeds rapidly in these patients, and the resulting hypoperfusion of the kidney leads to further deterioration in renal function. With a deteriorating glomerular filtration rate (GFR), less glucose is filtered, and blood levels rise dramatically. When these syndromes are fully manifested, there is total body depletion of water, sodium, potassium, magnesium, chloride, and bicarbonate. In DKA, the presence of large amounts of ketones creates an anion gap usually greater than 15 mEq, but this finding is not helpful in distinguishing between DKA and a hyperosmolar state with lactic acidosis.

CASE STUDY 1

A 48-year-old-white woman was brought into the emergency room unconscious. The patient had insulin-dependent diabetes mellitus since 21 years of age. She had a concurrent diagnosis of manic-depressive illness and had been admitted 12 times to the hospital previously for DKA primarily because of noncompliance with medication. Her medications at the time of presentation were lithium carbonate, 300 mg three times daily (TID); diazepam 0.5 mg twice daily (BID); and NPH U-100 insulin, 40 units subcutaneously in the morning and 20 units in the evening.

Examination in the emergency room revealed an unconscious thin white female with a pulse of 120/min and frequent premature beats, a temperature of 35.7°C, blood pressure of

80/40 mm Hg, and respirations at 20/min and deep. The patient was responsive to deep pain only. Her skin was dry and without evidence of trauma. Examination of the head and neck was unremarkable. Examination of the heart and lungs was unremarkable with the exception of the frequent premature beats. Abdominal examination revealed marked distension with hypoactive bowel sounds. There was no organomegaly. Her extremities were without edema. Central nervous system (CNS) examination revealed symmetrical hyper-reflexia of the lower extremities.

Discussion

These patients can be distinguished clinically both by history as well as laboratory data. Patients with DKA often present primarily with nausea, vomiting, Kussmaul respiration (i.e., deep and labored breathing), and alterations in mental status. The progression of symptoms usually occurs over a period of 12 to 48 hours, with a history of very rapid decompensation often present. Mucous membranes are dry, skin turgor is poor, and hypotension and tachycardia are the rule, although patients with severe acidosis may present with an underlying bradycardia. An odor of acetone on the breath is often detected. Many patients present with marked gastrointestinal pain, which may mimic an acute abdomen.

This is in contrast to the patient with HNC, whose illness may have evolved over a period of 3 to 7 days. Signs of nausea, vomiting, and gastrointestinal pain are rare and should lead one to suspect some underlying intra-abdominal process. Mental status may vary from drowsiness to coma, with the prognosis of the patient paralleling the depression of mental status. Hypotension and tachycardia again are found as well as marked dehydration. Kassmaul breathing may be present if the patient has a significant lactic acidosis.

CASE STUDY 1 CONTINUED

On admission the complete blood count revealed a hemoglobin concentration of 15.7 gm/dL, white blood cell (WBC) count of 18,000 mm^{-3} with a shift to the left, and a platelet count of 300,000 mm^3. Blood chemistry studies revealed a blood sugar level of 478 mg/dL, blood urea nitrogen (BUN), 47 mg/dL; creatinine, 5.1 mg/dL; sodium, 128 mEq/dL; potassium, 3.5 mEq/dL; and bicarbonate, 8 mEq/dL. Serum ketones were 1:8 in an undiluted sample. Arterial blood gas determination on room air revealed a Po$_2$ of 90 mm Hg, a Pco$_2$ of 24 mm Hg, and a pH of 7.09. Chest x-ray findings were unremarkable. Urinalysis revealed 4+ glucose and 3+ ketones. An electrocardiogram displayed sinus tachycardia with frequent aberrantly conducted beats felt to be of a supraventricular origin. In the emergency room a Foley catheter was inserted, and urine output averaged 70 cc/hr. Two liters of intravenous (IV) saline was infused during the first 2 hours. The patient was then given 10 units of regular insulin as an IV bolus, and an insulin drip of 7 units of insulin per hour was started.

Discussion

Laboratory studies differ as a rule between the two disorders[2] (see Table 22–1). In DKA blood sugar levels above 600 mg/dL are uncommon, whereas in the hyperosmolar state few cases have been reported in which the blood sugar was less

TABLE 22–1.

Laboratory Features of Diabetic Ketoacidosis and
Hyperosmolar Coma

Feature	DKA	HNC
Glucose (mg/dL)	300–600	>600
Osmolarity (mOsm/dL)	<320	>320
Sodium (mEq/dL)	130–140	140–160
BUN (mg/dL)	30–40	>60
pH	<7.25	>7.25–7.40
HCO_3 (mg/dL)	<15	Variable
Lactate	Usually nL	nL to increased
Amylase	nL to increased	Normal

than 600 mg/dL, and glucose levels are typically above 900 mg/dL. Serum osmolarity is usually greater than 350 mOsm/dL in the hyperosmolar state, whereas few patients with DKA will reach such levels. Uremia is usually manifested to a greater degree in nonketotic coma, with average BUN levels of 80 mg/dL as compared with approximately 30 mg/dL in DKA. This is due primarily to the decreased renal function seen in an older patient population. However, long-standing type I diabetes with nephropathy will present with an elevated BUN concentration. Serum sodium levels tend to be much higher in the hyperosmolar state despite the artifactual hyponatremia engendered by the elevation of blood glucose levels. (A rise in the blood glucose concentration of 100 mg/dL lowers the serum sodium level by 1.6 mEq/dL.[10]) Plasma ketones are positive in a 1:2 dilution or less in the hyperosmolar state, with higher levels being consistent with a diagnosis of DKA. Serum amylase levels are often elevated in the setting of DKA[11]; elevation in the setting of a hyperosmolar state should lead one to suspect underlying acute pancreatitis. One problem in the interpretation of serum ketones is that β-hydroxybutyrate, an organic acid present in high amounts, is not detected by routine assay. Once insulin treatment is initiated, β-hydroxybutyrate is converted to acetoacetate and may actually result in higher values for serum ketones after appropriate treatment has been initiated.

Diagnosis

Prompt diagnosis of these disorders is essential and should be suspected in all patients who present with mental status changes, dehydration, and in the case of ketoacidosis, vomiting and abdominal pain. The diagnosis of DKA can be made rapidly at the bedside with a fingerstick blood sugar level above 300 mg/dL, 4+ ketones in the urine, and an arterial blood gas showing a pH of less than 7.30.

The differential diagnosis of both of these disorders includes all types of metabolic coma. Alcoholic ketoacidosis can mimic both disorders.[12] This is caused by an accumulation of ketone acids in the absence of diabetes in poorly nourished alcoholic patients who are dehydrated from protracted nausea and vomiting. In this clinical setting, blood glucose levels are usually below 200 mm/dL, and plasma ketones values are only mildly elevated. Acidosis of uremia may also mimic this syndrome. Many diabetic patients have underlying renal dysfunction and may clinically appear identical to one of these hyperglycemic states. However, in uremic acidosis, ketosis is not present. Curiously, in diabetes spontaneous lactic acidosis is not uncommon and should be suspected among patients in coma with only mild elevations of blood sugar levels.

Treatment

The objectives of treatment are slightly different betwen DKA and hyperosmolar nonketotic coma. In the former, correction of the acidosis and electrolyte imbalance is primary, whereas in the hyperosmolar state correction of the dehydration, which is often severe, is paramount. Most patients require large amounts of fluid. Initial treatment with 0.9 normal saline is appropriate in both groups, with 1 to 2 L infused over the first 2 hours being appropriate management, especially if hypotension is present. The average fluid deficit in DKA is 6 L, whereas the average fluid loss in the hyperosmolar patient is between 9 and 12 L, and continued aggressive replacement with fluids is important. It has been shown that the fluid excreted by patients with hyperosmolar nonketotic coma is identical to 5% dextrose $(D_5)/0.45$ normal saline.[2] Therefore, when a normal blood pressure has been achieved, further fluid replacement with 0.45 normal saline is appropriate, with half of the calculated fluid deficit being replaced in the first 12 hours and the remaining half replaced in the subsequent 24 hours.

Because the primary morbidity in all of these patients is metabolic, establishment of a well-organized flowsheet to chart laboratory data is essential. All patients with DKA and most patients with the hyperosmolar nonketotic state will require insulin. In recent years, the therapeutic approach has involved the use of continuous infusion of IV insulin since impaired circulation due to dehydration and hypotension may prevent absorption of subcutaneously or intramuscularly administered hormone.[13, 14] In DKA, because of intense insulin resistance, an initial loading dose of 6 to 10 units of IV bolus followed by a continuous infusion of 0.1 to 0.15 units/kg/hr may be used. In the hyperosmolar state, insulin resistance is less intense because many of these patients have had no previous exposure to insulin therapy. The initial bolus treatment is identical, but subsequent infusions are at a rate of 0.05 to 0.1 units/kg/hr. Plasma glucose levels should be checked hourly, with serum electrolytes, arterial pH, and ketones being monitored at 2- to 4-hour intervals. The objectives are to lower blood glucose at a rate no more than 10% or 100 mg/dL/hr. A too-rapid decline in blood glucose may result in the development of rebound cerebral edema, especially in the patient with hyperosmolar nonketotic coma.[15, 16]

Infusion of bicarbonate is an area still open to much debate because appropriate institution of fluids and insulin results in the metabolism of serum ketone to bicarbonate.[17] Therefore, appropriate therapy often corrects the underlying acidosis without intervention with bicarbonate. Overly aggressive use of bicarbonate can rapidly lead to the development of a metabolic alkalosis with resultant cerebral edema. Current guidelines for the administration of bicarbonate suggest that a serum pH less than 7.10, a bicarbonate level less than 5 mEq/dL, or any compromise in myocardial function or arrhythmia would be an indication for the use of bicarbonate. Bicarbonate should be added to 0.45 normal saline because administration in 0.9 normal saline may further aggravate the hyperosmolar state. Because serum lactate levels are often elevated both in DKA and the hyperosmolar state, there is no justification for the use of Ringer's lactate in the treatment of these patients.

As a result of the osmotic diuresis and, in the case of DKA, ketonuria and frequent vomiting, body potassium stores are often markedly depleted. Because of the underlying acidosis, the serum potassium concentration is often normal to mildly elevated due to the shift of potassium from intracellular to extracellular fluid. With correction of the underlying dehydration and acidosis and the action of insulin stimulating cellular uptake of glucose, serum potassium levels decline rapidly. Potassium chloride should be administered at the onset of therapy if serum potassium levels are less than 4 mEq/dL and the patient is not anuric or 3 hours after initiation of therapy if the presenting potassium level is greater than 4 mEq/dL and the patient is not anuric. Average potassium replacement in the first 18 hours averages 120 to 160 mEq/dL. Although usually present, hypophosphatemia is not clinically significant. Replacement of phosphate has theoretical advantages because body phosphate stores are depleted and levels of 2,3-diphosphoglycerate (2,3-DPG) may be quite low. This has been postulated to impair oxygen release from hemoglobin to surrounding tissues. However, aggressive replacement of phosphate has been shown to have no clinical advantages in patients and may precipitate hypocalcemia.

CASE STUDY 1 CONTINUED

Two hours later the patient was arousable. The blood glucose concentration had fallen to 382 mg/dL; serum bicarbonate was at 10 mEq/dL. The nurse observed that the patient was in sinus tachycardia at a rate of 120 beats per minute, with frequent multifocal premature ventricular beats and occasional couplets and triplets. Her blood pressure was 90/60 mm/Hg. The serum potassium level was found to be 2.8 mEq/dL. A lithium level measured in the emergency room was 0.9.

Discussion

The complications in ketoacidosis are primarily related to the metabolic disorder. Cardiogenic shock may develop as a result of severe acidosis, especially in patients with underlying coronary artery disease. Cardiac arrhythmias due to hypokalemia or hyperkalemia are frequently seen. Irreversible fatal cerebral edema is the main complication we wish to avoid in the treatment of DKA. This is typically seen in the adolescent with no underlying illness who develops marked deterioration in consciousness after an initial period of clinical improvement. It usually occurs in the setting of too rapid a decline in blood glucose, with greater osmolarity in the CNS relative to the plasma.[16] In the clinical setting, cerebral edema has not been shown to occur until the plasma glucose has reached normal or near-normal levels of approximately 250 mg/dL. Accordingly, glucose-containing fluid should be administered when plasma glucose has fallen to this level. Fortunately, the incidence of this complication is quite low.

CASE STUDY 1 CONTINUED

After further hydration and replacement of potassium the patient's blood pressure rose to 110/60 mm Hg. Her rhythm remained sinus with only occasional unifocal premature ventricular contractions (PVCs). Two hours later her blood glucose concentration was 241 mg/dL, serum ketones were positive in a 1:16 dilution, serum sodium was 138 mEq/dL, serum potassium had risen to 3.6 mEq/dL, and serum bicarbonate was now at 11 mEq/dL. The patient's urine output remained at 100 cc/hr. At examination the patient was in sinus rhythm at a rate of 110/min. At that point, the patient received $D_5/0.45$ normal saline at a rate of 250 cc/hr, with 30 mEq/dL of potassium added to each liter. The insulin drip was stopped and the patient given 10 units of insulin subcutaneously. Two hours later the patient's blood sugar was 400 mg/dL.

Discussion

The most common error in managing insulin infusions is premature cessation of the insulin infusion. Subcutaneously administered insulin will not act significantly for 2 to 4 hours and results in rebound hyperglycemia. Appropriate management is reducing the infusion by 50% when subcutaneous insulin is given and adjusting the infusion rate further each hour until the blood glucose level is stable.

Many endocrinologists continue IV insulin at an infusion rate of 1 to 2 units/hr for 12 to 24 hours until serum bicarbonate levels have risen sufficiently and stabilized. This also prevents lability of blood glucose in the acute period.

CASE STUDY 1 CONTINUED

An infusion of IV insulin was restarted at a rate of 3 units/hr. One hour later the blood glucose had dropped to 328 mg/dL, and 1 hour after that it had fallen further to 218 mg/dL. At that time the infusion was reduced to 1.5 units of insulin per hour. The following morning the patient was awake and alert and able to tolerate breakfast. A regimen of 20 units of NPH insulin was started in the morning, 15 units of NPH insulin in the evening. The insulin infusion was continued through dinner time. At 6:00 P.M. that day, her plasma glucose concentration was 180 mg/dL; sodium, 135 mEq/dL; potassium, 4.1 mEq/dL; and bicarbonate, 19 mEq/dL. She was discharged from the hospital the following morning on her previous insulin regimen.

CASE STUDY 2

A 77-year-old white woman was brought to the emergency room unconscious. The patient had not been seen in 2 days but had spoken with her daughter 3 days previously complaining of diarrhea and stomach pain. She had been taking glipizide, 10 mg/day; hydrochlorothiazide, 50 mg each morning; and propranolol, 40 mg BID. Examination in the emergency room revealed an obese white female with a pulse of 120/min, a temperature of 38.4°C, blood pressure of 80/40 mm/hg, and respirations at 20/min and deep. The patient was responsive to deep pain only. Her skin was dry and without evidence of trauma. Examination of the head and neck was unremarkable. Lung fields revealed coarse rhonchi at the right base. Cardiac examination was unremarkable. Abdominal examination revealed abdominal distension with hypoactive bowel sounds. There was no organomegaly. Her extremities were without edema. The complete blood cell count revealed a hemoglobin content of 12.1 mg/dL, a white blood cell count of 15,000 mm^{-3} with a shift to the left, and a platelet count of 300,000 mm^{-3}. Blood chemistry studies revealed a blood sugar level of 952 mg/dL; BUN, 84 mg/dL; creatine, 5.5 mg/dL; sodium, 128 mg/dL; potassium, 3.9 mg/dL; and bicarbonate, 20 mg/dL. Serum ketones were faintly positive in an undiluted sample. Microscopic examination of the urine revealed 50 to 100 WBCs per HPF and 3+ bacteria. There were 3+ urine ketones. Arterial blood gas determination on room air disclosed a P_{O_2} of 70 mm Hg, a P_{CO_2} of 30 mm Hg, and a pH of 7.28. Chest x-ray films revealed clear lung fields and a minimally enlarged cardiac silhouette. An electrocardiogram displayed sinus tachycardia and nonspecific ST and T changes. In the emergency room a Foley catheter was inserted, and urine output averaged 100 cc/hr. Two liters of IV saline were infused during the first 2 hours. Appropriate antibiotics were started for presumptive urinary tract infection and possible aspiration pneumonia, and the patient was transferred to the ICU.

Discussion

This patient demonstrated the typical clinical history that we find in patients with hyperosmolar nonketotic coma, that is, a gradual onset in a geriatric patient with an underlying illness predisposing to dehydration. Additionally, the patient had been taking diuretics, further aggravating her dehydration. β-blockers have also been reported to precipitate hyperosmolar coma in rare circumstances by suppressing insulin secretion. On initial assessment, one may be tempted to diagnose this patient as having DKA. But the presence of trace amounts of ketones is not consistent with the diagnosis of DKA.

CASE STUDY 2 CONTINUED

Following the 2 L of fluid, infusion of 0.45 normal saline was begun at a rate of 250 cc/hr. Blood chemistry studies at this time revealed a blood glucose level of 750 mg/dL; BUN, 78 mg/dL; sodium, 132 mg/dL; and potassium, 3.8 mg/dL. The urine output over the next hour was 90 cc. The patient was given 10 units of human regular insulin as an IV bolus, and an infusion of 6 units of human insulin per hour was begun. Just prior to the next blood sugar reading, the patient began to have focal seizures in the right upper and lower extremities.

Discussion

This is typical and appropriate management of the patient with hyperosmolar nonketotic coma. The blood glucose level has fallen at a rate of approximately 100 mg/dL/hr, and there has been a slow stable improvement in serum electrolytes. Note that the continuous insulin infusion at a rate of 6 units of insulin per hour is at a somewhat lower hourly rate than would be used in a patient with DKA. Seizures are not an uncommon complication in a patient with hyperosmolar coma and are usually due to the hyperosmolar state. However, given the severe metabolic derangement seen in this illness, one must be suspicious not only of structural neurologic disease but also of abnormalities of serum calcium, magnesium, and sodium, which may precipitate seizure activity. In the absence of focal neurologic abnormalities such as a unilateral Babinski reflex, hyperreflexia, or a lack of spontaneous movement of an extremity, computed axial tomographic (CAT) scanning of the head would not be appropriate at this point in time.

CASE STUDY 2 CONTINUED

The patient was given 5 mg of diazepam by IV push, with cessation of seizure activity. Serum calcium and magnesium levels were within normal limits. Over the next 4 hours, her urine output continued to average 90 cc/hr. At the end of 4 hours, the patient's blood sugar level had dropped to 400 mg/dL. Serum lactate levels were found to be elevated. Serum ketones remained trace-positive. Two hours later, the patient's blood sugar levels were 250 mg/dL; BUN, 60 mg/dL; creatine, 4.8 mg/dL; and bicarbonate, 18 mg/dL. The IV infusion was then switched over to D$_5$/0.45 normal saline at a 4-hour rate, and the insulin infusion was cut to three units/hr. The patient was given 5 units regular insulin subcutaneously at this time.

Discussion

The therapeutic choice of diazepam is a correct treatment for seizures due to the hyperosmolar state. Diphenylhydantoin is not effective in this setting and may actually suppress insulin secretion.

The prime consideration when deciding to stop the continuous insulin infusion is that it is important to make the transition as gradual as possible. If IV insulin is stopped abruptly, there may be a significant rebound hyperglycemia while waiting for subcutaneously injected insulin to be absorbed and take effect. Therefore the insulin infusion should be cut in half at the time the subcutaneous insulin is injected and tapered as blood sugar levels decline.

CASE STUDY 2 CONTINUED

The following morning the patient's blood sugar level was 192 mg/dL; BUN, 40 mg/dL; and creatine, 3.4 mg/dL. Her serum bicarbonate was 22 mg/dL with an arterial pH of 7.35, and the urine output remained 100 cc/hr. The insulin drip was reduced to 1 unit/hr, and the patient was maintained on 6-hour infusions of D$_5$/0.45 normal saline with 30 mEq of potassium per liter of fluid.

Twenty-four hours later the patient was awake although disoriented. Blood sugar was well controlled on supplementation of insulin every 6 hours, and IV fluids were reduced to D$_5$/0.45 normal saline at 100 cc/hr. The patient was continuously moving and grasping her right leg. The right leg was mildly edematous to the midcalf and warm to touch, without evidence of palpable cords. Six hours later the patient suffered a cardiac arrest and expired.

Discussion

In the hyperosmolar patient, complications tend to be related to the precipitating illness or secondary to the marked hyperosmolarity. Venous thrombosis of the lower extremities, mesenteric plexus, or sagittal venous system in the brain have all been observed. Seizures may result from either the underlying metabolic derangement or from venous thrombosis in the brain.[20] This complication should be suspected in patients who have status focal seizures. Sepsis may often be disguised by the clinical presentation, and patients should be examined carefully for any potential source of infection. Surprisingly, despite profound dehydration and azotemia, acute renal failure and renal shutdown are quite uncommon, primarily because the continuous osmotic diuresis protects the renal tubules.

Since the advent of continuous IV insulin infusion, morbidity and mortality in these patients is no longer directly related to the degree of hyperglycemia. This patient, for example, apparently was suffering from a deep venous thrombosis of her right leg, her terminal event being a pulmonary embolism, a very common complication seen in the hyperosmolar state.

In the period several days following the original presentation, it is necessary to decide whether neurologic evaluation is appropriate. It is not uncommon for the geriatric patient to remain disoriented for several days following the original metabolic insult. Again, in the absence of focal neurologic findings or the clinical suggestion of head trauma, CAT scanning of the head should be deferred. One would not wish to use iodinated contrast media in this acute setting until adequate hydration and perfusion of the kidneys have been established.

EUTHYROID SICK SYNDROME

The euthyroid sick syndrome is not a true endocrine emergency; however, usually because of the underlying severity of these patients' illnesses, abnormalities suggestive of myxedema coma need to be evaluated and, if confirmed, treated rapidly. Frequently the decisions regarding treatment need to be made before all laboratory data are available. It is often quite difficult to distinguish between patients gravely ill due to underlying medical problems and those with myxedema coma because many physical signs are observed and few historical clues are available. Fortunately, the incidence of true myxedema coma is quite low relative to the frequency of euthyroid sick syndrome.

Pathophysiology

The thyroid pituitary axis is kept in delicate balance. Alterations in plasma thyroxine (T_4) concentration as little as 1 µg/dL above or below the pituitary set point will result in changes in plasma thyrotropin (TSH) levels.[21, 22] T_4 feeds back negatively at the level of the pituitary, with only a small negative-feedback loop at the level of hypothalamus. Elevated levels of T_4 suppress TSH secretion by the pituitary.[18, 19] Similarly, falling T_4 levels will stimulate TSH secretion by the pituitary.[20] Therefore, in patients with primary hypothyroidism and myxedema, marked elevation of TSH levels is the rule.

Two mechanisms are operative in the development of the euthyroid sick syndrome. The metabolic effects of T_4 in peripheral tissues usually occurs as a result of its monodeiodination to the more potent thyroid hormone triiodothyronine (T_3).[24] In the euthyroid sick syndrome, T_4 is preferentially deiodinated to reverse T_3, a metabolically inert hormone.[22] This may be a protective adaptation against starvation in severe systemic illness by the reduction of tissue metabolic demands. T_4 secretion is also decreased in the euthyroid sick state. This most likely is due to decreased secretion of TSH by the pituitary. Finally, impaired T_4 synthesis or decreased production of thyroid-binding globulin (TBG) may play a role.[23] This may be due to elevated levels of cortisol, dopamine, growth hormone, and neuropeptides, all of which are secreted in response to stress and inhibit the release of TSH by the pituitary.[23-25] More likely, the decreased TSH secretion is a normal physiologic response to normal levels of free T_4 in the plasma. Although measured total T_4 levels are low, there are circulating inhibitors of the binding of T_4 to TBG.[26, 27] Therefore, while small amounts of T_4 may be bound to the TBG reservoir (resulting in a low total T_3 by radioimmunoassay [RIA]), because of the presence of these circulating inhibitors, the level of *free* T_4 in the plasma remains normal, thereby keeping TSH secretion normal to low.

CASE STUDY 3

A 73-year-old male alcoholic was brought into the emergency room unresponsive and in respiratory distress. No further history was obtainable. Vital signs on admission were as follows: pulse, 130 beats per minute; temperature, 36.5°C; and blood pressure by cuff, 90/60 mm Hg. Respirations were 30/min and shallow. Physical examination revealed a pale malnourished male with poor oral hygiene. There was right anterior cervical adenopathy present. Examination of the lungs revealed rhonchi and wheezing at the right base posteriorly and at the left upper lobe posteriorly. Cardiac examination was normal. Abdominal examination was significant for a 15 cm liver and a palpable spleen. Laboratory studies revealed the following values: hemoglobin, 8.4 mg/dL; WBC count, 24,300 mm^{-3}; sodium, 128 mEq/dL; potassium, 3.7 mg/dL; BUN, 6 mg/dL; and creatinine, 1.1 mg/dL. Chest x-ray films revealed infiltrates in the right lower lung and left upper lung fields. The blood alcohol level was 270 mg/dL. Arterial blood gas analysis on room air revealed a Po_2 of 51 mm Hg, a Pco_2 of 39 mm Hg; and a pH of 7.33. While in the emergency room, the patient suffered a respiratory arrest and was intubated and transferred to the ICU. Subsequent to his intensive care admission, the patient became hypotensive and required infusion of dopamine at 5 μm/kg/min and large amounts of saline. On the third day of hospitalization, the patient's aspiration pneumonia had stabilized on appropriate antibiotic therapy. Although he was still unarousable, vital signs indicated a blood pressure of 90/60 mm Hg on a dopamine infusion of 8 μg/kg/min, respirations of 14/min, and a temperature 35.7°C. His pulse was 112 beats per minute. Further neurologic examination was noncontributory.

Discussion

The typical patient with euthyroid sick syndrome is often indistinguishable from the patient with myxedema coma. These patients are critically ill, are usually in an intensive care setting, and often are hypotensive and hypothermic. However, there are certain key distinguishing features. Patients with euthyroid sick syndrome typically have tachycardia, normal deep tendon reflexes, a nonpalpable thyroid gland, and none of the cutaneous stigmata of myxedema. Patients with myxedema coma usually have many of the signs of chronic hypothyroidism such as subcutaneous thickening, delayed deep-tendon reflexes, enlarged tongue, and goiter. Patients with euthyroid sick syndrome should have normal serum sodium, creatine phosphokinase (CPK), and cholesterol levels, whereas hyponatremia and elevations in total cholesterol and CPK levels are often seen in myxedema coma.[28] The hyponatremia results from impaired free water excretion seen in patients with myxedema.[29] Arterial blood gases in myxedema coma usually show signs of CO_2 retention and respiratory acidosis secondary to a depressed central respiratory drive.[30-32] In the euthyroid sick syndrome arterial blood gases vary only with the underlying illness (see Table 22–2).

Findings in this patient are typical of the euthyroid sick syndrome. The patient was malnourished before hospitalization and had stigmata of chronic alcoholism. He was suffering from a severe morbid state with multiple medical problems and refractory hypotension requiring inotropic support. In this critical setting the body is attempting physiologically to decrease metabolic demand in an accelerated starvation state and thereby reduce conversion of T_4 to T_3. Note that the hyponatremia, hypotension and hypothermia all suggest hypothyroidism. However, all these clinical findings can be seen in patients with congestive heart failure, alcoholic cirrhosis with hepatic coma, and severe Wernicke's syndrome.

CASE STUDY 3 CONTINUED

Because the patient was unarousable and hypothermic, thyroid function studies were performed, the results of which were as follows: T_4, 0.9 mg/dL; T_3 resin uptake, 45%; Free thyroxine index (FTI), 0.4. A clinical debate then ensued as to whether or not the diagnosis of myxedema coma was correct and thyroid supplementation would be necessary. Examination of the patient revealed normal skin turgor and no pretibial edema. The thyroid examination was not helpful, and deep-tendon reflexes were absent in the lower extremities. The TSH sample was then sent for assay. Arterial blood gas analysis revealed a pH of 7.27; pO_2, 96 mm Hg; pCO_2, 34 mm Hg; serum sodium, 138 mEq/dL; cholesterol, 147 mg/dL; and CPK, 340 units/L.

TABLE 22–2.

Comparison of Clinical and Laboratory Findings in Myxedema and Euthyroid Sick Syndrome

Physical Findings	Myxedema	Euthyroid Sick Syndrome
Goiter	Present	Usually absent
Hypothermia	Usually present	Often present
Bradycardia	Present	Absent
Hung-up reflexes	Present	Absent
Thinning of eyebrows	Present	Often present
Laboratory tests		
T_4 RIA	Low	Low
TSH	Increased*	Normal to increased
CPK	Increased	Normal to increased
Cholesterol	Increased	Normal to decreased
pCO_2	Increased	Variable

*Except in starvation, dopamine infusion.

Discussion

The thyroid functions are markedly abnormal, and because of the patient's failure to respond to appropriate medical management, the diagnosis of myxedema coma must be entertained. However, the clinical examination revealed no evidence of thyroid goiter, nor any stigmata of chronic hypothyroidism. Laboratory studies reveal no evidence of CO_2 retention, nor impaired free water excretion. Additionally one must be careful of misinterpreting low serum cholesterol values in the critically ill or malnourished patient, and in the critical care setting, CPK levels may be elevated for a number of reasons. In the alcoholic patient, for example, an elevated CPK value can suggest trauma or even rhabdomyolysis. In this patient there is no clinical urgency to initiate replacement thyroid hormone while awaiting the TSH results.

The traditional thyroid tests of total T_4 by RIA, free T_4 index, total T_3 by RIA, and TSH can be affected by a number of medical conditions, many of which are common to the patient with the euthyroid sick syndrome. Typically, total T_4 levels are decreased, and the calculated free T_4 index is similarly depressed. T_3 resin uptake in myxedema is decreased because of the large number of binding sites available on TBG. Radiolabeled T_3 added to the patient's serum will bind to TBG and result in a low amount of resin binding for assay. In the euthyroid sick syndrome, T_3 resin uptake is elevated because of circulating binding inhibitors that decrease the amount of binding sites available for radiolabeled T_3. More radiolabeled T_3 is available for resin binding, and this results in a high T_3 resin uptake. It is the low *calculated* free T_4 index that leads to frequent endocrine consultation and/or treatment for possible myxedema coma. The key discriminator between myxedema coma and the euthyroid sick syndrome is basal TSH levels, which should be elevated in all cases of myxedema due to primary hypothyroidism and normal in cases of the euthyroid sick syndrome. Tests such as reverse T_3 levels and free T_4 by dialysis are useful in confirming the diagnosis. However, these results are often available only long after the patient has clinically recovered or expired.

Further complicating interpretation of thyroid function in the critically ill are the effects of various medications on thyroid function testing. Dopamine infusion often used to treat hypotension can suppress TSH secretion.[33] It is possible in some patients that prolonged infusions of dopamine may even lead to a secondary hypothyroid state, further exacerbating these patient's poor clinical condition.[34] Glucocorticoids are often administered in pharmacologic doses to patients who are critically ill. Suppression of basal and thyrotropin-releasing hormone (TRH)-stimulated TSH secretion is common in this setting.[35, 36] Diphenylhydantoin will induce decreases in serum T_4 levels and occasionally will reduce T_3 levels as well. The basal serum TSH concentration is generally normal, but T_4 levels are usually significantly reduced.[37, 38] Amiodarone, an antiarrhythmic agent, has complex effects on thyroid hormone metabolism.[39, 41] Its high iodine content may actually raise T_4 RIA levels and the free T_4 index. However, TSH levels are often increased, not suppressed, as might have been expected with a high T_4 level. This drug apparently inhibits T_4-to-T_3 conversion and T_3 binding in the pituitary, thereby resulting in a false message and resultant stimulation of TSH secretion.

CASE STUDY 3 CONTINUED

While awaiting the TSH results, 100 μg/day of levothyroxine was started. In the interim, dopamine infusion had to be increased to 15 μg/kg/min due to increasing hypotension. Forty-eight hours later the patient's TSH came back at 1.1 mg/dL. Later that day the patient became increasingly hypotensive and expired, presumably of sepsis and cardiac failure.

Discussion

Differentiation between myxedema coma and the euthyroid sick syndrome is critical in establishing a treatment regimen. In the case of myxedema coma, treatment is lifesaving, but several studies indicate that inappropriate replacement of thyroid hormone in patients with euthyroid sick syndrome may actually increase morbidity and mortality. Despite the extremely low levels of total T_4 seen in the euthyroid sick syndrome, these patients do not require thyroid hormone because free hormone levels are normal. Indeed, the degree of lowering of total T_4 in the blood is an indicator of the patient's ultimate prognosis, with markedly decreased survival seen with those patients with total T_4 levels less than 3 μg/dL.[42, 43] Treatment should be initiated in those patients in whom respiratory failure, hypothermia, and poor free water excretion are demonstrated while awaiting laboratory studies to become available. However, conventional treatment plans for replacement of thyroid hormone in the setting of myxedema coma may actually be deleterious to the patient's clinical outcome. The previous treatment approach was to give the patient an initial dose of 500 μg of levothyroxine followed by 100 μg/day thereafter. However, following the initial 500-μg bolus, it was found that T_4 levels rise rapidly and to significantly high levels,[44] which predisposes the critically ill patient to potential cardiac arrhythmias.[45, 46] Currently, it is recommended that patients be given a dose of 100 μg of T_4 IV every day for 7 days while continuing physiologic support for ventilation and renal function. This regimen prevents any untoward cardiac complications while normalizing the physiologic derangements seen in myxedema coma after about 10 days of the onset of treatment.[47] In the truly myxedematous patient the earliest changes seen are improved free water excretion, improved respiratory drive, and a lowering of serum cholesterol levels. One potential complication is the precipitation of previously undetected adrenal insufficiency by correction of the thyroid status. Although it is usually not necessary, administration of hydrocortisone IV at the onset of thyroid treatment will help prevent this potential complication.[48] The key point to remember in treating myxedema coma is that the hypothyroidism developed over an extremely long period of time; thus correcting these abnormalities rapidly is usually not advisable.

This patient did indeed have the euthyroid sick syndrome. The patient's TSH was in the normal range, but had this value been obtained while the patient was receiving high levels of dopamine, one would have to interpret it with some caution. However, the 5-μg/kg/min infusion should not be sufficient to suppress TSH secretion, and therefore the patient is indeed euthyroid. Patients with T_4 levels less than 3 μg/dL deciliter have an increasingly higher morbidity and mortality, and those with levels less than 1 μg/dL are severely at risk. Thyroid replacement probably did not play a role in this patient's demise. However, some studies do suggest that there is increased morbidity in patients with euthyroid sick syndrome who are given thyroid hormone replacement, and therefore, aggressive replacement with T_4 should be withheld while awaiting definitive laboratory studies.

REFERENCES

1. Felig P, Baxter J, Broadus A, et al: *Endocrinology and Metabolism.* New York, McGraw-Hill International Book Co, 1981.
2. Arieff A, Carroll J: Nonketotic hyperosmolar coma with hyperglycemia: Clinical features, pathophysiology, renal function, acid-base balance, plasma–cerebrospinal fluid equilibria and the effects of therapy. *Medicine (Baltimore)* 1972; 51:73–94.
3. Wahren J, Felig P. Cerasi E, et al: Splanchnic and peripheral glucose and amino acid metabolism in diabetes mellitus. *J Clin Invest* 1972; 51:1870.
4. Larnerf J: Four questions times two: A dialogue on the mechanism of insulin action dedicated to Earl W. Sutherland. *Metabolism* 1975; 24:249.
5. DeFronzo R, Ferrannini E, Hendler R, et al: Influence of hyperinsulinemia, hyperglycemia and the route of glucose administration splanchnic glucose exchange. *Proc Natl Acad Sci USA* 1978; 75:5173.
6. McGarry JD: New perspectives in the regulation of ketogenesis. *Diabetes* 1979; 28:517.
7. Sherwin RS, Hendler RG, Felig P: Effect of diabetes mellitus and insulin on the turnover and metabolic response to ketones in man. *Diabetes* 1976; 25:776.
8. Felig P. Sherwin RS, Soman V, et al: Hormonal interactions in the regulation of blood glucose. *Recent Prog Horm Res* 1979; 35:501.
9. De Fronzo RA, Sherwin RS, Dillingham M, et al: Influence on basal insulin and glucagon secretion on potassium and sodium metabolism: Studies with somatostatin in normal dogs and in normal and diabetic human beings. *J Clin Invest* 1978; 61:427.
10. Katz JA: Hyperglycemia-induced hyponatremia. Calculation of expected serum sodium depression. *N Engl J Med* 1973; 289:843.
11. Vinicor F, Lehrner LM, Karn RG, et al: Hyperamylasemia in diabetic ketoacidosis: Sources and significance. *Ann Intern Med* 1979; 91:200.
12. Levy LJ, Duga J, Girgis M, et al: Ketoacidosis associated with alcoholism in nondiabetic subjects. *Ann Intern Med* 1978; 78:213.
13. Felig P: Insulin therapy: Rate and routes of delivery. *N Engl J Med* 1974; 291:1031.
14. Fisher JN, Shahshahani MN, Kitabchi AE: Diabetic ketoacidosis. Low dose insulin therapy by various routes. *N Engl J Med* 1977; 297:238.
15. Arieff AI, Kleeman CR: Cerebral edema in diabetic comas: II. Effects of hyperosmolarity, hyperglycemia and insulin in diabetic rabbits. *J Clin Endocrinol Metab* 1974; 38:1057.
16. Guisado R, Arieff AI: Neurologic manifestations of diabetic comas: Correlation with biochemical alterations in the brain. *Metabolism* 1975; 24:665.
17. Beigelman PM: Severe diabetic ketoacidosis (diabetic "coma"), 482 episodes in 257 patients; experience of three years. *Diabetes* 1971; 20:4980.
18. Vagenakis AG, Rapoport B, Azizi F, et al: *J Clin Endocrinol Metab* 1974; 54:913.
19. Saberi M, Utiger RD: *J Clin Endocrinol Metab* 1975; 40:435.
20. Fukuda H, Yasuda N, Greer MA: Acute effects of thyroxine, triiodothyronine, and iodide on thyrotropin secretion. *Endocrinology* 1975; 97:924.
21. Chopra IJ, Soloman DH, Chopra U, et al: Pathways of metabolism of thyroid hormones. *Recent Prog Horm Res* 1978; 34:531.
22. Gavin L, Castle F, McMahon PM, et al: Extrathyroidal conversion of thyroxine to 3,3'5'-triiodothyronine (reverse T_3) and 3,5,3'-triiodothyronine (T_3) in humans. *J Clin Endocrinol Metab* 1977; 44:733.
23. Wartofsky L, Burman K: Alterations in thyroid function in patients with systemic illness; The "euthyroid sick syndrome." *Endocr Rev* 1982; 3:164–217.
24. Wilber JF, Utiger RD: The effect of glucocorticoids on thyrotropin secretion. *J Clin Invest* 1969; 48:2096.
25. Morley JE: Neuroendocrine control of thyrotropin secretion. *Endocr Rev* 1981; 2:396.
26. Chopra IJ, Chua Teco GN, Nguyen AH, et al: In search of an inhibitor of thyroid hormone binding to serum proteins in nonthyroid illnesses. *J Clin Endocrinol Metab* 1979; 49:63–69.
27. Oppenheimer JH, Schwartz HL, Mariash CN, et al: Evidence for a factor in the sera of patients with nonthyroid disease which inhibits iodothyronine binding by solid matrices, serum proteins, and rate hepatocytes. *J Clin Endocrinol Metab* 1982; 54:757–766.

28. Surks M: Laboratory aids in the diagnosis of hypothyroidism. *Thyroid Today* 1977; 1:4.
29. Derubertis F, Michelis M, Bloom M, et al: Impaired water excretion in myxedema. *Am J Med* 1971; 51:41–53.
30. Wilson WR, Bedell GM: The pulmonary abnormalities in myxedema. *J Clin Invest* 1960; 39:42–55.
31. Nordquist Dhuner KG, Stenderg K, Orndahl G: Myxedema coma and CO_2 retention. *Acta Med Scand* 1960; 166:189–194.
32. Massumi RA, Winnacker JL: Severe depression of the respiratory center in myxedema. *Am J Med* 1964; 36:876–882.
33. Besses GS, Burrow GN, Spaulding SW, et al: Dopamine infusion acutely inhibits the TSH and prolactin response to TRH. *J Clin Endocrinol Metab* 1975; 41:985.
34. Kaptein EM, Spencer CA, Kamiel MN, et al: Prolonged dopamine administration and thyroid hormone economy in normal and critically ill subjects. *J Clin Endocrinol Metab* 1980; 51:387.
35. Duick DS, Wahner HQ: Thyroid axis in patients with Cushing's syndrome. *Arch Intern Med* 1979; 139:767.
36. Duick DS, Warren DW, Nicoloff JT, et al: Effect of a single dose of dexamethasone on the concentration of serum triiodothyronine in man. *J Clin Endocrinol Metab* 1974; 39:1151.
37. Heyma P, Larkins RG, Perry-Kenne D, et al: Thyroid hormone levels and protein binding in patients on long term diphenylhydantoin treatment. *Clin Endocrinol (Oxf)* 1977; 6:369.
38. Calvalieri RR, Gavin LA, Wallace A, et al: Serum thyroxine, free T_4, triiodothyronine, and reverse-T_3 in diphenylhydantoin treated patients. *Metabolism* 1979; 28:1161.
39. Jonckheer MH: Amiodarone and the thyroid gland: A review. *Acta Cardiol (Brux)* 1981; 36:199.
40. Jonckheer MH, Block P, Prockaert I, et al: Low T_3 syndrome in patients chronically treated with an iodine containing drug, amiodarone. *Clin Endocrinol (Oxf)* 1978; 9:27.
41. Burger A, Dinichert D, Nicod P, et al: Effects of amiodarone on serum triiodothyronine, reverse triiodothyronine, thyroxine and thyrotropin. *J Clin Invest* 1976; 58:255.
42. Kaptein EM, Weiner JM, Robinson WJ, et al: Relationship of altered thyroid hormone indices to survival in nonthyroidal illnesses. *Clin Endocrinol (Oxf)* 1982; 16:565–72.
43. Eisenberg D, Silberman H, Ryan J, et al: Prognostic significance of thyroid function tests in critically ill patients. *Surg Forum* 1980; 31:211–213.
44. Blum M: Myxedema coma. *Am J Med Sci* 1972; 264:433–441.
45. Bacci V: Cardiac arrest after intravenous administration of levothyronine. *JAMA* 1981; 245:920.
46. Georgitis WJ, Hofeldt FD: Myxedema coma and cardiac arrest. *JAMA* 1982; 247:980.
47. Ladenson PW, Goldenheim PD, Cooper DS, et al: Early peripheral responses to intravenous L-thyroxine in primary hypothyroidism. *Am J Med* 1982; 73:467–473.
48. Brown, ME, Refetoff S: Transient elevation of serum thyroid hormone concentration after initiation of replacement therapy in myxedema. *Ann Intern Med* 1980; 92:491–495.

23/Ethical Dilemmas in Critical Care Medicine

JAMES F. BRESNAHAN, Ph.D.

Other chapters in this book deal primarily with technical issues in critical care medicine. We turn now to troublesome human relations challenges, perplexities raised by differences of view among participants in medical decision making about the role of values in the practice of critical care medicine. We focus, then, on the effort to resolve ethical or moral dilemmas, and this for a very practical purpose, in order to achieve more effective patient care.

ETHICS IN CRITICAL CARE MEDICINE

Ethics in this medical context is nothing else than the effort of critical thinking to articulate "reasons why" some individuals affirm certain values very strongly and others, different values. Ethics aims, therefore, to explain how and why value conflicts arise about what to do. Better understanding of such conflict can often lead to mutually acceptable compromise in practice, if not always to agreement in principle. Ethical dialogue does not demand that any of the participants necessarily change their deeply held personal moral or ethical convictions. But it may enable more effective cooperation based on increased mutual understanding and respect.

Source Of Ethical Problems in Contemporary Clinical Medicine

Moral perplexity and dilemma in critical care medicine and thus the need for ethical reflection and discourse derive in our culture from two main sources: first, pluralism in the perception of and commitment to values on the part of the various participants and, second, the very complexity of the medical technology employed. These two sources more and more profoundly affect the human values' dimension of medical decisions that we cannot avoid making, especially in critical care medicine.

It is, first of all, important to recognize that moral dilemmas do not arise within a modern, culturally complex, and so morally pluralistic society because some participants in decision making are "evil," others "saintly." The need for ethical reflection on moral crises in critical care should not therefore be thought of as an exercise in moralistic "correction" of immorality, presumed or implied.

Complexity of Moral Pluralism

When we examine our varying experiences of value and our diverging interpretations of them, we find that people, care givers and patients, often agree that a particular value is truly "worthwhile" in shaping one's life, is truly important for decision making. However, we also find that in spite of such agreement at a very abstract, theoretical level, different people *prioritize* these shared values differently at another, more practical level where different values come into conflict with one another.

For instance, one person sees the primary value in the practice of critical care medicine to be *prolongation of biologic existence*. Another sees the controlling value in all medical practice to be *relief of human suffering*.[1, 2] These contrasting perspectives on which value takes priority and overrides competing values in a situation where prolongation of life and relief of suffering are in tension with one another lead to conflict about decisions to be made. And the disagreement is more acute precisely when the decision to be made involves a life and death situation.

On the one hand, shared professional and cultural experiences make it possible for us to understand what another person means by asserting a particular value. Ethical dialogue is possible—we do not simply live in "different worlds" of value.[3] But on the other hand, we can find ourselves puzzled, even put off, when confronted by the way a colleague gives a very different priority to shared values and so urges a very different resolution of a decisional challenge.

And yet, it can also happen that apparent theoretical agreement on values and their ranking will not necessarily produce agreement in practical application to a particular concrete situation. We can be surprised to find ourselves at odds with one another. Strangely too, we may often find that disagreement at a more theoretical level dissolves into agreement when we come to discuss practical cases together.[4] Ethics as critical reason giving enables us to explore these possibilities more deeply rather than attempt to resolve conflict by unreasoning imposition of a leader's authority.

Ethical dialogue, therefore, should be practiced as a quest for understanding. Its outcome often cannot be predicted, and the benefit of our surprise may be both new mutual understanding and discovery of alternative ways of resolving apparently intractable disagreement on what to do next. Where this can be achieved, everyone involved will contribute more effectively to patient care.

The Search to Subject Medical Technology to Human Purposes

Many of our disagreements about what to do next and how to do it in critical care medicine are even more perplexing to us because we are constantly confronted with technologic innovation. This creates previously unsuspected possibilities for both benefit and harm to desperately ill patients. The very novelty of many of the technical issues to which the rest of this book is addressed means that over and over again we find ourselves unprepared for the moral dimension of a decision that cannot be avoided. The novelty of the case outdistances our comfortably customary convictions about how to express moral values in medical diagnosis and treatment. And this kind of dilemma occurs widely in our high-technology culture, not in medical practice only.

Our ethical perplexity, therefore, is due not to some failure of moral fiber among modern medical care givers but rather to the success of our constantly advancing modern medicine in responding to acute crises.[5] Our moral imagination is constantly challenged. And this is especially true in the practice of intensive care medicine. How do we deal appropriately with the approach of human dying in this context of constant technologic innovation?[6] Our well-considered and customary answers frequently fail us. We have to think together anew about what we really intend, about how the new means we employ to achieve that intention may lead us to revise our understanding of the intention itself we thought was clear.

We perceive that our current skills and techniques of critical care can begin to fail, in some sense, to be effective in sustaining the humanity of patients. We encounter limit situations. Where patients cry out, "too much," we have to pause. Where "medical futility" in some sense becomes evident to one or another decision maker, we must take time to speak together of what we really intend and how we can achieve it.

Significant ethical perplexities can and do arise, of course, even during the more ordinary successful applications of techniques exemplified and described in earlier chapters. But, in this chapter we choose to deal with more dramatic situations— where death approaches—because these most vividly test our capacity for understanding one another's view of values and our ability to reconcile conflicting value concerns of all participants in decision making.[7, 8]

CASE STUDY 1: THE DYING PATIENT AND THE RELUCTANT ATTENDING PHYSICIAN

Mr. B., an 85-year-old retired business executive, has disseminated metastatic disease originating from prostatic cancer of 10 years' standing, as well as chronic obstructive pulmonary disease (COPD) and emphysema linked to a history of smoking. He is hospitalized from his home, where he resides with his wife, because of a pneumonia, and his fragile condition leads his attending physician of long standing, Dr. X.Y. to have him transferred to the intensive care unit (ICU). There, after consultation with the intensivists, it is proposed to Mr. B. by his physician that he be intubated and given support by a mechanical ventilator while antibiotic treatment continued.

Because Mr. B. is conscious and competent, before intubation Dr. X.Y. discusses with him the possibility, emphasized by consultants in the ICU, that should Mr. B. be intubated and placed on a ventilator, it might not be possible to wean him from it and return him to independent function. He is given to understand, as well, that this will probably also make impractical his return to life at home because his wife is not in good health and has shown confusion that suggests early signs of senility.

Mr. B. agrees to "try it." Mr. B. also agrees that a "do not resuscitate" (DNR) order be written that will forbid cardiac resuscitation beyond the use of pressors—should he experience life-threatening arrhythmias or cardiac arrest. He reiterates that he does not want full cardiopulmonary resuscitation (CPR), although he is willing to try the proposed intensive respiratory support.

Mr. B. is intubated and placed on the ventilator, and the regular course of antibiotic treatment of the pneumonia proves successful. But subsequently, careful and repeated efforts over 3 weeks to wean him from the ventilator fail. Preparations are made to transfer him from the ICU to a floor where chronic ventilatory support could be continued, pending placement in a skilled nursing home.

Discussion

In this case and in contrast to what frequently occurs, a competent patient is explicitly informed about problems of treatment that his attending physician and the intensive care consultants foresee.[9, 10] A relatively long-standing therapeutic alliance between the patient and his attending physician facilitates this. Awareness of the physician that there are burdens of treatment that the patient may well be unwilling to endure leads to maximum efforts from the beginning of intensive treatment to shape *reasonable goals of treatment* that respond to the patient's explanation of his hopes and desires for a continued life but only if burdens of treatment seem reasonable to him. Limits are set (limited "DNR") that appear to acknowledge this patient's own lifelong value commitments and that are sufficiently clear to be manageable by the ICU staff.

This would be desirable much more often in initiating intensive care treatment because the skills of intensivists in meeting minute-by-minute crises can sometimes obscure the overall aim or goal of these step-by-step interventions. Reasonable exercise of patient autonomy would then be impaired.

Dr. X.Y., Mr. B.'s attending physician, appears to agree to this experiment with intubation out of appropriate concern for wishes he believes his patient may have about limiting treatment and permitting death to occur, death now heralded by his fragile overall condition within the history of his declining health and advancing age.

This is *not* done because of Mr. B's chronologic age alone. That would raise questions about the *justice* of a decision to limit treatment, for instance, it might imply discriminating against the best interests of this aged patient because of concern for the best interests of other, younger patients who are making claim to resources being used to help him.[11, 12]

Here the question of limited treatment is raised because of his general condition and his age. Indeed, this competent patient's own reservations about the extent of treatment, previously expressed to his attending physician before being hospitalized as his health status deteriorated, indicate his own judgment that the limits of treatment tolerable for him at his age and in his condition are about to be reached. A judgment about "quality of life" is not being imposed upon Mr. B. by Dr. X.Y. Mr. B. makes the judgment himself.[13]

Yet, Mr. B.'s consent to ventilatory support seems reluctant. He seems to imply, at least, that he may change his mind about how tolerable treatment on the ventilator will be for him. He expresses a conditional willingness to go along with what his physician, Dr. X.Y., proposes "for now."

So far, the mutual trust and understanding of a relatively long-standing doctor-patient relationship appears effective in shaping the ongoing medical responses to the patient's illness.[14]

Appropriate and *clinically realistic* consultation among specialists and with Mr. B.'s attending physician appears to focus very appropriately on the interconnection between doubts about the success of the proposed treatment and the value commitments of this patient. Possible differences in perception and prioritization of values between care givers and Mr. B. are explicitly included in their critical care *clinical* analysis. Specifically, concern for the impact of "life-prolonging" treatment on the "quality of life" (which might produce "prolongation of dying," in Mr. B.'s view of it) demonstrates the appropriate concern of these professional care givers that their clinical judgment could become impaired by a "denial" of death and dying. They respond to Mr. B.'s awareness of the seriousness of his condition.

Also, appropriate resistance on the part of these care givers to the seductive impact of medical high technology and the aggressive action-oriented predispositions it can engender in them is also evident. This *patient's best interests* are being kept in the forefront of clinical judgment making at every moment. The DNR order does not prevent their aggressive technical response to his pneumonia and their willingness to help Mr. B. try out his ability to bear with intubation and treatment with the ventilator.

CASE STUDY 1 CONTINUED

Mr. B. is transferred from the ICU to a ventilator on the medical floor. After 10 days, Mr. B. communicates to his intern and to his nurses that he strongly desires to be removed from the ventilator. He shows too, what they interpret to be his clear although reluctant recognition that this will result in his dying. But, he writes, "This is too much to bear." When housestaff and nursing bring this up with Dr. X.Y., however, he expresses surprise and dismay—the patient has not communicated this to him at all. Moreover, Mr. B.'s wife appears confused about what Mr. B. is expressing to her and cannot make a clear decision when Dr. X.Y. brings this up with her.

Discussion

The agreement previously reached between Dr. X.Y. and Mr. B. included on Mr. B.'s part a proviso: "for now." Further investigation then might have revealed greater reluctance on the part of Mr. B. to undergo even initiation of ventilatory support in the ICU than was initially expressed by him or discerned by Dr. X.Y. and the ICU specialists. But, that "go ahead" satisfied Dr. X.Y. And, the ICU consultants assumed that an apparently more than usually nuanced understanding and agreement between patient and doctor existed. Now, Mr. B. has had well over a month of life on a ventilator, and he has been made aware that hope of weaning him has all but been eliminated. His real, time-tested experience of what this kind of living means to him, with his life goals and personal values, seems to be producing a wish for termination of treatment not really expected by Dr. X.Y.

Immediate care givers in constant and direct contact with Mr. B. are entrusted by him with a message that, apparently, he cannot give directly to his physician and that his wife in her present state cannot adequately grasp. These care givers remain open to hear his wishes and are concerned and ready to communicate it to Dr. X.Y. in spite of his reluctance to hear it.

From their interactions with Mr. B., these care givers appear convinced that Mr.

B. is not abnormally "depressed" (in a way that would be amenable to antipsychotic therapy), nor does Dr. X.Y. appear to think this is the case. Normal distress from enduring aggressive treatment and normal grief at the prospect of dying is accepted as inevitable and not usually psychologically disabling–not suicidal.[15] The response of the housestaff and nurses to the value judgment of Mr. B. concerning the excessively burdensome nature of his present course of treatment, especially given his advanced age and his expressed realism about the inevitability of his now dying (his wish for the limited "DNR"), supports the judgment that he appears entirely competent and "reasonable".[16]

Dr. X.Y.'s consultation with Mrs. B., although not unusual and not in general inappropriate, suggests some reluctance on his part to confront Mr. B. himself about his expressed wish to be taken off the ventilator.

Family members are appropriately consulted to help interpret what they believe the patient means and wants, at least when real doubts exist on the part of care givers. They do not, however, have any moral or legal "rights" to control treatment against the expressed wishes of a competent patient and should not be allowed to interfere between patient and physician. They do, of course, have a need and therefore a right to be informed of the approach of dying of their loved one and to be helped by care givers to deal with their anticipatory grief. And most patients expect this help for their loved ones from their care givers.

Thus, although Dr. X.Y. cannot deny the reasonableness of his competent patient's request, it now appears that he has great personal difficulty in accepting the appropriateness of discontinuing aggressive treatment once begun—although he might, perhaps, have been ready to more readily accept a decision not to begin it. Mr. B. seems to be well aware of this, too, hence his reticence with Dr. X.Y.

It is not unusual for patients to be solicitous of their physician's real although not directly expressed convictions and wishes and to act in a way that avoids provoking even the possibility of "abandonment" by their doctor, and this even though the particular physician does not even remotely hint at this and would never in fact do such a thing. This is particularly the case with dying patients who greatly fear a loss of support.

CASE STUDY 1 CONTINUED

The housestaff and nurses persuade Dr. X.Y. to request an "ethics consultation" from the Medical Staff Ethics Committee (which is available for that purpose only at the request of the attending physician). A panel of four persons appointed by the physician chair of this committee reviews the chart, speaks with Mr. B.'s immediate care givers, and then, with the explicit permission of Dr. X.Y., interviews Mr. B.

To the committee panel Mr. B. communicates in writing his deep respect and affection for Dr. X.Y., but also his perception that Dr. X.Y. really does not believe in stopping ventilatory support, which will result in Mr. B.'s dying. "He's full of ethics," writes Mr. B., smiling wryly. "But there are things worse than dying," Mr. B. writes with tears in his eyes. Further, Mr. B. writes that he fears to experience distress in breathing, that he desires to die in his sleep. He even writes that he would want "the big pill" that will let him die now without distress.

Mr. B. is reassured by the committee panel that his wish to be taken off the ventilator will be communicated to Dr. X.Y. and respected by him. The committee stresses above all that Mr. B. will be carefully and adequately medicated to prevent the distress and suffering he fears. The committee panel's physician chair communicates all of this to Dr. X.Y., and he accepts this account of his patient's wishes. He indicates, as well, his willingness to follow Mr. B.'s wishes. A patient care conference with the other care givers fills them in on these developments.

Mr. B. is brought back to the ICU at the request of Dr. X.Y., prepared with appropriate and adequate administration of sedatives, is taken off the ventilator, and is then extubated.

Mr. B. does not die immediately, and after a day is returned from the ICU to the regular floor and to the intern and nurses who have been taking care of him. With continued consultation of respiratory care he is kept comfortable with oxygen and analgesics, and he dies 48 hours later.

Discussion

In this case, the consultation, agreed to by the attending physician who was puzzled and upset about what other immediate care givers report his patient had expressed, resulted in increased mutual understanding among all participants. The Medical Staff Ethics Committee did not impose a treatment plan on Dr. X.Y; it confirmed to Dr. X.Y. the wishes of his patient reported by other care givers and at the same time reassured Mr. B. that what he was reluctant to express emphatically to his doctor had now been understood by Dr. X.Y. Dr. X.Y. retained primary responsibility for the decision but was given reassurance both that it was what Mr. B. wanted and that Mr. B. was not making an unreasonable request.

So finally, all agreed on a course of action. When the previously unarticulated conflict about the ethics of intensive treatment as death approaches was "out in the open," Mr. B. and Dr. X.Y. had a new basis for going forward toward a more precisely defined ultimate goal of treatment—"appropriate care of the dying." The other care givers were also fully informed and confirmed as well in their sense of having served both Mr. B. and Dr. X.Y. in this difficult moment.

A factor possibly clouding achievement of agreement is the request of Mr. B. for the "big pill" that would let him die in his sleep. Is this a request on his part for "euthanasia" (in the sense of "active euthanasia" by care givers), and does any particular care giver's agreement to remove ventilatory support and to administer adequate medication for comfort thereby become participation in the patient's suicide and, in effect, homicidal?

In these circumstances of prolonged and stressful aggressive intensive care treatment, Mr. B made an oblique suggestion ("a big pill") that something amounting to "active euthanasia" would be acceptable to him. Dr. X.Y. certainly seemed to oppose "active euthanasia" (understood to mean initiating a new lethal process to shorten the dying process, i.e., a lethal process distinct from and additional to the underlying disease processes that are causing Mr. B.'s demise). But the ethics consultants assured Dr. X.Y. that it was reasonable to interpret Mr. B.'s request to be for ending a treatment that he now perceived to be for him in his present circumstances *excessively burdensome*. Some would call this "passive euthanasia," but that need not deter Dr. X.Y. Such action ending what a patient judges excessively burdensome treatment has been declared to be morally acceptable by, among others, the Judicial Council of the American Medical Association.[17] Such action is consistently protected by U.S.

courts from being punished as homicide or assisting suicide, at least where, as here, a conscious and competent patient requests it.[18, 19]

After all, Mr. B. made this request that aggressive treatment now be ended after he had "given it a good try." Before his hospitalization, Mr. B. had already experienced the distress of air hunger as his COPD and emphysema worsened. It is not surprising that he feared a death gasping for breath. He was probably not aware of the medical capacity to titrate sedatives to ensure against such distress without deliberately aiming at death by overdose. So his words may be interpreted to indicate what he feared and to ask that it be forestalled.[20]

One need not suspect suicidal ideation or depressive desperation on the patient's part under these circumstances. One can easily interpret his request as reasonable because it merely asks physicians to no longer intervene to prolong his inevitably proximate dying—a dying that, in his view, had begun long since but was unduly delayed by the application of these intensive therapies.

Readjustment of the treatment plan here to emphasize comfort of Mr. B. in his dying therefore prevented overemphasis on prolonging biologic existence and an unthinking aggressive response to each developing medical crisis that sometimes can distort clinical judgment. The traditional hippocratic concern not to "do harm" by imposing "useless suffering" is brought to the forefront of attention and planning of therapy.

This responds to the rhetoric used by this patient whose words we may reasonably interpret to mean that he now wants desperately to make the simple point, "It's really time to stop now!" Thus, agreement by Dr. X.Y. not to continue respiratory support of Mr. B. need not be interpreted as an immoral and illegal participation in "active euthanasia" merely because the patient has spoken of a measure that might, ambiguously, suggest a readiness for active euthanasia.

If, however, Dr. X.Y.'s basic moral conviction is that biologic existence must always be prolonged by all medical means available, that no consideration of the patient's own judgment about his "quality of life" (even in the deep sense of intense suffering that cannot promise restoration of acceptable function) can justify withholding or withdrawing such treatment, then Dr. X.Y. should seek to transfer the final care of his patient to a physician who can accept Mr. B.'s, the other care givers' and the ethics committee panel's point of view. For in that case, deeply held moral convictions of the physician and of the patient would be hopelessly at odds with one another, and neither immoral compromise of the physician's sincerely held deep ethical commitment nor immoral compromise of the patient's sincerely moral autonomous request for cessation of treatment should be compromised.[21]

Pressures of "utilization review" simply to terminate or discharge Mr. B. were not reported in this case. Resources were not wasted, but rather Mr. B. was moved from the ICU to a medical floor, then back, and then to the floor again in response to real medical need. Mr. B. himself decided that further use of medical resources could not benefit him and asked for an end to their use. It is to be noted, however, that there exists no "DRG" for "dying" and yet that this course of treatment displays the need for sophisticated medicine in the service of pain control in a situation like Mr. B.'s.

An alternative approach might have been to transfer Mr. B. to a medically sophisticated "hospice" unit within the hospital.[22] In this case, such a transfer did not become feasible until more than a year after Mr. B.'s death, when such a hospice unit was established.

CASE STUDY 2: A PERMANENTLY UNCONSCIOUS, THEREFORE NOW INCOMPETENT, DYING PATIENT WITHOUT FORMAL "ADVANCE DIRECTIVES"

Mr. F., an 85-year-old retired commodities broker, has essentially the same medical problems as Mr. B., but with the additional factor that brain metastases have resulted in his becoming comatose while at home, before being brought to the hospital.

He is admitted immediately through the emergency room and brought to the ICU. When the same Dr. X.Y., who is also Mr. F.'s attending physician of long standing, arrived, he is asked by the resident in charge whether Mr. F. has prepared either a "living will" or a "durable power of attorney" (giving another person authority to make health care decisions on his behalf should he become incompetent). Dr. X.Y. says that they have never discussed together what Mr. F. would want at the stage of terminal care, so he does not know. Therapy is begun (essentially the same as for Mr. B, above), and it includes intubation and a ventilator. Also, a neurology consultation is requested.

Mrs. F. arrived and says that although Mr. F. did not prepare anything in writing about this, he very emphatically expressed his wishes both to her and to their son and daughter and their spouses on several occasions over the past 5 years since his prostate cancer was first detected. She admits that he was reluctant to execute a formal advance directive or speak of this to Dr. X.Y. because he thought Dr. X.Y., on whom he felt dependent, might object. Mr. F., she says repeatedly asserted that he wanted to be allowed to "die peacefully" when "the end comes," without "being put on a machine," especially should he become unconscious. And Mr. F. was particularly concerned that costs of his final hospitalization not compromise the modestly sufficient investments on which Mrs. F. would depend for her support after he should die.

The son and daughter and their spouses arrive, speak independently with Dr. X.Y. and the ICU intern caring for Mr. F., and confirm exactly what Mrs. F. has said their father had told them about his wishes for limited care when, in the future, he would become terminal.

On the second day, a neurologist conducts a thorough examination of Mr. F., including electroencephalography (EEG), and after consulting with Mr. F.'s medical oncologist as well as Dr. X.Y. about the course of Mr. F.'s mental deterioration before this hospitalization, writes a note indicating her strong opinion that Mr. F. is not brain dead (because brain stem function continues) but has now entered a permanent vegetative state because of cortical impairment from metasteses and that he cannot be expected to awake again to consciousness.

Both the neurologist and the medical oncologist orally expressed the opinion that Mr. F. might well continue in his present state for as much as a month or more if given aggressive support.

Mrs. F. and her children and their spouses meet with Dr. X.Y. and the ICU resident in charge on the third day and hear all of this information from them.

On the fourth day, they request of Dr. X.Y. that Mr. F. be extubated, be given whatever pain medication might be indicated to treat any residual capacity for pain he might have, and be allowed to die. They say that the ICU intern and nurse caring for Mr. F. discussed all of this with them and indicated they could make this request of Dr. X.Y.

Dr. X.Y. tells the ICU resident that he is reluctant to take this step, although he wishes he had not permitted Mr. F. to be intubated in the first place. He does not believe that Mrs. F. and the children are trying to entrap him into some kind of legal liability, but he also does not believe, personally and professionally, in stopping treatment once begun—at least not unless a patient, like Mr. B., is competent to tell him to do so. But, Dr. X. Y. agrees that no plans should be made to initiate medically engineered nutrition, whether by nasogastric tube, by central line, or by percutaneous endoscopic gastrostomy. In a patient care conference attended by all ICU personnel who have contact with Mr. F., all immediate care givers, when informed by the ICU resident of these plans, agree that new intensive measures should not be instituted and that removal of the ventilator and extubation would be appropriate.

Dr. X.Y. wonders, however, whether the prosecuting attorney of the city, known to have ambition for higher office, may accuse him of homicide should word be passed about their discontinuing Mr. F.'s ventilatory support under these circumstances.

Discussion

An examination of the ethical considerations in this case should precede all discussion of legal problems that may arise. In fact, a clear understanding of the ethical issues will be the best grounds for whatever argument may have to be made to avoid or defend against legal complications—for instance, to deflect action by a prosecuting attorney or to forestall it by seeking legal guardianship of Mr. F. for purposes of making medical decisions on his behalf that insulate care givers and family from criminal indictment.[23]

It should be noted, of course, that the execution of a living will in which the patient says what his wife and family testify to now, or better, appointment of a person other than his wife (whose financial interest might exclude her) with power of attorney that will survive the patient's becoming incompetent (if that is provided for in state law) would have prevented the concern of care givers (and, perhaps, family) about unwanted interference of the law in this situation.[24]

From an ethical point of view, then, what Mr. F.'s wife and family testify to gives solid grounds for the care givers, including Dr. X.Y., to believe that Mr. F. would now want them to extubate him on the fourth or fifth day while providing as well whatever sedation seems reasonable to prevent his possibly experiencing any pain. His family emphasize what Mr. F. wanted rather than what they themselves want. They do not so much substitute their judgment for his as clarify what he himself would request if he could.

The medical situation of Mr. F., as it can be judged from the convergence of the various perspectives of his attending physician, Dr. X.Y., his oncologist, and the consulting neurologist, is grim. He is at the terminal or immediately preterminal stage of his disease (depending on how one defines these terms, the period of time a patient would be able to survive *without* treatment should be used to define "terminal"). Death is surely "near" for Mr. F. due to advanced and incurable disease.

And Mr. F. has entered a final stage of unconsciousness that excludes reasonable expectation of his awakening even temporarily to inform care givers personally of how much further attempt at cure he wants.

Mr. F.'s present condition, therefore, corresponds to his relatively long-standing expression of his value convictions about enduring continued strenuous treatment and about dying. He has not therefore mandated help with suicide but only limitation of "curative" treatment when it will be useless or unreasonably burdensome because it will merely prolong a dying process. It is implicit in that Mr. F. has indicated that mere biologic survival without a capacity for interaction with his family and friends is of no interest or benefit to him.

His family has heard him state this repeatedly over a period that precedes the metastatic involvement of the brain and any signs of dementia.

Although care givers may wish to exclude financial considerations from their own decision making in favor of what they understand to be the patient's best medical interests, the patient should be able to define his own best interests to include limiting expense of medical care. Many reasonable persons consider that an important factor in deciding to limit treatment because it is judged by them excessively burdensome.

The fact that Mr. F. does so here for his wife's sake should not disable her from testifying to his wishes (otherwise "Catch 22" results). And possibly suspicions about improper motives and possible misrepresentation by her are here laid to rest by the independent testimony of their children. No reasonable suspicions are raised here about their or his wife's possibly malicious motives.

While it is generally emotionally easier for physicians not to begin treatment than to terminate it once it has been begun, the basic decision is of the same kind in either case. Treatment that is no longer more beneficial than harmful to this patient, given his reasonable preferences, should not be begun or, if begun, should be stopped.[25, 26]

The personal moral convictions of Dr. X.Y. may lead him to resign care to another physician who can follow Mr. F.'s wishes but should not lead him to oppose ending treatment. He admits he wishes he had not begun it. Dr. X.Y. would, of course, have to take more vigorous action to oppose ending treatment if he were really convinced that all other parties involved are unreasonable and/or bent on murderous harm to his patient.[27]

The belief of some persons that whenever the digestive tract remains viable medically engineered feeding and hydration must be instituted and continued as "basic comfort care" is flatly contradicted by many reasonable people.[28] This results in two at least equally plausible views of moral obligation with respect to medical means of nutrition and hydration. There is, therefore, no moral obligation to institute such measures when the parties involved are convinced that this is medical treatment that would only prolong a "normal" or "natural" dying process.

The various communications between medical and nursing staff and the family do not appear to be aimed at undermining the authority of the attending physician, Dr. X.Y., but rather are good faith attempts to help Mrs. F. and the children understand the significance for them and Mr. F. of information being given them. Attempts to artifically restrict such good faith communication usually increase the possibiity of misunderstanding and potential conflict.

It is generally undesirable that the decision-making process here be reviewed by a law court. Where all of the parties are agreed that dying would be prolonged, that further aggressive measures are excessively burdensome, appropriate compassionate care of the dying should be able to be provided without public interference.

At the foundation of the common law right to control one's medical treatment, and thus to refuse treatment unless there is a clear instance of suicidal action, there is very probably a constitutional right of privacy. And there is probably, as well, the specific constitutional right to free exercise of religion, to determine how one should deal with medical treatment in the all-important moment in living in which one enters upon dying, and to do so according to each one's deepest convictions. The privacy involved in such "extralegal" decision making as these parties must undertake will therefore ultimately be protected by court decisions in most jurisdictions. Or at least where death is clearly near due to inexorably progressing disease processes, such basic human right to act without intervention of courts will generally be conceded by courts. Where the destructive disease process is slower, however, or where real doubts are raised about the true desires of the dying patient, some courts may be reluctant to grant permission to terminate treatment.

It seems both morally appropriate and also clinically desirable to fully explain to all care givers involved directly or indirectly with Mr. F. what is to be done and why. This prevents uninformed dissent, and so the danger of inappropriate intrusion by public officials in the care of this dying man is minimized.

CASE STUDY 2 CONTINUED

While discussion among care givers and family about whether and when to remove Mr. F. from the ventilator continues, on the sixth day in intensive care as Dr. X.Y.'s reluctance to take this step seems to wane, Mr. F. suffers a cardiac arrest. Continued use of pressors does not counteract this event, and in accord with the "DNR" order Mr. F. is not subjected to further cardiac stimulation.

Subsequent to his death no one contacts the prosecuting attorney. The family of Mr. F. expresses appreciation to Dr. X.Y. and to the staff of the ICU. Mrs. F. appears both grieved and relieved.

Mr. F.'s daughter and her spouse confide to one of the principal nurses who care for Mr. F. that they are convinced they must execute durable powers of attorney. They assert that they intend to discuss with their own internist their plans to avoid the difficulties in limiting treatment in a terminal care situation that they experienced with their father and Dr. X.Y. in order to be sure that their own doctor does not have this kind of reluctance.

Discussion

Not all outcomes are managed by family and care givers, especially in situations where death takes a hand in the game.

Preparation of effective advance directives by everyone likely to be cared for in the contemporary North American health care milieu demands consultation with persons likely to be involved as well as fulfillment of legal formalities of the living will or durable power of attorney.

CASE STUDY 3: A PERMANENTLY UNCONSCIOUS, THEREFORE NOW INCOMPETENT DYING PATIENT WHOSE WISHES ARE CLEAR BUT A RELATIVE OF WHOM IS IN DISSENT ABOUT FOLLOWING THOSE WISHES

Mr. H., an 87-year-old retired automobile dealer, also a patient of Dr. X.Y., is in substantially the same clinical situation as Mr. F. Also like Mr. F., Mr. H. has a wife and daughter who testify to his expressed wishes about limiting aggressive medical treatment when he should become terminally ill. But Mr. H. has a son who has been estranged from his father for many years. This son now appears in the ICU on the third day of his father's hospitalization and hears all of the information about his clinical state and the testimony of his mother and sister about Mr. H.'s wishes.

On the fourth day this son states that he does not deny anything his mother and sister have said about his father's wishes. Nor does he doubt the accuracy of the collective judgment of Dr. X.Y., the medical oncologist, and the consulting neurologist that his father is now irreversibly dying and in a permanent vegetative state. This son insists, however, that he simply cannot and will not consent either to cessation of support by ventilator or to noninitiation of medical efforts to supply nutrition.

Mrs. H. and the daughter are greatly distressed. Dr. X.Y. is frankly afraid of being sued by the son or of being indicted by the prosecutor on the complaint of the son. The decision-making process completely stalls.

The immediate care givers, housestaff and nurses, are appalled at the aggressive measures now being continued and even to be added to. They view this virtually as medical torture that they must inflict on a fellow human being known not to want it and who is unconscious but may or may not have some vestigial experience of pain. At least, they insist to Dr. X.Y. and the attending chief of the ICU, this constitutes a meaningless and wasteful medical charade that demeans them and their profession.

Discussion

Some resolution of the son's problem is necessary for effective appropriate care of the dying father, Mr. H., along the lines recommended for Mr. F. Loyalty to his patient and fidelity to his patient's reasonable wishes is Dr. X.Y.'s (and also, all the other care givers') primary professional medical obligation, to be sure. But this son's apparently unreasonable, quite possibly guilt-ridden obstructionism cannot successfully be simply brushed aside, that is, his interference cannot be ignored without grave danger of making things even worse for the dying patient and for his wife and daughter.

This is one of the most distressing experiences that medical care givers can face.

Generally speaking, dying persons wish their care givers to take care of their family and loved ones, to help them through the stress of grief and loss. Seldom would a dying person simply demand that such needs be utterly ignored. Thus Dr. X.Y. and all doctors and nurses involved are implicitly empowered by the patient's probable implied wishes (in spite of his alienation from his son), as well as by the practical need to avoid probably grave interference with good care of this dying patient, to take all reasonable measures to help the son change his mind and consent to terminating treatment. This demands a combination of professional patience with imaginative approaches of every kind likely to help the son deal with his grief and anger in another, more fruitful way.

The intervention of liaison-consultation psychiatry may be of great help in fulfilling this obligation. Calling upon the consulting ethics committee, too, may open possibilities for helping the son to better understand what the medical situation of Mr. F. really is—a dying situation.

Only when such measures are seen to have failed and make recourse to a court of law inevitable in order to prevent a fully extended dying of Mr. H. should Dr. X.Y. and the other care givers strongly urge Mrs. H. to seek guardianship and explicit court authorization to order aggressive treatment of Mr. H. be terminated.

Of course, Dr. X.Y. and the other care givers should support Mrs. H. should she seek court action sooner rather than later. Since her and her daughter's grief and, indeed, the son's grief, too, will be increased by adversary proceedings at law, this support, although firm, will have to be carefully modulated. It should continue to aim at helping the son change his mind.

Should the son be adamant but the wife and daughter finally be unwilling to seek guardianship to contradict his wishes but fulfil those of Mr. H., then Dr. X.Y. and the other care givers may be faced with the need themselves to seek court approval of a transfer of Mr. H. to another facility that may be willing to care for him. This would be their moral duty if it appeared to be the only way to break the impasse preventing appropriate care of Mr. H. in his dying. But in any case, the longer Mr. H.'s dying is prolonged, the greater the care that Dr. X.Y. and the other care givers must exercise to be sure that any possible awareness of suffering in Mr. H. is medically alleviated by appropriate use of sedatives.

CASE STUDY 3 CONTINUED

All efforts over 2 weeks to help Mr. H.'s son to recognize the inevitable dying of his father fail. Morale of the ICU nurses and housestaff reaches a low point for the year. Dr. X.Y. consents to order modest doses of pain medication to ensure that Mr. H. is not aware of pain.

Mr. H.'s condition stabilizes, and he is transferred on ventilatory support to a medical floor. Turmoil builds on this unit as well but is contained by contracting for special extra nursing care for Mr. H. His family vacillates about legal action. Dr. X.Y. adopts a "wait-and-see" policy.

After another month, transfer of Mr. H. is successfully arranged to a public long-term care institution that accepts ventilator-dependent, permanently comatose patients—although with more limited personnel than are required in acute care hospitals. Three days after the transfer, Mr. H. dies.

Nothing more is heard from Mr. H.'s family.

With the help of the hospital lawyer, efforts are begun, involving both hospital administration and care givers, to interest the state legislature in a bill to establish nonjudicial procedures for resolving such disputes in the future, for instance, by empowering the spouse in consultation with the attending physician to determine to implement the expressed or implied wishes for termination of treatment of a now-incompetent patient against dissent of another family member. The state bar association convenes an interdisciplinary committee to draft such a statute, and a state legislator is found to sponsor it.

No immediate results of this initiative are reported.

Discussion

A struggle must be made to avoid resolution of problematic cases like this through what might be called "allowing to die by transfer." But an adequate consummation of this struggle requires that experienced care givers move out from the confines of the ICU and hospital, that they engage in efforts at advocacy within society, legislature, and law courts to change expectations and decisional procedures. The prevailing presumption in favor of continuing aggressive treatment must be given sane limits in situations where continued aggressive treatment aimed at "prolonging life" but in fact merely prolonging a dying process is unreasonably demanded at great expense—both in human attrition and medical resources. Only experienced care givers can really inform and persuade people at large and political leaders to change this prevailing presumption.

REFERENCES

1. Cassell E: The nature of suffering and the goals of medicine. *N Engl J Med* 1982; 306:639–645.
2. Cassell E: The relief of suffering. *Arch Intern Med* 1983; 143:522–523.
3. MacIntyre C: *XIX Tradition and Translation, Whose Justice? Which Rationality?* Notre Dame, Ind, University of Notre Dame Press, 1988.
4. Jonsen A, Toulmin S: *The Abuse of Causistry. A History of Moral Reasoning.* Berkeley, Calif, University of Californai Press, 1988.
5. Gaylin W: Modern medicine and the price of success. *Bull Amer Coll Surgeons* 1983; 68:4–7.
6. Reiser S: *Medicine and the Reign of Technology.* New York, Cambridge University Press, 1978.
7. President's Commission for the Study of Ethical Problems in Medicine and Biomedical and Behavioral Research: *Deciding to Forego Life-Sustaining Treatments. A Report on the Ethical, Medical, and Legal Issues in Treatment Decisions. March 1983.* Washington, DC, US Government Printing Office, 1983.
8. McCormick R: To save or let die: the dilemma of modern medicine. *JAMA* 1974; 229:172–176.
9. Cassem N: Treatment decisions in irreversible illness, in Hackett T, Cassem N (eds): *Massachusetts General Hospital Handbook of General Hospital Psychiatry.* St. Louis, CV Mosby Co, 1978, p 32.
10. Cassem N: The dying patient, in Hackett T, Cassem N (eds): *Massachusetts General Hospital Handbook of General Hospital Psychiatry.* St Louis, CV Mosby Co, 1978, p 16.
11. Thomasma D: Ethical judgments of quality of life in the care of the aged. *J Am Geriatr Soc* 1984; 32:525–527.
12. Callahan D: Terminating treatment: Age as a standard. *Hastings Cent Rep* 1987; 17:21–25.
13. McCormick R: The quality of life, the sanctity of life. *Hastings Cent Rep* 1978; 8:30–36.
14. President's Commission for the Study of Ethical Problems in Medicine and Biomedical and Behavioral Research: *Making Health Care Decisions. The Ethical and Legal Implications of Informed Consent in the Patient-Practitioner Relationship,* vol 1: *Report.* Washington DC, US Government Printing Office, 1982.
15. Cassem N: Depression, in Hackett T, Cassem N (eds): *Massachusetts General Hospital Handbook of General Hospital Psychiatry.* St Louis, CV Mosby Co, 1978, p 10.
16. Cassem N, Hackett T: The setting of intensive care, in Hackett T, Cassem N (eds): *Massachusetts General Hospital Handbook of General Hospital Psychiatry.* St Louis, CV Mosby Co, 1978, p 17.
17. Council on Ethical and Judicial Affairs, Dickey N, et al: Withholding or withdrawing life-prolonging medical treatment, in *Current Opinions on Ethical and Judicial Affairs of the American Medical Association.* Chicago, American Medical Association, 1986.
18. Council on Ethical and Judicial Affairs, Dickey N, et al: Withholding or withdrawing life-prolonging medical treatment—patients' preferences, in *Current Opinions on Ethical and Judicial Affairs of the American Medical Association.* Chicago, American Medical Association, 1986.
19. Bresnahan J: Suffering and dying under intensive care: Ethical disputes before the courts. *Crit Care Nurs Q.* 1987; 10:11–16.
20. Schneiderman L, Spragg R: Ethical decisions in discontinuing mechanical ventilation. *N Engl J Med* 1988; 318:984–988.
21. Bresnahan J, Drane J: A court divided: The Brophy decision. A challenge to examine the meaning of living and dying. *Health Prog* 1986; 67:32–37, 98.
22. Bulkin W, Lukashok H: Rx for the dying: The case for hospice. *N Engl J Med* 1988; 318:376–378.
23. Rhoden N: Litigating life and death. *Harvey Lect* 1988; 102:375–446.
24. *Handbook of Living Will Laws. 1987 Edition.* New York, Society for the Right to Die, 1987.
25. Wanzer S, Federman D, et al: The physician's responsibility toward hopelessly ill patients. *N Engl J Med* 1984; 310:955–959.
26. Wanzer S, Federman D, et al: The physicians's responsibility toward hopelessly ill patients. A second look. *N Engl J Med* 1989; 320:844–849.
27. Kass L: Neither for love nor money: Why doctors must not kill. *Public Interest* 1989; 94:25–46.
28. Steinbrook R, Lo B: Artificial feeding—solid ground, not a slippery slope. *N Engl J Med* 1988; 318:286–290.

Index